T0180435

Religion and Spirituality in Psychiatry

Although medicine is practiced in a secular setting, religious and spiritual issues have an impact on patients' perspectives regarding their health and the management of disorders that may afflict them. This is especially true in psychiatry, because spiritual and religious beliefs are prevalent among those with emotional or mental illness. Clinicians are rarely aware of the importance of religion and understand little of its value as a positive force for coping with the many difficulties that patients and their families must face. This monograph addresses various issues concerning mental illness in psychiatry: the relationship of religious issues to mental health; the tension between theological and psychiatric perspectives; the importance of addressing these varying approaches in patient care and how to do so; and differing ways of treating patients using Christian, Muslim, and Buddhist principles. This is a book specifically addressing the challenges that mental health professionals face when seeking to consider and integrate spiritual, religious, and cultural issues relevant to patient care.

Philippe Huguelet, MD, is lecturer in the Department of Psychiatry, University Hospital of Geneva and University of Geneva, Switzerland.

Harold G. Koenig, MD, is professor of psychiatry and behavioral sciences and associate professor of medicine at Duke University Medical Center and at the Geriatric Research, Education, and Clinical Center, Veterans Administration Medical Center, Durham, North Carolina.

Religion and Spirituality in Psychiatry

Edited by

Philippe Huguelet

University Hospital of Geneva and University of Geneva, Switzerland

Harold G. Koenig

Duke University Medical Center and Veterans Administration
Medical Center, Durham, North Carolina

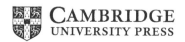
CAMBRIDGE
UNIVERSITY PRESS

CAMBRIDGE UNIVERSITY PRESS
Cambridge, New York, Melbourne, Madrid, Cape Town,
Singapore, São Paulo, Delhi, Mexico City

Cambridge University Press
The Edinburgh Building, Cambridge CB2 8RU, UK

Published in the United States of America by Cambridge University Press, New York

www.cambridge.org
Information on this title: www.cambridge.org/9781107405868

© Cambridge University Press 2009

First published 2009
Reprinted 2010
First paperback edition 2012

A catalogue record for this publication is available from the British Library

Library of Congress Cataloguing in Publication Data
Religion and Spirituality in Psychiatry / [edited by] Philippe Huguelet, Harold G. Koenig.
   p. ; cm.
Includes bibliographical references and index.
ISBN 978-0-521-88952-0 (hardback)
1. Psychiatry and religion.   I. Huguelet, Philippe.   II. Koenig, Harold George.
[DNLM: 1. Religion and Psychology.   2. Mental Disorders – psychology.
3. Mental Disorders – therapy. WM 61 R3825 2009]
RC455.4.R4R453   2009
616.89–dc22   2009001264

ISBN 978-0-521-88952-0 Hardback
ISBN 978-1-107-40586-8 Paperback

Contents

Contributors

Laurence Borras, MD
Department of Psychiatry, University Hospitals
of Geneva and University of Geneva, Geneva,
Switzerland

Elizabeth S. Bowman, MD
Clinical Professor of Neurology, Indiana
University, Consulting Psychiatrist, Indiana
University Epilepsy Clinic, Indianapolis,
Indiana

Arjan W. Braam, MD
Department of Psychiatry and the Institute
of Research in Extramural Medicine, Vrije
Universiteit Amsterdam, Amsterdam,
The Netherlands

Pierre-Yves Brandt, MD
Faculty of Theology and Religious Studies,
University of Lausanne, Lausanne,
Switzerland

Armando R. Favazza, MD
Department of Psychiatry, University of
Missouri–Columbia, Columbia, Missouri

Alyssa A. Forcehimes, PhD
Center on Alcoholism, Substance Abuse, and
Addictions, University of New Mexico,
Albuquerque, New Mexico

Claude-Alexandre Fournier
Faculty of Theology and Religious Studies,
University of Lausanne, Lausanne,
Switzerland

René Hefti, MD
Department of Psychosomatic Medicine,
Klinik SGM Langenthal, Langenthal,
Switzerland

Philippe Huguelet, MD
Department of Psychiatry, University Hospitals
of Geneva and University of Geneva, Geneva,
Switzerland

Charles Knapp MA, LPC
Co-Director, Windhorse Community Services,
Boulder, Colorado

Harold G. Koenig, MD
Department of Psychiatry, Duke University
Medical Center, and Geriatric Research,
Education and Clinical Center (GRECC),
Veterans Administration (VA) Medical
Center, Durham, North Carolina

Marcus M. McKinney, Dmin, LPC
Department of Psychiatry, University
of Connecticut School of Medicine,
Farmington, Connecticut, and Pastoral
Counseling, Saint Francis Hospital and
Medical Center, Hartford, Connecticut

Sylvia Mohr, PhD
Department of Psychiatry, University Hospitals
of Geneva and University of Geneva, Geneva,
Switzerland

Nader Perroud, MD
Department of Psychiatry, University Hospitals
of Geneva, Geneva, Switzerland

Samuel Pfeifer, MD
Psychiatric Clinic Sonnenhalde, Basel-Riehen,
Switzerland

Ralph L. Piedmont, PhD
Department of Pastoral Counseling,
Loyola College in Maryland, Columbia,
Maryland

Joel James Shuman, PhD
Center for Ethics and Public Life, King's College,
    Wilkes-Barre, Pennsylvania

Samuel B. Thielman, MD, PhD
Department of Psychiatry and Behavioral
    Sciences, Duke University School of
    Medicine, Durham, North Carolina

J. Scott Tonigan, PhD
Center on Alcoholism, Substance Abuse, and
    Addictions, University of New Mexico,
    Albuquerque, New Mexico

Sasan Vasegh, MD
Assistant Professor of Psychiatry, Department
    of Psychiatry, Ilam University of Medical
    Sciences, Ilam, Iran (Islamic Republic of)

William P. Wilson, MD
Professor Emeritus of Psychiatry, Duke
    University Medical Center, Distinguished
    Professor of Counseling, Carolina Evangelical
    Divinity School, Greensboro, North Carolina

1 | Introduction: Key Concepts

PHILIPPE HUGUELET AND HAROLD G. KOENIG

1. WHY THIS BOOK?

Patients facing illnesses may often use religion as a way to cope with the illness. What is problematic, however, is that sometimes symptoms have religious elements (e.g., delusion with religious content). However, clinicians involved in psychiatric care may have noticed that for patients with mental disorders, religion/spirituality *also* represents an important way of making sense of and coping with the stress that the illness causes. Despite these observations, clinicians often fail to inquire about the religious beliefs, practices, and experiences of patients, sometimes missing an opportunity to help relieve the suffering that psychiatric disorders cause. Some clinicians may have expertise in the religious aspects of psychiatric illness and are knowledgeable enough in this area to integrate it into their clinical practices; others may not know much about religion, may be reluctant to discuss issues related to it, and may completely avoid it in their encounters with patients. Thus, it is necessary to build a bridge between these two groups. This book tries to comprehensively and synthetically address such issues and seeks to give psychiatrists and other clinicians the tools they need to integrate religious and spiritual issues into their daily work with patients. A growing number of texts address religion, psychology, and psychiatry. The present book, however, seeks to give practical knowledge to clinicians who are not familiar with these issues and who may not a priori consider religion/spirituality when they take care of patients. To provide a foundation for the chapters to follow, this chapter briefly discusses definitions of key concepts in this area.

2. DEFINITIONS

There are many definitions for the words *religion* and *spirituality*. The scientific and theological communities are divided on how they define these terms.(1) In this book, the term *religion* is used to indicate specific behavioral, social, doctrinal, and denominational characteristics. In particular, it involves belief in a supernatural power or transcendent being, truth or ultimate reality, and the expression of such a belief in behavior and rituals.

Spirituality is concerned with the ultimate questions about life's meaning as it relates to the transcendent, which may or may not arise from formal religious traditions (but usually does). One may notice that spirituality's definition is more subjective, less measurable. From a clinical perspective, having a term that is broad and diffuse is good because this allows patients to define what it means for them. Using the language of spirituality helps to establish a dialogue with persons who may or may not consider themselves religious. From a research perspective, however, such lack of conceptual clarity is not permitted.

Some authors (2) distinguish *extrinsic* religion, that is, a means to nonsacred goals, such as increasing social contacts or attaining other external benefits, and *intrinsic* religion, that is, religion that is lived, internalized, and motivated for religion's sake, rather than for external benefits.

3. NEW PARADIGM

Religion is unique in the sense that it may involve beliefs that a supernatural being has influence on

1

how things are. Research on religion and mental health does not address the question of whether God exists. Rather, research on psychological processes involving religion is neutral with respect to the existence or nonexistence of God or any other supernatural being. In the context of care, clinicians should have the same attitude: Facing a patient addressing a religious issue, the question is not to determine whether it is true or false, but rather to consider it in terms of meaning, coping, and its relationship to current therapeutic goal(s). Addressing religion in the care of patients, one should recognize that religion involves multiple dimensions, for example, religious beliefs, religious affiliation, organized religious activity, "private" religiosity, religious commitment, religious experience, and religious coping i.e., religious behaviors or cognitions designed to help people adapt to difficult life situations.(3) A paradigm is needed to serve as a framework for research and patient care activity. Palouzian and Park(4) define a "multilevel interdisciplinary paradigm" as a framework that allows an accurate description of religious phenomena by recognizing "the value of data at multiple levels of analysis while making non-reductive assumptions concerning the values of spiritual and religious phenomena." As an example of the usefulness of this paradigm, Palouzian and Park describe the case of religious conversion, which can be examined both at a neuropsychological level and at a social-psychological level.

The multilevel interdisciplinary paradigm can accommodate subdisciplines of psychology, but also other domains such as evolutionary biology, neurosciences, anthropology, philosophy, other allied areas of science, and pastoral care.

Clinicians need to keep this paradigm in mind, because many disciplines may have something to offer depending on the specific clinical situations.

4. MODEL OF CARE

Psychiatric care often involves a multidisciplinary/multilevel model of care. The overarching paradigm that should be considered in the care of patients with psychiatric conditions is the bio-psycho-social model,(5) which aims at addressing the whole person. This model underscores the need to consider disorders from a holistic perspective, thus avoiding a reductionistic view that considers only biological (e.g., pharmacological treatments) or psychological aspects of the person. Appling this model includes integrating religion/spirituality into the social part of this model or, preferably, including this dimension in all three areas, thus approaching patients from a bio-psycho-social-religious/spiritual model. This is recommended because religion/spirituality affects social, psychological, and even biological aspects of human life, and all domains affect each other, including the spiritual.

5. PLACE OF RELIGION/SPIRITUALITY

Research suggests that religion/spirituality can be helpful for persons with physical disorders. For instance, outcomes of heart disease have been related to religious involvement.(6) This may be due to the relationship between religious beliefs and cardiovascular risk factors such as high blood pressure, cigarette smoking, and diet and to the stress-reducing effects of religious coping. Religion may also influence cancer incidence,(7) notably through dietary and health practices fostered by certain religious groups. The course and outcome of cancer may also be favorably influenced by religious involvement through improved health behaviors, but also by the use of religious coping that may instill hope and reduce anxiety.

In the field of psychiatry, partly for "historical" reasons, the general attitude toward religion has been ambivalent. Religious belief, practice, and experience have often been considered neurotic by mental health professionals, at least in the past. Religion offers a different way of viewing psychiatric illness that may conflict with that of psychiatrists. Evidence also exists showing that religion may offer help to patients with psychiatric conditions, particularly those with substance use disorders. This led to the implementation of 12-step programs to facilitate the treatment of patients with alcohol or drug problems (see Chapter 9). More recently, religious coping has been shown to influence the outcomes of bereavement and major depressive disorders (see Chapter 8). Concerning patients with psychosis, the diagnosis of "mystical delusion" has hindered clinicians from recognizing the positive influences of religion.(8) However, recent research from Switzerland and other countries has documented the powerful benefits in terms of coping that religion/spirituality can have for psychotic patients.(9, 10)

Thus, although further research on this topic is greatly needed, growing evidence demonstrates that religion/spirituality is important for patients with psychiatric conditions and may be beneficial or detrimental to their illness. We hope that providing updated information to clinicians about the research in this area and describing sensible clinical applications will help to overcome the reluctance among clinicians to address these issues with patients. At a minimum, this book will make mental health professionals more aware of an important area of patients' lives that is rarely addressed in clinical settings.(11)

6. THE ROLE OF CLINICIANS

The role of the clinician is not an easy one. Clinicians involved in psychiatry have many reasons for their reluctance to address spiritual/religious issues with patients.

First, clinicians' own religious involvement (or lack thereof) may influence the value they place on religious/spiritual issues. We are generally less involved in religious activities than our patients are (12) and are thus less likely to be interested in discussing these issues.

Second, there is widespread lack of knowledge about how to address religion or spirituality in clinical practice. Psychiatric training rarely devotes much time to such issues, as described later in this book (see Chapter 22).

Third, as mentioned earlier, there has been historical conflict between psychiatry and religion.

Some authors (Freud) have referred to religion as an "illusion," merely a neurotic defense against life's vicissitudes.(13) Antagonism remains today between clergy and psychiatrists, because their domains overlap and they often share the same "customers."

Fourth, some clinicians may fear that addressing issues pertaining to religion may represent walking into unknown territories, thus risking harm to patients. In some areas of the world (e.g., in Europe), clinicians may fear offending patients by bringing up such issues, which patients may not wish to address.

Fifth, psychiatrists may feel uncomfortable being involved in a social/care network in which roles are not well defined between clinicians, chaplains, and clergy. This is likely to be the case in areas where clinicians and clergy have not worked together before.

A common factor at the root of most of these concerns is a lack of knowledge and tools, which this book is intended to help correct.

7. WHO SHOULD READ THIS BOOK?

This book seeks to give knowledge and practical tools to clinicians taking care of patients with psychiatric disorders. The goal is to cover issues pertaining to psychiatry and religion/spirituality in a way likely to engage and maintain the interest of readers who may not be particularly interested in religion. There is a large gap between those who are interested in religion, consider it when treating their patients, and are drawn by books or papers on this topic, and those who have little or no interest in religion, do not broach this topic in clinical settings, and feel reluctant to "waste time" learning about this topic. The present text is designed to fill this gap by providing concise, detailed information that will help clinicians consider integrating spirituality into the care of patients, even if the clinician is not religious.

This book is written by psychiatrists, psychologists, theologians, and pastoral care experts and will be of use to all clinicians treating patients with psychiatric disorders.

8. WHAT THIS BOOK IS NOT

First, this book does not address claims about the supernatural (i.e., whether God exists), whether any particular religion is "true" or "false," or whether one religious tradition is healthier than another. Rather, religion is considered to be an important way of shaping human experience in the context of psychiatric disorders.

Second, this book is not a textbook on the psychology or sociology of religion. We do not emphasize concepts, definitions, or particular models of care. This has been addressed elsewhere.(3, 4) Rather, this book is focused on issues that are directly related to patient care.

9. CONTENT OF THE BOOK

This book presents (1) an overview of theoretical (2) a systematic description of specific psychiatric conditions and their relationship to religion/spirituality, and (3) psychosocial and curricular aspects of religion/spirituality in psychiatry, with an emphasis on clinical applications throughout.

First, we consider historical and theological factors relevant for clinicians, neuropsychiatric aspects of religion/spirituality, and a brief commentary on the Bible from a particular view regarding its "psychological" aspects.

Second, we discuss specific psychiatric disorders to provide a comprehensive update on recent research. This will include "Axis I" disorders, but also conditions such as identity disorders, religious delusions, and personality disorders. These chapters have been written from a multicultural perspective. Spiritual assessment will also be described.

Third, authors will address treatment in the community, which may involve coordination between clinicians, chaplains, and clergy. We include here three examples of treatment approaches involving Christian, Muslim, and Buddhist principles. Including these chapters does not mean that we share or endorse all the views presented here. The goal is to provide the reader with information on various religious ways of approaching the psychological needs of patients. As clinicians, we are confronted with patients who wish to engage in these treatments. Therefore, although many of us may not adopt such approaches, we should at least have knowledge about them so that we can advise patients about their merit. Finally, an overview is presented on what needs to be taught in psychiatric residency programs about religion/spirituality to enhance the competency of future psychiatrists (and other clinicians) in this area.

Thus, we welcome you on an informative and fascinating journey into a critical area of our patients' lives that may represent a powerful resource for healing or be intricately interwoven with psychopathology, requiring both professional psychiatric care and pastoral care to resolve and disentangle.

REFERENCES

1. Larson DB, Swyers JP, McCullough ME: *Scientific research on spirituality and health: A consensus report.* Rockville, MD: National Institute for Health Research, 1997.
2. Allport GW, Ross JM: Personal Religious Orientation and Prejudice. *Journal of Personality and Social Psychology* 1967;5:432–443.
3. Koenig HG, McCullough ME, Larson DB: *Handbook of Religion and Health.* Oxford: Oxford University Press, 2001.
4. Palouzian RF, Park CL: *Handbook of the Psychology of Religion and Spirituality.* New York: Guilford Press, 2005.
5. Engel GL: The need of a new medical model: A challenge for biomedicine. *Science* 1977;196: 129–136.
6. Goldbourt U, Yaari S, Medalie JH: Factors predictive of long-term coronary heart disease mortality among 10,059 male Israeli civil servants and municipal employees. A 23-year mortality follow-up in the Israeli Ischemic Heart Disease Study. *Cardiology* 1993;82:100–121.
7. Enstrom JE: Health practices and cancer mortality among active California Mormons. *Journal of the National Cancer Institute* 1989;81:1807–1814.
8. Mohr S, Huguelet P: The relationship between schizophrenia and religion and its implications for care. *Swiss Medical Weekly* 2004;134:369–376.
9. Mohr S, Brandt PY, Gillieron C, Borras L, Huguelet P: Toward an integration of religiousness and spirituality into the psychosocial dimension of schizophrenia. *American Journal of Psychiatry* 2006;163:1952–1959.

10. Yangarber-Hicks N: Religious coping style and recovery from serious mental illness. *Journal of Psychology and Theology* 2004;32:305–317.

11. Huguelet P, Mohr S, Brandt P-Y, Borras L, Gillieron C: Spirituality and religious practices among outpatients with schizophrenia and their clinicians. *Psychiatric Services* 2006;57:366–372.

12. Neeleman J, King MB: Psychiatrists' religious attitudes in relation to their clinical practice: A survey of 231 psychiatrists. *Acta Psychiatrica Scandinavica* 1993;88:420–424.

13. Gay P: *A Godless Jew: Freud, Atheism, and the Making of Psychoanalysis.* New Haven: Yale University Press, 1987.

2 Spirituality and the Care of Madness: Historical Considerations

SAMUEL B. THIELMAN

SUMMARY

Spiritual and religious issues are sometimes neglected or misrepresented in histories of psychiatry. This chapter outlines a historical approach to understanding how spiritual and religious ideas are expressed in medical and religious writings dealing with madness. Sacred writings, inscriptions, ancient architecture, commentaries, pastoral letters, medical texts, and religious and spiritual publications all reflect a range of ideas about the role of spirituality and the supernatural in the etiology and treatment of mental disorders. Beginning with ancient pagan and Jewish writings, and continuing with the writings of the early church fathers, medieval physicians and Puritan divines, the chapter describes ways in which spirituality influenced the care of emotionally distressed patients. The chapter discusses the ways in which both naturalistic and supernaturalistic views of madness are reflected in practice in the roots of modern medicine in the eighteenth century and how psychiatrists and others dealt with religious issues during the more secular nineteenth and twentieth centuries. The chapter argues against the position that there has been steady progression from a supernatural to a naturalistic understanding of madness and shows how religious and spiritual ideas continue to affect the psychiatric approach to mental disorders.

INTRODUCTION

The history of psychiatry has often been written as though the emergence of psychiatry involved a transition from superstition to reason, from religion to science, and that only in the modern era have we come to understand that madness is not the result of the influence of spirits, demons, and curses. In fact, the relationship among ideas of madness and religion, medicine and theology, treatment and ritual is complex and varied. Although natural explanations seem to compete with religious explanations, in fact, people actually caring for the mad often (although not always) held these explanations in mind concurrently, and doctors, clergy, and families used this understanding as a basis for managing those for whom they cared.

Different religious traditions, of course, have had different approaches to the mad. This chapter focuses primarily on care given in the Christian tradition in Europe and North America because it is this tradition that has shaped modern psychiatry's way of dealing with religious and spiritual issues. Historical accounts of the Islamic approach to the mad indicate a variety of ways of dealing with madness – from the traditional Islamic methods that involved casting out the devil, to Koran-based methods, to an approach that involves a naturalistic understanding.[1, 2] Hinduism and Buddhism have their own approaches to madness as well.[3–5]

I. THE BIBLE AND MADNESS

For a variety of reasons, including missionary activity, European colonialism, and the adaptable nature of Christian belief, Christians are present in significant numbers in most parts of the modern world.[6] The Bible is, arguably, the most globally influential of ancient religious texts, and it has influenced the West, both physicians and lay people, since the time of Constantine, so it is important to understand how the Bible presents madness. The Bible has several sections that have shaped views of madness – although in different ways at different times.

The Bible was written and edited over many centuries. The Old Testament (or Hebrew Scriptures), assumed its present form in about 90 AD.(7) The New Testament canon was established at the Council of Nicea in 325 AD. All Christian groups accept the parts of the Old Testament that Jews regard as canonical. Roman Catholic, Eastern Orthodox, and Coptic Christians, variously, include additional edifying Jewish writings that were not accepted as canonical by Jews.

Madness is portrayed in the Old Testament in several ways, sometimes in naturalistic terms, sometimes otherwise. Illustrative of the various ways madness is viewed in the Bible are the accounts of madness in 1 Samuel. In Chapter 21, the young David, not yet king of Israel, finds himself in a dangerous situation in the presence of Achish, a Philistine king, and his comrades. According to the Bible, "he changed his behavior before them, and pretended to be insane in their hands and made marks on the doors of the gate and let his spittle run down his beard" (1 Sam. 21:13, NRSV). Achish was disgusted and declared, "Do I lack madmen, that you have brought this fellow to play the madman in my presence? Shall this fellow come into my house?" (21:15). David was able to escape and carry on unharmed. In this setting, madness is presented as a natural phenomenon that is not unusual.

The same book of the Bible, five chapters earlier, includes an account of Saul that describes a supernatural cause of madness or, in Saul's case, despair. The writer records, "Now the Spirit of the Lord departed from Saul, and an evil spirit from the Lord tormented him" (1 Sam. 16:14). In this story, David was summoned to play his lyre for Saul, because David had musical talent, and David's music greatly consoled Saul. Saul hired David to work for him, and "whenever the evil spirit from God was upon Saul, David took the lyre and played it with his hand. So Saul was refreshed and was well, and the evil spirit departed from him" (16:23).

In the New Testament, madness is sometimes attributed to demons. In the Gospel of John, Jesus's opponents at one point say, "He is demon possessed and raving mad. Why listen to him" (John 10:20). In another incident, Paul tells the recipients of one of his letters, to make a point, that he is speaking as though he is mad, with no implication of a supernatural aspect at all.

These examples illustrate something that is true throughout the Old and New Testaments: when madness is portrayed, it is often seen in naturalistic terms, but the Lord often has something to do with the madness (for example, Deut. 28:28, Jer. 25:16 and 51:7, and Zech. 12:4).

Not only does the Bible contain information on an ancient way of viewing madness in spiritual terms, but it also contains large portions of wisdom literature that is analogous to modern self-help literature, although religious readers would consider it help from God. Wisdom literature exists in many writings from the ancient world, and there are parallels in the Bible to Egyptian wisdom literature. The books of Proverbs, Ecclesiastes, Wisdom, and Sirach all contain advice on how to live life and how to understand life's difficulties.

2. MADNESS AND RELIGION IN THE ANCIENT WORLD

The ancient world presents a wide range of worldviews and a number of philosophies of healing. Religion, psychology, and medicine were intertwined, for example, in the ancient healing cult, the cult of Asclepius. The cult of Asclepius was the most widespread healing cult in the ancient world, originating with the ancient Greeks and lasting until after the time of Christ. Asclepius was a god of healing whose temples were places of healing. One of the principal methods of healing in the temple was making a votive offering of a small replica of the diseased organ and waiting for healing. Healing often came through dreams in which Asclepius would appear. The Asclepian physicians were practitioners of rational medicine who, when they could not heal through rational medicine, directed the sick to the Asclepian temple (p. xviii).(8) Certain psychological methods were attributed to the god Asclepius. Galen of Pergamum (c. 130–216 AD), the well-known physician of the second century, offered this insight into how Asclepius, the deity, ordered psychological means to cure disordered emotions:

> And not a few men … we have made healthy by correcting the disproportion of their emotions. No slight witness of the statement is also our ancestral god Asclepius who ordered not a few to [write] odes … he ordered hunting and horse riding and exercising in arms…. For he not only desired to awake the passion of those men because it was weak, but also defined the measure by the form of exercises" (pp. 208–209).(8)

More significant for religion in the West were the Hippocratic writings and Plato and Platonism. Hippocratic medicine is highly valued in modern accounts of medical history because it encouraged observation over theory, and because it generally eschewed supernatural explanations of madness.(9)

Early church writers generally respected the work of physicians and had a view of madness that incorporated a spiritual perspective, while acknowledging the physical influences that cause mental distress as well. The writings of John Chrysostom (c. 347–407 AD) reflect this approach. John Chrysostom was bishop of Constantinople, a highly regarded preacher, and a person with considerable skills as a pastor. In a series of letters to Olympias, a deaconess who apparently suffered from bouts of despair, Chrysostom provided a wealth of information about his views on despair and its relationship to physical illness. Melancholia per se is not mentioned. Instead, Chrysostom referred frequently to *athumia* and its relationship to illness. Olympias apparently suffered from a chronic complaint of unclear origin, and this condition was accompanied by a sense of despair and gloom. Chrysostom at times tried to comfort her by assuring her that physical illness often caused despair. "[Job] was not tortured by despondency [until] he was delivered over to sickness and sores, then did he also long for death" (p. 294).(10)

As his correspondence with Olympias progressed, however, Chrysostom began to become somewhat more impatient. In rebuking her for persisting in her state of dejection he told her that he believed that her physical illness was caused by her sense of dejection:

> You lately affirmed that it was nothing but despondency which caused this sickness of yours…. I shall not believe that you have got rid of your despondency unless you have got rid of your bodily infirmity (p. 296).(10)

He then went on to rebuke her for taking pride in her sorrow:

> I … reckon it as the greatest accusation that you should say 'I take a pride in increasing my sorrow by thinking over it': for when you ought to make every possible effort to dispel your affliction you do the devil's will, by increasing your despondency and sorrow. Are you not aware how great an evil despondency is? (p. 301) … Do not then now desire death, nor neglect the means of cure; for indeed this would not be safe (p. 296).(10)

Finally, Chrysostom offered pastoral advice for her dejected state: he suggested that she pray, that she read his earlier letter, and even that she memorize it. He also suggested that she compare the blessings God had given her to her adverse circumstances to help her obtain consolation for her feelings of despair (p. 297).(10)

To the despondent, John Chrysostom recommended the Christian faith as a remedy in his homily on St. Ignatius: "If any is in despondency, if in disease, if under insult, if in any other circumstance of this life, if in the depth of sins, let him come hither with faith, and he will lay aside all those things, and will return with much joy."(11) Yet his letter to Olympias, directed as it was to a more specific case of despondency, is nuanced and humane.

Not all of the early church writers held a balanced view. Tatian (c. 160) was a disciple of Justin Martyr, a skilled speaker and theologian. In *Oration to the Greeks*, Tatian asserted a view that demons follow sickness.(12) The cure of madness is from God, not from the amulets that madmen were apparently supposed to wear.

> A disease is not killed by antipathy, nor is a madman cured by wearing amulets. These [cures from amulets result from] visitations of demons. … How can it be right to ascribe help given to madmen to matter and not to God? [The] skill [of those who use such means to cure] is to turn men away from God's service, and contrive that they should rely on herbs and roots.(12)

Tatian, however, did not always hold views consistent with orthodoxy, and his view of "herbs and roots" was probably not shared by many early church leaders.

3. RELIGIOUS APPROACH TO MADNESS IN THE MIDDLE AGES IN EUROPE

Of the few extant sources for learning about the spiritual side of the treatment of madness during the Middle Ages, perhaps the Leechbook of Bald is the most interesting. The Leechbook consists of three books owned by Bald, presumably a physician, and compiled in the ninth century in England.(13) The Leechbook contains remedies for all sorts of ailments. Many of the remedies are plant remedies, but the book also contains incantations and rituals to be used in the treatment of disease. Book I of the Leechbook of Bald contains several references to madness and interestingly distinguishes between demon possession and lunacy. Even for demon possession, the physician is to treat the demon-possessed man with an herbal concoction: "For a fiendsick

man, or demoniac, when a devil possesses the man or controls him from within with disease; a spew drink, or emetic, lupin, bishopwort, henbane, cropleek; pound these together, add ale for a liquid, let it stand for a night, add fifty libcorns, or cathartic grains, and holy water" (p. 137).(14) This mixture is put into every drink that the possessed man will drink, and he is then directed to sing Psalms 99, 68, and 69, then drink the drink out of a church bell and let a priest say mass over him. For the lunatic the writer prescribes another herbal concoction of costmary, goutweed, lupin, betony, attorlothe, cropleek, field gentian, hove, and fennellet. A mass is to be sung over it, and the lunatic is to drink the mixture for nine mornings, then give alms and earnestly pray to God for mercy (p. 139).(14)

There is an additional instruction for lunatics in Leechbook III, thought to be the most rooted in contemporary Anglo-Saxon medicine.(13) "In case a man be a lunatic; take skin of a mereswine or porpoise, work it into a whip, swinge [beat] the man therewith, soon he will be well. Amen" (p. 335).(15) There was also a formula for dealing with temptation: "Against temptation of the fiend, a wort hight red niolin, red stalk, it waxeth by running water: if thou hast it on thee, and under thy head bolster, and over thy house doors, the devil may not scathe thee, within nor without" (p. 343).(15) Clearly, Anglo-Saxon medicine incorporated a religious worldview, and they used for treatment both material means (the herbal remedies) and religiously symbolic means (drinking a concoction out of a church bell, saying masses as part of the treatment, and singing psalms as a means of receiving healing).

4. EMERGENCE OF A MORE NATURALISTIC CLINICAL APPROACH TO MADNESS AMONG ENGLISH PURITANS

Although in some spheres there was an increased interest in the occult and the supernatural during the Renaissance, those dealing with the mad moved even further away from relying on supernatural explanations. Reginald Scott's (d. 1599) book, *Discoverie of Witchcraft* (1584) reflects a point of view that grew in the sixteenth century: that people who are sad or distressed suffer from a natural malady and not from supernatural influences. Scott was a surveyor, not a physician, and was active in the county government of Kent, England. *Discoverie of Witchcraft* is primarily an extended and entertaining argument against the notion that witches actually have supernatural powers. In the process, Scott reveals a lot about charlatanism in the sixteenth century, and the book even explains a number of card-and-ball deceptions that in our time are considered to be magic tricks. Scott also touches on the treatment of the insane and, in so doing, reveals how religious reasoning was used by families to help those suffering from religious delusions.

Scott recounts the case of Ade Davie, wife of Simon Davie, a farmer from Scott's home county of Kent, and a person known to Scott. At some time in her early adulthood, Ade, who had no prior history of any sort of melancholy or madness, "grew suddenlie (as her husband informed me ...) to be somewhat pensive and more sad than in times past." Simon was worried, but did not tell anyone for fear that he would be thought guilty of "ill husbandrie." But Ade became worse. She could not sleep, she cried, she began sighing and "lamenting," and although her husband pressed her, Ade would not provide any reason for her sadness. Finally, Ade fell to her knees and confessed to Simon that she was depressed because she had sold her soul to the devil. Her husband replied, "Thou has sold that which is none of thine to sell ... Christ ... paid for it, even with his bloud ..., so as the divell hath no interest in it." The husband reasoned with her in this fashion. His wife then told him, "I have yet committed another fault and done you more injurie: for I have bewitched you and your children." But her husband reasoned with her, "Be content ... by the grace of God, Jesus Christ shall unwitch us: for none evill can happen to them that feare God." With time, Ade recovered, "and remaineth a right honest woman ... shamed of hir imaginations,

which she perceiveth to have growne through melancholie" (pp. 31–32).(16)

Scott's account and his general view of melancholy and the supernatural indicate that by the latter part of the sixteenth century, naturalistic explanations for mental disorders were prevalent even among educated laymen. In fact, naturalistic explanations for melancholy were prevalent among physicians throughout the Middle Ages, although spiritual/religious factors were acknowledged as playing a role in mental distress as well.(17)

By the seventeenth century, a rather sophisticated practical way of dealing with psychological distress emerged from the thinking of Puritan writers. These writers, because of their concern with spiritual experience, conversion, and the inner spiritual life, were often very attuned to the existence of states of mental distress and despair. Many offered pastoral advice that reflects a concern for the psychological well-being of the individual and provides a variety of spiritual explanations and remedies.

Among the most influential of the Puritan writers on emotional distress was Richard Baxter (1615–1691), an Anglican priest who, in those tumultuous times, became a "dissenter." Because he could not in good conscience comply with the British Act of Uniformity, he could not preach, and so he had a lot of time to write. Baxter wrote prolifically about many aspects of living a Christian life, and he also wrote about depression. During the 1660s, Baxter wrote *A Christian Directory* (1673), a gigantic compendium of thoughtful and well-organized spiritual counsel on a range of topics, including marriage, business ethics, lawsuits, government, dealing with sickness and dying, church government, recreation, and, most of all, how to lead a spiritual life.(18)

In *A Christian Directory*, Baxter wrote a lengthy set of instructions on identifying and treating melancholy. He thought of melancholy as a "diseased craziness, hurt or error in imagination and consequently of the understanding" (p. 294).(19) It was characterized by preoccupation with having irreparably sinned, perplexing thoughts, and the inability to divert thoughts to pleasant subjects. He, like many other Puritan writers, rejected the idea that the devil was primarily responsible for melancholy.

Baxter counseled that those who were melancholy reduce the time spent in religious exercises so that religious duties would become less burdensome. He advised the melancholy to seek cheerful company, to oppose blasphemous thoughts with reason, and to avoid "thoughts upon your thoughts." In addition to many other similar pieces of advice, Baxter advised, "Commit yourself to the care of your physician and obey him" for "I have seen [many people] cured by physic; and till the body be cured, the mind will hardly ever be cured, but the clearest reasons will be all in vain" (p. 267).(19)

Timothy Rogers (1658–1728) took a similarly medically oriented approach to depression, which nonetheless incorporates the religious worldview of Christianity in a nonmagical way. Rogers was a Presbyterian minister in England who became depressed in his early twenties. Although he subsequently was very effective as a preacher, he wrote extensively on the proper spiritual approach to melancholy.(20) Not surprisingly, his most well-known book, *Trouble of Mind and the Disease of Melancholy* (1691), contains practical wisdom shaped by his own experience. In Rogers' estimation, melancholy was a condition like gout or a gallstone, because it created great misery for the sufferer and the sufferer was helpless against it. Rogers advised those who cared for the melancholy person to educate those who suffered about the nature of the "disease" (his term). Empathy was also important:

> Look upon those that are under this woeful Disease of Melancholy with great pity and compassion. And pity them the more, by considering that you yourselves are in the body and liable to the very same trouble; for how brisk, how sanguine, and how cheerful soever you be, yet you may meet with those heavy Crosses, those long and painful and sharp Afflictions which may sink your spirits. (p. v)(21)

He counseled against harshness, which only poured oil on the flames and would chafe and exasperate them. He advised reassuring the patient that people recover from melancholy. He also pointed out that, although the devil was at work in melancholy,

> Do not attributed the effects of meer Disease, to the Devil; though I deny not that the Devil has an hand in the causing of several Diseases.... [I]t is a very overwhelming thing, to attribute every action almost of a Melancholly man to the Devil, when there are some unavoidable Expressions of sorrow which are purely natural, and which he cannot help, no more than any other sick man can forbear to groan (p. xv).(21)

Like Richard Baxter, he valued medical treatment, writing, "I would never have the Physician's Counsel despised." But he believed that the physician and the minister should work together, because both the soul and the body need attention in depression (p. iv).(21) The physician, by physic and diet and "harmless diversions" would prepare the troubled soul for the more complicated task of dealing with spiritual troubles. Clearly the Puritans, like many Christian writers before them, valued both medical and spiritual methods of treatment and believed that the two together were needed to treat melancholy.

Patients wrote of spirituality and the care of madness as well. The way in which spirituality was incorporated into thinking about madness in the seventeenth century emerges clearly from the account of George Trosse (1631–1713) of his own madness. Trosse was a Presbyterian clergyman who left a very readable autobiography that was published posthumously in 1714. Born in Exeter, he purposed early on to travel, make money, and live a life of luxury. He drank a lot, flirted a lot, and had very little use for religion. (22) Then, in 1656, when he was 25 years old, he began to experience emotional distress and hallucinations.

If I walked in the *Garden*, (as there sometimes I took many distracted turns) I
would fancy all about me *Places* of *Burning*,
and *Torments*, and *Devils*.... Thus I discovered the *Confusion* and *Distraction* of my
Mind where ever I went [Italics added].
(pp. 98–99)(23)

He was taken by friends to the house of a physician who specialized in the treatment of mad
people.

But at length, thro' the *Goodness of God*, and
by His *Blessing* upon *Physick*, a *low Diet*,
and *hard keeping*, I began to be ordered
and *civil* in my *Carriage* and *Converse*, and
gradually to regain the use of my *Reason*
[Italics added]. (p. 101)(23)

Trosse read the Scriptures, memorized portions of Scripture, began to "favor somewhat
matters of *Religion*," and prayed with a Christian
woman who was one of the employees of the
mad-house (p. 181).(23) He began to improve.
Trosse suffered two relapses shortly afterward,
but he recovered, attended university, and had an
active career as a Presbyterian minister until his
death at age 81.

5. DEVELOPMENT OF A MORE SECULAR MEDICAL APPROACH TO MADNESS DURING THE ENLIGHTENMENT

During the seventeenth and eighteenth centuries, philosophers and physicians began to think
of the soul less in religious terms and more in
philosophical or scientific terms. Likewise,
those dealing with the mad began separating
religious causes from other causes and religion/
spirituality became a category of madness.
This way of thinking about madness is most
clearly laid out in Robert Burton's *Anatomy of
Melancholy* (1621), in which Burton coined the
term "religious melancholy" and wrote at length
describing the condition and offering recommendations for cure.

In the eighteenth century, Enlightenment
thought permeated the philosophical aspects of
medicine, and the Reformation had created religious change all over Europe. A reform was also
taking place within madhouses and asylums in
Europe where the asylum began to be viewed as
having a therapeutic as well as a custodial purpose. Although management and medicine had
been part of the regimen of madhouses for some
time (p. 8),(24) several physicians for the mad
began outlining the need for a particular regimen
of management in the asylum and began to present the asylum as a therapeutic institution.(25)

Several individuals instituted extensive reforms for institutions for the mad. Sometimes
these reforms were driven by a religious motive,
as in England at the York Retreat. Sometimes
it was driven by a rationalist/secular reform
motive, as in the case of Philippe Pinel and his
reforms in France at the Salpetrière and other
hospitals. Sometimes the motives for humane
reforms were a mixture of these things, as they
were at the South Carolina Lunatic Asylum in
Columbia, South Carolina and at the Eastern
Lunatic Asylum in Williamsburg, Virginia.(26)
But whether reform motives were secular or religious, patients and their religious views had to be
considered.

In France, Philippe Pinel (1745–1826) instituted reforms at Bicêtre and Salpetrière, and
these reforms sprang from an Enlightenment/
rationalistic motive (pp. 9, 47, 53, 78–81).(27)
In fact, like his revolutionary contemporaries in France, Pinel did not have much use for
religion. Pinel was very much motivated by the
pursuit of knowledge and by the need to treat
mad patients humanely and with a degree of
respect. He criticized physicians' reliance on
contemporary theories of inflammation to
understand the brain, advocating instead that
they focus on the "management of the mind,"
that is, moral therapy (pp. 4–5).(27) Pinel's
approach to "religious enthusiasm" was to separate the religiously delusional patient from
others; encourage physical activity; remove
from view every book, painting, or other object
that could remind them of religion; order them

to devote time during the day to philosophical readings; and instruct them by "drawing apt comparisons between the distinguished acts of humanity and patriotism of the ancients, and the pious nullity and delirious extravagances of saints and anchorites" (p. 78).(27) Pinel recounts one instance when the directors of civil hospitals, in 1795, ordered that all religious objects be removed from hospitals. Although Pinel viewed this act as extreme, he did notice that, when implemented with goodwill and evident good intention on the part of hospital managers, it resulted in seeming improvement of many of the religiously delusional patients (pp. 80–81).(27)

But in other places, asylum reforms grew out of religious motives, especially among the Quakers and the hospitals under their influence in England and America, and religious exercises were an integral part of asylum management. The story of the reforms at the York Retreat is well known but inspiring. In 1790, a 42-year-old Quaker widow, Hannah Mills, died in the York Asylum in England six weeks after she had been admitted for melancholy. Local Quakers, who had tried to visit her to offer spiritual consolation, were denied access to her by officials at the asylum. William Tuke, one of those concerned about the death, was so moved by the way the case had been handled that he decided to establish a place of treatment for the mentally distressed that would provide care for Quakers. Although a physician was employed to provide medical treatment at the Retreat, laymen offered a gentle but religiously oriented therapy intended to calm those with mental disorders. Harsh management was not allowed, and patients were treated with dignity. In contrast to the authoritarian approach used by Pinel, Tuke's approach harnessed the gentle religious outlook of Quakerism to push patients toward wellness.

In 1813, Samuel Tuke published an account of the way the Retreat was managed, *A Description of the Retreat*, that became highly influential in inspiring similar reforms elsewhere (pp. 24 ff). (28, 29)

The Tukes believed that religious influences could be very helpful to the mad, and they were straightforward in stating their view. Samuel Tuke wrote:

> To encourage the influence of religious principles over the mind of the insane, is considered of great consequence, as a means of cure. For this purpose, as well as for others still more important, it is certainly right to promote in the patient, an attention to his accustomed modes of paying homage to his Maker. (p. 161)(30)

In the United States, especially, the model provided by the Retreat served as an inspiration for many of the early asylum superintendents as they established public and private institutions for the insane throughout the country in the early decades of the nineteenth century.

6. EMERGENCE OF THE MODERN MEDICAL APPROACH TO RELIGION AND MADNESS

By the nineteenth century, any notion that psychiatric disorders were directly the result of supernatural influence had vanished from medical writings and from most records of treatment. But interest in the influence of religion in mental disorders was prevalent, and there was an interest in both the positive and negative aspects of religion.

Indisputably, the most influential American physician who wrote about madness during the late eighteenth and early nineteenth century was Benjamin Rush (1746–1813). Not only was Rush an experienced general physician, but he was a prolific writer, a signer of the Declaration of Independence, and a firm advocate for reform of the care of mad people. Rush's book, *Medical Inquiries and Observations Upon the Diseases of the Mind* (1813), was in some ways an American counterpart of Pinel's *Treatise on Insanity* (1801; English version 1806). Both books were concerned with the classification and treatment, medical and "moral," of madness. Both books advocated humane treatment of patients. But philosophically, they differ significantly in their treatment of religion, because Rush, unlike Pinel, was a devout Protestant Christian.

Rush, like many physicians of his day, adopted a view of disease that placed heavy emphasis on the role of inflammation as a primary cause of many diseases. In the case of madness, Rush believed that disordered blood vessels were to blame. But this did not exclude the possibility of other influences, and religion was, in general, a positive influence.

Rush's book is sprinkled throughout with references to the Bible and to God and assumes throughout the correctness of his mildly Calvinistic perspective. For Rush, religion could influence patients both for ill and for good. On the one hand, a patient's madness might be precipitated by overstudy of Biblical end-time prophecies (p. 37)(31) or by incorrect doctrine (pp. 71, 83, and 115–116).(31) On the other hand, religion was in many instances helpful to patients. "Let not religion be blamed for these cases of insanity," Rush wrote. "[Its] tendency is to prevent [insanity] from most of its mental causes; and even the errors that have been blended with [religion] produce madness less frequently than love" (p. 45).(31)

Rush believed that there was a mental "believing faculty" that was disordered, for example, when people would "propagate stories that are probable, but false," a sort of paranoia (p. 272). (31) He thought this faculty was impaired in "persons who refuse to admit human testimony in favor of the truths of the Christian religion, [while] believing in all the events of profane history" (p. 274).(31)

As to treatment, Rush recommended, among many other things, reading the Bible as a way for patients suffering from hypochondriasis (or depression) to help themselves. Rush found that when hypochondriacal patients obsessed about having committed the unpardonable sin, reasoning with them seemed to help. In fact, Rush thought physicians should educate themselves about common religious problems of patients: "It is of consequence to a physician, to be fully prepared upon the subjects of the two errors

[of belief: unpardonable sin, and creation for misery] that I have named, for they are the two principal causes of religious hypochondriasm" (pp. 115–116).(31) He also advised that physicians enlist the support of the clergy in such instances because "erroneous opinions in religion … must be removed, by advising the visits of a sensible and enlightened clergyman" (p. 115).(31)

Rush's views reflect the general respect in America for religious patients that existed throughout most of the nineteenth century. Although some American asylum superintendents and others who treated madness held to a broader view of religion, others held views very similar to those of Rush, and religion and experienced clergy who were bereft of extremism were welcome in American asylums.

During the nineteenth century, the focus on religion began to disappear from most of European and American psychiatry, even in the countries that had been affected by religious reform.

Johann Christian August Heinroth (1773–1843), a German physician, who wrote on mental disorders, viewed psychiatric disorders as conditions resulting from sin, but his approach was exceptional.(32) More typical were the views of physicians such as Wilhelm Griesinger (1817–1868) who wrote:

The aid of religion in the treatment of insanity is not to be lightly estimated; the application of this remedy requires, however, great caution. Religious instruction should not be withheld from any patient who desires and requires it; it would, however, oppose the first principles of mental treatment to enforce such instruction, or attempt to interest in it any one who has no religion at heart. It would show total ignorance of the nature and circumstances of those diseases to aim at direct recovery by reforming or converting the patient by religious instruction. All such means should only aim at imparting quietude, trust, and hope to direct attention from the morbid representations to an earnest and remarkable theme to revive the modes of thought and sensation of his healthy state. (p. 347)(33)

In fact, Griesinger was concerned about the possibility of developing various forms of psychiatry that were religiously oriented.

Several medical psychologists would have the whole treatment of the insane to be specifically Christian. But Jews also require the aid of the alienist and his science, and there is no abstract, only a confessional Christianity. Therefore there would require to be a special Protestant, Catholic, etc., and again a Jewish, heathen, psychiatrie. Possibly even this may be yet desired (p. 348).(33)

Griesinger's concern was that physicians needed to treat patients who came their way regardless of religious background, and a form of psychiatry that was too sectarian would not serve the field of psychiatry, or patients, well.

There were those who had concerns about the relationship of religion to mental health for other reasons as well. While Benjamin Rush, writing at the beginning of the nineteenth century, believed that religion tended to be a positive influence, others, even in the United States, did not share his view. Amariah Brigham (1798–1849), an American asylums superintendent and the first president of the American Psychiatry Association (then known as the Association of Medical Superintendents of American Institutions for the Insane), wrote an entire book about the effect of religion on mental health, *Observations on the Influence of Religion upon the Health and Physical Welfare of Mankind* (1835). He was particularly concerned about the effects of "religious excitement" on mental health, observing, "It should, however, never be forgotten, that of all the sentiments imparted to man, the religious, is the most powerful," and, therefore, like other "exciting influences," could cause insanity (p. 285).(34)

Similarly, Isaac Ray (1807–1881), an American alienist known, among other things, for his expertise in forensic psychiatry, wrote in *Mental Hygiene* (1863) that religious excitement could be a powerful force in creating mental imbalance in those predisposed to insanity. Because religion involved nothing less than a person's eternal destiny, it was bound to have a negative effect on people who were emotionally unstable (p. 190). (35) So Ray counseled that people should "carefully avoid all scenes of religious excitement, and indulge their religious emotions in quiet and by ordinary methods, always allowing other emotions and other duties their rightful share of attention" (p. 193).(35)

7. LATE NINETEENTH AND TWENTIETH CENTURY

During the latter part of the nineteenth century, psychiatry itself in Europe and the United States tended toward a view of mental illness that was more pessimistic and focused on heredity and biology. The number of people in psychiatric hospitals increased substantially. In the late nineteenth century, however, there was also an increased interest in hysteria and the effect of the mind on the unexplainable presentations of disease. This period also saw the increased professionalization of medicine, medical specialization, and the beginnings of outpatient psychiatric practice and psychotherapy. With the interest of physicians in milder forms of mental disorder and in psychotherapy came a concurrent interest in the role of religion in psychological development. In the United States, psychologist William James (1842–1910) of Harvard explored, in *Varieties of Religious Experience* (1902), the role of religion in the life of ordinary individuals seeking to make sense of existence. James saw religious experience as a major way through which human beings dealt with the emotional complexities of their lives. It was also the way people made sense of the good and the evil that they experienced as they lived their lives.(36)

For medicine, however, the most important influence of the late nineteenth and early twentieth centuries was the work of Sigmund Freud (1856–1939), who, more than anyone else, was responsible for bringing psychiatrists out of the hospital and into the psychotherapy consulting room. Freud was an unabashed atheist, and his later works make very clear that he viewed religion as a shared delusion, helpful for some, harmful for others, but ultimately something that was an indicator of psychological immaturity. It was a way through which humans came to terms with the fear of death and the concern about meaninglessness.

Freud's thinking embodied the materialistic conception of medicine that continues to be influential and that, during Freud's time, was taught to him in London, Vienna, and Berlin. (37) In *The Future of an Illusion* (1927), Freud proposed that religion was a common but false belief and that God was a projection of internal desires. In *Civilization and Its Discontents* (1929), he wrote that religion was a delusion of the masses that could relieve some anxieties, but that fostered immaturity and restricted choice. Freud's view of religion set the tone for the psychiatric view of religion in the West, particularly the United States, during much of the twentieth century.

But some analysts were uncomfortable with Freud's hostility to religion (notably Carl Jung, but also Gregory Zilboorg) and, in fact, Freud's thought could be adapted to the purposes of religionists. A number of American Protestant clergy, interested in applying the insights of Freud to pastoral work, used psychoanalytic thought to enrich pastoral work. In 1906, the Reverend Elwood Worcester (1862–1940) and the Reverend Samuel McComb, both clergymen, set up an education and psychotherapy program through the Emmanuel Church in Boston and collaborated with an early psychoanalyst, Isidor Coriat, as well as prominent Boston physicians Joseph Pratt, James Jackson Putnam, and Richard Cabot. This effort, which became known as the Emmanuel Movement, continued until 1929. The program was intended to counter the influence of the new "healing cults" that were sweeping the United States. However, as it developed, it foreshadowed the modern pastoral counseling movement.(38–41)

Psychiatry itself tended to relegate religion to the province of hospital chaplains and clergy. In the United States, psychoanalytic thought and psychoanalytic psychotherapy, usually somewhat hostile to religiosity, became a major force in psychiatry through the 1960s.(42) Psychoanalysis, which in its early days had included practitioners from a range of disciplines, came to be comprised largely of psychiatrists, especially after 1938 when the American Psychoanalytic Association made psychiatric training part of the requirements for membership.(25) (In Europe, psychoanalysis was less influential, but more professionally inclusive.)

During the latter part of the twentieth century, the influence of psychoanalysis on clinical practice waned as psychiatry came to be influenced much more directly by the neurosciences and cognitive psychology. In addition, the spiritual, yet nonsectarian perspective of Alcoholics Anonymous, which came to national prominence in the 1940s and 1950s, highlighted the potential therapeutic benefits of spiritually oriented programs.(43) With the lessening philosophical opposition to religion, some psychiatrists and others interested in mental health explored more fully the role of religion in mental health. In 1968, the Committee on Psychiatry and Religion of the Group for the Advancement of Psychiatry published a report noting the positive as well as the negative influences of religion on mental health.(44) In 1986, the *American Journal of Psychiatry* published a seminal review article by Larson and colleagues documenting the lack of adequate literature on the mental health effects of religion.(45) During the 1990s and early 2000s, interest in religion and spirituality grew substantially and was evident in many geographical regions. The Royal College of Psychiatrists began the Spirituality and Psychiatry Special Interest Group in 1999, the World Psychiatric Association recently established a Section on Religion, Spirituality and Psychiatry, a journal of Muslim mental health has been founded, and the number of articles on religion in peer-reviewed journals has grown substantially.

It seems likely that interest in religion and spirituality will continue to be a focus of psychiatry, even if it is not a central focus. The United States continues to be a religious country. Europe, though much more secular, has been indelibly shaped by its religious heritage, and South America, Africa, Asia, and the Middle East all have populations for whom religion is a vital part of the fabric of life. As a result, it is very likely that psychiatric patients will often have psychopathology shaped by their religious beliefs and will frame their understanding of their life and inner concerns in religious or spiritual terms. Physicians for the mad have been dealing with religious problems for centuries, trying to reassure patients, offer comfort, and work out ways to use their own religious/spiritual/philosophical perspective to bring healing to their patients.

The opinions expressed in this chapter represent the personal views of the author and do not represent the views of the U.S Department of State.

REFERENCES

1. Dols MW, Immisch DE. *Majnun: The Madman in Medieval Islamic Society.* Oxford: Clarendon Press; 1992.
2. Sengers G. *Women and Demons: Cult Healing in Islamic Egypt.* Leiden, Netherlands: Brill; 2003.
3. Pach A. Narrative constructions of madness in a Hindu village in Nepal. In: *Skinner D, Pach A, Holland D, eds. Selves in Time and Place: Identities, Experience and History in Nepal.* Lanham, Md.: Rowman & Littlefield Publishers, Inc.; 1998:111–128.
4. Bhugra D. Hinduism and Ayurveda: Implications for managing mental health. In: Bhugra D (ed.), *Psychiatry and Religion: Context, Consensus and Controversies.* New York: Routledge; 1997:97–111.
5. Obeyesekere G. Depression, Buddhism, and the work of culture in Sri Lanka. In: Kleinman A, Good B, eds. *Culture and depression: Studies in the Anthropology and Cross-Cultural Psychiatry of Affect and Disorder.* Berkeley: University of California Press; 1985:134–152.
6. Barrett DB, Kurian GT, Johnson TM. *World Christian Encyclopedia: A Comparative Survey of Churches and Religions in the Modern World.* New York: Oxford University Press; 2001.
7. Metzger B. *The Canon of the New Testament: Its Origin, Development, and Significance.* Oxford: Oxford University Press; 1997.
8. Edelstein EJL, Edelstein L. *Asclepius: Collection and Interpretation of the Testimonies.* Baltimore: Johns Hopkins University Press; 1998.
9. Temkin O. *Hippocrates in a World of Pagans and Christians.* Baltimore: Johns Hopkins University Press; 1991.
10. Chrysostom J. Letters to Olympias. In: Schaff P, Wace H, eds. *A Select Library of Nicene and Post-Nicene Fathers of the Christian Church.* Grand Rapids, Mich: Eerdmans; 1978:2d series, vol. 9.
11. Chrysostom J. Homily on St. Ignatius. In: Schaff P, Wace H, eds. *A Select Library of Nicene and Post-Nicene Fathers of the Christian Church.* Grand Rapids, Mich.: Eerdmans; 1978:2d series, vol. 9.
12. Whittaker M, ed. *Tatian: Oration ad Graecos and Fragments.* Oxford: Clarendon Press; 1982.
13. Cameron ML. *Anglo-Saxon Medicine.* Cambridge: Cambridge University Press; 1993.
14. Leechbook I. In: Cockayne O, ed. *Leechdoms, Wortcunning, and Starcraft of Early England.* Bristol: Thoemmes Press; 2001:vol. 2.
15. Leechbook III. In Cockayne O, ed. *Leechdoms, Wortcunning, and Starcraft of Early England.* Bristol: Thoemmes Press; 2001:vol. 2.
16. Scot R, Summers M. *The Discoverie of Witchcraft.* New York: Dover Publications, Inc.; 1972.
17. Gowland A. The problem of early modern melancholy. *Past and Present.* 2006;191:77–120.
18. Keeble NH. Richard Baxter (1615–1691). Oxford Dictionary of National Biography. Oxford University Press; 2004. Available at: http://www.oxforddnb.com/view/article/1734. Accessed 6/26/08.
19. Baxter R. *The Practical Works of Richard Baxter.* Morgan, Pa.: Soli Deo Gloria Publications; 2000.
20. Wright S. Timothy Rogers (1658–1728). Oxford Dictionary of National Biography. Oxford University Press; 2004. Available at: http://www.oxforddnb.com/view/article/24002. Accessed 6/27/08.
21. Rogers T. *A Discourse Concerning Trouble of Mind, and the Disease of Melancholy.* London: Thomas Parkhurst and Thomas Cockerill; 1691.
22. Wright S. George Trosse (1631–1713). Oxford Dictionary of National Biography. Oxford University Press; 2004. Available at: http://www.oxforddnb.com/view/article/27758. Accessed 6/27/08.
23. Trosse G. *The Life of the Reverend Mr. George Trosse.* Montreal: McGill-Queen's University Press; 1974.
24. Parry-Jones WL. *The Trade in Lunacy: A Study of Private Madhouses in England in the Eighteenth and Nineteenth Centuries.* London: Routledge & Kegan Paul; 1972.
25. Shorter E. *NetLibrary Inc.: A History of Psychiatry from the Era of the Asylum to the Age of Prozac.* New York: John Wiley & Sons; 1997:xii, 436 p.
26. Thielman SB. *Madness and Medicine: The Medical Approach to Madness in Antebellum America, with Particular Reference to the Eastern Lunatic Asylum of Virginia and the South Carolina Lunatic Asylum.* Department of History, Duke University, 1986:244.

27. Pinel P, Davis DD. *A Treatise on Insanity*. New York, published under the auspices of the Library of the New York Academy of Medicine by Hafner Publishing Co.; 1962.

28. Cherry CL. *A Quiet Haven: Quakers, Moral Treatment, and Asylum Reform*. Rutherford, NJ: Fairleigh Dickinson University Press; 1989.

29. Digby A. *Madness, Morality, and Medicine: A Study of the York Retreat, 1796–1914*. Cambridge: Cambridge University Press; 1985.

30. Tuke S. *Description of the Retreat, an Institution near York, for Insane Persons of the Society of Friends. Containing an Account of Its Origin and Progress, the Modes of Treatment, and a Statement of Cases*. York, England: W. Alexander; 1813.

31. Rush B. *Medical Inquiries and Observations upon the Diseases of the Mind*. New York, published under the auspices of the Library of the New York Academy of Medicine by Hafner Publishing Co.; 1962.

32. Steinberg H. The sin in the aetiological concept of Johann Christian August Heinroth (1773–1843). Part 1: Between theology and psychiatry. Heinroth's concepts of "whole being," "freedom" "reason" and "disturbance of the soul." *Hist Psychiatry*. 2004;15(3):329–344.

33. Griesinger W, Robertson CL, Rutherford J. *Mental Pathology and Therapeutics*. London: New Sydenham Society; 1867.

34. Brigham A. *Observations on the Influence of Religion upon the Health and Physical Welfare of Mankind*. Boston: Marsh, Capen & Lyon; 1835.

35. Ray I, Curran FJ. *Mental Hygiene*. New York, published under the auspices of the Library of the New York Academy of Medicine by Hafner Publishing Co.; 1968.

36. Holifield EB. *A History of Pastoral Care in America: From Salvation to Self-Realization*. Nashville, TN: Abingdon Press; 1983.

37. Gay P. *A Godless Jew: Freud, Atheism, and the Making of Psychoanalysis*. New Haven, Conn.: Yale University Press; 1987.

38. Stokes A. *Ministry after Freud*. New York: Pilgrim Press; 1985.

39. Worcester E, McComb S. *Body, Mind and Spirit*. Boston: Marshall Jones Company; 1931.

40. Worcester E, McComb S, Coriat IH. *Religion and Medicine: The Moral Control of Nervous Disorders*. New York: Moffat Yard; 1908.

41. Cunningham RJ. The Emmanuel Movement: A variety of American religious experience. *A Q.* 1962;14(1):48–63.

42. Hale NG. *The Rise and Crisis of Psychoanalysis in the United States, 1917–1985: Freud and the Americans*. New York: Oxford University Press; 1995.

43. Cheever S. *My Name Is Bill: Bill Wilson: His Life and the Creation of Alcoholics Anonymous*. New York: Simon & Schuster; 2004.

44. Committee on Psychiatry and Religion. The psychic function of religion in mental health and illness. In Reports and Symposiums, Group for the Advancement of Psychiatry; 1968;642–725.

45. Larson DB, Pattison EM, Blazer DG, Omran AR, Kaplan BH. Systematic analysis of research on religious variables in four major psychiatric journals, 1978–1982. *Am J Psychiatry*. 1986;143(3):329–334.

3 Theological Perspectives on the Care of Patients with Psychiatric Disorders

JOEL JAMES SHUMAN

SUMMARY

The inclusion of religious considerations in psychiatry and clinical psychology affords both clinicians and patients an important resource in understanding and therapeutically addressing mental illness. Yet that inclusion also presents potential difficulties that may be avoided only by careful theological reflection; that is, by critical consideration of religious belief and practice from the perspective of one or more of those historical traditions we call "religions." To avoid theological reflection is to risk reducing religion to a technique valued only for its therapeutic utility, which clearly threatens the integrity of most religious traditions. In this chapter, I

1 offer an account of tradition and explain what it means to think theologically from within a religious tradition;

2 suggest the ubiquity of theological and atheological assumptions in the worldviews of every patient and clinician;

3 follow theologian George Lindbeck in likening thinking theologically to being part of a "cultural-linguistic" system constituting an entire way of life;

4 discuss two significant theological difficulties likely to arise at the intersection of psychiatry and clinical psychology for persons shaped by participation in the Jewish and Christian biblical narratives;

5 suggest the therapeutic significance of some religious communities as resources to be cultivated by clinicians.

A cursory glance at recorded history suggests that conditions like those we now call "mental illnesses" have been with us for a very long time, as have the attempts of various cultures to accommodate and care for their mentally ill members.(1) And while modern psychiatric medicine has made great strides in the recognition and effective treatment of mental illness and the destigmatization of the mentally ill, the discipline arguably has also followed a pattern typical of the applied sciences in modernity, a pattern characterized by an escalating spiral of specialization, reductionism, fragmentation, and alienation.(2) Just so, while medicine now knows more than ever about the neurochemical aberrations associated with depression, anxiety, psychosis, and so forth, these conditions are increasingly regarded as individualized pharmacological problems to be resolved clinically, as efficiently as possible. This slide toward reductionism is one reason the reintroduction into psychiatry and clinical psychology of religious considerations is, from my perspective as a theologian, so promising, for it calls into question the ready division of life, so characteristic of our time, into the respective domains of ostensibly discrete disciplines. It has become possible once again to see mental illness as more than a matter to be dealt with by the clinician and the individual patient in relative isolation. Clinician and patient alike, along with the members of their respective communities, may now understand psychiatric illness as a theological matter as well, one that may be addressed fully only in light of a measure of theological reflection.

Psychiatrists and other mental health professionals who wish to take seriously their patients' religious faith need to develop some sense of the theological issues at stake in such consideration.

By "theological" I mean first of all having to do with disciplined, critical reflection on religious belief and practice. Properly theological questions about matters at the intersection of religion with psychiatry are not primarily questions about the plausibility of religious belief from the perspective of current psychiatric theories, nor are they questions about the psychotherapeutic efficacy of religious belief and practice. Questions of both these sorts are clinically important and often theologically interesting, but neither accounts adequately for what it means to think theologically about psychiatry and religion. Rather, theological questions about psychiatric matters should begin by critically examining a patient's beliefs and dispositions in light of his or her association (or lack thereof) with the particular religious tradition of which she counts herself a member. A theologically sensitive clinician, that is, attempts to see and interpret a patient's condition not simply from the perspective of what course of action might be therapeutically effective in the short term, but also from the perspective of what would, to the greatest extent possible, respect the integrity of the particular religious tradition of which a patient is a member. This is not to say that the clinician should feel compelled to make the internal coherence of her patient's religious tradition the sole or even the primary arbiter of her judgment of that tradition or of her care for that patient; clearly some religious traditions have better stood the test of time, are more plausible, and more conducive to human flourishing than others. Yet to make clinical judgments about a religious tradition based solely on its therapeutic utility or its perceived threats to mental health is to avoid thinking theologically and risk doing violence, both to a particular patient and her religious tradition.

I. THEOLOGY AND TRADITION

I have suggested that theological reflection is always informed with reference to a particular religious tradition. A tradition, in the sense I am using the notion here, is best understood as a long-standing communal conversation that is both synchronic and diachronic, which is simply to say that it is a conversation among members of an historically continuous community that has for generations engaged voices from its past with respect to matters of enduring significance, while never failing to ground itself in the present or look toward the future.(3) A theological tradition is thus an enduring, never-completed argument about the nature of both proximate and ultimate reality and about the proper relationship of humanity to divinity, which is to say a theological tradition is to a significant extent also an extended conversation about the human condition and the best way for women and men to live. The possibility of such a conversation presumes the sharing of what might be called *canonical narratives* – that is, venerable stories about the origins of things, the way things are, and the way things ought to be – by the conversants. To the extent people live under the authority of the same canonical narratives, look to the same exemplars of virtue, and engage in the common practices evoked by those narratives, they may engage as well in intelligible theological discourse.(4) As such, theology is a discipline usually undertaken *from within* a tradition, at least in the sense that the theologian – I use the word here loosely to refer to anyone engaged in informed theological reflection – has an adequate working knowledge of the language, logic, and way of life characteristic of the tradition in question.(5)

And yet, a somewhat-more-than cursory understanding of a patient's faith tradition is only one part of the theological task of the clinician. The clinician should also be aware of his own theological situation, for even when the clinician does not count himself a member of a religious tradition or has no faith in anything resembling a god, his view of the world and of his patients is *nolens volens* based on theological (or atheological) suppositions. Every person, religious or not, lives with certain tacit and explicit assumptions about the way things are and the way they should be. A significant part of what it means to be human is consciously to consider the world one understands oneself to inhabit, and to order one's desire for the various goods one finds in that world. Such assumptions and ordering are acquired and develop along with the languages we use to describe our worlds; together, they constitute what are commonly called *worldviews*, all of which are in some sense theological. As Nicholas Lash puts the matter, "It is taken for granted, in sophisticated circles, that no one worships God these days except the reactionary and the simpleminded. This innocent self-satisfaction tells us little more, however, than that those exhibiting it do not name as 'God' the gods they worship."(6)

Just so, clinicians should practice their craft not only with a sensitivity to their own commitments and an awareness that the languages and logic of their discipline are in a broad sense "theological," but also with a conscious awareness of the genealogical connections of modern psychiatry and psychology to the Jewish and Christian faiths, especially as those faiths were understood and called into question by Continental thinkers of the mid to late nineteenth century, including Feuerbach, Nietzsche, and Freud. Freudian psychology has long since died the death of a thousand qualifications, but the specter of Freud's account of religion continues to haunt psychiatry and clinical psychology, such that even those mental health professionals who are themselves religious believers often carry with them the influence of Freudian categories, at the very least assuming a clear boundary between the realms of clinic and congregation. Yet, a clinician attentive to such matters will see that these presumed boundaries are not so clear. She may even recognize significant family resemblances (to borrow a phrase from the philosopher Wittgenstein) among the modern taxonomy of psychiatry and the recorded spiritual struggles of innumerable women and men of faith over the past three thousand years, discovering that religion has historically been far more than wish fulfillment, reality avoidance, or a less-than-optimal form of coping.(7)

The possession of an informed theological perspective on a patient's beliefs and dispositions may help the clinician better understand how such beliefs and dispositions relate to a particular patient's religious tradition. Those beliefs and dispositions may follow "naturally" from the patient's religious commitments, or they may be pathological in nature. As I have indicated above, these are not mutually exclusive alternatives. Religious belief and mental health (or the lack of either) may coexist in a wide range of complex and ever-changing arrangements, very few of which correspond in any uncomplicated way to the traditionally pejorative psychotherapeutic view of religion, which maintains that religious faith is both a cause and sometimes a sign of maladaptive thinking. Religious faith may not be a prerequisite for mental health, but neither is it an indicator *in se* of mental illness; people of faith are by no means all delusional, neurotic, or socially disabled.

More, active mental illness of various kinds is not incompatible with generally orthodox religious belief. A patient may be or desire to be profoundly faithful to his tradition even as he is at the same time profoundly sick; in many cases mental illness is an occasion for or even a cause of theologically problematic assumptions that factor into a patient's inability to live well. At the same time, a theologically orthodox faith may for many patients prove powerfully effective in a broadly (albeit unconventionally) therapeutic sense, offering them the means, often in conjunction with more conventional therapies, to cope with even serious mental illnesses. One thinks here of the protagonists in the novels of the American writer and physician Walker Percy; those characters' struggles with melancholy and other disturbances of the mind proved notoriously resistant to the interventions of psychiatry but were often responsive to the characters' immersion (or sometimes reimmersion) as a catechumens in an unfashionably orthodox Christian faith. One might also consider the role of the Christian Daily Office – a traditional regimen of daily liturgical prayer – as a useful adjunct to medication and therapy in Kathryn Greene-McCreight's chronicle of her struggles with major depression and bipolar disorder, or of Jeffery Smith's discovery of the writings of ancient Christian monastics on the "Dark Night of the Soul," which offered him an ultimately satisfying way of understanding and coping with his long history of serious depression.(7–12)

2. RELIGION AND RELIGIONS

I have advocated shifting the focus on matters at the intersection of religion and psychiatry from the individual patient's beliefs and the therapeutic utility of those beliefs to the ways her beliefs are shaped by her membership in or association with a religious tradition. My advocacy is based on the conviction that it is more descriptively accurate, not to mention more clinically useful, to talk about psychiatry and a particular religion, such as Judaism, Christianity, or Islam, than to talk about psychiatry and religion in general. The truth is that it is impossible to say very much about psychiatry and religious faith in general, because there really isn't any such thing as religious faith *in general*. The notion of a generic "religion," as Nicholas Lash has shown, is in essence an epiphenomenon of the shifting philosophical ground of early modern Europe, one aspect of which included an emerging suspicion of what traditionally had been a conspicuously "public" Christianity.(13) This is not to say that there are no resemblances among the traditions we call "religions." Certainly there are commonly held beliefs and practices among the adherents of various traditions (or those of no tradition who still call themselves religious or spiritual). More, the faiths we commonly call "Abrahamic" (Judaism, Christianity, and Islam) share a common historical heritage and comparable canonical narratives.(14) Still, too easily associating the beliefs, practices, and narratives of even these traditions avoids, rather than encourages, theological scrutiny. It has become fashionable in recent years in a wide variety of medical specialties, psychiatry not excepted, to investigate and in some cases even to commend the therapeutic effects of actions and dispositions broadly regarded as "spiritual" or "religious."(15) The operational assumption in most of this work has seemed to be that the subjective act of belief is more significant than the objective content of what is believed, insofar as the various historical

religious traditions are but ways of referring to a universal characteristic of human subjectivity, which we might name religious feeling or religious belief. The traditions, that is, are but species of a common *genus* named "religion," or now, more commonly, "spirituality." As such, they may be exchanged or hybridized according to therapeutic effectiveness and the needs of the religious consumer.(13, 15)

Such a view of "religion" corresponds to what the theologian George Lindbeck has called "experiential-expressivism," wherein the theological focus is on interpreting the always personal, usually inward, and often private experience of the believer. The content of the believer's experience, the raw material informing what theologians typically call *doctrine*, is seen from this perspective as "noninformative or nondiscursive symbols of inner feelings, attitudes, or existential orientations."(16) This way of understanding religion not only fits, but also emerges as part of, the contemporary North Atlantic sociopolitical context. The world inhabited by most mental health professionals and their patients is characterized by radical individualism and a sharp egalitarian impulse, a paradoxically reactionary suspicion toward traditional authority, and a belief that some form of scientific reason is the only legitimate arbiter of public truth. Subsequently, we tend to assume the existence of a deep division between the public and private realms, whereby we suppose that religious belief is a private, individual matter that cannot and should not be critiqued with respect to its content.(15, 17)

Yet such a highly individuated, private, experientially grounded understanding of religion falls decidedly short of accounting for what it has for most of history meant to "be religious." Lindbeck argues that the traditions we call "religions" are better understood as entire ways of life, which may be participated in properly only through initiation, extensive training, and life-long ritual reinforcement. Here he draws on the work of Wittgenstein in arguing that religions are not unlike languages, in that they *make possible* "the description of realities, the formulation of beliefs, and the experiencing of inner attitudes, feelings, and sentiments." Moreover, insofar as languages emerge from and are made intelligible by their association with the ways of life of particular communities, theological language cannot be dissociated from the practice of a common life. A religious tradition's "doctrines, cosmic stories or myths, and ethical directives are integrally related to the rituals it practices, the sentiments or experiences it evokes, the actions it recommends, and the institutional forms it develops. All this is involved in comparing a religion to a cultural-linguistic system."(16) Just so, a clinician can often assess the relationship of her patient's illness to that patient's religious faith only by taking into account not simply the fact that her patient believes, but also the entire cultural-linguistic framework within which that belief is acquired and exercised. In accounting for the cultural and linguistic history of her patient's faith, the clinician may be surprised to discover that her patient is part of a tradition that historically has afforded a generous space to those we today call the mentally ill and that also possesses abundant resources for wrestling with the particular theological and existential questions raised by mental illness.

3. PSYCHIATRY AND THEOLOGY IN TENSION AND IN CONVERSATION

The kinds of theological challenges mental health professionals are likely to face with respect to their patients' religious commitments depend to a significant extent on the particular religious tradition with which the patient is affiliated. Mental illness and its treatment will present different kinds of theological challenges to different religious traditions. In what follows I want to discuss what I take to be two ultimately inseparable challenges that mental illness and its contemporary treatment present to my own tradition, Christianity. Although adherents of other traditions, Judaism in particular, may recognize analogies with my account, I do not presume to speak here on behalf of any tradition other than my own.

A first type of theological challenge the clinician is likely to encounter at the intersection of psychiatry and religion is with the connotation elicited by the very category "mental" illness. Psychiatry's traditional suspicion of religion is often greeted with a corresponding antagonism by religious believers. Psychiatrists and other mental health professionals may have to contend with religious patients who are suspicious of and even hostile toward the very idea of modern psychiatry. Although this suspicion is clearly in part a defensive reaction, it is more complex than that. Judaism and Christianity have for centuries recognized and wrestled with the existence of melancholia, anxiety, and other conditions that bear undeniable resemblances to what modern psychiatry identifies as disorders of mood, affect, and personality. In the world of the Bible, such conditions are generally and for the most part understood as "spiritual" challenges, or perhaps as "sicknesses of the soul," the appropriate responses to which are similarly "spiritual," which is to say, religious. The psalms and prophetic writings in particular are replete with both communal and individual laments made by women and men confronted by the apparent absence of God from their lives and those of their communities. The "absences" lamented in these texts range from existential despair over the apparent meaningless of life, to expressions of the real or imagined fear of imminent death, to expressions of remorse over the commission of sins, to protests against God's failure to meet his covenant obligations to the psalmist's or prophet's community. In many cases, these laments include nothing less than pointed demands that God give an account of godself. And yet in spite of their introductory tone, these texts linger neither in anger nor despair, but transition without fail to expressions of praise and gratitude in response to anticipated liberation by the very God who at the time seems totally absent. Given the undeniably liturgical character of much of this literature (that is, the fact that it appears to have been written to be performed in the gathered public worship of the community), these transitions appear to correspond to declarations of forthcoming salvation by "a trusted, authorized official… not unlike the 'fear not' formula of Isaiah 43:1":

> But now says the Lord,
>> he who created you, O Jacob,
>> he who formed you, O Israel:
> Do not fear, for I have redeemed you;
>> I have called you by name, you are
>>> mine.(18)

This suggests that the public, communal performance of these texts was an important resource that sustained the community and its membership, not simply in extraordinary times, but also in the difficult conditions that characterize the ebb and flow of everyday life. The psalmists and prophets seem to understand that, even at its most pedestrian, life frequently presents us with tragic circumstances that we cannot imagine resolved to our satisfaction, apart perhaps from the extraordinary intervention of God, which in the short term, as the poet Michael Blumenthal says, is "oblique and obscure and not even assured."(19) One might argue, of course, that it is the sense of penultimate pathos characteristic of the psalmists' and prophets' worldview that is the problem, and that it is not necessary, much less healthy, to experience the ebb and flow of everyday life as fundamentally tragic.(11) Yet in the view of the biblical authors, this objection itself might be part of the problem. One prominent scholar of the Old Testament goes so far as to claim that one of the primary purposes of the prophetic writings is to call a people numbed by the comfortable social and economic stability typical of life in a politically powerful state to move beyond their superficial contentment and "engage their experience of suffering to death." The solution to the tragic and sometimes apparently absurd human condition is not blissful sleepwalking, but a hopeful engagement with an emerging reign of peace and righteousness secured by the love of God. Such an engagement can be sustained only by an imaginative countercultural community devoted to the mutual well-being of its entire membership.(20)

But how is any of this threatened by the modern notion of "mental" illness? There appears to be a trajectory within modern psychiatry that calls into question the biblical embrace of pathos, and in particular the undeniably social character of that embrace. On the one hand, this questioning takes the form of identifying religious belief, and communal religious practice in particular, as collective delusion; religious practice in this view is, at best, a less-than-optimal means of coping with the Sturm und Drang of life and, at worst, a dangerous avoidance of reality that needs to be unlearned by a rigorous course of therapy.(7) A more contemporary and much more common form of questioning, however, comes from the recent ascendancy of applied neuroscience and psychopharmacology, which tends to reduce the experience of mental illness to aberrations in the particular brain chemistry of the individual. I do not wish to take issue with the efficacy of contemporary psychopharmacology, which has proven itself, notwithstanding thoughtful social and philosophical interlocution; rather, I wish to visit the question of the theological significance of this efficacy.(10, 11) What are the implications for biblical faith of psychoactive medications that can, in a remarkably short time, effect deep changes in mood, behavior, and even personality?(21) What does it mean to have a "soul" so profoundly susceptible to chemical manipulation that personality itself appears to be transformed, quite apart from a change in circumstance or the mutual help and support of a faithful community?

Inarguably, neuroscience and the diagnostic and therapeutic interventions it has spawned challenge much conventional thinking about the soul. Some neuroscientists have gone so far as to claim that, since what was once identified as "soul" can now be accounted for largely in terms of brain chemistry, the very notion of "soul" is no longer tenable and should be regarded as one more decrepit member in the crumbling edifice of an outdated biblical worldview.(22) As it turns out, however, neuroscience and psychopharmacology are much more serious threats to the legacy of Plato and Descartes than to Judaism or Christianity.

Descartes, who is sometimes called the "father of modern philosophy" because of his emphasis on the human subject as the ultimate arbiter of meaning, is best known for his *Discourse on Method* (1637). In response to the emergence of a widespread dissatisfaction with the Aristotelian methodology undergirding the intellectual discourse of that day, Descartes sought to develop an alternative philosophical method based on a foundation of absolute certainty.(23) Beginning with a determination to "reject as absolutely false everything in which I could suppose the slightest reason for doubt," Descartes set out to establish an "entirely indubitable" remainder on which certain knowledge might be established. (24) Descartes believed he had found such a foundation in the human *psyche*; his conclusion was that he, Descartes, was "a substance, of which the whole essence or nature consists in thinking, and which, in order to exist needs no place and depends on no material thing."(24) Hence we have Descartes' nearly universally recognized dictum: "I think, therefore I am."

Perhaps because much of what he says echoed the then two-thousand-year-old legacy of Plato, Descartes' *ego* – the "I" – came over time to be identified with the soul. The human essence – the thing that made humans unique – was an ineffable, immaterial, and immortal *res cogitans*, a "thinking thing." The body, meanwhile, was ultimately nothing more than a temporary, passive extension of the soul, a *res extensa*. In part because of its explanatory power and in part because of its surface resemblance to some strands of biblical anthropology, Cartesian dualism became the dominant paradigm for thinking about what it meant to be human. Some version of Descartes' anthropology became axiomatic for all fields of inquiry, including theology and, less directly, medicine. The suppositions of the Cartesian model also shaped the translation and interpretation of scripture and popular piety, such that it became common for Christians to assume that the biblical account of the human person was essentially dualistic – that humans were immortal, immaterial souls temporarily inhabiting mortal, material bodies.

Yet, as biblical scholarship and theological scholarship have shown, Christianity has virtually no stake in defending Cartesian (or any other

variety of) dualism. Dualism was in fact at the center of some of the earliest and most persistent heresies faced by nascent Christianity. These heresies are collectively referred to as varieties of *Gnosticism*, which, generally speaking, maintains that the material creation, including the human body, is unimportant except in a temporary, strictly utilitarian sense. The limits inherent in material corporeality are to be ignored, struggled against, or fled, as often, as intensely, and as soon as possible. This earthly life is ultimately illusory; many Gnostics have gone so far as to liken it to a fleshy prison. But Gnosticism is patently inconsistent with the biblical narrative, which from the beginning insists on the goodness of creation and the significance of *embodied* human life, which the second-century Church Father Irenaeus called "the glory of God." Contrary to the Gnostic insistence that women and men ultimately are immaterial souls, the biblical portrayal of humanity is conspicuously corporeal; from the perspective of scripture, we are in this life and the next never less than our bodies. As Wendell Berry so succinctly explains the biblical story of the creation of Adam:

> The formula given in Genesis 2:7 is not man = body + soul; the formula there is soul = dust [earth] + breath. According to this verse, God did not make a body and then put a soul into it, like a letter in an envelope. He formed man of dust [earth]; then, by breathing His breath into it, he made the dust live. The dust, formed as man and made to live, did not *embody* a soul; it *became* a soul. "Soul" here refers to the whole creature. Humanity is thus presented to us, in Adam, not as a creature of two discrete parts temporarily glued together but as a single mystery.(25)

Thus, the categories so typical of modern thought, such as the distinction between the spiritual and the physical, or the body and the soul, or the natural and the supernatural, are from the perspective of scripture deeply problematic and useful only in a limited heuristic sense. The mystery we name "human" (from the Latin *humus*, "earth") is from the perspective of scripture altogether consistent with what neuroscience and the philosophy of mind call "non reductive physicalism" in which the notions "soul and mind are physiologically embodied," and yet not exhausted by neurophysiological explanation. "Human mind and behavior have new emergent properties that cannot be exhaustively explained by lower level physical phenomena. Thinking, deciding, willing, etc., are real and efficacious properties of embodied human life."(26) As Berry puts the matter, "Creation is one continuous fabric comprehending simultaneously what we mean by 'spirit' and what we mean by 'matter'.… The body, 'fearfully and wonderfully made,' is ultimately mysterious both in itself and in its dependences. Our bodies live, as the Bible says, by the spirit and breath of God, but it does not say how this is so. We are not going to *know* about this."(27)

Just so, the worldview of those who stand within the biblical-Christian traditions should not feel that the plausibility of their faith is threatened by the fact that their illness has a neurophysiologic aspect that responds to psychoactive medication. Because we are never less than our bodies, we are never less than an extraordinarily complex constellation of chemical reactions. More, we are no less real, less human, because of this.(28) Although there may in rare cases be good theological reasons to question the pharmaceutical manipulation of the human mind, members of the biblical traditions may generally and for the most part view them as gifts provided by God to facilitate human flourishing.

4. SUFFERING: WHAT IS THEOLOGY GOOD FOR?

As important as such assurances may be, they do not address an older and more intractable theological question with respect to mental illness, namely, the question of why such suffering afflicts good and faithful people. In philosophy, this is one version of what is typically called the problem of theodicy (from the Greek *theos*, "god"

and *dikē*, "justice"), which is typically posed in the form of a question: "Why does a benevolent, all-powerful God allow the innocent to suffer?" In a therapeutic culture like our own, which teaches us to value individual happiness above all other goods, the long-standing human tendency to reduce God to the role of being a dispenser of whatever we happen to want is multiplied. (15) Our bent is simplistically to assume that God wants us to have what we want and that religious behavior of various kinds is but a means of achieving what has already been afforded. Insofar as suffering of various kinds is an impediment to this kind of happiness, suffering becomes a problem to be solved rather than a mystery to be contemplated or an affliction to be ministered to by friends and neighbors. Thus, when we suffer, we are likely to begin by asking what we have done wrong to deserve suffering or what we need to do differently to rid ourselves of it.

Of course, it is perfectly appropriate not to want to suffer and so to ask whether we may be able to do something to escape or alleviate whatever suffering we might be experiencing. More, the God revealed by the biblical narrative is accessible and active as a healer. Yet from the perspective of scripture, "why" questions about sickness and suffering are almost always the wrong place to begin. For while it is absolutely the case that the God revealed in scripture intends the redemption of all creation, including the life of every person, that redemption must be viewed from the perspective of what theologians oftentimes call "salvation history," which includes an irreducibly *eschatological* (oriented toward an ideal future consummation) component. The human experience of suffering demands a theological response. From the perspective of Christian tradition, such a response focuses on the past, present, and future history of God's saving activity, which does not attempt to explain, but does account for, human suffering.

It is important to note that scripture does not offer a single, univocal account of why we suffer or what can be done about suffering. Yet neither are the scriptural voices addressing suffering cacophonous. It is possible to discern a kind of harmony among the scriptural accounts of suffering, which consists in five parts:

1 Suffering is not part of God's original or ultimate intention for any member of God's creation.
2 The world as we experience it is not the world God ultimately intends. Humanity has willfully alienated itself from God, from itself, and from the rest of creation, one typically inscrutable consequence of which is suffering.
3 God's activity toward creation is nonetheless fundamentally redemptive. God is sovereign over history – including the history of every person – and will ultimately consummate history to the benefit of God's creatures.
4 Christians therefore must cultivate an "apocalyptic sensibility" with respect to suffering, knowing that suffering has the penultimate, rather than the ultimate, word in their lives.
5 In the interim, suffering should not surprise us; indeed, it is in a broken creation in some sense inevitable. As such, it is an opportunity for Christians to serve those who suffer *and* a possible means by which God may further God's purposes in history.

Any account of suffering in light of the biblical narrative must begin with the insistence that suffering is part neither of God's original nor ultimate intention for the creation. Rather, creation exists as an expression of the fundamental goodness of God, for God is, according to scripture, love (1 John 4:8). A central tenet of Christian theology is that God is an *aseity*, which is to say that God is fully sufficient in and of godself (*a se*). God alone is self-sufficient; creation is therefore contingent, rather than necessary. All that is has been brought into existence and continues to exist by virtue of God's generous, playful, and totally gratuitous creative act – the overflowing of God's immeasurable love. All of creation, women and men in particular, exist joyfully to participate in God's love, to be God's friends.(29)

That God is love, and that God intends our flourishing and the flourishing of all creation, is to most of us far from self-evident. The world is full of suffering, as observation and personal experience plainly demonstrate. This antinomy, between the prevalence of suffering and the presumed goodness of God, evokes the theodicy question in its traditional forms. Yet this is a mistake precisely because it presumes that the existence of suffering is evidence of some defect in God. In fact, it is possible to see the existence of suffering as a function of God's *regard* for humanity. Insofar as humans are created in God's image and likeness, we possess a measure of freedom. It is by way of this freedom, Thomas Aquinas insists, that God "moves" us, which is to say that God is fundamentally noncoercive with respect to the human will; God's activity toward us is to entice us by attraction rather than to push us from behind. Of course, the correlative to the human capacity to choose God's intention is the freedom to choose against God's intention. Christian tradition calls the free human opposition to God's intention *sin* and suggests that it is sin that is the cause of various forms of suffering.

This is not so simple a claim as it would first seem, for "sin" here describes the state of a creation alienated from its Creator more than it describes any one person's discrete acts of opposition to God and God's intention. The two are of course not unrelated; as the biblical story of the "fall" indicates, creation's alienation from God has its origins in specific acts of human disobedience. More, certain "sinful" choices are quite obviously self-destructive and so contribute in relatively straightforward ways to the suffering of the sinner and those around him. Yet the biblical narrative, from the book of Job to the teaching of Jesus, for the most part rejects the idea that a given instance of suffering in a person's life is the result of a particular sin or sins that person has committed. Rather, the cumulative effect of generations of human disobedience is portrayed as a kind of collective centrifugal force that flings all of creation away from God toward disorder and chaos, such that even in the presence of the best of human intentions, nothing works quite the way it is supposed to.

Thus, suffering is one of the most obvious effects of sin, not in the sense that God punishes sinners by making them suffer, but in the sense that sin is in a variety of ways its own punishment. Insofar as it not only separates the person from God, but also distorts and renders dysfunctional his relationships to other persons and to the earth on which his life depends, sin makes him an often unwitting participant in the violent brokenness of the world we all inhabit. As the twentieth-century Protestant theologian Dietrich Bonhoeffer explains, with the first act of human disobedience, "Man's life is now disunion with God, with men, with things, and with himself…. Instead of seeing God man sees himself."(30) Alienated from God and the creation, women and men are destined to suffer.

And yet, in spite of appearances to the contrary, God's activity toward creation is fundamentally redemptive, which is to say it is in opposition to chaos and suffering. God is sovereign over history, including the history of each person, such that although God allows innumerable proximate contingent circumstances that can and do cause suffering, God ultimately consummates history to a good that includes the restoration of all creation's original well-being. Although this pattern pervades the biblical narrative, God's activity in this regard is both ideally exemplified and perfectly established in the life, death, and resurrection of Jesus of Nazareth. Subjected to the humiliation of false accusation, verbal and physical abuse, and a sham trial, Jesus was eventually sentenced by Roman authorities to death by crucifixion. From the cross he cried out the opening lines of Psalm 22, an extended, desperate lament of God's absence which begins, "My God, my God, why have you forsaken me?" In spite of his persistently having rejected the view that God visits the pious with prosperity and the sinner with suffering, Jesus's declaration indicates that he associated his experience not simply with injustice, but also with his having been abandoned by the very God whose imminent reign he had come to proclaim and make present. Thus, there is in the narrative of the cross a dramatic tension created by the disparity between the tenor of Jesus's life and teaching and his fate at the hands of imperial power. This narrative tension is resolved by Jesus's resurrection from death on the third day. According to John Howard Yoder, the resurrection is to be understood as a vindication of Jesus's life and teaching and an assurance of the sovereignty of good in history, such that "the triumph of the right… is sure because of the power of the resurrection and not because of any calculation of causes and effects …. The relationship between the obedience of God's people and the triumph of God's cause is not a relationship of cause and effect but one of cross and resurrection."(31)

Jesus's patient faithfulness in suffering is regarded by Paul as an example made possible by the theological hope that his resurrection foreshadows the general resurrection of the dead at the consummation of history (1 Cor. 15). In the interim, Christians are invited to cultivate an "apocalyptic sensibility" with respect to suffering, knowing that God is active in particular and unexpected ways invisible except to the eyes of faith. (15, 32) Thus, the biblical story, and the story of Jesus's death and resurrection in particular, "inserts into our present setting a fulcrum capable of being leaned on to pry us away from the assumption that the world as we see it is the only way it can be."(33) Suffering of whatever kind is not generally an indication that the sufferer has done something wrong, nor is it a sign that if she did things differently her suffering would cease or never have occurred. Suffering is simply one of the inevitable consequences of our habitation of a broken creation. As Paul puts the matter, "The sufferings of this present time are not worth comparing with the glory about to be revealed to us. For the creation waits with eager longing … in hope that the creation itself will be set free from its bondage to decay and will obtain the freedom of the glory of the children of God."(34) In the meantime, it is inevitable that most of us suffer and that some of us have the misfortune to suffer the pain of mental illness.

5. SUFFERING, HEALING, AND THE PEOPLE OF GOD

It is extremely important at this point to note that an acknowledgment of the ubiquity of suffering is neither fatalism nor an abandonment of the significance of this life in favor of a better life to come. Rather, from the perspective of the biblical narrative, the significance of suffering is shifted, such that suffering becomes, in spite of its potential horror, an opportunity for ministry and a means of faithful witness. According to the German theologian Gerhard Lohfink, the central theme in the biblical narrative is that God works in the world through a particular people whom God calls together for the purpose of bearing witness.(35, 36) This suggests that one of the, if not the most prominent, places where God's healing work may be seen is in and through the social ecology of God's people. In and through their common life, which proclaims God's love to the world, the people of God form a new society that makes possible a distinct way of dealing with suffering. They are given one another as friends pledged to share all manner of burdens, including, and perhaps especially, illness.(37) Suffering thus paradoxically becomes an opportunity for the people of God to care for each other in a way analogous to God's care for the creation: by patiently and lovingly being present to the brokenness and isolation suffering creates, by working to overcome the alienation endemic in a broken creation, and by proclaiming in so doing the emerging reign of God.

Thus, a mentally ill person who wants to know why God is allowing him to suffer or who is frustrated that his prayers for healing seem ineffectual may have his question redirected in the same way that Jesus redirected the questions of those who demanded to know whose sin was responsible for one man's congenital blindness: "Neither this man nor his parents sinned; he was born blind so that God's works might be revealed in him"(38). God is infinite not simply in mercy and compassion, but also in creativity. By bringing into existence a new community whose *telos* is to make God present to the world through their common life, God gives to those whose work is healing a powerful resource. By the provision of various forms of caring hospitality, the religious community becomes a locus of healing. Without assuming that every clergyperson and every religious community might

be legitimate therapeutic resources, the clinician should at least be free cautiously and judiciously to cultivate partnerships among the religious communities of consenting patients.

6. CONCLUSION

By necessity this chapter is incomplete and fragmentary. I have tried here to account for some of the things at stake theologically in the incorporation of religious matters into the treatment of the mentally ill. In so doing, I hope that I have achieved a medium somewhere between the trite simplistic view that religious practice is a means of getting what we want (whether God exists or not) and the hopelessly difficult perspective that because God (whether he exists or not) is beyond our control, we are alone in the world with our medication and psychotherapy. For although it is true that God is certainly wild and uncontrollable, it is also the case that God is at work effecting our redemption. In the words of the morning prayer from the *United Methodist Hymnal*, "New every morning is your love, great God of light, and all day long you are working for good in the world"(39).

REFERENCES

1. Foucault M. *Madness and Civilization: A History of Insanity in the Age of Reason.* New York, Random House; 1965 (1988).
2. Berry W. Discipline and hope. In: *A Continuous Harmony.* San Diego: Harcourt Brace and Company; 1970:95.
3. Wainwright G. *Doxology: The Praise of God in Worship, Doctrine, and Life.* New York, Oxford University Press; 1980.
4. MacIntyre A. *After Virtue: A Study in Moral Theory,* 2d ed. Notre Dame, Ind., University of Notre Dame Press; 1984:204–225.
5. MacIntyre A. *Whose Justice? Which Rationality?* Notre Dame, Ind., University of Notre Dame Press; 1988:370–388.
6. Lash N. Reality, wisdom, and delight. In: *The Beginning and the End of "Religion."* Cambridge: Cambridge University Press; 1996:49.
7. Greene-McCreight K. *Darkness Is My Only Companion: A Christian Response to Mental Illness.* Grand Rapids, Mich., Brazos Press; 2006:112–127.
8. Percy W. *Love in the Ruins.* New York, Ballantine Books; 1971 (1989).

9. Percy W. *The Second Coming.* New York, Ballantine Books; 1980 (1990).

10. Elliot C. Pursued by happiness and beaten senseless: Prozac and the American dream. *Hastings Center Report.* 2000;30:2, 7–12.

11. Kramer P. The valorization of sadness: Alienation and the melancholic temperament. *Hastings Center Report.* 2000;30:2, 13–18.

12. Smith J. *Where the Roots Search for Water: A Personal and Natural History of Melancholia.* New York, North Point Press; 1999.

13. Lash N. The beginning and the end of "religion"? On what kinds of things there are, hollow centres and holy places. In: *The Beginning and the End of "Religion."* Cambridge: Cambridge University Press; 1996:10–13, 93–111, 188–191.

14. *The Journal of Scriptural Reasoning.* Available at: http://etext.lib.virginia.edu/journals/ssr/ (last accessed 6/18/08); *A Common Word Between Us and You.* Available at: http://www.acommonword.com/ (last accessed 6/18/08).

15. Shuman J, Meador K. *Heal Thyself: Spirituality, Medicine, and the Distortion of Christianity.* New York, Oxford University Press; 2003;38, 19–43, 80–93, 71–111, 109.

16. Lindbeck G. *The Nature of Doctrine: Religion and Theology in a Postliberal Age.* Philadelphia, Westminster Press; 1984:16, 33.

17. Brooks D. The neural Buddhists. *The New York Times* Available at: http://nytimes.com/2008/05/13/opinion/13brooks.html (last accessed 5/20/08).

18. Brueggemann, W. *An Introduction to the Old Testament: The Canon and Christian Imagination.* Louisville, Ky., Westminster John Knox; 2003: 280–282.

19. Blumenthal M. *The Wages of Goodness.* Columbia, University of Missouri Press; 1992:54.

20. Brueggemann, W. *The Prophetic Imagination.* 2d ed. Minneapolis, Minn., Fortress Press; 2001: 39–57.

21. Kramer P. *Listening to Prozac: A Psychiatrist Explores Antidepressant Drugs and the Remaking of the Self.* New York, Viking; 1993.

22. Wolfe T. Sorry, but your soul just died. *Forbes.* 1996;158(13):210–223. Available at: http://www.orthodoxytoday.org (last accessed 5/20/08).

23. Sutcliffe F. Introduction. In: Descartes R. ed. *Discourse on Method and the Meditations.* New York: Penguin; 1968:7–23.

24. Descartes R. *Discourse on Method and the Meditations;* 1968:53, 54.

25. Berry W. Christianity and the survival of creation. In: *Sex, Economy, Freedom & Community.* New York: Pantheon; 1991:106.

26. Brown W. Human nature, physicalism, spirituality, and healing: Theological views of a neuroscientist. *Ex Auditu.* 2005;21:114.

27. Berry W. Health as membership. In: *Another Turn of the Crank.* Washington: Counterpoint; 1995:91.

28. Flanagan O. *The Science of Mind,* 2d ed. Cambridge, Mass., MIT Press; 1991.

29. Waddell P. *Friendship and the Moral Life.* Notre Dame, Ind., University of Notre Dame Press; 1989.

30. Bonhoeffer D. *Ethics.* New York, Collier; 1949 (1986):20.

31. Yoder J. *The Politics of Jesus.* Grand Rapids, Mich., Eerdmans; 1972:238.

32. Toole D. *Waiting for Godot in Sarajevo: Theological Reflections on Nihilism, Tragedy, and Apocalypse.* Boulder, Colo., Westview; 1998:205–266.

33. Yoder J. Ethics and eschatology. *Ex Auditu.* 1990;6:119; Quoted in Shuman and Meador, p.110.

34. Romans 8:18–21, NRSV.

35. Lohfink G. *Does God Need the Church?* Collegeville, Minn., Liturgical Press; 1999.

36. Yoder J. A people in the world. In: *The Royal Priesthood: Essays Ecclesiological and Ecumenical.* Grand Rapids, Mich.: Eerdmans; 1994:65–101.

37. Shuman J. God does not wear a white coat: But God can, does, and will heal us all. In: Laytham B. ed. *God Does Not.* Grand Rapids, Mich.: Eerdmans; Forthcoming 2009.

38. John 9:3, NRSV.

39. The United Methodist Hymnal, United Methodist Publishing House; 1989:877.

4   The Bible: Relevant Issues for Clinicians

ARMANDO R. FAVAZZA

SUMMARY

The Bible is the most globally influential and widely read book ever written. Both directly and indirectly, it has been a major influence on the behavior, laws, customs, education, art, literature, and morality of Western civilization. This chapter presents basic facts about the Bible itself because it is such a vast and complicated book that is confusing to many readers. The concept of the biblical God is explored because it is not uncommon for manic, schizophrenic, and depressed psychiatric persons to proclaim the delusion that they are God or Jesus Christ and to put themselves in harm's way. Further, high-functioning charismatic patients who believe they are God can do enormous damage by becoming cult leaders. Many religions, including those based on the Bible, use sin and guilt as methods that control their members' behavior but may result in depressive and obsessive-compulsive disorders; also, the notion that women must be submissive to their husbands may be used by men to rationalize abusive behavior. The chapter discusses homosexuality, an issue that divides societies and families because the Book of Levitical Laws condemns homosexual behavior. Christians are not obligated to follow these laws, yet many continue to despise homosexuality even though psychiatry no longer considers it to be a mental disorder. The history of Christian religious healing is reviewed and demonstrates that sick persons who participate in religious healing rituals may feel better temporarily and that some self-proclaimed Christian healers may be charlatans. Despite its complexity, the Bible has for more than two millennia provided solace and hope to the vexed and the hopeless. Psychiatrists should know about the Bible because of its importance in the lives of so many mentally ill persons and their families.

The Bible is the most globally influential and widely read book ever written. Judaism and Christianity are Bible-based religions, and neither could have survived by oral tradition alone. Judaism's impact on the world mainly has come through the brilliant accomplishments of individual Jews. Christianity's impact has been much greater because of its mission to convert all persons into Christians and because it became the main religion of the European continent whose soldiers, merchants, settlers, explorers, and priests traveled throughout the world bringing their Bibles and their religion with them.

Both directly and indirectly, the Bible has been a major influence on the behavior, laws, customs, education, literature, art, and morality of Western civilization. Its views on topics such as God, sin, guilt, gender, sexuality, homosexuality, and healing are especially relevant to psychiatrists in their clinical interactions with patients and are the subject of this chapter.

The United States is unique in the world for having both a high level of religious belief and of formal education. An estimation from numerous sources is that one-third of Americans watch religious television each week, and one-third believes that God speaks to them directly. A majority say they are church members, attend religious services at least once a month, and read the Bible at least once a week, while 25 percent attend weekly Bible study groups.(1) The world's largest publisher of Bibles found that most readers are frustrated in reading the Bible because it is difficult to understand, too long, boring, and contains contradictory messages. In fact, most readers hold false beliefs about the Bible.

I. BASIC FACTS ABOUT THE BIBLE

The Bible is composed of many individual books written by men whom Jews and Christians believe were divinely inspired. Each book was written to stand alone with no mention that one day they would be brought together to form one book. The Bible is divided into two parts. The first part, properly called Hebrew Scripture, was renamed the Old Testament (O.T.) by second-century Christians. None of the authors, with one exception, is known. Neither Moses, nor David, nor Solomon wrote any Biblical books; their names were used to lend authority to the texts.(2)

Jewish Scripture was written on multiple scrolls starting in 900 BC using sources from past millennia. The order in which they are presented is not the chronological order in which they were written. It is divided into the Torah (the first five books), the Books of the Prophets, and the Writings. All the books have been edited many, many times until they reached a form that is very like what appears in modern Bibles in 150 BC. It was not until about 90 AD that a council of rabbis decided exactly which books were holy enough to be included in the O.T. Jewish Scripture was originally written in Hebrew but was translated into Greek starting in 250 BC. It was translated into Latin by St. Jerome in 400 AD, and his version became the official O.T. portion of the Bible of Christianity for more than a thousand years.

Between 150 BC and 50 AD, no religious material was written that entered into the Bible. The New Testament (N.T.) was written between 50 AD and 150 AD, and the content was derived from multiple sources such as thousands of Greek manuscripts and material written on pieces of pottery. In fact, the text of the N.T. contains more variations than any other body of ancient literature. It was not until 367 AD that a final official list of books was compiled as the N.T. by

an influential bishop. None of the Gospel writers, with the possible exception of John, knew Jesus personally. In fact, evidence for the existence of Jesus is based solely on the Bible (the same is true about Moses, the central character of the O.T.), and the biblical Gospels about the life of Jesus were written more than twenty-five years after his death. He is not mentioned in any official Roman documents, and there are no drawings, coins, statues, letters, or any artifacts about Jesus from the time in which he lived.

Because there never has been a single original set of biblical scrolls or books, there is great variability in the thousands of editions of the Bible. This problem is complicated further because of the translations of the Bible into almost every language of the world and into versions that cater to special audiences, for example, people with limited vocabularies, politically correct persons, and teenagers. Despite these obstacles, Christian Fundamentalists and Evangelicals – who, according to a Gallup poll conducted in May 2006, comprise 30 percent of the American population – believe that every word in their version of the Bible is literally true and that the earth, for example, was created in 4004 BC, that the sun revolves around the earth, and that a pair of every animal on the earth was rescued on Noah's boat during a worldwide flood.(3) Christians regard both the O.T. and the N.T. as divinely inspired sacred Scripture but believe that the N.T. fulfills the O.T.

2. PROBLEMATIC BIBLICAL THEMES

The Bible is a vast, complicated, and often confusing book.(4) For more than two thousand years, scholars have continued to debate the meaning of many passages and even entire books. The Book of Job, for example, has been interpreted in many ways but none is convincing. Job was an honest, God-fearing, and moral person about whom God inquired during a heavenly counsel. A satan, a type of prosecutor as well as an agent of God, said that Job was righteous only because he was so prosperous. God agreed to test Job by causing the loss of his possessions and the death of his children. God was pleased that Job remained righteous. The satan then urged God to take away Job's health by covering his entire body with scabs and wounds, betting that he would then curse God. God agreed, and Job sat in a pile of dung ash and was so thoroughly miserable that his wife urged him to "curse God and die!" Some of Job's friends told him that he must have sinned because God is just and only punishes sinners. Yet Job proclaimed his innocence, begged for mercy, and said that he would remain righteous even though God had made his soul bitter. God then spoke with Job and listed his mighty works. Job replied, "Behold, I am vile: how shall I answer you?" God again humbled Job with more examples of his power. Job said, "I abhor myself, and repent in dust and ashes." God then restored Job's possessions by twofold and allowed him to have seven sons and three daughters and to live for 140 years. The story ends well for Job. But why would a just God punish such a righteous man? It puzzled Job, and it still puzzles readers.

Many people turn to the Bible for solace and for both spiritual and behavioral guidance, especially in difficult times. It is not surprising that mentally ill persons may be influenced by what they have read in the Bible and by what they have been taught about it. Sometimes this turning to the Bible has positive results, but at other times, the opposite occurs. This chapter considers some problematic Biblical themes that may affect the lives of patients.

2.1. God

When the O.T. was written, there were many gods in the area we now call the Holy Land. For the Jews, however, the God Jehovah emerged as the supreme God. In the passage of time, the other gods disappeared, were forgotten, or were changed into different supernatural beings such as angels, principalities, powers, Sons of God, cherubim, and seraphim. God selected the Jews as his chosen people and made a covenant that he would look after them, allow them to prosper, and to rule the Holy Land as long as they kept his commandments and followed his laws.

In the O.T., God intervened many times in the lives of the Jewish community and often punished them when they did not follow the rules of the holy covenant. In the beginning, God appeared to Moses at Mount Sinai, but afterwards only sometimes revealed himself in visions and dreams. He then let his prophets speak for him until, finally, at the end of the O.T., he totally disappeared. He let his chosen people be forced into exile in Babylon, but then he allowed them back home to rebuild the destroyed Holy Temple. His people vowed again to follow his commandments and laws. He made no appearance but simply had the prophet Ezra read from a scroll that contained everything of importance that he had to say.

Throughout the centuries, Jews have been persecuted, especially by Christians who hated them for their role in Christ's crucifixion. In fact, the N.T. contains many anti-Semitic passages. Throughout all the terrible persecution of the past two thousand years, however, the community of Jews has demonstrated to the world that suffering can be made redemptive and a promise of better things to come. Then came the Holocaust where the Nazis methodically exterminated millions of Jews. This led to a crisis of faith not only among Jews but also among Christians who could not understand why God did not intervene. Many persons felt that God was no longer a real presence, that maybe he was dead, and that human beings were responsible for their own fate.

In the N.T., the God of the Jews is still present but is composed of three "persons": the Father, the Son, and the Holy Spirit, each one being uncreated, omnipotent, eternal, co-equal, and unalterable. Jesus Christ, the Son of God, was sent to earth in human form to educate the masses and then to be crucified to wash away the sins of the world and to save humankind. Jesus on the Cross of the Crucifixion is the most iconic image of Western civilization. His voluntary suffering, crucifixion, and resurrection, according to Christians, both fulfilled and transcended the prophecies of the O.T.

It is not uncommon for manic, schizophrenic, and depressed psychotic persons in Christian culture areas to proclaim the delusion that they are

God or Jesus Christ. Many of these patients are alienated from their families, have no home, and are penniless. Their delusion elevates them from a downtrodden to an exalted state, from being powerless to being the most powerful person in the universe. Psychiatric treatment that consists of bringing these patients back to their often-miserable reality is usually unwanted by them. Their reluctance is understandable, but they must be committed to a mental institution in many cases and treatment must be forced on them to protect them from harming themselves or others. Because God is all powerful, patients who believe themselves to be God may jump off high buildings thinking that they can fly, or they may put themselves fearlessly in perilous situations, or they may rarely kill innocent people (although killing is more often the result of a perceived vocal or visual command message from God).

High-functioning, charismatic patients who believe they are God can do enormous harm by becoming cult leaders. Over the centuries, it has been impressive that so many people have come under the influence of delusional leaders who relentlessly twist the words of the Bible to justify their beliefs. In 1993, American federal forces tragically burned the ranch of a Christian cult called the Branch Davidians. Fifty-four adults and twenty-one children died in the fire. The cult leader had convinced the cult members that he was Jesus Christ and that he was entitled to 140 wives as queens and concubines and to have sex with as many young girls as he could get his hands on. The destruction of the cult was a botched attempt to rescue its members, especially when it became known that the cult leader was sexually abusing female children. On a much larger scale, Jim Jones, a delusional, charismatic leader of a Christian Apocalyptic cult convinced his followers to move from San Francisco to the remote jungles of Guyana, South America. In this captive setting, he played the role of God, demanded total allegiance, and preached that the American government was trying to exterminate African-Americans. His delusional grandiosity and abusiveness escalated. He forcibly drugged many members of his cult. When a U.S. congressman

came to inspect Jones's camp and four members of the cult decided to leave with him, Jones became floridly psychotic. He convinced more than nine hundred cult members to drink poison and to die by telling them that they would be "translated" to another planet where they would live blissfully.

Some patients consciously, but often unconsciously, feel a strong identification with the suffering Christ of the Passion. Indeed the N.T. states that "Christ also suffered for you, leaving you an example, that you should follow in his steps. … Do not be bewildered by the fiery ordeal that is upon you. … It gives you a share in Christ's sufferings, and that is cause for joy" (1 Pet. 2–4). This identification may be encountered in patients who repeatedly self-injure themselves. The psychiatrist, Edward Podvoll (5) was correct in noting that

> The self-mutilator can incorporate into his actions patterns which, to a greater or lesser degree, remain unarticulated in most of us. That is, such patterns already exist in muted intensities within the patient's social field. As such, he may even perform a service to his culture in his dramatic expression of those patterns which are felt to be intolerable within the self. Still other patterns invoked are those which elicit silent levels of admiration and envy. The history of these images reaches at least as far back as the Passion of the Cross and has prevailed among some of the most respected members of our culture. (p. 219)

In the N.T., Jesus established several rules for Christian behavior that have resulted in relatively rare but horrible acts of major self-mutilation.(6) The Gospel of Matthew 5:28–30 states, "Anyone who looks lustfully at a woman already has committed adultery with her in his thoughts. If your right eye is your trouble, gouge it out and cast it from you. … And if your right hand causes you to sin, cut it off and cast it from you; for it is more profitable for you that one of your body parts perish, than for your whole body to be cast into hell." Almost the exact words appear in the Gospel of Mark 9:43–48.

Case Example

A 39-year-old single man took out his right eye with his fingernail in obedience to Matthew's biblical injunction. He claimed that voices of devils, angels, and persons he had formerly known commented on his behavior in an accusatory tone and commanded him to injure his remaining eye. He believed that he had stolen the soul of a nurse seven years previously and that she exerted great control over him. He also believed that he possessed both male and female sexual organs and that he produced numerous babies daily.(7)

In another passage, Jesus told his disciples that divorce was permissible only in cases of adultery. They commented that if a man's wife committed adultery, "It is better not to marry." Jesus replied, "All cannot accept this saying, but only those to whom it has been given. For there are eunuchs who were born thus from their mother's womb, and there are eunuchs who were made eunuchs by men, and there are eunuchs who have made themselves eunuchs for the kingdom of heaven's sake. He who is able to accept it, let him accept it" (Matt. 19:11–12). What exactly is meant by this passage has been debated for two millennia. A small number of Christian groups have used it historically to justify the castration of its members (within the Eastern Orthodox tradition, for example, the sect known as the Skoptsi, or eunuch, was widespread in eighteenth and nineteenth century Russia, and the Catholic Church's practice of castrating young boys to preserve their high-pitched voices for the Vatican choir endured until 1880), and some psychotic patients have used it to justify their self-castration.

Case Example

A shy, withdrawn man with an excellent work record was constantly afraid that people would consider him a homosexual because of his gentleness. At the age of 35 years, he suddenly developed deep religious feelings. His work deteriorated as his religious preoccupations increased. He was hospitalized and received electroshock treatment. He dwelled on the Bible and on outer space. He then decided that he must renounce "the sex life of the world." After reading passage 19 in the Gospel of Matthew, he castrated himself with a razor in the belief that this act of purification would qualify him to serve as the pilot who would carry the godly to outer space.(8)

Although it is difficult to anticipate acts of major self-injury, ominous signs in a psychotic or pre-psychotic person include intense religiosity, a focused interest in the Bible, and a marked change in physical appearance such as cutting off all of one's hair or dressing bizarrely. It should be noted clinically that one act of major self-injury puts a patient at very high risk for a second act.

2.2. Sin and Guilt

In both Judaism and Christianity, sin refers to any behavior that violates the moral codes of conduct established by God primarily in the Bible but also in theological works by esteemed rabbis, priests, and church councils. The O.T. Book of Leviticus contains 613 laws revealed by God to Moses concerning offerings, the priesthood, purification, the Day of Atonement, feasts, the tabernacle, blasphemy, the Sabbath years, and blessings for obedience and curses for disobedience. Although the laws refer mainly to priestly legislation, all Jews were expected to know and obey them. A major theme in Leviticus is atonement through animal sacrifice. "For the life of the flesh is in the blood, and I have given it to you upon the altar to make atonement for your souls; for it is the blood that makes atonement for the soul (17:11). Those persons who atoned for their sins achieved holiness. "You shall be holy; for I am holy" (11:44). The O.T. also contains the Ten Commandments. Punishment for not keeping the laws and commandments include death, humiliation, loss of possessions, and all sorts of bodily ills such as insanity, scabs, boils, and famine.

Animal sacrifice has long been abandoned by Jews who note that the O.T. prophets said that atonement and a return to holiness were also possible through prayers and repentance. Thus, Samuel 15:22 states, "Does the Lord delight in burnt offerings and sacrifices as much as in obeying the voice of the Lord? To obey is better than sacrifice, and to heed is better than burnt offerings." And Hosea 6:6 states, "For I desire mercy, not sacrifice, and acknowledgment of God rather than burnt offerings."

In the N.T. Jesus overthrew the Levitical laws and expanded on the Ten Commandments in his Sermon on the Mount (Matt. 5–70) as well as on the concept of sin. For him, the one unpardonable sin was blasphemy against the Holy Spirit. The N.T. Epistle of Paul to the Romans notes, "For the wages of sin is death, but the gift of God is eternal life in Christ Jesus our Lord." The N.T. firmly established the concepts of hell and heaven. Differing interpretations of the N.T. by various Christian groups hold that heaven can be reached only by the grace of God, or by a combination of good works in addition to the grace of God, or by being fortunate enough to be a person predetermined by God for heaven. People can be reconciled with God through baptism, following his rules, prayers, and acts of contrition.

A common result of sin is guilt, the remorseful feeling of having done something wrong leading to self-reproach and even self-hatred. Because human beings are imperfect, it is impossible for them to consistently fulfill the expectations of Judaism or Christianity, for example, one of the Ten Commandments states that it is sinful to covet a neighbor's wife or possessions. Thus, even fantasies may be sinful. Both religions rely partly on a guilty conscience to control the behavior of its members. People regard their conscience, which in psychodynamic terms is the conscious part of their superego, as if it were a guide or a judge that is better than themselves and even separate from themselves. It reflects a society's ethical and moral standards that, in great part, derive from religious teachings. Behaviors, such as committing a sin, that are disapproved of by one's conscience result in anxiety, guilt, and lowered self-esteem. A saying commonly attributed to the Jesuit Order of Catholic priests is, "Give

us control of a child until he is six years old and he will be ours forever." The reasoning here is that the basic structure of the conscience is set in early childhood but will affect people for the rest of their lives.

The conscience is an important stabilizer in people's lives. Persons with a limited conscience are sociopaths and moral monsters, but persons with an overly strict conscience may experience chronic guilt. Dythymic persons experience their guilt by feelings of inferiority, depression, and worthlessness, while obsessive-compulsive persons experience their guilt by attempting to deny and to magically counteract it through their symptomatic rituals that, like a religious service, must be performed flawlessly. People whose consciences are unbearably harsh may develop a psychotic depression with suicidality and come to regard themselves as truly great sinners who are condemned to hell.

Because the conscience reflects a society's moral and ethical standards, cultural changes over the past century have diminished the potency of sin as a regulator of behavior and of hell as an actual, eternal reality. True sin is based on the notion of a free will choice, but this notion has been undermined by alternative explanations for behavior, for example, genetics, chemical imbalances in the brain, defective neural circuitry, child-rearing practices, peer pressure, and the influence of advertising. As far back as 1850, the incredulous congregation in Nathaniel Hawthorne's novel *The Scarlet Letter* had already lost its ability to comprehend the heartfelt confession of their adulterous minister. "Ye, that have deemed me holy! Behold me here, the one sinner of the world."

The reality of hell was based on the visions and accounts of persons who claimed to have seen it, but this was undermined when the two greatest evocations of hell were described centuries ago in Dante's *Inferno* and Milton's *Paradise Lost,* which were published as poems that sprang from the writers' imaginations. Today, sin has been transformed into mental illness and criminality, while hell has been transformed into accounts of toxic dumps and drug-induced stupors, and in the

Nazi concentration camps there was much wailing and gnashing of teeth.

2.3. Women's Issues

The Judeo-Christian tradition has been the most significant force in defining the "natural" role of Western women. The unifying core of this tradition is the Bible, which provides numerous examples of proper and improper female comportment. Unfortunately the Bible was written and edited over the course of more than a thousand years so that no consistent "model" woman emerges. Although the Catholic Church has long offered Mary, the mother of Jesus, as the ideal woman because of her attributes of virginity and suffering, the Protestant Revolution did away with veneration of Mary, and the twentieth century feminist revolution devalued both female virginity and suffering. Additionally, for several thousand more years, rabbis, priests, and ministers in endless writings and sermons have provided sometimes contrary interpretations of biblical statements about women. Many Orthodox Jews, for example, demand that a woman's head should be practically bald and that wigs should be worn, while some Fundamentalist Christian groups demand long, uncut tresses on female members. St. Paul clearly states that women should cover their heads while in church; some congregations follow this thinking, others don't. If such diverse interpretations of the Bible exist on the simple matter of a woman's hair, then there is little chance that more significant and complex issues will be understood identically by all readers.

Creation stories usually have great prestige in a culture. The story of Adam and Eve surely has enormous implications for male-female relationships, yet, once told, it is never mentioned again in the Old Testament except for a momentous interpretation in the apocryphal book of Ecclesiasticus (about 180 BC): "From a woman sin had its beginning, and because of her we all die. Allow no outlet to water and no boldness of speech in an evil wife. If she does not go as you direct, separate her from yourself" (25:24–26). Ecclesiasticus appears in the Greek Orthodox and Catholic Bible but not the Protestant. Neither is it included in the Jewish Bible, although its exposition of traditional Hebrew wisdom and advice for men made it a favored text by many rabbis. What advice and wisdom about women were offered? From a woman's perspective, the high point comes early in Chapter 3: "Whoever honors his father atones for sin, and whoever glorifies his mother is like one who lays up treasure." Everything then rapidly goes downhill. "Do not give yourself over to a woman so that she gains mastery over your strength" (9:2); "Taking hold of an evil wife is like grasping a scorpion" (27:7); "Keep strict watch over a headstrong daughter lest, when she finds liberty ... she will sit in front of every post and open her quiver to the arrow" (26:10–12); "A wife's charm delights her husband, and her skill puts fat on his bones. A silent wife is a gift to the Lord. ... Like the sun rising in the sign of the Lord is the beauty of a good wife in her well-ordered home" (26:13–16); "He who acquires a wife gets his best possession, a helper for him and a pillar of support" (36:24).

The portrayals of woman as a man's possession whose role is to cook, keep a neat house, and be silent and of woman as the seductive scorpion who can make men miserable are found throughout the "wisdom" literature of the Hebrews. This popular type of literature, found in many cultures and often offering the same advice, was developed by sages who spoke from experience; priests and prophets ended *their* comments with the definitive phrase "thus saith the Lord." The biblical book of Proverbs, several centuries older than Ecclesiasticus, contained many of the same ideas. "For the lips of an immoral woman drip honey, and her mouth is smoother than oil; but in the end she is bitter as wormwood, sharp as a two edged sword. Her feet go down to death, her steps lay hold of hell" (5:3–5); "The mouth of an immoral woman is a deep pit; he who is abhorred by the Lord will fall there" (22:14); "Do not give your strength to woman" (31:3). The virtuous wife (31:10–31) arises before dawn to prepare food, helps the poor, brings in money by investing in land and by selling the garments that she makes, is wise and kind, and does not eat the bread of idleness.

Overall, women in the Old Testament were valued primarily as mothers. Some of the most poignant moments describe the grief of mothers for their dead children, especially their sons. "A voice was heard in Ramah; lamentation and bitter weeping, Rachel weeping for her children, refusing to be comforted for her children, because they are no more" (Jer. 31:15). After the Gibeonites hanged her sons, "Rizpah took sackcloth and spread it for herself on the rock, from the beginning of the harvest until the late rains poured from heaven on their bodies. And she did not allow the birds of the air to rest on them by day nor the beasts of the field by night" (2 Sam. 21:10).

Secondarily, women were valued as wives. In the early days, polygamy was the norm. By the eighth century BC, monogamy was standard and was a metaphor for Jewish acceptance of one God. Women could not file for divorce, but men had little problem. "When a man takes a wife and marries her, and it happens that she finds no favor in his eyes because he has found some uncleanliness in her," the husband merely had to hand her a written certificate of divorce (Deut. 24:1). Because a woman, even after marriage, owed some allegiance to her family of birth, the problem of divided loyalty was always present. Also, wives could become contentious, spider-like, and even bovine. Amos 4:1 refers to them as cows. The presence of concubines – unmarried women who lived with the family at the pleasure of the husband – undoubtedly made life easier in some ways by taking the edge off things. The ultimate state of degradation into which women might descend is depicted during a famine in Samaria. One woman says to another, "Give me your son, that we may eat him today, and we will eat my son tomorrow" (2 Kings 6:29).

In contrast to images of women as mother and wife, the O.T. contains a bevy of prostitutes and adulteresses who intrigued the Israelites. The expression "to play the harlot" is used throughout the O.T. to describe the act of abandoning one's faith. "Yet they would not listen to their judges,

but they played the harlot with other gods, and bowed down to them" (Judg. 2:17). In a powerful metaphor Israel, the bride of God, became a prostitute. "You have polluted the land with your harlotries and your wickedness. … You have had a harlot's forehead; you refuse to be ashamed" (Jer. 3:2–3). An elaboration of this theme forms the drama of the book of the prophet Hosea who was ordered by God to marry a prostitute and have children of prostitution "for the land commits great harlotry by forsaking the Lord" (1:2). Hosea obeyed. Just as his wife pursued her lovers, so too did Israel pursue false gods. But Hosea reclaimed his wife and God reclaimed Israel.

In the N.T., Jesus stirred up problems in his dealings with women. He broke one of the Ten Commandments when he neither honored nor even acknowledged his mother when she called out to him, concerned for his safety. Rather, he looked at the crowd around him and said, "Here are my mother and my brothers! For whoever does the will of God is my brother and my sister and my mother" (Mark 1:30–31). He even healed a woman with a chronic vaginal flow – the essence of Jewish uncleanliness – who touched his robe. He elevated the status of women by declaring that the only legitimate reason for divorce was adultery. Until then a man was free to divorce his wife, according to the great Rabbi Hillel, even if her major fault was that she spoiled the soup. His relationship with Mary Magdalen was distorted by interpreters of the Bible who made her out to be a penitent prostitute instead of venerating her as the first person to see the resurrected Christ. In the Gospel of Thomas, one of the many gospels not selected for inclusion in the Bible, Peter the disciple said to Jesus, "Let Mary Magdalen leave us, for women are not worthy of life." Jesus replied, "I myself shall lead her in order to make her male, so that she may become a living spirit like you males."

She became the perfect foil for Mary, the virgin mother of Jesus, the greatest woman in Christendom.(9) The Bible actually says little about Mary but the early church fathers made her out to be the perfect model of womanhood even though, when a woman in a crowd called out to Jesus, "Blessed is the womb that bore you and the breasts that you suckled," he replied, "Blessed rather are those who hear the word of God and keep it" (John 11:27–28). The church's vehement defense of her virginity is based on a mistranslation of the word for "a young woman" in Matthew's Gospel. Virginity was a major theme in early Christianity and was seen as a pathway to heaven. In the fourth century, St. John Chrysostom noted that virgins did not have to worry about being "split apart by labor pains and wailings," and that "the virgin is not obligated to involve herself tirelessly in the affairs of her spouse and she does not fear being abused."

In order to buttress their argument for the ideal of virginity, the church fathers declared that women were problematic because they inspired men to lust. St. Bernard, for example, wrote that a beautiful woman was like a temple built over a sewer. *The Witch's Hammer*, an erudite, medieval guide book about the detection and persecution of witches that influenced European witch trials for several centuries, concluded, "All witchcraft comes from carnal lust, which in women is insatiable. See Proverbs 30. The mouth of the womb never says 'enough.' Wherefore for the sake of fulfilling their lusts they consort even with devils."

Attitudes such as these posed great problems for Catholic women. The closest approximation to being like the Virgin Mary was to become a nun and to marry Christ. Thus, in the fourteenth century, the pious Margery Kemp wrote what Jesus supposedly told her when she went to bed, "Take me as thy wedded husband, as thy dear-worthy darling, and as thy dear son, for I will be loved as a son should be loved by the mother, and I will that thou lovest me, daughter, as a good wife ought to love her husband." With dazzling virtuosity the virginal, ascetic Margery simultaneously became Christ's mother, daughter, and spouse.

Married women were in a bind because it was impossible to be both a virgin and a mother. The compromise that resulted in a great deal of marital discord was for a wife to fulfill her marital sexual obligations but not to enjoy them. Another problem was that the Virgin Mary was venerated for her maternal sufferings. In many images she is shown as Our Lady of Sorrows with seven swords piercing her breast. In trying to emulate the suffering Mary, female ascetics, such as St. Catherine of Siena, whipped themselves, pressed thorns in their skin, ate cat vomit and dead rodents, and even developed skin wounds like the stigmata of Jesus. However, the foremost method of suffering was self-starvation, whose deepest goal was to facilitate a divine union with Jesus by subsisting on a diet of communion wafers. Thus, anorexia was approved as a saintly behavior. Some modern anorexics believe that there is no fat in heaven because the gate to enter paradise is very narrow (Matt. 7:14).

2.4. Marriage

The most common type of marriage in the Bible is the patriarchal kind in which the father/husband is the supreme authority as established in Genesis. God said to Eve, "In pain you shall bring forth children; your desire shall be for your husband, and he shall rule over you." David's and Solomon's many wives exemplify polygamy, although usually just two wives was more typical. By the eighth century, monogamy had become the prevalent form of marriage. The bride and groom entered into a covenant that involved not only them but also their families. On a larger scale, monogamy represented the covenant between God and Israel. Isaiah's chapters 61 and 62 compared the bride's and bridegroom's clothing with "the garments of salvation" and "the robes of righteousness" and promised that the desolate forsaken land of Zion would attain salvation through marriage with the Lord, and just as the bridegroom rejoices over the bride, "so shall God rejoice over you." In 2 Corinthians 2, Paul betrothed the church to Christ "as a pure bride to her one husband."

Marriage in Christianity has been somewhat problematic beyond the issue of the husband's domination over the wife. Although the Catholic catechism states that Jesus established marriage as a sacrament, most scholars disagree. In fact, both Jesus and Paul tolerated marriage but hardly gave it glowing reviews. Marriage for them was "a form of this world [that] is passing away" because the end of the world was approaching, "So that he who marries his betrothed does well; and he who refrains from marriage does better" (1 Cor. 7). That Jesus attended a wedding at Cana, where he performed his first miracle by changing water into wine, is not particularly significant. It would be a totally different story if he had consecrated the couple's marriage with a nuptial blessing.

With a few exceptions, the early church fathers were not terribly high on marriage. Ambrose wrote, "Even a good marriage is slavery. What, then, must a bad marriage be?" For Jerome, "Marriage is only one degree less sinful than fornication." The church adopted the Roman concept that a valid marriage simply required the consent of the bride and groom. Marriage was a secular contract and the church recognized the validity of all marriages, including those among slaves, that followed local civil laws. A priest could attend a marriage as a witness. At the Council of Elvira in 309 AD, many rulings were made about the necessity for control over sexual matters; it was in this century that priests began to intrude cautiously into the marriage ceremony by blessing the newlyweds. In the sixth century, marriages were often associated with a mass but their validity was still based on a secular contract. It wasn't until the Council of Trent in 1563 that the church officially proclaimed marriage to be a sacrament. The current Catholic catechism states, "In the Latin Church, it is ordinarily understood that the spouses, as ministers of Christ's grace, mutually confer upon each other the sacrament of matrimony by expressing their consent before the Church."

In modern times, just about all Christian churches, some more reluctantly than others, have modified their position on divorce because secular divorce is so prevalent. Even in those churches that might excommunicate persons who get divorced, members of the church usually will accept divorced persons as new members. The Catholic Church still has a hard-line policy about divorce, but each year new records are being set by couples who have their marriages annulled by the church, sometimes on a flimsy pretext. Many parish priests do not withhold communion from remarried persons even though they technically are acting against church policy. I might add that, for a long time, psychiatrists considered divorce a sign of emotional immaturity. However, when enough psychiatrists themselves divorced their spouses, they changed their position. Now, divorce may indicate a mentally healthy action depending on the circumstances. Psychiatry reflects the times in which we live and the customs of the people.

The period of the exile of many Jews in Babylon (587–538 BC) marks an important historical division. Before the exile, women, although subordinate to men, had a certain status. Along with concubines, slaves, precious metals, and animals, wives belonged to a man, but they could not be purchased or sold. Women could participate in religious ceremonies. They could be prophetesses or wise persons or sorceresses. They could be heroines, like Deborah, or agitators, like Jezebel.

When the Israelites returned from their exile, they were determined to avoid the circumstances that caused God to treat them so harshly. Their solution was a back-to-the-basics focus on purity, which meant keeping within the boundaries of divine order. There was a renewed emphasis on the covenant established between Abraham and God. "And you shall be circumcised in the flesh of your foreskins, and it shall be a sign of the covenant between me and you" (Gen. 17:11). Because circumcision was an option only for men, females could enter into the covenant only through their relationship with men. To emphasize the importance of sacrificial blood, which made atonement possible, other forms of blood were deemed impure. Thus, a menstruating woman was unclean and so was everything she sat on. Slowly but surely, the social and religious status of women declined. A special court was constructed in the temple to keep women in their place away from the sanctuary. The period of a woman's impurity was seven days following the birth of a boy, but fourteen days after the birth of a girl. Ecclesiasticus noted that only one man in a thousand is wise, "But a woman among these I have not found" (7:28). A man could have a trial marriage with a female captive. "And it shall be, if you have no delight in her, then you shall set her free" (Deut. 21:14).

Ezra was so distressed by the iniquities of his fellow Jews that he tore his clothes and pulled out his hair. At a great assembly he said that the wrath of God would continue until they rid themselves of impure, pagan wives. Shechaniah spoke up, "Let us make a covenant with our God to put away all these wives and those who have been born to them, according to the advice of my master and of those who tremble at the commandment of our God; and let it be done according to the law" (10:3). Nehemiah was even more zealous: he slapped people around, cursed a lot and forced them to swear by God that they would not intermarry (13:25). In modern times, polls show that half of American Jews marry outside their faith and that only one-third of their children are being reared as Jews.

In the N.T., Jesus recognized that people marry but noted that "those who are considered worthy of participating in the coming age, which means in the resurrection from the dead, do not marry" (Luke 20:35). On the road to the crucifixion he said to the daughters of Jerusalem, "Behold, the days are coming when they will say, 'Blessed are the barren, and the wombs that never gave birth, and the breasts that never nursed an infant'" (Luke 23:29). Paul never met Jesus, yet developed a working theology based on his interpretation and development of Jesus's words. In 1 Corinthians he wrote, "It is good for a man not to touch a woman … I say to the unmarried and to the widows … if they cannot exercise self-control, let them marry. For it is better to marry than to burn with passion … but he who refrains from marriage does better." He also wrote, "The head of every man is Christ, and the head of every woman is her husband." The Letter to the Ephesians, which has been attributed to Paul, contains the warning, "Wives, submit to your husbands, as to the Lord. For the husband is the head of the wife. … Just as the church is subject to Christ, so let the wives be subject to their own husbands in everything." The warning is softened by requiring husbands to love their wives as their own bodies. Paul was very clear about the inferior status of women, even forbidding them to speak in church but rather to speak to their husbands at home if they wanted to know something.

This attitude has persevered throughout the centuries and has been used by men to condone spousal abuse. It is not uncommon for psychiatrists to encounter women who believe they must endure abuse because the Bible commands them to submit to whatever their husbands do.

Case Example

A psychiatrist was asked to examine an attractive woman who had been hospitalized following a life-threatening overdose. She reported that she was a devout Christian but her husband was an alcoholic who often beat her. On weekends he would bring home women he had met in a bar and have sex with them after forcing his wife to leave the bedroom and to sleep on a couch. She had complained to her pastor but was told that she needed to become a better wife who could sexually meet her husband's needs. After years of enduring such abuse and deciding that she was stuck in a hopeless situation, she had tried to kill herself. The psychiatrist, after determining that she had a great deal of personal strength and that she was demoralized but not mentally ill, utilized a forceful therapy. He told her that since her husband did not respect her, as stated in the Bible, she was not obligated to submit to him. He urged her to stand up for herself and to leave her husband immediately and to go to a local women's shelter. When she expressed dismay over what the church members would think of her, he advised her to find a new church. She followed his advice, divorced her abusive husband, moved to another city, and decided that she would wait before seeking another church. A year later she wrote to tell the psychiatrist that she was doing well, had made new friends, found a job, and was enjoying her freedom.

Unfortunately, not all such cases turn out so well. Many abused women may give in to guilt-evoking pressure from their husband, their family, their pastor, and even members of their religious congregation to return to the abusive situation because "it's against the Bible not to submit to your husband." This argument is most commonly encountered among Orthodox Jews, Fundamentalist Christians, and Mormons.

The rise of secular feminism and of female biblical scholarship in the twentieth century has elevated the status of women in both Judaism and Christianity. In many cases, women can now be ordained as ministers and rabbis, but the Catholic Church still reserves the priesthood only for men. Women today often hold prominent positions in their congregations and are more apt to receive support for the decision to leave abusive relationships, although some orthodox and fundamentalist religious groups still hold on to the belief of female submission to their husbands in every circumstance.

2.5. Homosexuality

Condemnation of homosexuality, a socially divisive issue, is often based on several biblical citations. The Book of Leviticus contains myriad laws, such as prohibitions against trimming one's beard, eating shellfish or pork, and wearing garments made of a mixture of linen and wool; in addition, adulterers, fortune tellers, and male homosexuals should be put to death. Although Christians are not obligated to follow the Levitical laws, most groups have selectively chosen to uphold the prohibition against homosexual behavior.

Another source commonly cited in favor of this prohibition is from the book of Genesis, which tells the story of two angels dressed as men who came to the city of Sodom. A man named Lot allowed them to stay in his home. A group of townsmen surrounded the home and asked about the two men, saying, "Bring them out to us that we may know them." Frightened, Lot told them to leave his guests alone and offered his virginal daughters in their place. The townsmen failed

to break down the door and left. The next day, God rained fire and brimstone on the city, killing all its inhabitants, although Lot and his children escaped. The earliest interpretations of this story focused on the Sodomites' arrogance and rudeness to strangers; God killed them for incivility to his angels. The theme of sexuality emerged full force in the first century BC writings of Philo of Alexandria, a Jewish historian. Rabbinical writings about Sodom generally did not mention homosexuality. Although some church fathers agreed with Philo, others did not, pointing to a parallel story in Chapter 19 of the Book of Judges in which homosexuality was not implicated. The Sodomite townsmen wanted "to know" the men; the verb "to know" is used 943 times in Jewish Scripture, and in only ten places does it clearly refer to sexual intercourse. However, over time, the homosexual interpretation won out: the King James Bible translates the townsmen's request, "that we may know them carnally," whereas the New English Bible says, "so that we can have sexual intercourse with them." Some scholars refute these translations and note that Lot was not a full citizen of Sodom. The townsmen were suspicious because he had allowed two strangers to stay in the city at night without asking permission of the proper officials and, thus, they wanted "to know" who the two men were.

Jesus does not mention homosexuality. However, he did link Sodom with the inhospitality that his disciples might encounter when preaching (Matt. 10:14–15). St. Paul, who barely tolerated marital sexuality, seems to have disapproved of homosexual behavior, but the exact meaning of the specific words he used is unclear. In 1 Corinthians 5:11, for example, he includes in his list of the unrighteous who will not go to heaven people who are *malakoi* and *arsenokoitai*. The translations of these words vary widely and include effeminate, child molesters, homosexual, masturbators, immoral, sexually immoral, depraved, and male prostitutes.

Paul's other reference to homosexuality occurs in chapter one of his Epistle to the Romans. Paul's major points here are that the just shall live by faith and that the worship of idols in the image of corruptible humans, birds, animals, and creeping things has resulted in God's wrath as manifested by decaying moral standards and vile passions. Paul then lists examples: same-sex sex *para phusin* (against or in excess of nature), sexual immorality, wickedness, covetousness, envy, murder, strife, deceit, evil mindedness, back-biting, hating God, violence, pride, boasting, inventing evil things, disobedience to parents, and being undiscerning, untrustworthy, unloving, unforgiving, and unmerciful.

Paul clearly disapproves of homosexual acts, but what does the phrase *para phusin* mean? In 11:24, Paul says that God could *para phusin* graft a wild olive tree onto a cultivated olive tree. God surely could not act immorally, but he could act in a way that is "unexpected, unusual, or different from what would occur in the natural order of things."(10) Even the conservative Interpreter's Bible notes that Paul's purpose in this section "is to point not at sins, but to judgment." It is likely that Paul is not condemning homosexuality itself but rather mainstream Gentile men and women who had overstepped their normal sexual practices. In fact, St. John Chrysostom's fourth-century homily on Romans stated that Paul's disapproval of homosexual practices pertained only to people who fall in lust and not to those who fall in love.

Although homosexual behavior was common throughout the ancient world, the designation of a person as a *homosexual* did not occur until the eleventh century AD when St. Peter Damian coined the word *sodomia*, thus establishing an abstract essence. Persons who indulged in *sodomia* were thereafter referred to as sodomites (homosexuals).

Homosexuality was listed as a mental disorder in the early editions of the American Psychiatric Association's Diagnostic and Statistical Manual until 1973. In that year, a vote was taken by the association's members, and a majority decided to remove homosexuality from the official list of mental disorders. Despite this action, the overwhelming majority of Christian churches have maintained their positions that homosexual behavior is sinful and a threat to social morality. In contrast, the general public has become much more tolerant as demonstrated by broad acceptance of homosexuality on popular television shows and movies. Although some Christian churches have ordained homosexuals as priests, the issue remains troublesome and has caused major conflicts. While the Catholic Church has been disgraced in recent years by revelations about widespread priestly pederasty, it has been long known that many priests have a homosexual orientation. A study of homosexual priests found that 4 percent were celibate while the others averaged 227 partners each.(11) In another study, of 62 percent of priests who responded, 32 percent had exclusively male sexual partners.(12)

Case Example

An agitated, anxious, and guilt-ridden 18-year-old man sought psychiatric help. He and all his family were born-again Christians. The patient confessed a lifelong attraction to men. He knew that this was wrong and said that he prayed and cried to Jesus for help but that his feelings did not change. When he told his family members they became furious with anger and his mother even called him an abomination who had given himself over to the devil. The psychiatrist reassured the patient that his feelings did not constitute a mental illness and discussed various interpretations of the biblical passages regarding homosexuality with a particular focus on the fact that Jesus overthrew the Levitical laws, including the one ordering the death of homosexuals. The psychiatrist also met with the patient's parents who, after discussing the matter, were somewhat less angry. He told them that their son's homosexuality was inborn and not a deliberate choice, and that there was no treatment that could change a person's sexual orientation. The parents agreed to send their son to a distant college and to allow him to return home for holidays as long as he did not mention his homosexuality. They said that they would try to show him Christian love but that it would be difficult.

2.6. Healing

The O.T. attributed most disease to God's revenge against sinners. In Deuteronomy, God threatened the disobedient with all sorts of physical ills including insanity, blindness, severe fever, tumors, boils, and scabs. Because God caused diseases, it seemed only logical to look to God for cures. Exodus 15:17 is the definitive Old Testament statement on God the healer. "If you diligently heed the voice of the Lord your God and do what is right in his sight, give ear to his commandments and keep all his statutes, I will put none of the diseases on you which I have brought on the Egyptians. For I am the Lord who heals you."

The most common acceptable "treatment" for sick Hebrews was prayer. The Hebrews led a spiritualized life in which God's handiwork was implicit in every event. He was seen as the prime mover in everything from famine and war to family discord and diseases. Because they diminished God's position, formal medical practice and magic were disdained by the early Hebrews. To remain healthy and to have a good heart, the best approach was to follow God's rules as written in the code of Moses. Many of the rules were, in fact, incidentally beneficial to public health. Rest one day a week. Eat vegetables with impunity but avoid pork (pigs probably were sacred to some Semitic group; Moses didn't know that pork is often infested with parasites). Don't pollute the water supply. No incest. Wash frequently. Bury human excreta. Obey these rules and you not only stay on God's good side, but you also decrease the possibility of getting sick.

Things started to change in about the fourth century BC after the Hebrews returned from their exile in Babylon. The priestly writers who reedited the Bible put such an emphasis on purity that physically "impure" humans, such as lepers, the blind, and the lame, were treated badly and excluded from the Holy Temple (Lev. 13–14; 2 Sam. 5–7). Perhaps it is purely coincidental, but the attitude toward physicians began to change as handicapped and chronically ill persons were increasingly stigmatized by the priests.

By 180 BC, Jesus the Son of Sirach wrote that physicians are needed and should be honored (Ecclus. 38). Likewise, sensible persons should take medicines that heal and take away pain. When you are sick, you should pray to the Lord for healing, but "there is a time when success lies in the hands of a physician."

In the N.T., Jesus revolutionized the approach toward the sick. He actually welcomed the sick as well as socially marginal and even despised persons such as the blind, eunuchs, hunchbacks, dwarfs, cripples, tax collectors, and prostitutes. He immediately healed all the sick people who approached him, even on the Sabbath day. He did not take a medical or social history and didn't require confessions or a therapeutic relationship. Most important, he didn't blame the sick for being sick. The early Christians accepted Christ as the Messiah in great part because of his healings, which fulfilled O.T. prophecies.

Almost 20 percent of the Gospels are devoted to Christ's forty-one healing encounters. His usual technique was to say a few words and to touch the sick person. What types of illness did he heal? The list includes the fever of Peter's mother-in-law; eleven lepers; a man with palsy, and one with dropsy or edema; the severed ear of the High Priest's servant who had arrested him; a crippled man; a boy and a girl on the brink of death; the woman with vaginal bleeding; a man's withered hand; a centurion's paralyzed servant; the dead son of a widow; four blind men; the blind and lame in the Temple; a blind, mute man; and, most of all, people who were possessed with demons. He passed on the power to cast out (exorcise) demons to his twelve disciples and to all believers.

For several centuries, healing through both exorcisms and prayer was common in early Christianity and was effective in recruiting members to the new church. However, once the church was officially recognized by the Romans, healings greatly diminished. This change was facilitated in 400 AD when St. Jerome made an error in his translation of the Bible into Latin. The classic N.T. model for healing was the text from James 5:13–26. James wrote that sick people should call the elders of the church to pray at their bedside and anoint them with oil in the name of the Lord. They should confess their sins and pray for one another and "they will be healed." Jerome made a mistake and translated the phrase as "they will be saved." Thus, spiritual salvation displaced the healing of illness.

Another major factor in the church's neglect of healing was the increasing importance given to the biblical writings of Paul, who basically reclaimed the old Jewish concept that sick persons are sinners. Sickness itself was a consequence of demons, idols, false gods, and all the hosts of wickedness in the universe. Paul himself had a sickness (probably epilepsy). He asked God to cure him three times but God refused. According to Paul, God then said, "My grace is sufficient for you, for my power is made perfect in weakness." This was truly a brilliant, new idea: a handicap was transformed into an asset by perceiving it so. Instead of regarding an infirmity merely as a defect or liability, declare it an opportunity to receive the power of Christ and make the most of it. The upside of this reformulation is the enhanced sense of self-worth that it provides to the disabled and chronically ill. The downside is the potential for persons to accept their infirmities with passivity or even to harm themselves deliberately in pursuit of a higher, spiritual goal.

The glorification of suffering has influenced Christian attitudes toward illness for almost two thousand years, and medical treatment was devalued until the eighteenth century. However, the church did encourage devotion to sacred relics such as the bones of saints and ascribed healing powers to them. Specific saints were associated with differing body organs and diseases. St. Lucy, for example, supposedly enucleated her eyes to calm the ardor of a suitor who had praised their beauty and, thus, became the patron saint of persons with eye diseases. St. Dymphna of Belgium was the patron saint of the mentally ill. Churches were built to display these relics and became healing shrines that attracted pilgrims.

Relics lost their power to heal as medical practice became more scientific and effective. The only major healing shrine today is in Lourdes, France.

It was established in 1858 when a young girl had visions of a lady subsequently identified as the Virgin Mary. Several million pilgrims each year travel to Lourdes in search of healing, although the Catholic Church has certified only about 100 miraculous cures. Sick visitors to Lourdes return home uncured but usually feeling better. Patients benefit from the support of the family members who accompany them on their pilgrimage; from sharing expectations for improvement with thousands of like-minded patients; from participation in emotionally charged and spiritually uplifting ceremonies that include fervent praying, hymn singing, and a formal parade of children, priests, nuns, bishops, nurses, and physicians; and from a sense of expectant excitement. In the words of Jerome and Julia Frank (1991),(13) "The improvement probably reflects heightened morale, enabling a person to function better in the face of an unchanged organic handicap. Fully documented cures of unquestionable and gross organic disease are extremely infrequent – probably no more frequent than similar ones occurring in secular settings." Improvement seems to be linked with the intensity of the faith of patients. According to Cranston (1995),(14) those who feel better are "almost invariably simple people – the poor and the humble; people who do not interpose a strong intellect between themselves and the Higher Power."

The rebirth of interest in healing began in New England at the end of the nineteenth century with the development of the mind-cure movement. In 1875, Mary Baker Eddy founded the Church of Christian Science, which preached that sickness is only a belief that can be destroyed by the divine Mind, and that disease is simply fear made manifest on the human body. She considered medications, surgery, and hypnotism to be examples of false beliefs and mortal illusions. Harvard psychologist William James published his masterpiece, *The Variety of Religious Experience*, in 1902.(15) He noted that mind-cures replaced morbid beliefs with healthy-minded attitudes. "The whole matter can be summed up by one sentence: God is well and so are you. You must awake to the knowledge of your real being."

The actual rebirth of Christian healing started in Topeka, Kansas, in 1900 when a Methodist minister rediscovered the practice of speaking-in-tongues (glossalalia) and was able to heal sick people. His inspiration was a passage in the Gospel of Mark (16:17), which states that believers will not only speak in tongues but also lay hands on the sick who will recover. His experience was warmly embraced by the Pentecostal Church and led to the rise of preachers who became famous for their healing sermons. Eventually, televangelists took over the movement, which has grown to enormous proportions not only in the Untied States but also throughout Christian cultural areas around the world. Today it is not uncommon for 100,000 people to attend faith healing services at large arenas. While some of the so-called healers undoubtedly believe they are doing God's work, many are charlatans who make a lot of money. Originally they focused on demon possession, but as people have become more sophisticated, they now focus on demonic *oppression,* especially for persons with impulse control disorders. Follow-up studies have not found any long-lasting practical results from this type of "healing."(16, 17)

Many persons, including the mentally ill, engage in intercessory prayers to overcome their illness. On three occasions in the Gospels Jesus promises, "Whatever things you ask in prayer, believing, you will receive" (Matt. 21:22); "Ask, and it will be given to you" (Luke 11:9); and "Whatever you ask the Father in My name, He will give you" (John 16:23). Unfortunately, intercessory prayers are rarely, if ever, effective. If a person does recover from an illness, it is impossible to prove that prayers are responsible. Studies comparing sick persons who are prayed for at a distance and without the knowledge of the patients have failed to show better results than for control groups for whom no prayers are offered. A problem with such studies is that people in the control group may pray for themselves or may be prayed for by relatives or hospital staff. When prayers are not answered, patients may be told that even Jesus's prayer to his Father asking to be spared from the crucifixion was not answered. In other words, God's will takes precedence over individual desires. He only answers prayers that are part of his own plan, which cannot be known in advance. Thus, whatever happens is God's will.

There is no harm in praying for healing, and participation in prayer-healing ceremonies fosters hope and positive feelings that may help both patients as well as family members and friends feel better. This, in turn, may energize a sick person's natural recuperative powers, perhaps by affecting the immune system or by increasing motivation in a rehabilitation program.

Case Example

An obviously depressed woman sought psychiatric help. She described herself as a devoutly Christian woman whose 10-year-old daughter had died six months earlier in an automobile accident. She said that she had prayed at her daughter's bedside daily asking for God to cure the girl. She had a Bible and even read aloud to the psychiatrist the passages cited above in which God promises to give believers what they ask for. She was angry with God and with her religion. She had already heard the usual clichés, for example, "She's in a better place now"; "God had a special plan for her"; "The good die young." The psychiatrist acknowledged her loss and then told her that she was depressed. He urged her to take antidepressant medications and to enter therapy so that she could overcome her depression and honor her daughter's memory appropriately. He explained that depression is an illness that interferes with clear thinking. He explained that she should not come to any major decisions about God, her religion, or the apparent senselessness of her daughter's death until her depression had lifted and she could then enter into meaningful dialogues with God and her pastor.

3. SOLACE

In the dullness of a fool, the Bible can seem foolish. In the grips of a zealot, it can suffocate the human spirit. In the hands of a psychopath, it can rationalize greed, lust, and all the antisocial vices. It has been used to justify religious wars, slavery, racism, self-castration, anti-Semitism, and countless other behaviors. But artists, authors, architects, and composers have been moved by the Bible to produce some of the most sublime, beautiful, and marvelous works ever created by humankind. Countless deeds of mercy and charity have been performed over the centuries in the pursuit of biblical holiness and in imitation of Christ. And for more than two millennia, the Bible has provided solace and hope to the vexed and the hopeless.

Because the Bible is so vast and complicated, it can be interpreted to suit many purposes. If it were an easy text, there would not be so many divisions among both Christian and Jewish groups. Yet many persons, including the mentally ill, often read the Bible to reaffirm their faith in a God that personally cares for them and is always present for them. In their reading, they may discover a passage or bit of wisdom that has special meaning and allows them to continue living and to follow a certain course in life. Some patients attend Bible study groups through their church or through online or correspondence courses. For some, just holding the Bible in their hands or looking at it on their bed table offers some measure of reassurance.

Psychiatrists should have some knowledge of the Bible because it may be so important to some of their patients. It may be useful to remind religious patients who are noncompliant with their treatment that Jesus healed everyone who sought help, and that it is their Christian duty to recover from their illness.

REFERENCES

1. Wurthnow R. *Sharing the Journey: Support Groups and America's New Quest for Community*. New York, Free Press; 1994.
2. Fox RL. *The Unauthorized Version: Truth and Fiction in the Bible*. New York, Knopf; 1992.
3. Wills G. A country ruled by faith. *New York Times Book Review* Nov. 16, 2006;53.
4. Favazza A. *PsychoBible: Behavior, Religion, and the Holy Bible*. Charlottesville, VA, Pitchstone Publishing; 2004.
5. Podvoll E. Self-mutilation within a hospital setting. *Br J Med Psychol*. 1969;42:213–221.
6. Favazza A. *Bodies Under Siege: Self-Mutilation and Body Modification in Culture and Psychiatry*. Baltimore, MD, Johns Hopkins; 1996.
7. Ananth J, Kaplan HS, Lin K-M. Self-enucleation of the eye. *Can J Psychiatry*. 1984;29:145–146.
8. Kushner AW. Two cases of auto-castration due to religious delusions. *Br J Med Psychol*. 1967;40:293–298.
9. Warner M. *Alone of All Her Sex: The Myth and the Cult of the Virgin Mary*. New York, Random House; 1976.
10. Boswell J. *Christianity, Social Tolerance, and Homosexuality*. Chicago, University of Chicago Press; 1980.
11. Wagner R. *Gay Catholic Priests*. San Francisco, CA, Institute for the Advances Study of Homosexuality; 1980.
12. Murphy A. *Delicate Dance: Sexuality, Celibacy and Relationships Among Catholic Clergy*. New York, Crossroads; 1992.
13. Frank JD, Frank JB. *Persuasion and Healing*, 3d ed. Baltimore, MD, Johns Hopkins University Press; 1991.
14. Cranston R. *The Miracle of Lourdes*. New York, Popular Library; 1955.
15. James W. *The Varieties of Religious Experience*. New York, Modern Library; 1902.
16. Nolan W. *Healing: A Doctor in Search of a Miracle*. New York, Random House; 1974.
17. Pattison EM, Lapino NA, Doerr HA. Faith healing. *J Nerv Ment Dis*. 1977;157:397–400.

5   Religion/Spirituality and Neuropsychiatry

NADER PERROUD

SUMMARY

In this chapter, we review the neurobiological basis of spirituality and related religious experiences. We first focus on regions of the brain associated with mystical and spiritual experiences showing that increased activity in the frontal and temporal lobes is a key component of such practices. We then explore serotonergic and dopaminergic systems in measures of spirituality. In this field, we mainly explore association studies between genetic polymorphisms and spirituality as a personality trait. These studies strongly suggest a higher activity of serotonergic and dopaminergic systems in individuals with high spirituality. We then propose a model encompassing both religious activities and measures of spirituality in connection with serotonergic and dopaminergic systems. This explanatory model could help to understand the complex link between psychiatric disorders and spirituality.

1. INTRODUCTION

Spiritual experiences, religion, and rituals may be viewed as the result of the evolutionary changes in the brain that have led humans to socialize and to form communities and societies. Within the evolutionary perspective, spirituality or religiousness could be seen as an advantageous tool for human beings over other species. This could be understood as a complex neurochemical process occurring in the brain. This view has led researchers to explore the brain's neurochemical activity to explain some of the spiritual processes we experience. However, dealing with the neurobiology of religious and spiritual experiences is a complicated and difficult task. A new way of looking at the above would perhaps give us an opportunity to draw a biological picture. Here, we will discuss the neurobiological basis of spiritual experiences and spirituality and also the role played by neurotransmitters. We will focus on the serotonergic and dopaminergic systems. The effect of genes and their possible interaction with environmental factors in the understanding of spirituality will be tackled. As clinicians, our thinking is driven by an attempt to understand the possible impact of spirituality and its neurobiological and genetic effect on psychiatric diseases. Within this perspective, we will also link spiritual neurobiological hypotheses to these disorders.

Research has sought to understand spirituality and religious experiences through two main approaches: One has been concentrated on religious practices and meditation and their relationship with activities in the brain. The second has been based on the relationship between genes and spirituality as a personality trait. In this chapter, we will briefly discuss both approaches.

But first we will discuss serotonin and dopamine neurotransmitters, which have been specifically investigated in terms of spirituality.

2. SEROTONIN (5-HT) AND OTHER NEUROTRANSMITTERS

Neurotransmitters are chemicals that relay messages between the neurons in the brain across a gap called a synapse. These neurotransmitters are distributed widely in the brain and cover specific regions. They are synthesized in the pre-synaptic neuron and are released from this neuron into the synaptic gap to act on a specific neurotransmitter receptor. They can bind only to this specific receptor, and their effect is determined by this receptor. Several types of neurotransmitters cause either excitement or inhibitory impulses. For example, glutamate is the most important excitatory neurotransmitter in the brain, whereas gamma-aminobutyric acid (GABA) and glycine are inhibitory ones. However, we will focus on serotonin and dopamine, because they are the most investigated of the neurotransmitters in our subject area. They cover the brain activities of both those who are involved in religious practices and those involved in spiritual activities.

2.1. Serotonin or 5-hydroxytryptamine (5-HT)

If both sympathetic (norepinephrine, adrenaline) and parasympathetic (acetylcholine) systems have been shown to be stimulated in meditation and other related experiences (see below), serotonin (5-HT) and to a lesser degree dopamine have been the focus of geneticists and neuroscientists. The involvement of the 5-HT system in spiritual-like experiences is supported by observations that drugs (LSD, psilocybin) can induce spiritual experiences. These drugs are known to perturb the 5-HT system in several brain regions. They produce perceptual distortions, illusions and hallucinations, and sometimes a sense of insight and spiritual awareness, mystical experiences, and religious ecstasy. These effects can resemble the perceptions and ideation described by subjects who have experienced spirituality. Some benefits or "side effects" of praying and meditation on psychiatric disorders could be explained by a modulation of this neurotransmitter (see below).

Although 5-HT can be found mainly in the gastrointestinal tract, 5-HT is also a monoamine that serves as a neurotransmitter in the brain. Serotonergic neurons that synthesize 5-HT are located in the brainstem in an area called the raphe nuclei. Their axons project in many areas of the brain, notably the cerebral cortex, hypothalamus, limbic system, and the striatum. These neurons modulate the activity of several brain regions by their inhibitory or excitatory action on brain receptor subtypes. In addition, 5-HT is believed to play an important role in several psychiatric conditions including depressive disorders, anxiety disorders, suicidal behaviors, aggression and anger-related traits, and even schizophrenia and similar disorders. Particularly, low levels of 5-HT have been associated with aggression, violent behavior, suicidal tendency, and clinical depression in human studies. As we will discuss below, 5-HT has also been directly implicated in meditation and religious experiences.

2.2. Dopamine

Dopamine is produced in several areas of the brain. It is the primary neurotransmitter involved in the reward pathways and is commonly associated with the pleasure system of the brain. Drugs that increase dopamine signaling (like cocaine), particularly in the nucleus accumbens, may produce euphoric effects. Psychostimulants, such as amphetamine and cocaine, induce dramatic changes in dopamine signaling; large doses and prolonged use can induce symptoms that resemble schizophrenia. Moreover, in the mesolimbic pathway, dopamine increases arousal and goal-directed behaviors.

Given its importance in many personality traits or dimensions such as anger-related traits (1) and the main role of this neurotransmitter in the function of the frontal lobes, dopamine has also been investigated in spirituality. Moreover, from a psychiatric point of view, perturbation of dopaminergic systems has been suggested in psychiatric disorders including schizophrenia, Parkinson's disease, and drug and alcohol dependence. Of note, dopaminergic neurons are also under the control of the 5-HT system.

3. NEUROBIOLOGICAL BASIS OF MEDITATION AND SPIRITUAL EXPERIENCES: ANATOMICAL PATHWAYS AND STRUCTURES

Many of the major sources concerning the neuroanatomy of spirituality in humans are studies that measure brain activity during deep religious or transcendental practices such as meditation. For instance, the neuroscientist Andrew Newberg studied the brain functions of subjects as they were meditating or praying using several imaging techniques.(2–4) Based on neuroimaging, neurochemical, hormonal, and physiological studies, he examined several types of spiritual experiences and practices. He proposed that mystical and meditative experiences are measurable processes, and could be described a complex anatomical pathway that he implicated in spiritual and meditative experiences. Newberg found several regions and pathways involved in meditative actions (defined as a specific state characterized by sustained attention, focus on an object, a change in the body's spatial orientation and deafferentation, arousal, emotion, and relaxation). Some key cognitive functions such as abstraction of generals from particulars were, from his point of view, crucial in the experience of meditation and spiritual experiences. As a result, Newberg stated, "These functions allow us to automatically generate a causative construct such as spirits, god or power when no 'observational or scientific' causal explanation is found." He suggested that construction of myths, spiritual powers, or gods is the only choice human beings have to explain their world or understand their environment when no other explanation exists.

3.1. Frontal Lobe, Limbic System, and Parietal Lobe

The frontal lobe is one of the regions that has been most implicated in religious activity.(5) Newberg (2–4) focused on the prefrontal cortex and its connections with the thalamus, posterior superior parietal lobe, and limbic system (mainly the amygdala and hippocampus). By measuring

cerebral blood flow, he determined that the deeper people descend into meditation or prayer, the more active the frontal lobe and the limbic system become. His observation was consistent with other studies that found a higher activity of the frontal lobe during meditation or religious recitation.(6–9) The frontal lobe is the seat of concentration and attention; the limbic system is where feelings, emotions, and behavioral emotional states such as ecstasy are processed. Interestingly, it seems that, at the same time the frontal lobe and the limbic system are activated, the parietal lobe, which is responsible for temporal-spatial orientation, becomes less activated. (2, 6, 10, 11) Taken all together, these findings give us a nice picture of a profound meditative practice.

3.2. The Temporal Lobe

To a lesser extent, the medial temporal lobe has also been involved in religious activity, and individuals who were more spiritual have reported stronger beliefs in paranormal phenomena. (12–15) These studies were in agreement with four other studies (measuring brain activity either by topographical electroencephalogram, cerebral blood flow, or cerebral metabolism) that found an activation of the temporal lobe during religious practice.(6, 11, 16, 17) The medial temporal lobe comprises the hippocampus, which seems to be particularly important for memory function and is also part of the limbic system.

3.3. Autonomic Nervous System and Other Related Systems

Systems such as the autonomic nervous system (sympathetic and parasympathetic systems) were also found to go through a significant change in terms of activity during meditation and spiritual experiences.(18) Activation of the autonomic system creates a reduction in heart and respiratory rates, which in turn brings about a sense of relaxation. Although there have been many studies on the effect of religious and spiritual activity on the parasympathetic and sympathetic systems, it is not clear if both systems are affected equally or not.

It has also been proposed that the activation of the autonomic nervous system has an impact directly on the 5-HT level in the brain as demonstrated by higher urinary excretion of metabolites of 5-HT during meditation.(19) This observation could be linked to a higher level of 5-HT during these practices. However, in other studies it appears that inhibition of 5-HT activity or at least 5-HT deficiency is associated with spirituality and religious beliefs and practices.(20, 21) Noradrenalin is also involved in such experiences and is highlighted by a decrease in stimulation of the locus coeruleus, which produces and distributes the noradrenalin throughout the brain.(22)

Some studies also found increased activity in serum GABA (the main inhibitory neurotransmitter in the brain) during meditation. This possibly reflects increased GABA activity in the brain linked to the deafferentation observed during meditation practice.(23) Finally, still other neurotransmitters have been shown to be involved during meditation, such as dopamine or glutamate.(22, 24) For example, Kjear et al.,(24) in a functional imaging study, found an activation of the dopaminergic receptors in the striatum during meditation, which reflected a much higher level of dopamine in this region. However, a clear picture does not seem to emerge from all these studies. Meditation and its related practices are probably too complex to be simply explained by the way neurotransmitters perform and change in the brain. Probably the main and most consistent findings in all the above studies are the increased activation of prefrontal temporal cortices and the limbic systems during meditation or religious experiences (versus parietal or occipital lobes). This should also be the easiest way to understand the possible link between psychiatry and spiritual experiences.

3.4. Meditation, Spiritual Experiences, and Psychiatry

Many studies have shown an association between aggressive behavior and frontal lobe brain damages.(25) Moreover, individuals showing a very high degree of aggression display low baseline activity in their frontal cortex.(26, 27) It is postulated that the frontal cortex provides inhibitory input to the circuits in the thalamus and amygdale that promote aggression.(28) Thus, higher activity in the frontal cortex is linked to reduced aggression. This observation is of particular interest in the possible link between religious practices such as meditation and psychiatric disorders.

It has also been shown that prayer and meditation can improve both physical and psychological states.(29) Recently Mohr et al.(30) found that religious practice was significantly correlated with better coping among schizophrenic subjects. This information may be useful for clinicians in psychiatric practice. In a recent study, Borras et al.(31) found that two-thirds of schizophrenic patients considered spirituality very important or essential in everyday life. They concluded that religion and spirituality contributed to the way their illness manifested itself and patients' attitude toward treatment. In another study, it was found that religion may play a protective role against suicide attempts among patients with schizophrenia and schizoaffective disorder.(32) These results could be linked to a reduced aggressiveness possibly associated with religious practice. This reduced aggressiveness may be caused by activation of the frontal lobe during religious practice. By helping individuals to meditate and so to increase the activity of their frontal lobe, we may reduce the risk or magnitude of aggressive behavior such as suicide attempts.

Of note, numerous studies have demonstrated that reduced levels of impulsivity and aggressiveness are associated with higher levels of 5-HT.(33) This observation could also be linked to the above-mentioned findings of higher levels of serotonin during meditation. If this were the case, spiritual practice (meditation or intense praying) could act as a selective-serotonergic antidepressant. The latter acts on a specific transporter (see below) in the brain to enhance the level of 5-HT. This not only can treat depressive disorders but also reduce aggressiveness. But serotonergic antidepressants are also known, because of their action on 5-HT levels and secondarily on dopamine systems, to enhance psychotic symptoms in schizophrenic patients. Does the intensive practice of meditation have the same effect on schizophrenic patients? This issue requires clarification, and further research is needed before encouraging patients to perform such practices.

Finally, as discussed above, other neurotransmitters have been involved in spiritual experiences, and most of them have been implicated in different psychiatric disorders or endophenotypes (see below) such as those associated with aggressiveness or suicidal behavior. We will here mention, for example, that dopamine and noradrenalin have been involved in aggression. It seems that blocking D2 receptors (for example, with risperidone, an antipsychotic used to treat schizophrenia) can reduce aggression. In the same way, noradrenalin by enhancing arousal seems to be linked to aggression. The reports of elevated dopamine levels during meditation or religious trances (22, 24) could also be linked to the dopaminergic hypothesis of schizophrenia. This hypothesis suggests that schizophrenia is the result of overactivity or at least disturbed regulation of dopamine in the frontal lobe. The observed increase of dopamine during religious activities may have a deleterious effect on these subjects, because it may highlight or enhance psychotic relapses.

What is really the link between religious practices and psychiatric disorders from the neuropsychiatric point of view is not very clear. It seems that, on one hand, it can reduce aggression. On the other hand, it can, as a side effect, enhance psychotic features in schizophrenic patients. Clinicians should consider this issue and always discuss with their patients their religious practices. It is important to know not only if they are believers, but also the intensity of their religious feelings.

4. GENES, PERSONALITY, AND SPIRITUALITY

God, spiritual powers, or spirits are concepts we can find all around the world in human culture.

This is a strong indication that this concept is somehow preloaded in the human genome. Within the neuroscience and evolutionary perspective, a provocative question can be raised: Were human beings inspired by gods, spirits, or messages sent from above to create religion or did evolution bring about a sense of spirituality or religiosity to bring together people in communities and societies to help the evolution of the species? If the second answer is the right one, there might be a genetic background behind this behavior. In other words, is it possible to find genes for spirituality in humans, because genetic selection will have chosen individuals with higher beliefs to hold groups together? Is it nature or nurture that makes some people more spiritual than others?

4.1. Spirituality as a Personality Trait or Endophenotype

The first step in genetic studies is to find intermediate traits called endophenotypes. An endophenotype is an intermediary measure between a gene-effect and a disorder. Endophenotypes are thought to be more influenced by genes than would be a complex disorder. For example, in the path leading from genes to schizophrenia, one could look at the association between one given gene and paranoid delusions, auditory hallucinations, or aggressiveness, which are all connected to endophenotypes. The association between DNA variants and psychological phenotypes give us the potential to find more easily which genes influence heritable psychological traits such as personality. For instance, in the path between genes and spirituality or religiousness, investigators focused on personality dimensions.

Classic genetic analysis emphasizes mendelian traits. In mendelian diseases, such as cystic fibrosis, there is a strong correlation between the genotype someone carries and his or her phenotype/disease. In other words, a single gene is responsible for that condition within a family. But most behavioral traits are multigenic; it means that they are determined by several genes interacting together and with environmental factors. In contrast to single-locus mendelian traits, multigenic traits do not have a simple recognizable pattern of inheritance, and thus the relative contributions of several genes to one trait are difficult to analyze. Nevertheless, determining which genes contribute to complex human traits has profound implications for the care and treatment of human diseases.

Convincing evidence shows that psychological traits, including spirituality, are stable in time and influenced by genetic factors to a significant degree. Indeed, several family, twin, and adoption studies have shown that genetic factors underlie at least some individual differences in personality traits. This heritability is estimated to be around 40 to 60 percent.(29, 34, 35) Most of these reports also suggested that genetic variation could contribute to as much as 40 to 50 percent of the individual variation in terms of a person's religiosity. Based on this assumption, some researchers focused their analyses on genes and genetic polymorphisms mainly related to 5-HT and dopaminergic systems. They postulate that religious belief could be genetically driven and consider spirituality as a personality component. Of note and contrary to spirituality, genetic analyses indicate that religious affiliation is primarily a culturally transmitted phenomenon.(34) In the same way, how faithfully an individual practices any religion (rituals such as attending services or the degree to which he observes it) is dependent more on environmental factors.

Of particular interest is Cloninger's description of personality.(36, 37) Using the Temperamental and Character Inventory (TCI), he described the main temperamental dimensions associated with human behavior. From his point of view, differences in temperament are thought to be associated with activity in specific central neurotransmitter systems. Among these, the self-transcendence scale encompasses several aspects of religious behavior, subjective experience, and the way an individual perceives the world. It has been found to be an important correlate with an individual's sense of coherence, self-esteem, hope, and emotional well-being in adults. It is considered as the most stable TCI

dimension over time. *Self-transcendence* consists of three subscales: spiritual acceptance, transpersonal identification, and self-forgetfulness. High scorers on *spiritual acceptance* (or openness to things not literally provable) endorse extrasensory perception and ideation, whether it has to do with named deities or a common unifying force. Low scorers, by contrast, tend to favor a reductionistic and empirical worldview. *Transpersonal identification* has to do with a tendency to feel connected to a larger universe, whereas *self-forgetfulness* refers to the ability to get entirely lost in an experience. Geneticists and neuropsychiatrists were therefore highly interested in this personality trait and tried to understand it either from a genetic point of view or from a biological one. In the next part, we briefly look at what a neurotransmitter receptor is and then focus on the 5-HT receptor and studies done with spirituality traits. Then we will turn to the genetic aspect of the link between genes and spirituality.

4.2. Neurotransmitter Receptor

A neurotransmitter receptor is a protein on the cell membrane that binds to a specific neurotransmitter and initiates the cellular response. There are a thousand different receptors in the human brain, each specific for one neurotransmitter: 5-HT, dopamine, cannabinoids, norepinephrine, and so on. For example, more than five different receptors have been discovered for dopamine: dopamine receptor 1 (DRD1), dopamine receptor 2 (DRD2), and others. Neurotransmitter receptors can be localized either postsynaptically, where their action is the recognition of specific neurotransmitters and the activation of effectors within the cell to give a specific message, or presynaptically, where they act as autoreceptors to modulate the firing of the neuron, either inhibiting or exciting it.

4.2.1. The Serotonin Receptor 1A (5-HT1A)

As for dopamine receptors, several 5-HT receptor subtypes have been identified in the brain. Among them, the 5-HT1A receptor has been the most studied. These receptors are located both post- and presynaptically. Presynaptic 5-HT1A autoreceptors are highly concentrated on cell bodies in the raphe and modulate the cell firing and release of several neurotransmitters in all brain areas. Thus, the 5-HT1A receptor may have a role as general regulator of neurotransmitter activity such as 5-HT and dopamine.

In a recent positron emission tomography (PET) study, Borg et al.(20) found an association between 5-HT1A receptor binding potential and self-transcendence scores (a personality trait associated with spirituality, see previously) in healthy, male subjects. This association, however, depended completely on the subscale spiritual acceptance, which measures an individual's apprehension of phenomena that cannot be explained by objective demonstration. Whether the low 5-HT1A receptor density observed in subjects scoring high on a measure of spirituality reflects low or high activity in 5-HT cortical projection areas is not clear, and literature provides support for both interpretations. Interestingly, several studies have found an abnormal density of brain and platelet 5-HT2A and 5-HT1A receptors in subjects suffering from some psychiatric disorders. For example, it has been proposed that 5-HT receptors may be up-regulated in depressive disorder or in subjects displaying suicidal behaviors as a compensatory response to chronic low levels of 5-HT.(38) Following this hypothesis, low 5-HT1A receptor density should reflect higher 5-HT activity in the brain of subjects with high spirituality or at least a high efficiency of the 5-HT system. The results could be linked to the observed higher activity of 5-HT system during meditation and related experiences. These findings could have important implications for the pathophysiology of many psychiatric disorders and the role of spirituality in these conditions. However, it also has to be stated that lower 5-HT1A receptor density has been linked to greater anxiety and chronic stress. The findings of Borg et al. are therefore also consistent with the notion that those who are more spiritual are biologically more prone to anxiety.(39, 40) Understanding the complex link

between spirituality, the 5-HT system, environmental factors, and symptoms such as psychotic features could help to find new ways to reduce the morbidity associated with several neuropsychiatric conditions. For example, activation of 5-HT1A receptors (by eltoprazine and other 5-HT1A-receptor agonists) reduces aggressive behavior.(41) Globally this observation adds to the possible effect of religious practice on aggression. This should be taken into account in clinical practice.

4.3. A Genetic Polymorphism

A polymorphism is a genetic variant that appears in at least 1 percent of a population, but in genetics, the term is reserved for variation in a population's DNA. Genetic polymorphisms provide us with the possibility to predict interindividual differences in susceptibility to clinical disease. There are several different types of polymorphisms. The single nucleotide polymorphism (SNP) refers to a variation of a single nucleotide (A, T, C, or G) within the DNA sequence between members of a species. For example, the following two DNA sequences from different individuals, ATTAGCC and ATCAGCC, differed by a single nucleotide, a C allele in place of a T allele. The other polymorphism we shall consider is the insertion-deletion polymorphism. An insertion-deletion polymorphism is an insertion or deletion of a part of the DNA that is found in some people but not in others. The sequence with the insertion is normally called the long allele, whereas the one with the deletion is called the short allele. Finally, short tandem repeat polymorphisms and/or variable numbers of tandem polymorphisms (VNTR) are short sequences of DNA that are repeated numerous times in a gene.

Polymorphisms may fall either within a coding region or in a non-coding region. In the same way they can change the amino acid sequence of the protein. However, even if these polymorphisms are located in a non-coding region or don't change the amino acid sequence, they could still have great impact on the expression of the protein. Given that, these variations in the DNA sequences can affect a number of diseases.

4.3.1. Insertion-Deletion in the Promoter Region of the Serotonin Transporter Gene (5-HTTLPR)

One important target of antidepressants, namely selective serotonin reuptake inhibitors (SSRIs), is the 5-HT transporter (5-HTT). It has therefore widely been studied in depressive disorders but also more broadly in several psychiatric conditions. Like many other neurotransmitters, 5-HT is removed from the synaptic cleft by neurotransmitter transporters in a process called *reuptake*. During the reuptake process, 5-HT is taken back into the axon terminal that released it so it cannot bind to its receptors. This reuptake is performed by the 5-HTT.

A forty-four-base pair (bp) insertion-deletion in the promoter region (a regulatory region of DNA located upstream from a gene, providing a control point for regulated gene transcription) of the 5-HTT gene (5-HTTLPR) has been described and shown to be functional (the short allele is associated with reduced expression of the 5-HT transporter and lower 5-HT reuptake activity). Nilsson et al. recently found that homozygosity for the long 5-HTTLPR allele was associated with high scores of spiritual acceptance. The associations, however, were only found in boys.(42) Interestingly, the long allele has been negatively associated with depression, anger- and aggression-related traits, suicidal behavior, and other psychiatric conditions. Furthermore, homozygosity for the long 5-HTT allele has been associated with high CSF levels of the 5-HT metabolite 5-HIAA in nonhuman primates.(43) This result adds weight to the hypothesis of a higher activity of the 5-HT system in spirituality. Interestingly, it has been recently shown that 5-HTTLPR modulates the effect of stressful life events in several psychiatric outcomes.(44) This polymorphism has also been found to modulate the neuronal activity of the amygdala in response to fearful stimuli in humans.(45) Indeed, homozygosity for the long allele of the 5-HTTLPR has been associated with a decreased amygdala reactivity and high capability to process environmental threat and to adaptively cope with persistent stress. The Nilsson et al. findings, therefore, suggest a better function of the 5-HT system in individuals with high spirituality. Given the role of this polymorphism and more generally of 5-HT in religiosity and spirituality, it could be interesting to further investigate genes involved in 5-HT systems and religious behaviors. Why this association was observed only in boys remains a question to be debated. It reminds us of the association between 5-HT1A binding potentials and spiritual acceptance that was carried in male subjects only. Gender differences in religious behavior have been reported in the literature.(46) Taken together, these results indicate that other uninvestigated variables such as environmental or hormonal factors could govern the phenotypic expression of spirituality differently among men and women. For instance, it has been recently found that the estrogen receptor alpha gene may influence various aspects of personality in women.(47)

Interestingly, Bachner-Melman et al.,(48) in an intriguing study analyzing genetic background of dancers, found that the 5-HTTLPR gene was associated with spiritual facets of creative dance. They found that dancers carrying the short allele of 5-HTTLPR scored high on the Tellegen Absorption Scale, a questionnaire that correlates positively with spirituality and altered states of consciousness. They unfortunately do not discuss why the short allele was linked to this scale. It is not unusual to see discrepant genetic associations with any one given trait in genetic studies. They mainly reflect some undetected bias such as ethnicity or gender. Nevertheless, these results, as well as those from Nilsson et al., suggest an involvement of the 5-HT system in manifestation of spirituality.

4.3.2. Single Nucleotide Polymorphisms in the 5-HT Receptors and Spirituality

Borg et al.(20) identified, as mentioned above, a relationship between self-transcendence and 5-HT1A receptor binding potential. Some investigators were therefore interested in single nucleotide polymorphism (SNP) within the gene's coding for 5-HT receptors. These authors reported associations of genotypes of the 5-HT1A receptor and the 5-HT2A and 5-HT6 receptors with self-transcendence. A functional variant in the promoter region of the gene coding for the 5-HT1A receptor has been reported. It is a C to G substitution, which was demonstrated to be involved in modulating the rate of transcription of the 5-HT1A gene.(49) The 5-HT1A G variant is supposed to result in an enhanced 5-HT1A auto-receptor expression, whereas the C variant results in a lowered 5-HT1A receptor expression and in consecutive enhanced 5-HT activity. Lorenzi et al. (50) found that individuals with two copies of the C allele had lower self-transcendence scores than carriers of the G allele. Their results support the involvement of 5-HT1A receptors in human spiritual implications. However, Borg et al. found lower 5-HT1A receptor binding potentials in subjects with high self-transcendence scores. Based on that finding and due to a lower 5-HT1A receptor density, they suggested that high self-transcendence scores were possibly linked to high 5-HT release. Given this hypothesis and the functionality of the 5-HT1A polymorphism, the C variant should normally have been found to be associated with high self-transcendence scores. These conflicting results are difficult to explain and several reasons could be given. We refer to the explanations given by Lorenzi et al. in their article. We will just say that the path between a given SNP in a gene and a given phenotype such as the 5-HT1A receptor density in the human brain is far more complex than in animal or laboratory studies. A polymorphism that is supposed to enhance 5-HT1A expression in cell culture could have totally different implications in the human beings. As highlighted by Lorenzi et al., "Molecular genetic studies cannot cover and explain subsequent biological, developmental, and environmental modulating process, which ultimately produce a definite phenotype." Nevertheless, taken together these results provide further evidence of the involvement of serotoninergic system in the self-transcendence character trait. Interestingly abnormal 5-HT1A receptor signaling in brains of psychiatric subjects including depressive subjects and suicide victims and/ or attempters has been found.(51) The functional 5-HT1A C-1019G (rs6295) variant in the promoter region of the gene has been associated with major

depression, anxiety-related traits, and suicide.(30) More broadly, 5-HT receptors haven been implicated in a large range of psychiatric conditions. Given the implication of 5-HT receptors in spirituality, researchers should try to better understand the complex links between spirituality and psychiatric conditions, not only from the clinical point of view, but also from the genetic perspective.

The function of the 5-HT6 receptor is not well understood. It is abundant in the limbic system and thus should have some involvement in mood disorders and personality traits. Ham et al.(52) studied two other polymorphisms: one in the gene coding for the 5-HT6 gene, a silent polymorphism that consists of a T to C substitution (C267T), and another functional one located in the promoter region of the 5-HT2A gene, the A-1438G. In a Korean sample, they found that subjects heterozygous for the A-1438G polymorphism of the 5-HT2A receptor and/or those carrying a C allele of the C267T scored significantly lower on the self-transcendence scale. Of note, the A allele of the A-1438G polymorphism has been associated with suicide and impulsive traits.

Interestingly, the psychotropic effects of LSD are attributed to its strong partial agonist on 5-HT2A receptors. Given the mystic-like experiences obtained when taking this drug and the implication of 5HT2A receptors in spirituality, a relative hyperactivity of the 5-HT system should be suspected.

4.3.3. Other Polymorphisms Associated with Measures of Spirituality: The Dopamine Transporter and the Activating Protein-2 (AP-2)

4.3.3.1. Dopamine receptors

Dopamine receptors are distributed throughout the central nervous system and are involved in many processes such as motor control, learning, pleasure, motivational behavior, and reward seeking. As mentioned above with 5-HT receptors, there is more than one dopamine receptor, and dopamine receptors are also located in pre- and postsynaptic levels. DR2 are, for instance, the target of antipsychotics.

4.3.3.1.1. Polymorphisms in the Dopamine Receptor 4 gene (DRD4)

The gene coding for the Dopamine Receptor 4 (DRD4) is highly polymorphic, although most of the research in psychiatry and personality focused largely on a variable number of tandem (VNTR) polymorphisms in exon 3. These polymorphisms have been shown to be functional. (53) Following the Cloninger hypothesis, which suggested an involvement of dopaminergic systems in some dimensions of personality,(36, 37, 54) Commings et al.(55, 56) were intrigued by the considerable role of dopamine genes, and the DRD4 gene in particular, in spiritual transcendence. As already said, dopamine receptors, and especially DRD4, play an important role in the function of the prefrontal cortex. The DRD4 gene is indeed expressed in a high level in the frontal area and the nucleus acumbens,(57–59) regions associated with affective and emotional behaviors.(57) Because spirituality may especially use the prefrontal cortex, it should use dopaminergic systems. From this perspective, Coming et al.,(55, 56) in two consecutive studies investigating several polymorphisms (including the VNTR) in the DRD4 gene, found a significant relationship between spiritual transcendence and DRD4 receptor polymorphisms. At a lesser level, Comings et al. also found other dopamine receptors to be associated with spiritual transcendence. Their results suggest an involvement of DRD4 in the personality trait of spiritual acceptance. Their authors concluded that this may be a function of the high concentration of the dopamine D4 receptor in the cortical areas, especially the frontal cortex. Dopamine is thought to increase creative drive of idea generation. This involvement in creativity could be linked to spirituality. Indeed, as previously mentioned, creative dance correlated positively with spirituality and altered states of consciousness. So better dopaminergic tone in people carrying particular genotypes of the DRD4 gene could lead people to seek spirituality and religious practices to give them pleasure or euphoria through higher effectiveness of DRD4 receptors and also because these practices have been shown to enhance dopamine levels

(see upstream). It has effectively been argued that the activation of the dopaminergic system during meditation and other religious activities may be related to the seeking of these activities.(4)

However, the link with spirituality is far more complex than this single association would tell us, because it has been shown that the dopaminergic system is under the control of 5-HT1. Indeed, stimulation of 5-HT2A and 5-HT1A receptors – half of the dopaminergic neurons in the medial prefrontal cortex (mPFC) express 5-HT2A receptors – can elicit dopamine release.(60, 61)

4.3.3.1.2. Activating protein-2 (AP-2)

Transcription factor AP-2 (activating protein-2 [AP-2]) is a specific DNA-binding transcription factor family. In one sense, it participates in and regulates specific neural gene expression and has been shown to be involved in neural survival, death, and development.(62, 63) In particular, gene coding for dopamine transporter and 5-HTT displays multiple AP-2 binding sites in their regulatory regions. It has been proposed that AP-2, by its regulation of monoaminergic genes (dopamine and 5-HT), could affect the release and metabolism of 5-HT and dopamine in the frontal cortex. Because dopamine receptors and 5-HTT have been implicated in personality traits and spirituality, one might speculate AP-2 could interactively influence these traits.

Different isoforms of the AP-2 family have been identified, including the AP-2β. One polymorphism of interest for spirituality in the gene coding for the transcription factor AP-2β is a four base-pair repeat polymorphism in the second intron (CAAA,) which has been associated with anxiety, binge-eating disorder, and levels of homovanillic acid. Homovanillic acid is a metabolite of major catecholamines like dopamine. Nilsson et al.,(42) in the same paper investigating 5-HTTLPR, found a significant association between this repeat polymorphism and Self-Transcendence. Again and as observed for 5-HTTLPR, this association was observed only in boys and showed that carriers of the short allele (less repeat) had higher self-transcendence scores. Interestingly, this observation was also completely explained by the subscale spiritual acceptance. However, in girls and not in boys, they found an interactive effect of the genotypes for 5-HTTLPR and AP-2β. Indeed the presence of the LL genotype of 5-HTTLPR and the short allele of the AP-2β polymorphism resulted in low scores in self-transcendence whereas high scores were associated with a short allele of 5-HT-TLPR and a short AP-2β allele. The inverse pattern was observed for the homozygous of the long allele of the AP-2β.

AP-2 and other transcription factors regulate the expression of a number of monoamine neurons during development and also a variety of candidate genes involved in psychiatric disorders. These transcription factors are therefore good candidates for explaining interindividual differences in temperament and psychiatric vulnerability. For instance, it has been proposed that homozygosity for the long AP-2β allele could be associated with low central 5-HT activity. In other words, the results of Nilsson et al. suggested that low self-transcendence/spiritual acceptance are linked to low central 5-HT activity through the AP-2β genotype. This hypothesis is concordant with the above results showing not only an involvement of 5-HT in spirituality but also the higher activity of 5-HT system during meditations and related experiences.

4.3.3.1.3. The cytochrome P450 2C19 (CYP2C19) polymorphism

The gene coding for the CYP2C19 enzyme mainly involved in the metabolism of sex hormones is also highly polymorphic. Of interest in our subject, this enzyme has been implicated in multiple brain functions and also catalyzes the metabolism of 5-HT.(64) One study in a Japanese sample (65) found that in females, scores of self-transcendence were lower in those considered as poor metabolizers (given their genotype) than those considered as extensive metabolizers. Because these results were based on women only, we may assume an involvement of sex hormones, and especially, a higher testosterone concentration.

Considering the progress in gene-environment interaction studies and its effect on complex traits

such as spirituality, it would be of interest to take into account environmental factors in further genetic studies on spiritual traits. The importance of gene-environment interactions in research and especially in psychiatric research will be discussed below.

5. GENE-ENVIRONMENT INTERACTION AND CORRELATION

5.1. Gene-Environment Interaction

Recently, research has paid attention to the gene-environment interaction as a new and different comprehensive model of psychiatric disorders. (66) Classical approaches in genetic psychiatric research assume a direct path between genes and behavior. The goal of this approach is to associate psychiatric disorders or intermediate phenotypes (or endophenotypes such as spiritual transcendence) with individual differences in DNA sequences. However, many studies have failed to replicate previous findings, and because of inconsistent findings, many scientists have abandoned this approach. A recent and promising approach is the understanding of complex disease and personality traits through the gene-environment interaction approach, or GxE. GxE typically occurs when the effects of one given environmental factor on one individual is dependant on his or her genotype background. For example, exposure to cannabis is a well-known environmental pathogen that elicits the development of schizophrenia. However, not all individuals smoking cannabis will develop schizophrenia, only those who have a genetic vulnerability will. Another classical illustration of GxE is the phenylketonuria. Children with two abnormal copies of the gene that codes for phenylanaline hydroxylase, a key enzyme that converts the amino acid phenylanaline to another amino acid thyrosine, express the disease. Accumulation of phenylanaline in the blood of children who lack both functional copies of the gene leads to abnormal development of the brain and mental retardation. However, a simple reduction of phenylanaline intake by a restricting regimen completely prevents the mental retardation. Phenylketonuria is a particularly clear example of GxE. The environmental factor (diet) is necessary for the expression of the disease. In contrast to the main-effects studies, GxE studies do not necessarily expect an association between gene and behavior/disorder in the absence of an environmental factor.

Measures of spirituality and religiousness are typical examples of complex traits that could be understood by GxE studies. As with complex diseases, the absence of perfect concordance in monozygotic twin studies indicates a nongenetic contribution to spirituality. Moreover, from the previous findings (see above), environmental factors such as hormonal levels (as a reflection of gender effect), diet, drugs, region of origin, and so on seem to play a key role in the comprehension of this trait.

A great deal has been learned about the role of genetic influences on personality in recent years, but this has raised many additional questions, including those concerning the influence of environmental factors and the nature of their interaction in spirituality. How environmental factors, such as diet, drugs, hormonal levels, and parental care, and developmental adversities, such as childhood trauma or stressful life events, interact with genes to modulate measures of spirituality should be a subject for further research.

5.2. Gene-Environment Correlation

Following recent findings of genetic sensitivity to environmental factors, most studies investigating gene-environment interplay focused on GxE. However, few of them were interested in gene-environment correlation (rGE) or even tried to identify one in their samples. rGE typically reflects genetic differences in exposure to particular environments. As mentioned above, GxE refers to the influence of environment on the expression of one given gene. rGE, in contrast, refers to the genetic influences on environmental exposure. As early as the 1960s, personality researchers discussed the role of the person in producing her or his environment.(67) The person's behavior was not seen as a consequence of solely situational contexts. In their view, it was suggested that people's personalities influence the way others respond to them and, in this way, influence the choice of how, where, and with whom they were going to interact. As previously discussed, and based on several studies showing the importance of the genetic component on individual differences in personality, we suggest that the genetically driven way an individual is going to behave will influence this individual's exposure to a particular environment. In the end, such interactions between gene and environmental influences could make certain environmental influences heritable. This is referred to as rGE.(68)

If we take the example of spirituality, there are three different types of rGE.

5.2.1. The Passive rGE

Passive rGE refers to the interaction between the environment in which a child is raised and the genes he inherits from his parents. For example, a child carrying a gene susceptible to spirituality may grow in a family with high spirituality, which will in turn elicit the expression of genes of spirituality in that child. Because parents who show a sense of spirituality (which has been shown to be heritable, see above) tend to elicit spirituality in their children, a highly religious environment might be a marker for the genetic vulnerability parents transmitted to their child rather than a causal risk factor for child spirituality.

5.2.2. The Evocative rGE

Evocative rGE refers to the association between the individual's genetically influenced behavior and the reaction of others to that individual's behavior. For example, an individual who is genetically driven to behave in a spiritual way will attract the attention of other like-minded people. The latter will then bring him into a spiritual environment.

For example, one can find that good coping among schizophrenic subjects is the result of an interaction between a genetic polymorphism and a religious environment. This interaction could be, in fact, the reflection of a hidden evocative rGE. In the latter, a schizophrenic subject may, by his behavior, elicit a spiritual environment because of his or her particular genotype. This in turn will enable the individual to cope better.

5.2.3. The Active rGE

Active rGE refers to the association between an individual's genetically influenced traits and the environmental niches selected by this individual. For example, individuals who are highly spiritual may seek out religious community to express their spirituality. Here the individual, because of his genetic background, will *actively* seek an environment that will enhance the expression of his genes. Contrary to the latter, with the evocative rGE, the individual will be "discovered" by those around him.

All these examples illustrate how, in some cases, a genetic effect can be detected or have a different impact on a trait only when an environmental variable is taken into account. The major question in studies dealing with spirituality is this: Which environmental factor should one study in relation to this trait? Personality seems to be influenced by parenting style. The intensity of parental care or the intrusiveness of parents should probably be important environmental candidates. Other environmental factors are presupposed. It has been found that religiousness has a large shared environmental component (that is, environmental factors shared by close relatives), especially in childhood and adolescence. For example, heritability factors for religiousness may have less influence in childhood than in adulthood, showing that age is an environmental moderator of the heritability and should be taken into account.(35) As mentioned above, hormonal levels (partially under genetic control also), ethnicity, and drugs are also putative environmental factors.

The demonstration that early environmental factors could considerably strengthen or even highlight associations between genes and personality is a promising new area of research in complex behavior. The publication by Caspi and his co-workers (66) showed what was widely hypothesized but rarely demonstrated. This important work stated that both nature and nurture contribute to the shaping of behavior. Many studies have since

tried to find such interaction in psychiatry. For example, it has been shown that individuals sexually abused in their childhood displayed higher risk of making a violent suicide attempt only if they were carrying a particular genotype.(69) Such studies should be promising in the understanding of spirituality. However, human personality and spirituality are complex traits and require a more encompassing view to understand their genetic and molecular architecture.

5.3. Religious Activity as an Environmental Factor?

Contrary to spirituality, religious activities, which are supposedly less heritable and so less under the influence of genes, could be seen as environmental factors. Given the impact of meditation on 5-HT, dopamine levels, and the functioning of the brain, it would be surprising if religious activities did not have an impact on the gene expression. Within this perspective, Timberlake et al.(70) investigated the moderating effects of three styles of religiosity (religious affiliation, organizational religious activity, and self-rated religiousness) on the genetic and environmental determinants of smoking initiation. They found that self-rated religiousness moderated genetic influences on the likelihood for smoking. This kind of study could also have a huge impact on psychiatric disorders. If we consider religious practice as an environmental factor, it would be interesting to know, based on an individual's genotype, which individual is susceptible to respond favorably and which is not.

6. CONCLUSION

The results from the present review might suggest that a high degree of spirituality is linked to 5-HT and dopaminergic systems. In the initial Cloninger hypothesis, it was proposed that different personality traits were influenced by genes related to 5-HT, and dopaminergic and noradrenalin-related genes. The above studies of 5-HT and dopaminergic genes suggest higher levels of activity in both systems, not only in individuals with a

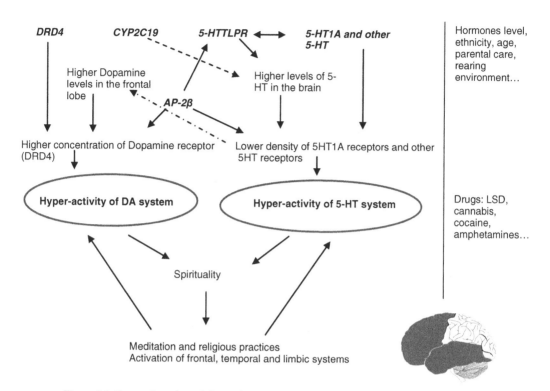

Figure 5.1. Serotoninergic and dopaminergic systems in spirituality and religious practices.

high sense of spirituality but also during religious activities such as meditation. It can be speculated that, during the development of the midbrain neurotransmitter systems, early genetically driven modulation of the 5-HT and dopamine systems participate in the formation of spirituality in adults. We can now try to draw a biological picture of spirituality and religious practices (Figure 5.1). In this model, individuals carrying particular genetic polymorphisms within 5-HTT, DRD4, CYP2C19, 5-HT1A, 5-HT2A, 5-HT6, and AP-2B genes (either directly or interacting together) will have, through different pathways, a relatively higher level of 5-HT and dopamine in specific areas of their brain. As a secondary side effect, this will enhance the sense of spirituality in individuals and possibly religious practices. To be complete, this model should also include environmental factors modifying either gene expression or 5-HT and dopamine levels.

These hypotheses are only speculations based on limited research. The reality of spiritual experiences and individual beliefs is far more complex than this simple model. Our purpose was only to review current knowledge on the biology of spiritual experiences. "God only knows" if one day we will be able to explain all our thoughts and feelings by neurobiology.

REFERENCES

1. Baud P, Courtet P, Perroud N, Jollant F, Buresi C, Malafosse A. Catechol-*O*-methyltransferase polymorphism (COMT) in suicide attempters: a possible gender effect on anger traits. *Am J Med Genet B Neuropsychiatr Genet.* 2007;144(8):1042–1047.
2. Newberg A, Alavi A, Baime M, Pourdehnad M, Santanna J, d'Aquili E. The measurement of regional cerebral blood flow during the complex cognitive task of meditation: a preliminary SPECT study. *Psychiatry Res.* 2001;106(2):113–122.
3. Newberg A, Pourdehnad M, Alavi A, d'Aquili EG. Cerebral blood flow during meditative prayer: preliminary findings and methodological issues. *Percept Mot Skills.* 2003;97(2):625–630.
4. Newberg AB, Iversen J. The neural basis of the complex mental task of meditation: neurotrans-

mitter and neurochemical considerations. *Med Hypotheses*. 2003;61(2):282–291.

5. Muramoto O. The role of the medial prefrontal cortex in human religious activity. *Med Hypotheses*. 2004;62(4):479–485.

6. Aftanas LI, Golocheikine SA. Human anterior and frontal midline theta and lower alpha reflect emotionally positive state and internalized attention: high-resolution EEG investigation of meditation. *Neurosci Lett*. 2001;310(1):57–60.

7. Jevning R, Anand R, Biedebach M, Fernando G. Effects on regional cerebral blood flow of transcendental meditation. *Physiol Behav*. 1996;59(3):399–402.

8. Lehmann D, Faber PL, Achermann P, Jeanmonod D, Gianotti LR, Pizzagalli D. Brain sources of EEG gamma frequency during volitionally meditation-induced, altered states of consciousness, and experience of the self. *Psychiatry Res*. 2001;108(2):111–121.

9. Azari NP, Nickel J, Wunderlich G, et al. Neural correlates of religious experience. *Eur J Neurosci*. 2001;13(8):1649–1652.

10. Herzog H, Lele VR, Kuwert T, Langen KJ, Rota Kops E, Feinendegen LE. Changed pattern of regional glucose metabolism during yoga meditative relaxation. *Neuropsychobiology*. 1990;23(4):182–187.

11. Lazar SW, Bush G, Gollub RL, Fricchione GL, Khalsa G, Benson H. Functional brain mapping of the relaxation response and meditation. *Neuroreport*. 2000;11(7):1581–1585.

12. Persinger MA. Preadolescent religious experience enhances temporal lobe signs in normal young adults. *Percept Mot Skills*. 1991;72(2):453–454.

13. Persinger MA. People who report religious experiences may also display enhanced temporal-lobe signs. *Percept Mot Skills*. 1984;58(3):963–975.

14. Britton WB, Bootzin RR. Near-death experiences and the temporal lobe. *Psychol Sci*. 2004;15(4):254–258.

15. MacDonald DA, Holland D. Spirituality and complex partial epileptic-like signs. *Psychol Rep*. 2002;91(Pt 1):785–792.

16. Lou HC, Kjaer TW, Friberg L, Wildschiodtz G, Holm S, Nowak M. A 15O-H2O PET study of meditation and the resting state of normal consciousness. *Hum Brain Mapp*. 1999;7(2):98–105.

17. Persinger MA. Striking EEG profiles from single episodes of glossolalia and transcendental meditation. *Percept Mot Skills*. 1984;58(1):127–133.

18. Jevning R, Wallace RK, Beidebach M. The physiology of meditation: a review. A wakeful hypometabolic integrated response. *Neurosci Biobehav Rev*. 1992;16(3):415–424.

19. Bujatti M, Riederer P. Serotonin, noradrenaline, dopamine metabolites in transcendental meditation-technique. *J Neural Transm*. 1976;39(3):257–267.

20. Borg J, Andree B, Soderstrom H, Farde L. The serotonin system and spiritual experiences. *Am J Psychiatry*. 2003;160(11):1965–1969.

21. Fallon BA, Liebowitz MR, Hollander E, Schneier FR, Campeas RB, Fairbanks J, et al. The pharmacotherapy of moral or religious scrupulosity. *J Clin Psychiatry*. 1990;51(12):517–521.

22. Kawai N, Honda M, Nakamura S, et al. Catecholamines and opioid peptides increase in plasma in humans during possession trances. *Neuroreport*. 2001;12(16):3419–3423.

23. Elias AN, Guich S, Wilson AF. Ketosis with enhanced GABAergic tone promotes physiological changes in transcendental meditation. *Med Hypotheses*. 2000;54(4):660–662.

24. Kjaer TW, Bertelsen C, Piccini P, Brooks D, Alving J, Lou HC. Increased dopamine tone during meditation-induced change of consciousness. *Brain Res Cogn Brain Res*. 2002;13(2):255–259.

25. Anderson SW, Bechara A, Damasio H, Tranel D, Damasio AR. Impairment of social and moral behavior related to early damage in human prefrontal cortex. *Nat Neurosci*. 1999;2(11):1032–1037.

26. Soloff PH, Meltzer CC, Becker C, Greer PJ, Kelly TM, Constantine D. Impulsivity and prefrontal hypometabolism in borderline personality disorder. *Psychiatry Res*. 2003;123(3):153–163.

27. Volkow ND, Tancredi LR, Grant C, et al. Brain glucose metabolism in violent psychiatric patients: a preliminary study. *Psychiatry Res*. 1995;61(4):243–253.

28. Davidson RJ, Putnam KM, Larson CL. Dysfunction in the neural circuitry of emotion regulation – a possible prelude to violence. *Science*. 2000;289(5479):591–594.

29. Koenig LB, McGue M, Krueger RF, Bouchard TJ, Jr. Religiousness, antisocial behavior, and altruism: genetic and environmental mediation. *J Pers*. 2007;75(2):265–290.

30. Mohr S, Huguelet P. The relationship between schizophrenia and religion and its implications for care. *Swiss Med Wkly*. 2004;134(25–26):369–376.

31. Borras L, Mohr S, Brandt PY, Gillieron C, Eytan A, Huguelet P. Religious beliefs in schizophrenia: their relevance for adherence to treatment. *Schizophr Bull*. 2007;33(5):1238–1246.

32. Huguelet P, Mohr S, Jung V, Gillieron C, Brandt PY, Borras L. Effect of religion on suicide attempts in outpatients with schizophrenia or schizo-affective disorders compared with inpatients with non-psychotic disorders. *Eur Psychiatry*. 2007;22(3):188–194.

33. Nelson RJ, Trainor BC. Neural mechanisms of aggression. *Nat Rev Neurosci*. 2007;8(7):536–546.

34. D'Onofrio BM, Eaves LJ, Murrelle L, Maes HH, Spilka B. Understanding biological and social influences on religious affiliation, attitudes, and behaviors: a behavior genetic perspective. *J Pers*. 1999;67(6):953–984.

35. Koenig LB, McGue M, Krueger RF, Bouchard TJ, Jr. Genetic and environmental influences on religiousness: findings for retrospective and current religiousness ratings. *J Pers*. 2005;73(2):471–488.

36. Cloninger CR, Bayon C, Svrakic DM. Measurement of temperament and character in mood disorders:

a model of fundamental states as personality types. *J Affect Disord.* 1998;51(1):21–32.

37. Cloninger CR, Svrakic DM, Przybeck TR. A psychobiological model of temperament and character. *Arch Gen Psychiatry.* 1993;50(12):975–990.

38. Gross-Isseroff R, Salama D, Israeli M, Biegon A. Autoradiographic analysis of age-dependent changes in serotonin 5-HT2 receptors of the human brain postmortem. *Brain Res.* 1990;519(1–2):223–227.

39. Ramboz S, Oosting R, Amara DA, Kung HF, Blier P, Mendelsohn M, et al. Serotonin receptor 1A knockout: an animal model of anxiety-related disorder. *Proc Natl Acad Sci U S A.* 1998;95(24):14476–14481.

40. Charney DS. Psychobiological mechanisms of resilience and vulnerability: implications for successful adaptation to extreme stress. *Am J Psychiatry.* 2004;161(2):195–216.

41. Ramboz S, Saudou F, Amara DA, et al. 5-HT1B receptor knock out – behavioral consequences. *Behav Brain Res.* 1996;73(1–2):305–312.

42. Nilsson KW, Damberg M, Ohrvik J, et al. Genes encoding for AP-2beta and the serotonin transporter are associated with the personality character spiritual acceptance. *Neurosci Lett.* 2007;411(3): 233–237.

43. Bennett AJ, Lesch KP, Heils A, et al. Early experience and serotonin transporter gene variation interact to influence primate CNS function. *Mol Psychiatry.* 2002;7(1):118–122.

44. Caspi A, Sugden K, Moffitt TE, et al. Influence of life stress on depression: moderation by a polymorphism in the 5-HTT gene. *Science.* 2003;301(5631):386–389.

45. Hariri AR, Mattay VS, Tessitore A, et al. Serotonin transporter genetic variation and the response of the human amygdala. *Science.* 2002;297(5580):400–403.

46. Kirk KM, Eaves LJ, Martin NG. Self-transcendence as a measure of spirituality in a sample of older Australian twins. *Twin Res.* 1999;2(2):81–87.

47. Westberg L, Melke J, Landen M, et al. Association between a dinucleotide repeat polymorphism of the estrogen receptor alpha gene and personality traits in women. *Mol Psychiatry.* 2003;8(1): 118–122.

48. Bachner-Melman R, Dina C, Zohar AH, et al. AVPR1a and SLC6A4 gene polymorphisms are associated with creative dance performance. *PLoS Genet.* 2005;1(3):e42.

49. Lemonde S, Turecki G, Bakish D, et al. Impaired repression at a 5-hydroxytryptamine 1A receptor gene polymorphism associated with major depression and suicide. *J Neurosci.* 2003;23(25):8788–8799.

50. Lorenzi C, Serretti A, Mandelli L, Tubazio V, Ploia C, Smeraldi E. 5-HT 1A polymorphism and self-transcendence in mood disorders. *Am J Med Genet B Neuropsychiatr Genet.* 2005;137(1):33–35.

51. Drevets WC, Frank E, Price JC, et al. PET imaging of serotonin 1A receptor binding in depression. *Biol Psychiatry.* 1999;46(10):1375–1387.

52. Ham BJ, Kim YH, Choi MJ, Cha JH, Choi YK, Lee MS. Serotonergic genes and personality traits in the Korean population. *Neurosci Lett.* 2004;354(1):2–5.

53. Munafo MR, Clark TG, Moore LR, Payne E, Walton R, Flint J. Genetic polymorphisms and personality in healthy adults: a systematic review and meta-analysis. *Mol Psychiatry.* 2003;8(5):471–484.

54. Cloninger CR. Neurogenetic adaptive mechanisms in alcoholism. *Science.* 1987;236(4800):410–416.

55. Comings DE, Gade-Andavolu R, Gonzalez N, et al. A multivariate analysis of 59 candidate genes in personality traits: the temperament and character inventory. *Clin Genet.* 2000;58(5):375–385.

56. Comings DE, Gonzales N, Saucier G, Johnson JP, MacMurray JP. The DRD4 gene and the spiritual transcendence scale of the character temperament index. *Psychiatr Genet.* 2000;10(4):185–189.

57. Emilien G, Maloteaux JM, Geurts M, Hoogenberg K, Cragg S. Dopamine receptors – physiological understanding to therapeutic intervention potential. *Pharmacol Ther.* 1999;84(2):133–156.

58. Oak JN, Oldenhof J, Van Tol HH. The dopamine D(4) receptor: one decade of research. *Eur J Pharmacol.* 2000;405(1–3):303–327.

59. Wedzony K, Chocyk A, Mackowiak M, Fijal K, Czyrak A. Cortical localization of dopamine D4 receptors in the rat brain–immunocytochemical study. *J Physiol Pharmacol.* 2000;51(2):205–221.

60. Bortolozzi A, Diaz-Mataix L, Scorza MC, Celada P, Artigas F. The activation of 5-HT receptors in prefrontal cortex enhances dopaminergic activity. *J Neurochem.* 2005;95(6):1597–1607.

61. Diaz-Mataix L, Scorza MC, Bortolozzi A, Toth M, Celada P, Artigas F. Involvement of 5-HT1A receptors in prefrontal cortex in the modulation of dopaminergic activity: role in atypical antipsychotic action. *J Neurosci.* 2005;25(47):10831–10843.

62. Moser M, Imhof A, Pscherer A, et al. Cloning and characterization of a second AP-2 transcription factor: AP-2 beta. *Development.* 1995;121(9): 2779–2788.

63. Mitchell PJ, Timmons PM, Hebert JM, Rigby PW, Tjian R. Transcription factor AP-2 is expressed in neural crest cell lineages during mouse embryogenesis. *Genes Dev.* 1991;5(1):105–119.

64. Fradette C, Yamaguchi N, Du Souich P. 5-Hydroxytryptamine is biotransformed by CYP2C9, 2C19 and 2B6 to hydroxylamine, which is converted into nitric oxide. *Br J Pharmacol.* 2004;141(3):407–414.

65. Ishii G, Suzuki A, Oshino S, Shiraishi H, Otani K. CYP2C19 polymorphism affects personality traits of Japanese females. *Neurosci Lett.* 2007;411(1):77–80.

66. Caspi A, McClay J, Moffitt TE, et al. Role of genotype in the cycle of violence in maltreated children. *Science*. 2002;297(5582):851–854.

67. Caspi A. Personality development across the life-course. In: Damon W, Eisenberg N, eds. *Handbook of Child Psychology: Social, Emotional, and Personality Development*. New York: John Wiley & Sons; 1998: pp. 311–388.

68. Jaffee SR, Price TS. Gene-environment correlations: a review of the evidence and implications

for prevention of mental illness. *Mol Psychiatry*. 2007;12(5):432–442.

69. Perroud N, Courtet P, Vincze I, et al. Interaction between BDNF Val66Met and childhood trauma on adult's violent suicide attempt. *Genes Brain Behav*. 2008;7(3):314–322.

70. Timberlake DS, Rhee SH, Haberstick BC, et al. The moderating effects of religiosity on the genetic and environmental determinants of smoking initiation. *Nicotine Tob Res*. 2006;8(1):123–133.

6 Religion/Spirituality and Psychosis

PHILIPPE HUGUELET AND SYLVIA MOHR

SUMMARY

Psychotic disorders such as schizophrenia are frequent around the world and account for a great amount of disability. Antipsychotic treatments improve symptoms, but do not often allow patients to regain their full social capacities. In this context, it is crucial to help patients recover, that is, to find ways to lead a fulfilling life and to develop a positive sense of identity founded on hopefulness and self-determination. In this perspective, it appears that religion/spirituality can be an important component of recovery. Additionally, it can be an essential coping mechanism, helping patients to deal with the symptoms of illness, social difficulties, and so on. Even if religion/spirituality may cause distress to patients with psychosis, studies show little evidence that religion/spirituality fosters or triggers psychotic relapses. Psychosocial approaches (both individual and group) can address religious issues through fostering social integration in patients' religious communities and working on identity and meaning. Individual treatments may also address spiritual crisis. Overall, the clinician's goal should be to negotiate a common worldview with patients in domains concerned with their care, integrating both their beliefs and secular psychiatric knowledge. This is particularly crucial in cultural contexts in which traditional and/or religious healing may be of more importance than in Western countries.

I. THE RELATIONSHIP BETWEEN PSYCHOTIC DISORDERS AND RELIGION/SPIRITUALITY

Religious issues have only recently been considered in relation to psychiatry. This may be due to several factors: an underrepresentation of religiously inclined professionals in psychiatry that can be observed among both North American [1] and European psychiatrists,[2, 3] a lack of education on religion or spirituality for mental health professionals,[4] and the tendency of mental health professionals to pathologize the religious and spiritual dimensions of life.[4, 5] The neglect of religious issues in psychiatry may also reside in the rivalry between medical and religious professions, which issues from the fact that both professions deal with human suffering.[6, 7] Things may be even more complicated when considering patients with psychotic disorders, mostly due to entanglement of religion with the illness. As described later, some patients may present with symptoms involving religious content; others (perhaps the very same patients) may consider religion the most important thing in their lives.

Many questions arise about the relationship between religion and psychiatry in individuals with psychotic disorders:

- Does religion affect the development of psychosis?
- Are there situations in which religion may be harmful to patients with psychosis?

- Are patients with psychosis more prone to engage in religious activities?
- Can religious coping help patients with psychosis?
- Does religion have an effect on patients' outcomes?
- What about delusions with religious content (this point will be discussed in Chapter 7)?
- How can clinicians deal with the religious issues brought forth by patients with psychosis?

The goal of this chapter is to answer these questions.

2. OUTLINE

After defining certain terms, the history of the relationship between psychosis and religion will be briefly described. Some of the medical aspects of schizophrenia and other psychoses will then be presented, that is, diagnostic and epidemiological issues, descriptions of known risk factors for schizophrenia, particularly the relative contribution of biological versus psychosocial factors. These aspects provide justification for the paradigms that shed light on psychosis as a construct. Given the advantages of a holistic approach to psychosis in its biological, psychological, and social dimensions, the role that religion/spirituality may play will be described.

Studies on psychosis and the role religion may play – negative or positive in terms of coping and outcome – will be described.

Practical notions of how to deal with religious/spiritual aspects of the care of patients with psychosis will be discussed, including assessment, individual and group treatments, and how to work with the clergy and religious leaders.

Finally, we will describe a multicultural perspective on ways that psychosis is understood and treated across countries, taking religious factors into account.

3. DEFINITIONS

Psychosis is not equivalent to schizophrenia. In fact, the term *psychosis* – and *psychotic* – is used either to describe symptoms (that is, psychotic symptoms) or diagnoses, which can be defined as "mental disorder[s] in which the thoughts, affective response, ability to recognize reality, and ability to communicate and relate to others are sufficiently impaired to interfere grossly with the capacity to deal with the reality."(8)

In the present chapter, we use the term *schizophrenia* when the aim is to discuss elements pertinent to this diagnosis. The term *psychosis* is used to refer to the broader group of psychotic disorders, that is, schizophreniform disorder, schizoaffective disorder, delusional disorder, brief psychotic disorder, and so on.

Some patients may present with psychotic symptoms such as delusions and hallucinations without suffering from psychotic disorders (for example, in mood disorders). That's why this book includes a special chapter, distinct from the present one, on delusions and hallucinations with religious content.

The definitions of religion and spirituality are found in the first chapter. To simplify the reading, the term *religion* will be used to refer to both religion and spirituality, unless both terms are necessary.

4. RELIGION AND PSYCHIATRY IN THE HISTORY OF PSYCHOSIS

Little is known about how psychosis was expressed in very ancient times. The lack of literature on this topic leads some authors to believe that psychosis was rare, if not absent, in antiquity. (9) This controversial view gives some weight to the argument that psychosis may be – at least partially – due to infectious causes, that is, factors that may have become more salient when humans began to move across continents.

Religions affect how the mentally ill are understood and cared for. In the early Christian churches, mental illnesses were thought to be caused by possession by demons, and sacramental healing and exorcism were practiced. The Christian notion of compassion for the poor and suffering led to the creation of hospitals for the mentally ill. However, during the Inquisition, Christian churches showed great cruelty toward the mentally ill. Overall, Christian views of mental illness oscillated between the biological and the spiritual. (10) In Islam, mental illness was considered to be a medical condition, and care for the mentally ill was an intellectual and academic tradition dating back to the Middle Ages. The illness was considered as a blessing to believers. The mystical tradition of Islam provided traditional religious healing. For instance, Islamic hospitals were built during the ninth and tenth centuries (11) that encouraged prayers and incantations as choice of treatment. The Koran's precepts were the source of medical practices that spread throughout the Islamic world.(12) This complemented Galenic approaches, together with music therapy. Eastern traditions (Hinduism, Buddhism, Confucianism, and Taoism) provided different models of mental illness, with a focus on existential and transpersonal issues. Buddhism emphasizes compassion and the importance of life in this world, which led to the care of the mentally ill in hospitals, monasteries, or families.(13)

In Europe, asylums were built across the nineteenth century, leading – at least at the beginning – to help protect individuals with serious mental disorders. Unfortunately, due to financial constraints (among other reasons), these asylums became places of seclusion, at least until the arrival of antipsychotic medications. These medications led to a "deinstitutionalization" which brought about real improvement in the living conditions of some patients and further neglect for others.

A nosological distinction between psychosis and affective states (mood disorders) was first made in 1874 by Kraepelin. In 1911, Bleuler introduced the term *schizophrenia*. These authors emphasized organic factors in the etiology of schizophrenia.(14) Later, due to Freud's work, schizophrenia was conceptualized as a psychological disorder in which religion could play a negative role. Today, a general consensus gives prevalence to a bio-psycho-social model that makes it possible to understand psychosis in various ways. Each of these approaches completes the other rather than excluding it. In this perspective, both the positive and negative facets of religion can be considered, complementing to other psychological, social, and biological aspects.

5. THE CAUSES OF PSYCHOSIS – THE RELATIVE CONTRIBUTIONS OF BIOLOGICAL VERSUS PSYCHOSOCIAL FACTORS

Most research and hypothesis testing related to the etiology of psychosis were conducted during the twentieth century. As mentioned above, we have moved beyond former controversies, and any valid model should include both psychological and biological factors. Biological factors include not only genetics and infectious factors such as influenza,(15) but also early brain damage related for instance to starvation of the mother. (16) Recently, more emphasis has been given to psychological factors, especially social deprivation.(17) This factor is illustrated by the increased risk linked to immigration, at least through its effect on social contacts. It appears (even if it is still controversial) that early abuse (that is, sexual) may increase the risk of developing psychosis as an adult.(18) Additionally, some potential risk factors, such as cannabis intake, include both biological and psychosocial components. There is evidence (19) that heavy cannabis intake may (1) foster acute psychotic episodes, (2) exacerbate chronic psychoses, and even (3) increase the risk for developing a chronic psychotic condition.

These elements related to the cause(s) of psychosis form the background for some hypotheses about religion's impact on the risk of psychosis.

In the biological domain, one could note that the healthy lifestyle recommended by most religions may improve health, thus diminishing the risk of disease. Psychosocial factors such as social contacts may be enhanced by religious involvement, particularly among immigrants. Finally, factors related to drug use/abuse may be diminished because religion discourages this behavior.(20)

6. THE IMPACT OF PSYCHOSES IN TERMS OF COST OF CARE AND HUMAN SUFFERING

Schizophrenia is a disorder characterized not only by hallucinations and delusions, but also by apathy and social withdrawal. Long-term outcomes vary greatly, ranging from full remission (about a fourth of patients are able to lead a "normal" life even after being diagnosed with schizophrenia at some point in time) to lifelong disorders that require continuing assistance from mental health services. Overall, the majority of patients suffer from persisting interpersonal and social disabilities. With a lifetime prevalence of about 1 percent, schizophrenia may account for 2.3 percent of all health-care costs in developed countries and 0.8 percent in developing economies.(21)

Before the arrival of antipsychotic medications, individuals with schizophrenia may have been considered "insane," that is, permanently incapable of thinking and behaving in appropriate ways. Unfortunately, this point of view has survived in some places, leading (among other causes) to abuse in the care of these patients. However, the past few decades have gradually witnessed the appearance of a more respectful attitude toward patients with psychosis. This position incorporates the observation that although patients may have *transient* symptoms altering their ability to make judgments (that is, the so-called "psychotic" symptoms), they are fully aware of what happens around them and what they wish to do most of the time. It is true that patients with psychosis often make erroneous choices, such as taking drugs or withdrawing from social interactions, but these decisions may be more accurately defined as ways to cope with emotional difficulties such as anxiety and discouragement. Moreover, subjects with psychosis are far from being the only individuals who resort to such behaviors.

The point is that most people with schizophrenia – as well as those who care for them– have to cope with a severe disease for many years (or in some cases, the rest of their lives). These individuals must often dramatically change their professional and personal plans in early adulthood, just as goals and dreams may be on the verge of becoming a reality. This disorder is associated with some degree of cognitive impairment, vulnerability to stressors, and also a great deal of stigmatization (22), and the critical question is how to help patients cope with such a weighty burden.

7. A PARADIGM FOR UNDERSTANDING PSYCHOSIS

Schizophrenia can be understood through the stress-vulnerability model.(23) This model perceives schizophrenia as the result of a psychobiological vulnerability (that is, genetic and early environmental factors; see above). The onset of the disorder and its course is determined by the interplay of biological and psychosocial factors. The most important biological factors are medication and substance abuse. Psychosocial factors influencing the course of schizophrenia are stress, coping skills, and social support.

Comprehensive care for patients with schizophrenia involves pharmacological treatment, which generally gets most "positive" symptoms under control, and psychosocial treatment, that is, psychotherapy, social skills training, family support, and orientation in the domains of living conditions, occupation, and other factors affecting day-to-day life.(21) In the field of psychopharmacology, the enthusiasm for new-generation antipsychotics has been shown to be partially unfounded.(24) In this context, it has become necessary to reemphasize psychosocial treatments, which remain the cornerstone of the treatment of patients with severe mental disorders. Thus, psychosocial approaches should be given more importance to provide patients with optimal chances for improvement. At this point, one may notice that this model can easily accommodate the bio-psycho-social model.(25) Additionally, it justifies an intervention based on the goal of recovery, which involves an action aimed at improving psychosocial factors. All these interventions are important, but they do not meet the most basic need of these individuals: like every other human being, these people need to find meaning in their lives.

This is the point at which the treatment of individuals with psychoses such as schizophrenia should intersect with other resources that aren't mentioned above. Resources such as involvement in peer support, work, art, and spiritual/religious activities can help patients. These goals, which focus on personal fulfillment rather than on a complete restoration of a prior level of functioning, are part of the concept of recovery. (26) Over the past few years, recovery has been-recognized as an organizing principle for the systems of care for the mentally ill that can replace paternalistic, illness-oriented services.(27)

8. INDIVIDUAL TREATMENT AND COMMUNITY PROGRAMS

Schizophrenia and other psychoses affect all areas of a patient's life. Consequently, treatments should comprehensively cover all affected areas. This should include individual, supportive, and cognitive approaches,(28) but it may also involve psychodynamic therapy (29) (even if it may be difficult to integrate both behavioral interventions and more psychoanalytically oriented approaches).(30)

A comprehensive treatment also involves a variety of actions, for example, aggressive community treatment, family and individual psycho-education, supported employment, social skill training, and integrated treatment for substance misuse.(21)

Recovery-oriented services should take these aspects into account to obtain a better understanding of the meaning of what patients are experiencing, and this from the perspective of their personal histories.(31) Guidelines have been developed to facilitate the development of services according to this paradigm.(27) Beyond the comprehensive approach briefly described above, treatment features should include a variety of services that support consumer self-sufficiency, encourage the use of advanced directives, provide culturally sensitive treatments, emphasize consumer choice, limit the use of coercive measures, and address barriers to access. This is the framework that allows us to study, assess, and intervene on spiritual and religious issues when treating people with psychosis.

9. THE ROLE RELIGION/SPIRITUALITY

We have described why religion/spirituality should be incorporated within a recovery-oriented approach to patients with psychosis.

But how can we integrate this part of treatment? This is not an easy question to address. Indeed, the answer depends on various factors, the main one being the cultural context in which clinicians work. Ultimately, the choice to be made will be whether the clinicians should deal with an issue by themselves, or whether it should be delegated to a trained religious professional.

In fact, we must admit that research is still needed on this topic to fully address some crucial questions. The first is to know what patients want us to do. Do they want us to discuss religion with them? If we hypothesize that the answer to this first basic question is affirmative, others arise beyond that. What can we do, what are the issues a clinician could broach with his or her patient? As mentioned before, some issues certainly fall within the domain of the clinician; others, however, may best be addressed by a specialist in religion – a chaplain, pastoral counsellor, or other member of the clergy trained in mental health care.

If research is lacking on these issues, common sense may suggest some indirect answers, which are described later in this chapter.

10. ASSESSMENT OF RELIGION/SPIRITUALITY

Before considering factors related to the interaction between religion/spirituality and psychosis in terms of coping and treatment, we briefly describe how to assess these elements in patients with psychosis. Although more general aspects of the assessment of religion and spirituality are discussed in Chapter 16, we emphasize here aspects specific to patients with psychosis. The main issue (and maybe the most difficult for clinicians) is that these patients may express themselves in ways that make it difficult to disentangle normal elements from pathological ones.

However, types of religious coping in schizophrenia and how they may affect clinical outcomes and adherence to psychiatric treatment must be assessed. No validated questionnaires exist that survey religion and religious coping for psychotic patients. Wulff (32) pointed out that no assessment could be adapted to every kind of religious belief and practice.

Mohr et al.(33) developed a semistructured interview, based on several different scales and questionnaires, including the "multidimensional measurement of religiousness/spirituality for use in health research,"(34) the "religious coping index,"(35) and a questionnaire on spiritual and religious adjustment to life events.(36) This clinical interview explores the spiritual and religious history of patients, their beliefs, their private and communal religious activities, and the importance of religion in their daily lives. It also explores the importance of religion as a way of coping with their illness and the consequences of illness, as well as the synergy versus incompatibility of religion with psychiatric care. The salience of religiousness (that is, the frequency of religious activities and the subjective importance of religion in daily life), religious coping, and synergy with psychiatric care is quantified by the patient by means of a visual analog scale.

This questionnaire can be used by clinicians who wish to get a comprehensive view of their patient's situation. For patients whose religion may be intertwined with their psychopathology, the most appropriate evaluation method is the clinical interview, which allows clinicians to adapt their language to the beliefs of each individual.

However, clinicians should act cautiously when dealing with patients for whom religion is not important and who currently have no or few religious practices. Any spiritual stance, including a professed absence of belief, should be respected. Addressing religious coping with patients with low religiosity could send the message that they are missing something, and thus be harmful. This may be the counterpart of the dismissive message about spirituality that is so frequently sent when the issue is not addressed with patients for whom it is central.

11. RELIGION AS A PRECIPITANT OF ACUTE PSYCHOTIC CONDITIONS

Classification systems describe disorders characterized by acute psychotic symptoms that cannot be accounted for by schizophrenia (for example, hallucinations or delusions that last no more than one month with eventual full return to premorbid functioning). It is possible that, at least in some cases, predisposed individuals could be destabilized by intense religious experiences, which may represent such a disorienting experience that it may serve as a precipitant.

Some case reports have shown that manic episodes may be induced by religious practices.(37) Concerning acute psychotic conditions, religious conversion may play a role in precipitating psychosis in vulnerable individuals.(38) Koenig (10) mentions the case of John Cuidad (considered the patron saint of psychiatric nurses) and Anton Boisen (founder of clinical pastoral education), who experienced episodes of psychosis following their religious conversions.

Further research is needed on the question of whether religion acts as a stressor involved in some brief psychotic disorders. Nevertheless, when clinicians are confronted with such a condition, they should examine religion as a possible stressor. The fact that such a cause may be masked by delusions with religious content warrants a careful assessment focusing on the temporal relation between events and symptoms.

12. STUDIES ON RELIGION AND PSYCHOSIS SHOWING A HARMFUL INFLUENCE

There is some evidence that religion and spirituality can be harmful for patients with psychosis. Indeed, spiritual and religious concerns may become part of the problem as well as part of the recovery: Some people recount that they experienced organized religion as a source of pain, guilt, or oppression. For some patients, it was a positive resource for recovery, and the faith community was welcoming and hospitable; for others, it was stigmatizing and rejecting. Some felt uplifted by spiritual activities; others felt burdened by them. Some felt comfort and strength in religiousness; others felt disappointed and demoralized.(39)

Religiousness may exert a harmful influence through religious movements/churches that discourage psychiatric care or amplification of morbid cognitions by religious considerations.

It is difficult to obtain an exact picture reflecting the extent to which patients with psychosis may be negatively influenced or abused by religious communities. On one hand, people with psychosis do not usually have much money, thus not much to be taken, and they may have unpleasant and disruptive symptoms that cause religious communities to reject them. On the other hand, their difficulties, both in terms of interpersonal ties and cognitive experiences, may lead them to try to cope with these issues through religion in a way that may be harmful to them. It is difficult to find medical literature quantifying this issue. Psychosis itself may precipitate a change in affiliation to a less traditional religious group (40). But abuse may occur within both traditional and nontraditional religious groups. Anthropology has illustrated some examples of patients who were negatively affected or abused by religious communities.(41) However, a cross-sectional study showed that among 115 patients, only 2 had been negatively influenced (for a limited time) by religious communities.(42)

The concern that religion exerts a deleterious influence on patients with delusions can be supported by the fact that patients who have delusions with religious content may experience a worse long-term prognosis.(43) However, it is not possible to conclude that a causal effect exists. Indeed, among other arguments, it appears unlikely that delusions with religious content constitute a unitary phenomenon, because delusions themselves proceed from different mechanisms. Research on medication-free individuals with schizophrenia indicates that delusions can be separated into three distinct factors: delusions of influence (for example, delusions of being controlled, thought withdrawal, thought insertion, or mind reading), self-significance delusions (delusions of grandeur, reference, religion, and guilt/sin), and persecutory delusions.(44) Religious content may be found in *each* of these categories: A patient may have the conviction that he or she is controlled by a god or that a god puts thoughts in his or her mind; he or she may think that he or she is a god;

or he or she may be convinced of being persecuted by the devil or some other religious figure. Delusions with religious content may be related to former personal and social experiences and thus understood in the context of a person's life and culture.(45) Rhodes and Jakes (46) suggest that religious experience could represent attempts made by patients to interpret their anomalous experiences, i.e. a way to cope when facing distressing events such as hallucinations. Delusions with religious content are encountered in 25 percent to 35 percent of patients with schizophrenia, although they are not specific to that population.

13. THE IMPACT OF RELIGION ON OUTCOME

As mentioned before, when considering the stress-vulnerability model,(23) every factor likely to increase support and/or relieve stress may improve a patient's outcome. Religion is likely to play roles in this regard. Indeed, it can provide assistance in coping with the illness, difficult life experiences, and existential issues, as well as provide interpersonal support through peers and clergy.

When considered in the light of the recovery model (that is, beyond aiming at symptom reduction), religion's impact becomes even more obvious. A vast majority of patients with schizophrenia do not have work, and their activities and social contacts are restricted. Clinicians are confronted with the need of these patients for hope, self-fulfillment, and personal growth. Farkas (47) argues that positive psychology (for example, dimensions such as personal accomplishment and self-esteem) is important for these patients. Keeping in mind the importance religion represents for these patients,(42) it must be examined as a resource for recovery. Qualitative research indicates that religion and spirituality can be a major resource in recovery,(48) as reported by patients. To our knowledge, there are still no outcome studies shedding light on the role religion may play in the prognosis of psychoses such as schizophrenia (either in terms of symptom relief or recovery). Neither is it known how religiousness alone evolves over time in patients with psychosis.

Preliminary results of a study we conducted in Geneva, Switzerland indicate that continuous positive religious coping improves the outcome in schizophrenia (in terms of symptoms, social functioning, and quality of life). While awaiting more data, cross-sectional studies can provide information pertinent to clinical practice.

14. THE ROLE OF RELIGION IN COPING

Cross-sectional studies have examined the role of religion/spirituality in the process of coping with mental illness.(49) Pargament (50) suggested that religious coping can serve five purposes: spiritual (meaning, purpose, hope), self-development, resolve (self-efficacy), sharing (closeness, connectedness to a community), and restraint (help in keeping emotions and behavior under control). Religious coping may be adaptive or not.

But what about patients with severe psychiatric disorders such as schizophrenia?

A qualitative study of Bussema and Bussema (51) found that patients with severe mental disorders (not only psychotic conditions) used all of these five coping strategies. However, the "restraint" factor, that is, a way to keep them from undesirable actions, was the least effective for symptom management. The authors also identified nonadaptive religious coping that caused feelings of guilt and hopelessness or of being ignored, judged, or condemned by the religious community, which at times hindered efforts to manage negative symptoms. Moreover, in the absence of fellowship, faith and hope were difficult to sustain when confronted with persistent illness.

In a recent quantitative and qualitative study,(42) we studied the role of religion/spirituality as a coping mechanism among 115 stabilized patients with schizophrenia or schizo-affective disorders. For almost half the patients (45 percent), religion was the most important element in their lives. Religion was used as a positive way of coping for 71 percent of subjects and as a negative way of coping for 14 percent of patients. Recently, we were able to replicate theses findings in 123 patients living in Quebec, Canada.(52) The subjective importance of religion, the religious practices, and the rate of positive/negative coping were remarkably similar to those found in the Geneva cohort.

14.1. Positive Religious Coping

At a *psychological level*, religion gave these patients a positive sense of self (for example, hope, comfort, meaning of life, enjoyment of life, love, compassion, self-respect, and self-confidence). For two-thirds of these patients, religion provided meaning to their illness, mainly through positive religious connotations (for example, a grace, a gift, God's test to induce spiritual growth, and spiritual acceptance of suffering), less frequently through negative connotations (for example, the devil, demons, and God's punishment). However, even if those meanings were negative in religious terms, they were positive in psychological terms by fostering an acceptance of the illness or a mobilization of religious resources to cope with the symptoms. For example, one patient said, "I think my illness is God's punishment for my sins; it gives meaning to what happened to me, so it is less unjust" (30-year-old woman, paranoid schizophrenia). For three-quarters of patients, religious coping had a positive impact on symptoms (for example, by lessening the emotional or behavioral reactions to delusions and hallucinations and/or by reducing aggressive behavior). A patient who suffered from delusions of persecution clearly expressed this by saying, "I always have a Bible with me. When I feel I am in danger, I read it and I feel I am protected. It helps me to control my actions of violence" (26-year-old man, paranoid schizophrenia). A patient who had delusions of control said, "At some time during every day, I feel that other people can control me from a distance and that they can do anything they want with me. However, I do not feel anxious like I did before. The Buddhist monk told me it was only my imagination and he teaches me how to meditate. In this way, I distance myself from this idea of control; I tell myself that it is just a symptom of an illness, that there is nothing true about it and it has no meaning" (20-year-old man, paranoid schizophrenia).

Religion may also help to reduce anxiety, depression, and negative symptoms. As one patient said, "I am spiritual in my heart. My way of meditating is to sing. There is a link between breath and spirit. When I sing, I don't feel as depressed and I am more enthusiastic about doing things" (44-year-old man, paranoid schizophrenia).

At the *social level*, religion provided guidelines for interpersonal behavior, which led to reduced aggression and improved social relationships. As this patient said, "Believing in Jesus helps me to control my actions. That means not striking my fellow man when he upsets me!" (31-year-old man, paranoid schizophrenia).

Unfortunately, in spite of the subjective importance of religion, only one-third of the patients who were using religious coping in a positive way actually received social support from a religious community. Some patients didn't receive any support from their communities due to their symptoms. As one patient said, "I've gone to church every Sunday since childhood; I listen to the sermon; I don't speak to anyone" (50-year-old man, paranoid schizophrenia). More often, symptoms hindered religious patients from practicing within their religious communities.

However, for some patients, religious communities provided social support. One patient said, "I am a single woman; I have a lot of problems. At church, I meet a lot of people. It comforts me. I participate in every church activity: the service on Sunday, the intercession prayer group and I sing in the choir. The pastor and church members pray for me" (39-year-old woman, paranoid schizophrenia).

Religion may also play a role in decreasing or increasing adherence to psychiatric treatment. (See Chapter 18 on this topic.)

14.2. Negative Religious Coping

Fourteen percent of patients reported negative effects of religious coping. For those patients, religion was a source of despair and suffering.

Four patients felt despair after the spiritual healing they had sought was unsuccessful. As one patient said "I didn't get any comfort from psychiatry. So I turned to Christian Science, which has healed many people. Prayer is an assertion that healing is already there and to see it. I tried for years. It comforted me when it was new, but I didn't succeed, so they told me that I was a negative person and a bad influence on others. I was not worth their attention. Since then, I've been drinking alcohol" (41-year-old woman, hebephrenic schizophrenia). Others used religion to cope, but with a negative outcome. As an example, one man said, "I suffer from being so isolated. I wasn't a believer, but I went to church in order to meet people. But when I read the Bible, it disturbs me. I begin to think I have behaved wickedly and then I believe I am the devil" (47-year-old man, schizo-affective disorder). Although religion was meaningful for these patients, it always carried negative religious connotations. In some cases, religious coping increased delusions, depression, suicide risk, and substance intake. One patient found community support, but this led to a loss of faith and increased medication compliance. "I went to church to be healed and to meet a woman. I believed Jesus would help me, but this is a lie. More problems came, like a curse. Evil has the power on earth. God is a cruel God. I want to die because I suffer too much. It is not Jesus who helps me, but people; at least, medication helps me for anxiety" (43-year-old man, paranoid schizophrenia).

14.3. Clinical Correlates

At the time of the study, sixteen of the patients with positive or negative religious coping presented religious beliefs mixed with their delusions or hallucinations. At a psychological level, they experienced religion either as negative (six cases) or positive (ten cases). However, none of these patients actually participated in community religious practices.

Overall, it appears that religion can serve as a powerful coping mechanism for patients with psychosis, as it can for other, "healthy" people. The main difference is that patients with psychosis may find it difficult to develop social contacts in this area. This has important therapeutic implications (see below).

15. RELIGION'S INFLUENCE ON OTHER BEHAVIORS

Coping may also be used to deal with other issues such as suicidal behavior and substance abuse. Religion may indeed play positive and negative roles in the frequent comorbidities associated with schizophrenia.

15.1. Suicidal Behaviors

Religion may protect against *suicide attempts*. The aforementioned research showed that 25 percent of all subjects acknowledged that religion played a protective role with regard to suicide, primarily through ethical condemnation of suicide and religious coping.(53) However, one out of ten patients reported that religion played an exacerbating role, not only due to issues with negative connotations but also due to the hope for something better after death.

15.1.1. Protective Role of Religion

One patient said, "When I feel such despair that I want to jump out of the window, I think about God. This helps me to live, even if life is so hard sometimes" (41-year-old man, paranoid schizophrenia).

For patients who had previously attempted suicide (fourteen patients), the positive role of religion included not only religious coping and ethical condemnation of suicide, but also rediscovery of meaning in life through religion and, for one patient, a mystical experience after a suicide attempt that restored hope and the courage to live.

Psychotic patients who had never attempted suicide (twenty patients) reported several aspects that played a protective role: religious coping that helped them fight despair and suicidal thoughts and restore hope, "finding the joy to live in God's love" (six patients), finding a reason to live in religion (three patients), and religious beliefs that condemn suicide (four patients).

15.1.2. Exacerbating Role of Religion

One patient said, "Spirituality is essential in my life; I know that there is a life after death. Once, I took medication to die in order to experience death and know what it's like afterwards" (36-year-old man, schizo-affective disorder).

The patients who had previously attempted suicide (nine patients) reported some negative aspects of religion: suicide attempts following a break with a religious community (three patients), suicide attempts involving religious delusions and hallucinations (three patients), wishing to die in order to be with God or to live another life after death (one patient), the loss of a faith which was the meaning of life (one patient), and a mystical experience of death (the patient believed in life after death and wanted to experience it) (one patient).

Two patients who had never attempted suicide reported negative aspects of religion: wishing to die in order to be with God and anger with God.

15.2. Substance Abuse

Religion provided guidelines for some patients that protected them from *substance abuse*.(54) Religious involvement was indeed significantly inversely correlated to substance use and abuse. A content analysis showed that religion may play a protective role in substance misuse in 14 percent of the total sample, especially for patients who had stopped substance misuse (42 percent). It played a negative role in 3 percent of cases. Patients' stories indicated how the various protective mechanisms of religion worked or how religion led them to use substances to cope. One patient said, "I felt bad. I smoked a lot of hashish every day. Once I had a religious conversion after a mystical revelation that the way I was behaving was not what God wanted for me" (34-year-old man, paranoid schizophrenia). Conversely, some patients who misused drugs may have been less likely to participate in private and/or collective religious practices than abstinent patients because of the social impairment, inappropriate affects, and reduced motivation to cope with the outside world brought about by both their illness and substance use and abuse. Some patients with schizophrenia who were drug abusers said they had been rejected by their faith community when they became ill, but others said that, even if they could have found help and support in religion, they lost contact because of their lack of motivation or because they lost their points of reference.

16. TOWARD AN INTEGRATIVE VIEW

Religion/spirituality can help patients with psychosis in the following ways:

First, spirituality/religion may be used to cope with current difficulties, that is, symptoms and social and interpersonal problems.

Second, it may help to prevent potentially harmful behaviors, such as interpersonal violence, substance abuse, and suicidal or parasuicidal attempts.

Third, it can be a key element in the recovery process that every individual with a severe psychiatric disorder should engage in. A person without long-term life goals is like a bicycle that isn't moving: It falls down. Religion and spirituality can play a role that goes beyond cognitive alterations, symptoms, and stigma by allowing even patients with severe forms of schizophrenia to experience personal growth (as part of the recovery process).

Examining these issues unearths some clues about what to consider when treating patients with psychosis. Before going into further detail, it must be emphasized that the context in which these elements are implemented should always be kept in mind. Indeed, cultural elements must be taken into account when considering religion/spirituality in the individual care of patients with psychosis, but the kind of therapeutic work underway is also important. A therapist engaged in a psychoanalytically oriented approach will not proceed in the same way as a cognitive therapist or a clinician practicing supportive therapy.

17. INDIVIDUAL TREATMENT

Specific therapies involving religion are discussed in Chapters 17 and 19 to 21. Aspects concerning illness representation and treatment adherence are discussed in chapter 18. We would like to focus here on elements to be considered principally when practicing behavioral-cognitive or supportive therapy with patients with psychosis.

To our knowledge, no specific guidelines exist in the scientific literature on how to incorporate religious issues in the individual care of patients with psychosis. In fact, we do not even know whether patients want to speak about religious issues or not. But, based on research on coping and religious involvement in patients who suffer from psychosis, we can tentatively examine some issues that may be relevant for them.

The first step is to *assess* the religiousness of the patient (see above and Chapter 16). The patient may report no participation in any religious activity or some extent of involvement in spirituality and/or religion. The spiritual assessment may also reveal a problem(s) warranting intervention.

The following section describes which issues could be components of individualized treatment.

Research on coping in patients with psychosis shows that the personal dimension of religion is not correlated with its social dimension, that is, that many patients have religious beliefs and pray alone but do not have social contacts related to their faith. In fact, they replicate what happens in other areas of their lives because they have problems creating and maintaining an interpersonal and social network. This area can be a focus of treatment; these deficits should be overcome (or at least the goal should be made to overcome them) through social skills training or individual counseling.

For any one of various reasons, patients may be in a period of spiritual crisis. This can happen to anyone, but in patients with psychosis, their crisis may be to some extent embedded in delusions or other "bizarre" thoughts. In such cases, the situation cannot be resolved by sending the patient to a chaplain or member of the clergy. A thorough assessment should make it possible to disentangle a "true" spiritual crisis from the expression of delusional thoughts. Finding the answers to the following questions can help in this process: Is the patient experiencing a relapse? Is he or she in a moment of his or her life suggesting the possibility of such a spiritual crisis? Things can be even trickier considering the fact that patients may be experiencing symptoms and a period of spiritual crisis as well. Generally, clinicians should assess and treat – if possible – such a situation before referring the patient to a chaplain or a spiritual leader. In this latter case, the clinician should discuss the patient's medical context with him or her (with the patient's consent).

Identity building is also an issue of importance. Indeed, patients with psychosis often have problems related to identity, at least partly due to the consequences of their disorder. Even if most of the therapeutic work with these patients is now behavioral-cognitive based, there is a growing trend to emphasize psychodynamic issues again.(30) In general, a psychodynamic approach may be helpful in resolving conflicts and identifying recovery goals. As mentioned in Chapter 12 on self-identity, both the individual and social aspects of religion/spirituality may be key components of identity. Depending on the time available and the skills and the orientation of clinicians, it should be possible to integrate these aspects into individualized treatment plans. Working on identity is not an easy process. The first step is to engage the patient in a narration of their story, making it possible to reappraise certain elements of their identity, including the spiritual/religious components. Further steps may be envisaged, but a thorough knowledge of the psychodynamic field is required at this point.

Another issue pertaining – at least partly – to psychodynamics is the quest for meaning, not in a religious perspective, but in the sense of understanding one's current reactions and emotions. In the field of religion, patients could begin to understand why they invest God as a paternal figure, in the light of the relationship with their parents. Different studies suggest higher levels of insecure attachment in patients with psychosis as compared to controls.(55) Based on research investigating attachment styles and spiritual coping in patients with psychosis, we identified a relationship between patients' compensation strategies in the process of constructing affective security and spiritual beliefs. The first analyses suggest that patients reproduce interpersonal parental experiences that are associated with a compensatory coping strategy in the context of a relationship to a spiritual figure.(56)

As mentioned below, all these interventions should be brought together with a common goal in mind: recovery. In particular, individualized treatment should help to provide culturally sensitive treatments, emphasize consumer choice, and address barriers to access.

18. IMPLICATIONS FOR GROUP THERAPY

Rehabilitation is often implemented to progress toward recovery. However, patients have reported that the services they received were least helpful in achieving goals in spiritual and religious domains.(57) Nevertheless, moving beyond individual treatment, group activities have been developed in some places, mostly in the United States. A group format has some advantages over individual treatment in terms of costs but also in terms of the opportunities for interaction among patients.

Some groups are less rigidly organized and/or psychodynamically oriented; others are more structured, based on behavioral-cognitive principles. Kehoe (58, 59) has been a pioneer in the field, having run such a group for decades. This activity consists in weekly sessions involving ten to twelve patients for two to three years in general. The groups aim to foster tolerance, self-awareness, and nonpathological therapeutic exploration of a value system. Each new member is asked to describe his or her religious/spiritual quest. Then, through interactions with peers, patients are given an opportunity to consider how their beliefs may help in their recovery and/or create conflicts. Interestingly, none of the patients decompensated during the group meetings, and staff concerns about this issue thus seemed unfounded.

Phillips et al.(60) developed a psychoeducational group, a more structured format involving seven sessions. This program is defined as semistructured; information is provided on specific topics such as spiritual resources, striving, and struggles, followed by discussions. Their research was based on the study of ten subjects, and the authors concluded that this intervention appeared to reach most of its objectives.

Wong-McDonald (61) described the outcome of an optional spirituality rehabilitation program, as compared with an ordinary program. This spirituality group, added to a psychosocial rehabilitation program, consists of discussing spiritual concepts, encouraging forgiveness, listening to spiritual music, and encouraging spiritual and emotional support among members. Compared to the usual treatment, this additional group allowed patients to achieve their goals in 100 percent versus 57 percent of cases.

Revheim & Greenberg (62) developed the Spirituality Matters Group (SMG) for hospitalized patients. SMG aims to offer comfort and hope through structured exercises focusing on spiritual beliefs and coping. These exercises involve more activities with a specific orientation, such as reading from the book of Psalms or reciting and writing prayers, in addition to cognitively oriented activities, such as emotion-focused coping. Created in the United States, this group is conducted both by clinicians and religious representatives. It involves a mixture of psychological and religious features, which should be implemented, at least in public facilities, with caution in other areas, such as Europe.

According to reports in the literature, group activities involving spirituality are bourgeoning, at least in the United States. Other programs may exist elsewhere, but without being reported. However, the development of such activities warrants a careful evaluation of the social and cultural context in which they are implemented.

19. A MULTICULTURAL PERSPECTIVE

Our goal is not to describe health systems in developing countries where western-style care is implemented. Rather, we highlight some alternative ways of conceptualizing and treating psychosis, that is, integrating spirituality into patient care.

The first point to clarify is that developing countries do not have a monopoly on attributing supernatural causes to psychiatric disorders. For example, Pfeifer (63) showed that in a rural area of Switzerland, more than a third of psychiatry outpatients believed that an evil influence was a possible cause of their problem. Moreover, 30 percent of patients sought help through rituals such as prayer and exorcism. Those patients suffering from schizophrenia reported the highest rate of rituals involving exorcism.

Conversely, some research has shown that mental illness may be recognized as such in developing countries. For example, Younis (64) reported that in Sudan, schizophrenia was identified in 76 percent of cases, both in urban and rural populations. Psychiatric treatment was advised for more than half of them.

Nonetheless, spiritual factors in the treatment of mental illness have a place of their own in developing countries, as shown by Campion & Bhugra.(65) These authors report that in South India, almost half the patients seeking treatment in a psychiatric hospital had previously solicited help from religious healers. The highest rate was in the group diagnosed with schizophrenia (58 percent). Less than a third of patients reported an improvement through these treatments, which consisted of chanting mantras, ingestion of holy water or ash, use of animal sacrifice, or other rituals. Ninety-nine percent of patients had stopped any religious treatment at the time of the psychiatric consultation.

In Uganda, Africa, Teuton et al.(66) carried out a qualitative investigation of the conceptualization of "madness" across indigenous, religious, and "allopathic" healers. For indigenous healers, "madness" is seen as a sign of a deviation or a form of harm instigated by a jealous party. For religious healers, it is attributed to the influence of Satan. "Allopathic" healers (that is, psychiatrists and specialized nurses) have few resources and provide limited services, usually psychotropic medication. The authors investigated healers' attitudes toward their peers who practice a different approach. Indigenous and religious healers were often tolerant of "allopathic" medicine. Psychiatrists' attitudes were characterized by both tolerance and conflict.

In Brazil, Redko (67) studied young people suffering from first episodes of psychosis in poor neighborhoods. Religion allowed them to express their personal and interpersonal reactions to psychosis through the manipulation of religious referents. Religious idioms and signifiers were useful to label or describe what they experienced, indicated attempts to cope with psychosis, and reflected the quest to reinforce one's own existence and sense of self. The authors discuss the fact that religion can heal, in terms of the descriptions above, but also can act in a "regressive" way, for instance, when patients remain absorbed by their delusions.

Bilu and Witztum (68) report their experience in Jerusalem with Jewish, ultra-orthodox, severely ill patients. These patients turn to the clinic as the very last resort, after having attempted – and failed – to employ religious healing. They try to incorporate religiously congruent elements into their secular treatment modalities. The authors found that medications such as antipsychotics, initially ineffective, turned out to be quite potent when accompanied by a religiously informed intervention, when "drugs are presented to create a mystical wall against demonic assault" (p. 208).

Interestingly, ethnic minority groups may search for spiritual methods of healing when being treated in Western countries. Khan & Pillay (69) reported that patients from South Asia with schizophrenia living in the United Kingdom preferred home treatment, primarily so they could practice their faith and retain the possibility of adding faith healing to their psychiatric treatment. The authors explain their motivations not only as a desire to maintain their cultural identity, but also as a means of having access to more holistic treatment.

Overall, it appears that in developing countries or in areas where religious paradigms may be applied to health issues, religious and "allopathic" care coexist for treating psychosis. Interestingly, some separation appears between these approaches, as it does in more developed countries (even if treatment of psychosis based on religious principles is less common in the occident). Without being naïve – by claiming that religious worldviews can perfectly fit into our medical model – there appear to be opportunities for dialogue between "modern" psychiatry and religious healers.(66) As in Western countries, this could be done while keeping in mind the principles of recovery. Both psychiatrists and religious healers should admit that patients need good medication, psychosocial counseling, and something more, something related to life goals but also to a sense of one's identity, which is sometimes strongly rooted in religion and culture.

20. CONCLUSION

Psychosis is often associated with persistent symptoms and/or social disabilities. In this context, recovery, which aims to achieve a life worth living rather than a "cure" for all symptoms, may be an important goal. That's where religion/spirituality can come into play in the lives of individuals with psychosis. Research has shown that religion/spirituality, rather than triggering psychotic symptoms, can provide powerful coping mechanisms. Indeed, it can help patients cope with symptoms such as hallucinations, depressive thoughts, and suicidal ideations; it may prevent substance abuse; and it can help patients to set life goals. Clinicians organizing individual and group treatments should integrate religion/spirituality in nonjudgmental and neutral ways. In particular, religious involvement may help patients to socialize, and they should be assisted in that pursuit. Therapy may include at least some religious components as they relate to identity, relationships, contextual issues, and so on. Globally, with patients suffering from psychosis, it appears crucial to understand illness in both scientific and spiritual terms, thus maximizing patients' compliance with treatment as well as enhancing the therapeutic relationship.

REFERENCES

1. Shafranske E. *Religion and the Clinical Practice of Psychology*. Washington, DC, American Psychological Association; 1996.
2. Neeleman J, King MB. Psychiatrists' religious attitudes in relation to their clinical practice: a survey of 231 psychiatrists. *Acta Psychiatr Scand*. 1993;88:420–424.
3. Huguelet P, Mohr S, Borras L, Gillieron C, Brandt PY. Spirituality and religious practices among outpatients with schizophrenia and their clinicians. *Psychiatr Serv*. 2006;57:366–372.
4. Lukoff D, Lu FG, Turner R. Cultural considerations in the assessment and treatment of religious and spiritual problems. *Psychiatr Clin North Am*. 1995;18:467–485.
5. Crossley D. Religious experience within mental illness. Opening the door on research. *Br J Psychiatry*. 1995;166:284–286.
6. Roberts D. Transcending barriers between religion and psychiatry. *Br J Psychiatry*. 1997;171:188.
7. Sims A. The cure of souls: psychiatric dilemmas. *Int Rev Psychiatry*. 1999;11:97–102.
8. Sadock BJ, Sadock VA. Comprehensive textbook of psychiatry. *Kaplan, Sadock*, ed. Philadelphia: Lipincott Williams & Wilkins; 2000:686.
9. Torrey EF, Miller J. *The Invisible Plague: The Rise of Mental Illness from 1750 to the Present*. New Brunswick, NJ: Rutgers University Press; 2001.
10. Koenig HG. *Faith and Mental Health*. Philadelphia, PA: Templeton Foundation Press; 2005.
11. Cloarec F. *Bimarestans: lieux de folie et de sagesse, la folie et ses traitements dans les hôpitaux médiévaux au Moyen-Orient*. Paris: L'Harmattan; 1998.
12. Dols MW. *Majnun: The Madman in Medieval Islamic Society*. Oxford: Clarendon Press; 1992.
13. Kinzie JD. The historical relationship between psychiatry and the major religions. In: Boehnlein JK, ed. *Psychiatry and Religion: The Convergence of Mind and Spirit (Issues in Psychiatry)*. Washington, DC: American Psychiatric Publishing, Inc.; 2000.
14. Wing JK: Concepts of schizophrenia. In: Hirsch SR, Weinberger DR, eds. *Schizophrenia*. Oxford: Blackwell Science; 1995:3–14.
15. Rapoport JL, Addington AM, Frangou S, Psych MR. The neurodevelopmental model of schizophrenia: update 2005. *Mol Psychiatry*. 2005;10:434–449.
16. St Clair D, Xu M, Wang P, et al. Rates of adult schizophrenia following prenatal exposure to the Chinese famine of 1959–1961. *JAMA*. 2005;294:557–562.
17. Hoffman RE. A social deafferentation hypothesis for induction of active schizophrenia. *Schizophr Bull*. 2007;33:1066–1070.
18. Morgan C, Fisher H. Environment and schizophrenia: environmental factors in schizophrenia: childhood trauma – a critical review. *Schizophr Bull*. 2007;33:3–10.
19. Hall W. Cannabis use and psychosis. *Drug Alcohol Rev*. 1998;17:433–444.
20. Kendler, KS, Liu XQ, Gardner CO, McCullough ME, Larson D, Prescott CA. Dimensions of religiosity and their relationship to lifetime psychiatric and substance use disorders. *Am J Psychiatry*. 2003;160:496–503.
21. Mueser KT, McGurk SR. Schizophrenia. *The Lancet*. 2004;363:2063–2072.
22. Crisp AH, Gelder MG, Rix S, Meltzer HI, Rowlands OJ. Stigmatisation of people with mental illnesses. *Br J Psychiatry*. 2000;177:4–7.
23. Nuechterlein KH, Dawson ME. A heuristic vulnerability/stress model of schizophrenic episodes. *Schizophr Bull*. 1984;10:300–312.
24. Lieberman JA, Stroup TS, McEvoy JP, et al. Clinical antipsychotic trials of intervention effectiveness (CATIE) investigators. Effectiveness of antipsychotic drugs in patients with chronic schizophrenia. *N Engl J Med*. 2005;353:1209–1223.
25. Engel GL. The need for a new medical model: a challenge for biomedicine. *Science*. 1977;196:129–136.
26. Andresen R, Oades L, Caputi P. The experience of recovery from schizophrenia: towards an empirically validated stage model. *Aust N Z J Psychiatry*. 2003;37:586–594.
27. Sowers W. Transforming systems of care: the American Association of Community Psychiatrists guidelines for recovery oriented services. *Community Ment Health J*. 2005;41:757–774.
28. Fowler D, Garety P, Kuipers E. *Cognitive Behaviour Therapy for Psychosis: Theory and Practice*. Chichester: John Wiley & Sons; 1995.
29. Martindale B. Psychodynamic contributions to early intervention in psychosis. *Adv Psychiatr Treat*. 2007;13:34–42.
30. Spaulding W, Nolting J. Psychotherapy for schizophrenia in the year 2030: Prognosis and prognostication. *Schizophr Bull*. 2006;32:94–105.
31. Huguelet P. Le rétablissement, un concept organisateur des soins aux patients souffrant de troubles mentaux sévères. *Schweiz Arch Neurol Psychiatr*. 2007;158:271–278.
32. Wulff DM. *Psychology of Religion: Classic and Contemporary*. New York: John Wiley; 1997.
33. Mohr S, Gillieron C, Borras L, Brandt PY, Huguelet P. Assessing spiritual and religious coping in schizophrenia. *J Nerv Ment Dis*. 2007;195:247–253.
34. Fetzer Institute. Multidimensional measurement of religiousness/spirituality for use in health research. U.S. Department of Health and Human Services, 1999.

35. Koenig HG, Parkerson GR, Meador KG. Religion index for psychiatric research. *Am J Psychiatry.* 1997;154:885–886.

36. Pargament KI, Koenig HG, Perez LM. The many methods of religious coping: development and initial validation of the RCOPE. *J Clin Psychol.* 2000;56:519–543.

37. Yorston GA. Mania precipitated by meditation: a case report and literature review. *Ment Health Relig Cult.* 2001;4:209–213.

38. Sedman G, Hopkinson G. The psychopathology of mystical and religious conversion experiences in psychiatric patients. *Confin Psychiatr.* 1966;9:1–19.

39. Fallot RD. Spiritual and religious dimensions of mental illness recovery narratives. *New Dir Ment Health Serv.* 1998;80:35–44.

40. Bhugra D. Self-concept: psychosis and attraction of new religious movements. *Ment Health Relig Cult.* 2002;5:239–252.

41. Nathan T, Swertvaegher JL. *Sortir d'une Secte.* Paris: Les Empêcheurs de Penser en rond; 2003.

42. Mohr S, Brandt PY, Borras L, Gillieron C, Huguelet P. Toward an integration of spirituality and religiousness into the psychosocial dimension of schizophrenia. *Am J Psychiatry.* 2006;163:1952–1959.

43. Thara R, Eaton WW. Outcome of schizophrenia: the Madras longitudinal study. *Aust N Z J Psychiatry.* 1996;30:516–522.

44. Kimhy D, Goetz R, Yale S, Corcoran C, Malaspina D. Delusions in individuals with schizophrenia: factor structure, clinical correlates and putative neurobiology. *Psychopathology.* 2005;38:338–344.

45. Drinnan A, Lavender T. Deconstructing delusions: a qualitative study examining the relationship between religious beliefs and religious delusions. *Ment Health Relig Cult.* 2006;9:317–331.

46. Rhodes JE, Jakes S. The contribution of metaphor and metonymy to delusions. *Psychol Psychother.* 2004;77:1–17.

47. Farkas M. The vision of recovery today: what it is and what it means for services. *World Psychiatry.* 2007;6:4–10.

48. Fallot RD. Spirituality and religion in recovery: some current issues. *Psychiatr Rehabil J.* 2007;30:261–270.

49. Pargament K, Brant C. Religion and coping. In: Koenig H, ed. *Handbook of Religion and Mental Health.* San Diego, CA: Academic Press; 1998:111–128.

50. Pargament KI, *The Psychology of Religion and Coping.* New York: Guilford Press; 1997.

51. Bussema EF, Bussema KE. Gilead revisited: faith and recovery. *Psychiatr Rehabil J.* 2007;30:301–305.

52. Borras L, Mohr S, Czellar J, et al. Religious coping among outpatients suffering from chronic schizophrenia: a cross-national comparison. International conference on spirituality, Praha, Czech Repub., September 21–23, 2007.

53. Huguelet P, Mohr S, Jung V, Gillieron C, Brandt PY, Borras L. Effect of religion on suicide attempts in outpatients with schizophrenia or schizo-

affective disorders compared with inpatients with non-psychotic disorders. *Eur Psychiatry.* 2007;22:188–194.

54. Huguelet P, Borras L, Gillieron C, Brandt PY, Mohr S. Influence of spirituality and religiousness on substance misuse in patients with schizophrenia or schizo-affective disorder. *Substance Use and Misuse* (in press).

55. Dozier M, Stovall KC, Albus KE. Attachment and psychopathology in adulthood. In: Cassidy J, Shaver PR, eds. *Handbook of Attachment: Theory, Research and Psychopathology.* New York: Guilford Press; 1999: 497–519.

56. Rieben I. Attachment styles and religious coping in schizophrenia. European Conference on Religion, Spirituality and Health, Bern, Switzerland, May 1–3, 2008.

57. Lecomte T, Wallace C, Perreault M, Caron J. Consumers' goals in psychiatric rehabilitation and their concordance with existing services. *Psychiatr Serv.* 2000;556:209–211.

58. Kehoe NC. A therapy group on spiritual issues for patients with chronic mental illness. *Psychiatr Serv.* 1999;50:1081–1083.

59. Kehoe NC. Spirituality groups in serious mental illness. *South Med J.* 2007;100:647–648.

60. Phillips RE, Lakin R, Pargament KI. Development and implementation of a spiritual issues psycho educational group for those with serious mental illness. *Community Ment Health J.* 2002;38:487–495.

61. Wong-McDonald A. Spirituality and rehabilitation: empowering persons with serious psychiatric disabilities at an inner-city community program. *Psychiatr Rehabil J.* 2007;30:295–300.

62. Revheim N, Greenberg WM. Spirituality matters: creating a time and place for hope. *Psychiatr Rehabil J.* 2007;30:307–310.

63. Pfeifer S. Belief in demons and exorcism in psychiatric patients in Switzerland. *Br J Med Psychol.* 1994;67:247–258.

64. Younis YO. Attitudes of Sudanese urban and rural populations to mental illness. *J Trop Med Hyg.* 1978;81:248–251.

65. Campion J, Bhugra D. Experience of religious healing in psychiatric patients in South India. *Soc Psychiatry Psychiatr Epidemiol.* 1997;32:215–221.

66. Teuton J, Dowrick C, Bentall RP. How healers manage the pluralistic healing context: the perspective of indigenous, religious and allopathic healers in relation to psychosis in Uganda. *Soc Sci Medi.* 2007;65:1260–1273.

67. Redko C. Religious construction of a first episode of psychosis in urban Brazil. *Transcul Psychiatry.* 2003;40:507–530.

68. Bilu Y, Witztum E. Working with Jewish ultra-orthodox patients: guidelines for a culturally sensitive therapy. *Cul Med Psychiatry.* 1993;17:197–233.

69. Khan I, Pillay K. Users' attitudes toward home and hospital treatment: a comparative study between South Asian and white residents of the British Isle. *J Psychiatr Ment Health Nurs.* 2003;10:137–146.

7 Delusions and Hallucinations with Religious Content

SYLVIA MOHR AND SAMUEL PFEIFER

SUMMARY

Delusions and hallucinations with religious content have been a subject of interest in psychiatry over the last two hundred years. The prevalence of these psychotic symptoms displays great variations across periods and cultural areas. Hallucinations and delusions with religious content are not restricted to schizophrenia. They can also be found in patients with mood disorders, that is, those presenting with depressive or manic states. In some studies, religious delusions have been associated with a poorer prognosis. We discuss psychological explanations of delusions and hallucinations to point out that religion and psychopathology may interact in complex ways.

In order to disentangle the two, we (1) critique the category of religious delusion, that is, it is not a valid theoretical category, it is a stigmatizing category for patients and a confusing category for clinicians; (2) provide guidelines to differentiate between functional or dysfunctional roles of religion to disentangle religion from psychopathology; (3) examine implications for the clinicians in the assessment of hallucinations and delusions with religious content; and (4) discuss treatment issues.

I. DESCRIPTION OF THE PHENOMENA

No area of psychopathology draws such public attention and morbid fascination as religious delusions. The discrepancy between grandiose revelations and disorganized behavior, between holy words and unholy demeanor, between mystical experiences and offensive conduct causes pitiful rejection at best and religious unrest at worst.

Historical accounts of "religious insanity" are found in a two-volume 1200-page textbook by German psychiatrist K.W. Ideler (1) who was medical director of the psychiatric department of the famous Berlin Charité. He attributes "religious insanity" to ancient mystics living in the desert, to the flagellants of the eleventh century, possession epidemics in medieval monasteries, as well as radical religious movements during Reformation, to name but a few examples. In 1879, Krafft-Ebing (2) described "paranoia chronica (acuta) halluzinatoria religiosa" (p. 293) and talked about "theomania." Historical accounts of religious delusions go back to the very first issues of the *American Journal of Insanity*, the precursor of the *American Journal of Psychiatry*.(3, 4) However, in their fascination with the often bizarre and grotesque religious content of delusions, the authors mostly failed to adequately express the respect for healthy religion and to address the difference between functional and dysfunctional aspects of religion.

Although William James did not directly address the topic of religious delusions in his seminal work on the varieties of religious experience,(5) he commented on religious mysticism to be only half of the great mystical stream, insanity being the other "diabolical" half.

Over the last thirty years, an increasing body of literature has tried to approach the topic of religious delusions in more "objective," scientific terms using psychopathology, anthropology, and cultural sociology on the one hand and neurobiological techniques on the other hand to explore the nature of this phenomenon.

1.1. Prevalence

Religious delusions have been described in all major cultures across the continents. However, prevalence varies greatly with countries and sociocultural contexts. Several studies have been conducted to compare the expression of symptoms in patients with schizophrenia in different cultures. Here are some examples: In Malaysia, religious delusions were far more common for Malay patients (44 percent) than for Chinese patients (5 percent).(6) The rate of religious delusion was 6 percent in Pakistan versus 21 percent in Austria.(7) Another study showed rates of 21 percent in Germany, 20 percent in Austria, and 7 percent in Japan.(8) The rate of grandiose and religious delusions was 19 percent for Africans; 9 percent for Europeans; 8 percent for North Americans, Australians, and New Zealanders; 6 percent for Middle Easterners; and 8 percent for Asians.(9) Gender and social class affect the rate of religious delusions in Pakistani patients with schizophrenia. Religious delusions were found more often in men than women and in higher social classes than lower ones.(10) A comparative study of the prevalence of religious delusions in Eastern and Western Germany shows a distinctly higher prevalence in the Catholic region of Regensburg, compared to very low prevalence rates in atheistic East Berlin.(11) The authors concluded that religious delusions are "above all, associated with cultural factors" and have to be viewed as a secondary phenomenon in schizophrenia, not inherent to the illness process.

The prevalence of religious delusions varies widely not only with geography, but also with time. For example, in Egypt, the rate of religious delusions rose from 5 percent to 21 percent during a twenty-two-year period when patterns of religious emphasis in Egyptian society changed.(12) In China, religion has been repressed by the communist government for decades. During that time, religious delusions were low with a rate of only 8 percent in Shanghai, contrasting with the 32 percent in Taiwan.(13)

Obviously, the content of delusions is influenced not only by the religious background but also by cultural and political particularities. Political change and technological progress have an impact on the content of delusions. For example, since the year 1997 when the Internet became available to the general public, cases of "internet delusions" are increasingly reported in the literature. Internet delusions are not considered as a new diagnostic entity but rather as a new type of delusional content for two well-known delusions: delusion of persecution and delusion of control (14)

1.2. Religious Delusions Not Restricted to Schizophrenia

Delusional phenomena are not limited to patients with schizophrenia. They may be found in all diagnostic categories that involve delusional thought. Already in 1931,(15) a detailed statistical analysis of delusional content in manic-depressive disorders was presented. Religious delusions were found in 5 to 8 percent of manic-depressive patients as compared with 12 to 15 percent of schizophrenic patients.

In a more recent study in the United States, among psychiatric patients hospitalized in an emergency ward, the rate of religious delusions was higher for patients with schizophrenia (36 percent), but these symptoms were also observed among patients with bipolar disorder (33 percent), other psychotic disorders (26 percent), alcohol or drug disorders (17 percent), and depression (14 percent).(16)

The content of delusions varies over diagnostic categories, however. Delusional thought often seems to be more bizarre and linked to disorganized actions in schizophrenic disorders.

Case Example

A 30-year-old man was arrested by the police when found lingering around an atomic power plant, being obviously disturbed. The man was not religious before the incident, but he reported that when visiting a church, he experienced an encounter with God in the shape of a light that shone through the stained-glass windows. He felt compelled to burn banknotes in the church. When he drove away, the oncoming cars and trucks gave him messages with their headlights. Finally, he left his car with the ignition key on and continued his pilgrimage on foot, spending two nights in the woods. He claimed to have received a mission from God to protect the people around the nuclear plant from harmful radiations. He therefore approached the fence around the power plant, carefully pacing up and down. Finally, he urinated into a bottle, deposing his urine in drops along the fence to create a protective wall.

In major depressive disorders with psychotic features the content is "mood congruent," underlining the basic feelings of worthlessness, guilt, and rejection.

Case Example

Sister Mary (not her real name), a member of a Catholic women's order, had a history of bipolar illness. When she lapsed into a depressive state, she was directed to a psychoanalyst and received antidepressant medication. After two serious suicide attempts, she was admitted to a clinic. "I developed feelings for my therapist which were not acceptable. It was infidelity against Jesus. I have fallen from grace. Bad things happen around me, and it is my fault. I have the terrible feeling of the evil using me. I am like a nuclear bomb, destroying and burning everything around me. I have no more right to live. It would be better to destroy my life than that of the community."

1.3. Religious Delusions Associated with a Poorer Prognosis

Religious delusions may lead to violent behavior. Aggression and homicide have been perpetrated by religiously deluded people.(17–19) Some religiously deluded people have literally taken statements from the Bible to justify plucking out offending eyes or cutting off offending body parts. This may lead to autocastration.(17)

Approximately half the cases of self-inflicted eye injury occur with psychotic preoccupations about sinfulness and higher deities.(18) Potentially lethal self-injuries could be perpetrated under religious delusion, as the following 30-year-old man with paranoid schizophrenia reported.

Case Example

One night, I was persecuted by voices. I drove a knife into my belly to kill the demons." Another example is a 23-year-old man with paranoid schizophrenia, who reported, "Once, during a crisis of anxiety, I was controlled by others, I believed myself to be in a relationship with God, I had to kill myself to save the children (playing in front of his house). It was an obligation. I took a leash to hang myself, the leash broke, I fell down, the children were still alive, and anxiety went away.

Religious delusions have been associated with poorer outcome more generally. In India for example, sexual, religious, and grandiose delusions and flat affect on admission predicted a poorer clinical outcome over a ten-year period.(19) In the United Kingdom, patients with religious delusions in one study appearred to be more severely ill.(20) In the United States, among hospitalized patients with schizophrenia, people with religious delusions were also more severely ill; they had more hallucinations for a longer period of time.(16) In a German study, the intensity of religious faith was associated with poorer outcome; however, religious delusions were not differentiated from normal religious faith.(21) Thus, the association between religious delusions and poorer outcome seems at least controversial. Is this relationship an artifact? Is it due to delusion or to religion? Or is religious delusion in itself a marker of the severity of the pathology?

2. MODELS OF DELUSION

2.1. What is Religious Delusion?

To answer the question, we have to consider both concepts: the concept of *religion* and the concept of *delusion*. The following case examples illustrate some of the questions involved.

Case Example

A 40-year-old man suffering from paranoid schizophrenia for fourteen years reported, "I am a Catholic. I believe in God, in paradise, in angels and also in the Sun God. Gods protect me. I listen to God, these are no voices. God gave me the mission to conquer a sacred land, for soon comes the end of the world. The Sun God gives me the power to do it. I have to prepare the war."

A 40-year-old man suffering from paranoid schizophrenia for ten years reported, "I have no problems in life. I am not sick. I have to put up with psychiatry because the good God does not forgive. Since I have done some stupid things, God has frozen my brain and made his puppet of me. From that time forward God speaks with me and I speak with him. It's great. I spend all of my time speaking with the good God. I would love to go to the movies, listen to music or find a woman, but I can't because God doesn't allow me and he is never silent."

Many researchers understood the two terms of religion and delusion together in a rather pragmatic way, resulting in a variety of definitions of the construct, mainly influenced by the *content* of the delusions. The heterogeneity of definitions is one of the factors influencing the different reported frequencies. Many studies have been conducted with the Present State Examination (PSE), a widely used structured clinical interview developed in collaboration with the World Health Organization to assess psychiatric symptoms. (22) This instrument was constructed to provide a reliable description of symptoms of mental illnesses, irrespective of the language and the culture of doctor or patient. Religious delusion, one of the 140 symptoms listed, is defined as follows: "Both a religious identification on the part of a subject (he is a saint or has special spiritual powers) and an explanation in religious terms of

other abnormal experiences (e.g., auditory hallucinations) should be included." A symptom called "subculturally influenced delusions" includes "specific idiosyncratic beliefs held with conviction by small subgroups within the community, e.g., sects, tribes or secret societies, but not by the community at large (such as Voodoo, witchcraft or special religious beliefs). If the subculturally derived beliefs are held with exceptional fervor and conviction, or are further elaborated by the subject, so that other members of the subgroup might well recognize them as abnormal, then the symptom is rated as severe."

Some of the studies cited above took the symptom of religious delusion as defined by the Present State Examination.(6, 9, 10, 19) In other studies, grandeur delusion and belittlement delusions with a religious theme were considered as religious delusions.(8) In one study,(12) "religious symptoms" were defined as any symptom with a religious content, such as, special knowledge or power from God, curse by black magic, control by an evil spirit, identification with a religious figure, relationship with a religious figure, being commissioned by God, possessed by an evil spirit, punished by God, a sinner, persecution related to religion, or evil eye.

In a final study, nine forms of delusions were differentiated (nihilistic, poverty, somatic, grandiose, persecutory, ideas of reference, guilt, being controlled, jealousy) for twenty-one themes. Among those themes, "religious/supernatural" was separated from "possession" and from "I am God/Jesus/Buddha/a heavenly being." Persecution by "religious leaders" and "supernatural beings" would also be identified as religious delusions.(13)

2.2. Defining Religion

There is no consensus in the literature as how to define religion, in spite of the many concepts to be found. In the present review, we favor a broad definition that includes both spirituality (which is concerned with the transcendent, addressing the ultimate questions about life's meaning) and religiousness (which refers to specific behavioral, social, doctrinal, and denominational characteristics). However, most studies have not used detailed inventories of personal religiosity such as the construct of religious centrality.(23, 24) Rather, emotional and behavioral aspects of religious life have simply been described and detailed. Interestingly, Siddle et al.(25) report that the dichotomous self-categorization of being religious or not used in their study was as valid as more complex measures. The broad definition of religion may include not only classical forms of religious life but also more exotic beliefs as described in the following :

Case Example

A 50-year-old man with paranoid schizophrenia, who regularly attends the meetings of a UFO association, reported, "I am a little strange. Since childhood, I have strange experiences. I regularly see UFOs. Once, I went too close to a saucer and was abducted by the aliens. This is why I have visions and I hear voices. These are not hallucinations. Since then I have a passion for UFOs, more than that – it is a priesthood. I believe in God, but I prefer to call him 'a highest benevolent entity.' Beside God, there are benevolent alien entities, i.e., Christ alien entities, and malevolent alien entities, i.e., satanic entities. With those entities, one does not have any liberty of choice, they influence us."

Indeed, the growing rate of people believing in UFOs and alien abductions has been analyzed in terms of the emergence of a new religious movement.(26)

In this context, the cultural background is important, being likely to influence both worldview and the contents of delusions. Thus, a clear definition of religious delusions is needed to allow the clinician to be sensitive to cultural diversity. For such a definition, we need to go back to the definition of what a delusion is per se.

2.3. What Is a Delusion?

Defining delusion is not an easy task. The diagnostic approach sets up qualitative differences between delusions and other beliefs. According to the *Diagnostic and Statistical Manual of Mental Disorders, Fourth Edition, Text Revision (DSM-IV-TR)*,(27) a delusion is a false belief based on incorrect inference about external reality, which is firmly sustained despite what almost everyone else believes and despite what constitutes incontrovertible and obvious proof to the contrary. The belief is not one ordinarily accepted by other members of the person's culture or subculture (for example, it is not an article of religious faith). When a false belief involves a value judgment, it is regarded as a delusion only when the judgment is so extreme as to defy credibility.

Delusional conviction occurs on a continuum and can sometimes be inferred from an individual's behavior. It is often difficult to distinguish between a delusion and an overvalued idea (in which case the individual has an unreasonable belief or idea but does not hold it as firmly as in the case of a delusion). Contents of the delusion may include a variety of themes (for example, persecutory, referential, somatic, religious, or grandiose).

This definition of delusion has frequently been criticized. The falsity criterion of delusions has been dismissed for being not applicable, not resolved, or even resolved in the sense that the content of the delusion was in fact true. (28) Especially, delusional religious beliefs lack any clear empirical content.(29) Indeed religious beliefs like delusions, lying outside the realm of objective falsifiability, subjective certainty, and incorrigibility.(30) The level of conviction may change with time.(31) Individuals can group and form a community based on delusional beliefs. (32) Notwithstanding, the categorical nature of the diagnostic approach underlines a core psychopathological feature indicative of substantial break with reality, which holds widespread clinical acceptance and shows reliability.(33)

The discontinuity between pathology and normality has been challenged by epidemiological studies with standardized diagnostic instruments that demonstrate the presence of delusions in persons without psychiatric disorders. It has been shown that 10 to 28 percent of the general population have delusions (depending on the broadness of criteria), whereas the prevalence of psychosis varies around 1 percent.(34, 35, 36) This leads us to consider delusions not as discrete discontinuous entities, but as a complex and multidimensional phenomenon. Assessing the presence of a delusion may then best be accomplished by considering a list of dimensions, none of which is necessary nor sufficient, but which, when adding one to the other, result in greater likelihood of a delusion. For instance, the more implausible, unfounded, strongly held, not shared by others, distressing, and preoccupying a belief is, the more likely it is to be considered a delusion.(37) Although the number and the nature of dimensions vary across studies, the most common dimensions are *conviction, preoccupation, pervasiveness, negative emotionality, and action-inaction.*(38)

When comparing delusions in depression and schizophrenia, the criterion mood-congruent versus mood-incongruent delusional beliefs appears as a specific dimension, "incongruence with affective state." The other dimensions are behavioral and emotional impact of delusional beliefs, cognitive disintegration, delusional certainty, and lack of volitional control. Delusions in depression display the same severity as delusions in schizophrenia with regard to delusional certainty and behavioral and emotional impact.(39)

The Peters Delusions Inventory (PDI) questionnaire was created to investigate delusions in general and in psychiatric populations.(40) This scale scans for a set of beliefs, questioning if people hold them and how much they are convinced, worried, and distressed by them. Those beliefs were mainly drawn from the symptoms list of the Present State Examination (22) and the Schneiderian's first rank symptoms of schizophrenia.(41) Several studies have been conducted with this scale, comparing delusional ideations in healthy and psychiatric populations. For example, in a study of primary-care patients without lifetime history of psychiatric disorder, the range of delusional beliefs ranged from 5 percent to 70 percent.(42) Of course, compared

to deluded psychiatric inpatients, healthy adults appeared to endorse fewer of those beliefs and to be less distressed, preoccupied, and convinced. Nevertheless, it is important to acknowledge the fact that, on average, healthy adults endorsed one-third of those delusional beliefs. Moreover, 11 percent of healthy adults endorsed more delusional beliefs than deluded psychiatric inpatients.(43) One study of particular interest is the comparison between deluded psychotic in-patients, new religious movements' members (Hare Krishnas and Druids), and two control groups (nonreligious and Christian). The new religious movements' members endorsed as much delusional ideation as psychotic patients, with the same level of *conviction*, but with levels of *preoccupation and distress* similar to the control groups.(40)

Another way to tackle this is to differentiate initial beliefs that are directly linked to observation and theoretical beliefs based on introspection and judgments. By comparing delusions among inpatients with schizophrenia and the religious belief ("God exists") of highly religious Christians acting as a control group, it appeared that the religious beliefs and delusions did not differ on levels of conviction, falsity, affect, nor influence on behavior.(44) Those studies point out that assessing the contents of beliefs is of little use to differentiate religious beliefs from delusions.

2.3.1. Formation and Conservation of Delusions

Another approach to better understand delusions is to focus on their formation and conservation. Three types of theoretical models try to explain the formation of delusions based, respectively, on motivation, cognitive deficit, and perceptual anomalies. Theories based on the motivation view of delusions suggest that they have a defensive, palliative function, being an attempt to relieve pain, tension, and distress. In this view, delusions provide a kind of psychological refuge and are understandable in terms of the emotional benefits they confer.

Theories based on the deficit view of delusions argue that they are the consequence of fundamental cognitive abnormalities. A set of theories emphasize the cognitive biases and cognitive deficits that have been found in deluded people, such as the jumping to conclusions, an external attribution style, an attention bias for threatening stimuli, source monitoring deficits, and deficits in theory of mind. Thus, delusions constitute disorders of beliefs. For example, the formation of the delusion of persecution has been explained by a motivational factor (to preserve self-esteem) and a cognitive factor (attributing negative events to external causes). The delusion of persecution is then upheld by a selective attention for threatening stimuli and a recall bias of threatening stimuli.(45)

A third type of theoretical model is based on the interpretation of abnormal perceptions or experiences. Delusions are viewed as normal and rational explanations of such phenomena. (46) This model postulates that the mechanisms of formation of delusional beliefs are the same as those of nondelusional beliefs.

Like any other beliefs, delusional beliefs aim at giving meaning to events, they are personal theories. Those personal theories are needed in the face of unexpected events. The data not fitting with the theory then will be either ignored or reinterpreted. So, unusual beliefs are understandable in the personal and cultural context of the individual and his or her way to give meaning to his or her experiences.

For Freeman et al.,(47) the formation and the maintenance of the delusion of persecution goes as follows. The delusion emerges after a precipitating event that occurs often in a context of anxiety and depression. For individuals prone to psychosis, stress induces confusion between internal and external events, which leads to abnormal experiences (for example, hallucinations and imposed thoughts and actions). The individual needs to explain those abnormal experiences. In this search for meaning, previous beliefs about self, others, and the world will be activated. Those explanations are also influenced by the cognitive bias associated with psychosis.

The conservation of the delusion is explained by the reduction of the cognitive dissonance

(selective bias for data confirming the delusion and avoidance of other data) and the disturbed affect associated with delusion (anxiety and depression). In summary, three components have been found in the formation and the conservation of delusion: cognitive deficits and bias, abnormal experiences, and emotions. However, there is no consensual model that explains the role of those dimensions in delusion, even if they are all necessary. Indeed, some authors consider only abnormal perceptual experiences as indispensable for the formation of delusion.(48) For other authors, although cognitive bias and deficits are essential for the formation of delusions, this is not the case for abnormal perceptual experiences.(45)

The role of emotion in the formation of delusion is conceptualized either as a defense to preserve self-esteem(45) or as an emotional state of anxiety and depression that contributes to delusion by a cognitive bias (for example, by the anticipation of the threat) and behavioral reinforcement (for example, by safety behaviors).(47) For Morrison,(49) delusions and hallucinations result from intrusions into consciousness of thoughts, perceptions, and bodily sensations that are misattributed to an external source, due to such thoughts being inconsistent with the person's beliefs about his or her own mental processes (metacognitive beliefs). This is the interpretation that causes despair and dysfunction. The root of negative metacognitive beliefs about self and others often lies in childhood traumatic events. Indeed, a robust association has been found between childhood negligence and abuses and the onset of psychosis.(50)

2.4. Hallucinations and the Role of Abnormal Perceptual Experiences

The debate about the necessary or contingent character of abnormal perceptual experience in delusion is still open. However, abnormal perceptual experiences, like delusional beliefs, are not restricted to psychiatric patients. For example, in an epidemiological study conducted in the United States with 15,000 adults, 4.6 percent reported having auditory hallucinations, with a third meeting the criteria for a psychiatric diagnosis.(51) Similar results were drawn from the United Kingdom: the annual prevalence of auditory or visual hallucinations is 4 percent in the general population, with only one out of eight people with hallucinations meeting criteria for a psychiatric diagnosis.(52) When taking into account hallucinations in the domains of sight, sound, taste, touch, and smell, about 11 percent of the general population score above that reported by psychotic inpatients.(53) Many delusional patients report abnormal perceptual experiences, yet not all of them.(54).

2.4.1. What Is a Hallucination?

According to *DSM-IV-TR*,(27) "Hallucinations are distortions of the perception. Hallucinations may occur in any sensory modality (e.g., auditory, visual, olfactory, gustatory and tactile), but auditory hallucinations are by far the most common. Auditory hallucinations are usually experienced as voices, whether familiar or unfamiliar, which are perceived as distinct from the person's own thoughts. Certain types of auditory hallucinations (i.e., two or more voices conversing with one another or voices maintaining a running commentary on the person's thoughts or behavior) have been considered to be particularly characteristic of schizophrenia. The hallucinations must occur in the context of a clear sensorium; those that occur while falling asleep (hypnagogic) or waking up (hypnopompic) are considered to be within the range of normal experience. Isolated experiences of hearing one's name called or experiences that lack the quality of an external percept (e.g., a humming in one's head) are also not considered to be hallucinations characteristic of schizophrenia. Hallucinations may also be a normal part of religious experience in certain contexts." So, the *DSM-IV-TR* (27) defines delusion as false beliefs and hallucinations as false perceptions. How is it possible to experience false perceptions?

The origin of a false perception may be attributed to biological deficits in brain functioning that produce psychotic experiences. Indeed,

for Frith,(55) the basic mechanism lies in the incapacity to differentiate an internal from an external source of action (that is, confusion of the source of intended actions). Hence, people do not feel they control their own actions. Moreover, the incapacity to understand the mental state of other people (theory of mind) leads to the incapacity to understand them, to confusion in relationships, and then wrong inferences and suspicion.

For Hemsley,(56) hallucination results from a confusion between memory and perception. The subject is unable to differentiate essential elements from accessory elements in a situation. As thoughts are automatically retrieved through memory, when these are alien to his or her expectancies, they are attributed to an external source. For Slade and Bentall,(57) five factors are required to produce a false perception: stressful events, cognitive deficits, external stimuli, reinforcement by the reduction of emotional tension, and expectancies (the subjects hallucinate what they know).

Indeed, raised anxiety was found just prior to a hallucinatory report, as well as a decrease of anxiety while hallucinating. Mood state reduction is then experienced as rewarding and increases the frequency of hallucinations. (58) Several hypotheses come from cognitive psychology to explain the misattribution of an internal event to an external source. For Bentall,(59) the ability to distinguish between interior and exterior, between reality and imagination, is a metacognitive ability. Some individuals would slide more easily from interior to exterior, and then would interpret internal stimuli as external. Garety and Freeman(60) explained the phenomenon by a data-gathering bias (no use of situational and cognitive clues) and by motivational factors (avoidance of negative affects and need to give meaning to incomprehensible events).

For Morrison,(49) metacognitive beliefs concerning both positive beliefs about worry and negative beliefs about uncontrollability and danger associated with thoughts lead the subject to attribute intrusive thought to the exterior; the hallucinatory experience is therefore favored by the reduction of cognitive dissonance.

The most common type of hallucination is auditory. About 60 percent of patients with schizophrenia experienced auditory hallucinations.(57) However, most people experiencing minor auditory hallucinations have no psychiatric disorder and are not in need of psychiatric treatment.(51, 61, 62)

So, what are the factors that differentiate voice-hearers with psychiatric disorder from voice-hearers without psychiatric disorder? Two related factors are at stake: the characteristics of auditory hallucinations and how the subject reacts toward them. Romme and Escher developed a therapeutic approach for voice-hearers based on the differential functioning of patient and nonpatient voice-hearers. As for the characteristics of the hallucinations, both patients and nonpatients hear positive and negative voices. But the big difference between them is the effect of the voices. *Nonpatients* (i.e., those without psychiatric disorder) feel their experiences as mainly positive, whereas *patients* are scared, upset, and disrupted in their daily life by those voices. For patients, they present a social-emotional problem that they are not able to solve. This leads to emotional distress, social isolation, and behavioral problems. Voice-hearers produce many different theories to explain their experience, which vary according to their own view on life and religion and their cultural background. Psychiatry and psychology consider the voices as within the person. But to the hearers, it better describes their experience to say the voices lay outside of themselves. Some may view them as a symptom of disease, but for others, they come from other living people, from spiritual entities (God, ghosts, angels, evil spirits) or may indicate special spiritual powers (gift of mediumship or, telepathy). The attribution of the source of the voices leads to specific coping strategies. Some of those theories are shared by various subcultures.(63)

According to Chadwick and Birchwood,(64) auditory hallucinations are a trigger. The person gives a meaning to his or her hallucination, which then leads to emotional and behavioral reactions. What causes despair and maladjusted behavior is a dysfunctional meaning attributed to the voices in terms of malevolence and omnipotence.

2.5 Association of Delusions and Hallucinations

Delusions and hallucinations often go together both in patients and in the general population.(65) This association may be partly due to some delusions generated to give meaning to hallucinations. Another hypothesis for this association lies in their common underlying psychological mechanisms: a basic cognitive disturbance leads to an anomalous conscious experience (for example, heightened perception, actions experienced as unintentional, racing thoughts, thoughts appearing to be broadcasted, thoughts experienced as voices, two unconnected events appearing to be causally linked). Such anomalous experiences are puzzling and associated with anxiety and depression, and they required explanations. Those explanations are influenced by cognitive bias and metabeliefs. Hence, delusions are dysfunctional attempts to make sense of anomalous perceptual experiences. (66) For Morrison,(49) metacognitive beliefs are an underlying factor for both delusions and hallucinations.

All psychiatric and psychological theories of hallucinations postulate the misattribution of an internal event to an external cause. In that, clinicians, like voice-hearers, develop strong convictions about the meaning of such experiences – meaning rooted in their culture. The *DSM-IV-TR* (27) points out the role of culture in the definition of hallucination – "Hallucinations may also be a normal part of religious experience in certain contexts" – and delusion – "The belief is not one ordinarily accepted by other members of the person's culture or subculture (e.g., it is not an article of religious faith)." We will now explore how to make sense of these studies for application to clinical practice.

3. CLINICAL IMPLICATIONS: HOW TO DEAL WITH RELIGIOUS DELUSIONS

3.1. Disentangling Religion and Psychopathology

A number of studies have tried to establish the influence of premorbid religiosity on the formation of religious delusions. Thus, Getz et al.(67) examined patients from Catholic, Protestant, and non-religious backgrounds regarding the frequency of religious delusions. They did not find any difference in the severity of religious delusions across the various groups. In conclusion, they wrote, "Religious affiliation may influence the frequency of religious delusions…, but religious affiliation appears to be independent of religious delusion severity." Siddle et al.(20) found 68 percent of their patients to have some sort of religion, but only 23 percent showed some form of religious delusion.

From the studies on delusions and hallucinations, we have emphasized the continuity between normality and psychopathology, the multidimensional character of those symptoms, and their common ground due to the key role of beliefs for giving meaning to strange experiences. Sometimes, this meaning takes a religious flavor. Culture provides a framework of symbols that allows for meanings to be created, and among them religious symbols. Religion has even been reduced by some to a system of meanings.(68) The clinician is confronted by a sensitive problem: how to distinguish a religious belief from a religious delusion.

3.2. Delusion as a Dysfunctional Belief

Sims (69) gave three criteria to distinguish a religious belief from a religious delusion:

1 The experience reported by the patient gives the impression of a delusion.
2 Other psychiatric symptoms are present.
3 The outcome of the experience seems more like the evolution of a mental illness, rather than a life-enhancing experience.

For studying religious delusions in patients with schizophrenia, the acceptability of the beliefs by their religious community had to be added. However, this criterion is not sufficient in itself.

Magico-religious beliefs are a major source of confusion for the clinician. Two examples from different cultural backgrounds may illustrate this fact. About a third of Protestant Christians in Australia endorse a demonic etiology of major depression and schizophrenia.(70) Among religious Protestant patients in Switzerland, 82 percent with psychotic disorders believed that a possible cause for their problems was influence of evil spirits. But 50 percent of patients with nonpsychotic disorders (mood disorders, anxiety disorders, personality disorders, and adjustment disorders) also attribute their disorders to demonic influences.(71)

Similar figures have been found in a study in North India in a non-Christian context, where the ancient belief in magic is embedded in the prevailing religious context. In a study of magico-religious beliefs in schizophrenia conducted in India,(72) the authors found a high prevalence of magico-religious beliefs (75 percent of patients with schizophrenia). However, these were understood primarily as a guideline to treatment, rather than in terms of identification of pathology. Belief in supernatural influences was common among patients' relatives (even from an urban background and with adequate education), and treatment based on such beliefs was sought to a considerable extent.

Hence, the belief in demons or magical forces as the cause of auditory hallucination is not sufficient to define a religious delusion. It has to go along with other signs of mental illness, for example, disorganized behavior and other behavioral features that are not seen in those who may share some odd religious convictions. Moreover, demonic attributions to symptoms may even have some beneficial effect, albeit in a rather unusual way as the following case example illustrates:

Case Example

A 33-year-old man with paranoid schizophrenia who was a "born again" Christian, giving Christ a central position in his life, reported, "I am a schizophrenic. I have to take regularly my medication, otherwise I speak with trees. I still hear voices, but I have the discernment. As I believe in God, I believe in evil. I know that voices are from the enemy who wants to destroy me with insults and belittlements. I don't listen to those voices, since the evil is a liar. There is nothing true in it. So I pray to Jesus who heals my soul. Sometimes, I hear the voice of God. He gives me strength, peace and courage."

In this case, the patient's religious frame of reference provides him with effective religious coping strategies, such as selective attention to positive voices and reduction of the emotional impact of the negative voices. Voice-hearers often give meaning to their voices, not as auditory hallucinations, but as a form of communication with another plane, with a spiritual realm, or access to different levels of consciousness.(63) Belief in demons as the cause of mental health is not restricted to Christianity. Intensive religious practices are often associated with increased religious delusion rates (40, 67); however, they are not necessary for the onset of religious delusions.(20)

The first step to disentangle religious beliefs from religious delusions lies in the *functionality* of the belief. If the religious belief is a source of emotional distress or impaired behavior and social functioning, then it is a delusion. This perspective is documented by studies on content-free dimensions of delusions. This approach allows the clinician to distinguish a religious belief from a delusion, but does it mean that the delusion is "religious" (when it is)?

3.3. Religious Delusion: A Confusing Category for Clinicians

We have already seen that the category of religious delusion includes or excludes the same contents depending on the classification criteria. The list of themes for delusions is infinite, with some delusions specific to subcultures. New delusions

appear in relationship with socio-political events and new technologies.

The general themes for delusions (such as persecution, grandiosity, or belittlement) are filled with a diverse set of cultural and idiosyncratic content. Religion is one of the many sources of "color." In factor analysis, "delusion of persecution" is a factor by itself.(73) However, typical themes of religious delusions are persecution (often by the evil or demons), grandiosity (believing oneself to be God, Jesus, or an angel), belittlement (to have committed some unforgivable sin), and being controlled (possession). Then religious contents may be found in delusions of influence (possession), self-significance delusions (to be Jesus, to have committed the unforgivable sin), and persecution (by the evil or demons).

So, to disentangle religious beliefs from religious delusions, one has to substitute the category "religious delusion" by a more valid typology of delusions (as, for example, delusions of influence, self-significance delusions, and delusion of persecution), and specify the presence (or not) of religious content. This approach reverses the way to handle religious delusion by identifying first the presence of a delusion by its severity, then the type of delusion, and finally the presence or absence of religious content.

As an illustration of this strategy, we cite a study focused on the content of persecutory delusions that showed that in 19 percent of cases the agent of persecution was a spiritual entity. (74) The content of grandiose delusion was of religious nature in 55 percent of the cases.(75) The agent of control in delusions of influence may be another person, an anonymous group of persons, a nonhuman device such as a satellite or computer, but it can also be a supernatural entity.(76)

3.4. Religious Delusion: A Stigmatizing Category for Patients

Suppressing the category of religious delusion will not only lead to a better understanding of the psychopathology of delusion, but also to a more respectful attitude toward the spirituality and religiosity of the persons involved. To label a delusion as "religious" often leads to an attribution of pathology to the spiritual and religious life of patients; this labeling is indeed stigmatizing. Like many people who turn toward religion to cope with stressful events in their life, psychiatric patients often rely on religion to cope with their symptoms and the consequences of their illness. (24) However, the spiritual needs of psychiatric patients are often neglected.(77) Just because someone displays delusions with religious content does not mean that all his or her spiritual and religious life is symptomatic of psychiatric illness.

3.5. Functional Impact of Delusions

According to Pierre,(30) deciding whether religious experience is pathological should depend on its functional impact (if it causes distress and dysfunction). "Delusional" therefore refers not to the content of a belief per se, but to how a belief is held and its consequences (that is, with excessive preoccupation, conviction, and emotional valence, and resulting in functional impairment). When looking for the content-free dimensions of delusions (conviction, pervasiveness, preoccupation, action, inaction, and negative affect) across types of delusions, delusions with religious content seem to be accompanied by more intense suffering than other forms of delusions.

Do these approaches, focused on the dimensions of delusions and the process of formation and conservation of delusion, imply that the content may be ignored? Definitely not. The great variation of delusional themes across cultures is evidence of their importance for the individual. Culture gives words and images for the expression of suffering. The content of delusions is also related to the person's history.

3.6. Psychodynamic Considerations

Therapy for delusions and hallucinations with religious content requires a broad understanding of the underlying processes. It is not enough to give medication to treat the pathological symptoms.

Understanding the delusional person in the initial phase of the treatment is equally important.

In a Swiss study,(78) four functions of delusions with religious content were described: explanation, context, exculpation, and wish fulfillment/significance.

Explanation refers to the interpretation or cognitive reframing of threatening hallucinations, psychotic experiences, and delusional perceptions. What is vaguely perceived as an evil, life-threatening, and overwhelming threat to a person's existence, obtains a new significance if it is labeled "demonic." "Why me?" is one of the most tormenting questions of the delusional person. Whereas normal life would give no explanation for singling out an individual in such a destructive way, the events receive significance in the light of religious writings, where the just is threatened and attacked, even in the absence of personal wrong-doing. But there are also positive connotations, such as identifying a comforting voice as the voice of Jesus or an angel in the midst of puzzling and threatening events.

Context refers to the ultimate human desire to understand individual suffering in a larger framework of reference. Culture is a major source for such contextualization. For the religious person, accounts in the Bible, the Koran, or other holy books can serve as the over-arching scenario for his or her personal revelations, sensations, and fears. The end of the world, the apocalypse, is a common theme, but so is the advent of a new era or of a savior. In grandiose religious delusions, the person ascribes such meaning to herself, which is logical for her in the delusional context but offensive to the religious surroundings, resulting in rejection and social isolation. Delusional context can serve as a coping mechanism in persecutory delusions: The more powerful the subjects feel in the face of their persecutors, the less depressed they are and the greater their self-esteem.(74)

Exculpation or "*dis-egoification*" refers to the psychodynamic mechanism of guilt reduction. Some patients report sexual desires and erotic sensations that they would never acknowledge in their healthy ego state. The delusion of Jesus coming to them in their sultry dreams exempts them from guilt. Others may commit self-mutilations or aggressive acts against their family – if it was ordered by an evil (delusional) power or a (delusional) logical necessity. It is not their fault. Thus, the religious delusion helps them to keep some ego-stability, albeit fragile and deceptive, in the midst of personal failure and a behavior that would not be compatible with their healthy religious convictions.

Finally, *wish-fulfillment and significance* may come out of delusional experiences. In a study on the stressful events preceding the initial onset of psychosis, grandiose delusions were often triggered by loss.(79) Patients with schizophrenia often are socially isolated, poor, and rejected. Delusions, however, can give them significance beyond their external misery. Thus, a single woman, living on a farm together with the family of her brother, developed the delusion of pregnancy. She was convinced that she had conceived the baby from the Holy Spirit. Now she was a worthwhile woman, soon to have a baby like her sister-in-law, even more than that – a chosen woman like the Virgin Mary. Unfortunately, the pleasant delusion was accompanied by sleeplessness and disorganized behavior that finally required the patient to be hospitalized.

3.7. Treatment Considerations

In this context, clinicians need cultural sensitivity, to be respectful and to differentiate between functional and dysfunctional beliefs. The question is not if the belief is true or false, because this is not the central question in delusions with religious content. Rather, the clinician has to decide if the behavior associated with the delusions and hallucinations requires care or not. In other words, is the belief a source of suffering; does it increase distress and impair social and occupational functioning? If so, the treatment of the delusional condition has to be standard treatment for such symptoms, including medication, psychotherapy, and social support. Psychotherapy can draw on the psychodynamics described above, helping to find out what the belief means to the person in his or her current life situation.

Religious beliefs (as well as ecological convictions and other prejudices) can be an obstacle for the acceptance of medication and professional help. Delusions with religious content have been associated with a poorer outcome, which could be associated with greater refusal of psychiatric treatment.(20) Religious beliefs – delusional or not – may be in contradiction with psychiatric care.(80) Patients may prefer to seek help in a religious context, for example, miraculous healing or visiting the grave of a prophet or a religious shrine. Others are brought to magical practitioners or exorcists by their relatives – often without sufficient improvement.(71, 72) Wisdom is needed to convince patients and their families to accept medical treatment. This wisdom may come from the religious community, as illustrated in the two following vignettes:

Case Example

A 24-year-old man with paranoid schizophrenia reported, "Two years ago, I began to hear voices of demons; I believed I was Jesus Christ. I escaped from the psychiatric clinic to consult a priest for an exorcism. He told me that I could not be Jesus Christ and he taught me the gospel. Since that time, I met with him every week. The voices told me not to take any medication. He told me not to listen to them, since demons are liars. He told me that the medication could help me. Since then, I've agreed to take it."

A 20-year-old man with paranoid schizophrenia reported, "I didn't trust the psychiatrist; I believed I had no mental disorder but rather had some supernatural power, being able to see and hear people others could not. Those hallucinations had meaning. So I went to consult a Buddhist monk to get his advice. The Buddhist monk told me it was only my imagination and he taught me how to meditate. He also told me that he could not heal me and that I had to go to a psychiatrist. It's he who caused me to adhere to the Western biomedicine."

Social support should also include relatives or peers who must be informed about the nature of delusional disorder. Respect for religious beliefs and traditions could be combined with an explanation of neurobiological processes leading to a distortion of otherwise functional religious beliefs. Winning the trust of family and peers is a major way to ensure long-term compliance and recovery.

But more is needed with regard to the role of spirituality and religiosity in patients' lives. In patient-centered care, the clinician needs to proceed with a spiritual assessment (see Chapter 16). Hence, the clinician will know if the patient belongs to a religious community, if his/her religious beliefs are shared by other people, how salient religion is in his or her life and for coping, if there are unmet religious needs, and if he or she may benefit from religious support.

REFERENCES

1. Ideler KW. *Versuch einer Theorie des religiösen Wahnsinns* [Attempt of a theory of religious paranoia] Vol. 1 and 2. Braunschweig, Germany: Schwetschke; 1848.
2. Krafft-Ebing, R. *Lehrbuch der Psychiatrie.* Stuttgart, Germany: Enke; 1879.
3. Workman J. Insanity of the religious-emotional type, and its occasional physical relations. *Am J Insanity.* 1869;26:33–48.
4. Farr CB, Howe RL. The influence of religious ideas on the etiology, symptomatology and prognosis of the psychoses: with special reference to social factors. *Am J Psychiatry.* 1932;88:845–865.
5. James W. *The Varieties of Religious Experience.* 1902; repr. New York: Longmans, Green; 1916.
6. Azhar MZ, Varma SL, Hakim HR. Phenomenological differences of delusions between schizophrenic patients of two cultures of Malaysia. *Singapore Med J.* 1995;26:273–275.
7. Stompe T, Friedman A, Ortwein G, et al. Comparison of delusions among schizophrenics in Austria and in Pakistan. *Psychopathology.* 1999;32:225–234.
8. Tateyama M, Asai M, Hashimoto M, Bartels M, Kasper ST. Transcultural study of schizophrenic delusions. Tokyo versus Vienna and Tubingen (Germany). *Psychopathology.* 1998;31:59–68.
9. Ndetei DM, Vadher A. Frequency and clinical significance of delusions across cultures. *Acta Psychiatr Scand.* 1984;70:73–76.
10. Suhail K. Phenomenology of delusions in Pakistani patients: effect of gender and social class. *Psychopathology.* 2003;36:195–199.
11. Pfaff MQ, Quednow BB, Bruene M, Juckel G. Schizophrenia and religiousness – a comparative study at the time of the two German states. *Psychiatr Prax.* 2008; in press.
12. Atallah SF, El-Dosoky AR, Coker EM, Nabil KM, El-Islam MF. A 22-year retrospective analysis of the changing frequency and patterns of religious symptoms among inpatients with psychotic illness in Egypt. *Soc Psychiatry Psychiatr Epidemiol.* 2001;36:407–415.
13. Kim K, Hwu H, Zhang LD, et al. Schizophrenic delusions in Seoul, Shanghai and Taipei: a transcultural study. *J Korean Med Sci.* 2001; 16:88–94.
14. Lerner V, Libov I, Witztum E. "Internet delusions": the impact of technological developments on the content of psychiatric symptoms. *Isr J Psychiatry Relat Sci.* 2006;43:47–51.
15. Bowman KM, Raymond AF. A statistical study of delusions in the manic-depressive psychoses. *Am J Psychiatry.* 1931;88:111–121.
16. Appelbaum PS, Robbins PC, Roth LH. Dimensional approach to delusions: comparison across types and diagnoses. *Am J Psychiatry.* 1999;156:1938–1943.
17. Waugh A. Autocastration and biblical delusions in schizophrenia. *Br J Psychiatry.* 1986;149:656–659.
18. Patton N. Self-inflicted eye injuries: a review. *Eye.* 2004;18:867–872.
19. Thara R, Eaton WW. Outcome of schizophrenia: the Madras longitudinal study. *Aust N Z J Psychiatry.* 1996;30:516–522.
20. Siddle R, Haddock G, Tarrier N, Faragher EB. Religious delusions in patients admitted to hospital with schizophrenia. *Soc Psychiatry Psychiatr Epidemiol.* 2002;37:130–138.
21. Doering S, Muller E, Kopcke W, et al. Predictors of relapse and rehospitalization in schizophrenia and schizoaffective disorder. *Schizophr Bull.* 1998;24:87–98.
22. Wing JK, Cooper JE, Sartorius N. *Measurement and Classification of Psychiatric Symptoms.* London: Cambridge University Press; 1974.
23. Huber S. Are religious beliefs relevant in daily life? In: Streib H, ed. *Religion Inside and Outside Traditional Institutions.* Leiden, Netherlands: Brill Academic Publishers; 2007:211–230.
24. Mohr S, Brandt PY, Borras L, Gillieron C, Huguelet P. Toward an integration of religiousness and spirituality into the psychosocial dimension of schizophrenia. *Am J Psychiatry.* 2006;163:1952–1959.
25. Siddle R, Haddock G, Tarrier N, Faragher EB. The validation of a religiosity measure for individuals with schizophrenia. *Mental Health Relig Cult.* 2002;5:267–284.
26. Appelle S, Lynn SJ, Newma L. Alien abduction experiences. In: Cardena E, Lynn SJ, Krippner S, eds. *Varieties of Anomalous Experience: Examining the Scientific Evidence.* Washington, DC: American Psychological Association; 2000.

27. American Psychiatric Association. *DSM-IV-TR: Diagnostic and Statistical Manual of Mental Disorders*. Washington, DC: American Psychiatric Association; 2000.

28. Spitzer M. On defining delusions. *Compr Psychiatry*. 1990;31:377–397.

29. Leeser J, O'Donohue W. What is a delusion? Epistemological dimensions. *J Abnorm Psychol*. 1999;108:687–694.

30. Pierre J. Faith or delusion ? At the crossroads of religion and psychosis. *J Psychiatr Pract*. 2001;7:163–172.

31. Myin-Germeys I, Nicolson NA, Delespaul PA. The context of delusional experiences in the daily life of patients with schizophrenia. *Psychol Med*. 2001;31:489–498.

32. Bell V, Maiden C, Munoz-Solomando A, Reddy V. "Mind control" experiences on the internet: implications for the psychiatric diagnosis of delusions. *Psychopathology*. 2006;39:87–91.

33. Bell V, Halligan PW, Ellis, HD. Explaining delusions: a cognitive perspective. *Trends Cogn Sci*. 2006;10: 219–226.

34. Eaton WW, Romanoski A, Anthony JC, Nestadt G. Screening for psychosis in the general population with a self-report interview. *J Nerv Ment Dis*. 1991;179:689–693.

35. Kendler KS, Gallagher TJ, Abelson JM, Kessler RC: Lifetime prevalence, demographic risk factors, and diagnostic validity of nonaffective psychosis as assessed in a US community sample. *The National Comorbidity Survey. Arch Gen Psy*. 1996;3:1022–1031.

36. Van Os J, Hanssen M, Bijl R, Vollebergh W. Prevalence of psychotic disorder and community level of psychotic symptoms. *Arch Gen Psy*. 2001;58:663–668.

37. Freeman D. Suspicious minds: the psychology of persecutory delusions. *Clin Psychol Rev*. 2007;27:425–457.

38. Combs D, Adams S, Michael C, Penn D, Basso M, Gouvier W. The conviction of delusional beliefs scale: reliability and validity. *Schizophr Res*. 2006;86:80–88.

39. Oulis P, Lykouras L, Gournellis R, Mamounas J, Hatzimanolis J, Christodoulou GN. Clinical features of delusional beliefs in schizophrenic and unipolar mood disorders: a comparative study. *Psychopathology*. 2000;33:310–313.

40. Peters E, Day S, McKenna J, Orbach G. Delusional ideation in religious and psychotic populations. *Br J Clin Psychol*. 1999;38:83–96.

41. Schneider K. *Clinical Psychopathology*. New York: Grune Stratton; 1959.

42. Verdoux H, Maurice-Tison S, Gay B, Van Os J, Salamon R, Bourgeois ML. A survey of delusional ideation in primary-care patients. *Psychol Med*. 1998;28:127–134.

43. Peters E, Joseph S, Day S, Garety P. Measuring delusional ideation: the 21-item Peters et al. Delusions Inventory (PDI). *Schizophr Bull*. 2004;30:1005–1022.

44. Jones E, Watson JP. Delusion, the overvalued idea and religious beliefs: a comparative analysis of their characteristics. *Br J Psychiatry*. 1997;170:381–386.

45. Bentall RP, Corcoran R, Howard R, Blackwood N, Kinderman P. Persecutory delusions: a review and theorical integration. *Clin Psychol Rev*. 2001;21:1143–1192.

46. Maher BA. Delusional thinking and perceptual disorder. *J Individ Psychol*. 1974;30:98–113.

47. Freeman D, Garety PA, Kuipers E, Fowler D, Bebbington PE. A cognitive model of persecutory delusions. *Br J Clin Psychol*. 2002; 41:331–347.

48. Davies M, Coltheart M, Langdon R, Breen N. Monothematic delusions: towards a two-factor account. *Philos Psychiatr Psychol*. 2001;8:133–158.

49. Morrison AP. The interpretation of intrusions in psychosis: an integrative cognitive approach to hallucinations and delusions. *Behav Cogn Psychother*. 2001;29:257–276.

50. Read J, van Os J, Morrison AP, Ross CA. Childhood trauma, psychosis and schizophrenia: a literature review with theoretical and clinical implications. *Acta Psychiatr Scand*. 2005;112:330–350.

51. Tien AY. Distributions of hallucinations in the population. *Soc Psychiatry Psychiatr Epidemiol*. 1991;26:287–292.

52. Johns LC, Nazroo JY, Bebbington P, Kuipers E. Occurrence of hallucinatory experiences in a community sample and ethnic variations. *Br J Psychiatry*. 2002;180:174–178.

53. Bell V, Halligan PW, Ellis HD. The Cardiff Anomalous Perceptions Scale (CAPS): a new validated measure of anomalous perceptual experience. *Schizophr Bull*. 2006;32:366–377.

54. Bell V, Halligan PW, Ellis HD. Are anomalous perceptual experiences necessary for delusions? *J Nerv Ment Dis*. 2008;196:3–8.

55. Frith C. The neural basis of hallucinations and delusions. *C R Biol*. 2005;328:169–175.

56. Hemsley D. Perceptual and cognitive abnormalities as the basis for schizophrenic symptoms. In: David AS, Cutting J. eds.. *The Neuropsychology of Schizophrenia*. Hove, UK: Lawrence Erlbaum Associates Ltd; 1993.

57. Slade P, Bentall, R, *Sensory Deception: A Scientific Analysis of Hallucination*. London: Croom Helm; 1988.

58. Delespaul P, deVries M, van Os J. Determinants of occurrence and recovery from hallucinations in daily life. *Soc Psychiatry Psychiatr Epidemiol*. 2002;37:97–104.

59. Bentall R. *Reconstructing Schizophrenia*. London: Routledge; 1990.

60. Garety PA, Freeman, D. Cognitive approaches to delusions: a critical review of theories and evidence. *Br J Clin Psychol*. 1999;38:113–154.

61. Bentall R, Slade, P. Reliability of a measure of disposition towards hallucinations. *Personal Indiv Diff*. 1985;6:527–529.

62. Posey T, Losch, ME. Auditory hallucinations of hearing voices in 375 normal subjects. *Imagination Cogn Personal*. 1983;2:99–113.

63. Romme M, Escher, S. *Making Sense of Voices*. London: Mind Publications; 2000.

64. Chadwick PB, Birchwood M. The omnipotence of voices. A cognitive approach to auditory hallucinations. *Br J Psychiatry*. 1994;164:190–201.

65. Laroi F, Van der Linden, M. Metacognitions in proneness towards hallucinations and delusions. *Behav Res Ther*. 2005;43:1425–1441.

66. Garety PA, Kuipers L, Fowler D, Freeman D, Bebbington PE. A cognitive model of the positive symptoms of psychosis. *Psychol Med*. 2001;31:189–195.

67. Getz GE, Fleck DE, Strakowski SM. Frequency and severity of religious delusions in Christian patients with psychosis. *Psychiatry Res*. 2001;103 :87–91.

68. Park CL. Religiousness/spirituality and health: A meaning systems perspective. *J Behav Med*. 2007;30:319–328.

69. Sims A. *Symptoms in the Mind: An Introduction to Descriptive Psychopathology*. London: WB Saunders; 1995.

70. Hartog K, Gow KM. Religious attributions pertaining to the causes and cures of mental illness. *Mental Health Relig Cult*. 2005;8:263–276.

71. Pfeifer S. Belief in demons and exorcism in psychiatric patients in Switzerland. *Br J Med Psychol*. 1994;67:247–258.

72. Kulhara P, Avasthi A, Sharma A. Magico-religious beliefs in schizophrenia: a study from North India. *Psychopathology*. 2000;33:62–68.

73. Kimhy D, Goetz R, Yale S, Corcoran C, Malaspina D. Delusions in individuals with schizophrenia: factor structure, clinical correlates, and putative neurobiology. *Psychopathology*. 2005;38:338–344.

74. Green C, Garety PA, Freeman D, et al. Content and affect in persecutory delusions. *Br J Clin Psychol*. 2006;45:561–577.

75. Smith N, Freeman D, Kuipers E. Grandiose delusions. An experimental investigation of the delusion as defense. *J Nerv Ment Dis*. 2005;193:480–487.

76. Pacherie E, Green M, Bayne T. Phenomenology and delusions: who put the "alien" in alien control? *Conscious Cogn*. 2006;15:566–577.

77. Fitchett G, Burton LA, Sivan AB. The religious needs and resources of psychiatric inpatients. *J Nerv Ment Dis*. 1997;185:320–326.

78. Gasser R. *Religiöser Wahn. Eine katamnestische Untersuchung zu Verbindungen zwischen religiösem Wahnerleben, belastenden Lebensereignissen und Überzeugungen religiöser Gemeinschaften* [Religious Delusions. A catamnestic study on the relations between religious delusional experience, traumatic life events, and beliefs in religious communities]. Lizentiatsarbeit an der Philoso-phischen Fakultät: Psychologisches Institut II der Universität Zürich; 2007.

79. Raune D, Bebbington P, Dunn G, Kuipers E. Event attributes and the content of psychotic experiences in first-episode psychosis. *Psychol Med*. 2006;36:221–230.

80. Borras L, Mohr S, Brandt PY, Gilliéron C, Eytan A, Huguelet P. Religious beliefs in schizophrenia: their relevance for adherence to treatment. *Schizophr Bull*. 2007;33:1238–1246.

8   Religion/Spirituality and Mood Disorders

ARJAN W. BRAAM

SUMMARY

The spectrum of mood disorders is extensive, ranging from melancholia and bipolar disorder at the clinical end to milder depression, adaptation reactions, and mourning at the other end. In empirical studies, several aspects of religiousness are often found to be associated with lower levels of depressive symptoms. The findings generally pertain to community-based studies. Although the studies rarely address clinical samples, there is evidence that religiousness predicts a better recovery from depression. However, more and more studies demonstrate that depressive symptoms are often accompanied by religious discontent manifested as negative feelings toward God or a sense of having been abandoned by God. There is hardly any evidence of how religiousness is related to the presentation and course of bipolar disorder. It is hypothesized that religiousness itself may become a subject of mood swings, but could also evoke disillusionment in the patient, and suspicion in the clinician. Religiousness has been reported to be associated with better outcomes among those suffering from grief. Studies of suicide statistics show that, to a limited extent, religiousness can protect people from suicide. One initial aim of a clinical approach involving religion is to include spirituality and religiousness in the examination of psychiatric symptoms. Another aim is to establish a mutual understanding of how spirituality and religiousness are relevant, which in the case of some patients can be a meaningful investment in the therapeutic relationship.

Depression is common throughout the life course. With a lifetime prevalence in the United States of 16.6 percent [1] and a twelve-month prevalence of 6.7 percent, [2] it is one of the mental health problems with the highest prevalence in the population, second to anxiety disorders – although there is a considerable overlap between depression and anxiety. Moreover, studies indicate that people who recover from a depressive episode are still at risk for recurrence. The World Health Organization (WHO) [3] notes that depression is one of the major causes of disability worldwide in all age groups and accounts for about 12 percent of all disability. Melancholia is the most typical and classical presentation of depression with several compelling features such as impoverishment of emotional life and delusions of nihilism or guilt. Milder depressions and subthreshold levels of depression known to be persistent and to easily develop into depressive disorder are, however, much more frequent.

Manic episodes that occur in bipolar disorder are among the most dramatic presentations in clinical psychiatry. Although the lifetime prevalence (3.9 percent) and twelve-month prevalence (2.6 percent) of bipolar disorder are much lower than of unipolar depression, [1, 2] the core features are well known, such as delusions of grandiosity, marked euphoric states, severe sleep deprivation, and continuous agitation sometimes leading to humiliating and socially devastating situations. The subsequent depressive episodes are characterized by painful efforts to reverse the social effects of the manic episodes, the acceptance of psychiatric vulnerability, a tendency to demoralize, and problems with side effects from medication.

This chapter offers an overview of how religion is related to depression and bipolar disorder. In addition to the results of empirical research, prototypical findings are presented on depression, bereavement, influence of life course on depression, bipolar disorder, and suicide. The basic implications for clinical practice are then addressed, with special attention devoted to efforts to bridge the differences in style between mental health workers and patients regarding religious and spiritual beliefs.

1. RELIGION AND DEPRESSION: A CHESSBOARD IN BLACK AND WHITE

The relationship between religion and depression gives rise to ample speculation. Is religion the last spark of hope in times of darkness? Might religion provide sources of effective coping? Or could religion even prevent depressive episodes? If research findings about religion capture the interest of the press, it can lead to headlines like *Religion Helps*. But other questions deserve equal attention. Do certain types of religious convictions induce a depression if guilt feelings are disproportionately emphasized? If religious convictions are conceived as irrational cognitions, would the assumed potential for coping always be disappointing because illusions fail to offset the effects of adversity? These are some questions posed by skeptics, but skepticism should not be confused with clinical observations about the relationship between religion and severe depression. In cases of melancholia, depression seems to turn the patient away from religious life as well as from any other positive emotions or goal-directed behavior. Once even negative emotions are out of reach, the anesthesia of emotional life is complete, resulting in a state of hopelessness and emptiness that is hard to imagine. Patients describe it as a state of profound darkness, a state sometimes resembling death or even hell, and at this point an existential aspect seems inevitable. Given these very different points of view, clinicians need to seek venues in this landscape of religion and depression. But what venues make

sense? To gain greater understanding of the relationship between depression and religion, one common way to describe associations with depression is summarized. Furthermore, some discussion is focused on the many dimensions by which religion may be conceptualized.

Epidemiological insights into the emergence of depression have been strongly influenced by the theoretical and empirical work of Brown and Harris.(4) These sociologists demonstrate how various social factors influence the development of depression. They distinguish three factors in their *vulnerability-stress model*: (1) provoking factors, including the stressors directly preceding the depression; (2) vulnerability factors reflecting poor social resources such as a lack of intimate relationships, poor personal resources such as a pessimistic attribution style, or personality traits such as a high level of neuroticism; and (3) symptom-formation factors determining the severity and type of depression symptoms.

The vulnerability-stress model can be complemented by two types of protective factors.(5) If a factor mitigates the effects of stress, it is referred to as a protective factor with a stress-buffering effect. This stress buffer is closely related to the nature and timing of a provoking agent. Stress buffers can be viewed as ways of coping successfully. The second type of protective factor is defined as acting independently of stress and is viewed as a protective factor with a main effect. It exerts a background effect counterbalancing the effects of long-standing vulnerability factors.

None of the factors noted above sufficiently explain the possible types of effects that promote or inhibit the recovery from depression. Therefore, depression-maintaining and recovery-promoting factors should be incorporated in the model as well.

2. RELIGIOUSNESS AS A MULTIDIMENSIONAL CONSTRUCT

For decades there has been a consensus about the multidimensionality of religiousness,(6) and many varieties can be distinguished within the behavioral, cognitive, affective, and motivational dimensions. The behavioral dimension pertains to organized religious behavior such as church attendance as well as nonorganized religious behavior such as private prayer. The cognitive dimension pertains to religious beliefs and convictions and traditions of religious beliefs representing the context of socialization. The motivational dimension pertains to the relative importance or salience of religion in personal life. Here, one concept often emerges in the literature: that is, intrinsic religious motivation defined as the extent to which people live from within their religion, with faith as a supreme value in its own right, permeating life with motivation and meaning. Another variation is extrinsic religious motivation, defined as the utilitarian type of religiousness, useful to the self in granting safety and social standing.

With respect to the relationship between religiousness and depression (an affective disorder), one may assume that the affective dimension of religiousness is of crucial importance. This affective dimension, however, did not receive much attention in empirical studies until recently. Glock (6) conceptualized the affective dimension as *religious experience*. Although unintended by Glock, the term *experience* bears a connotation of relatively eccentric or, at any rate, very private emotions, as are linked to conversion, mysticism, or exaltation. These sudden emotions may come up less in daily life and presumably do not apply to all religious believers. Thus, the question remains as to how basic religious feelings in common life should be interpreted.

From a psychodynamic perspective, the affective domain of religiousness also includes object-relational aspects of the God image as conceptualized by Ana-Maria Rizzuto.(7) Object relations are ongoing, internalizing representations of relationships with significant others, especially with regard to the emotional functions of the relationships. Rizzuto elaborated on psychoanalytic ideas on the mental representation of the relationship with God. This special type of object relation bears some resemblance to relationships with early attachment figures, but the God object relation also firmly relates to cultural traditions.(8) The God object relation or *God image* may nurture a sense of basic trust, but can also arouse a sense of awe, anxiety, discontent, or anger.

Another domain of religiousness pertains to religious coping. Initially, the conceptualization of religious coping followed fairly random patterns. Pargament,(9) however, contributed to a deeper understanding. He distinguished between religious destinations – objects of significance related to the sacred – and religious pathways – religious attitudes and behaviors. Pargament argued that religious coping is determined by how an individual either conserves or transforms religious destinations and religious pathways.

By no means does religiousness represent a monolithic concept. It involves a system with various dimensions, various aspects within each dimension, and a range of positions and varieties for each aspect. Moreover, aspects of religiousness not only belong to various dimensions, they can also change over time. Of course the aspects of religiousness are interrelated, but here again a range of combinations can be discerned. One should bear in mind that statements about associations between religiousness and mental health always require specification about the dimensions or specific aspects of religiousness.

All the aspects of religiousness can be assumed to act as factors related to depression in various ways ranging from vulnerability factors to recovery-promoting factors. The integral examination of the relationship between religiousness and depression can thus be depicted as a matrix, a chessboard with numerous combinations (Table 8.1). In the columns, the types of factors related to depression can be distinguished, and in the rows, the dimensions of religiousness appear with their main aspects. For example, religious cognitions such as the conviction that every human carries guilt throughout life may give rise to exaggerated feelings of guilt in times of depression, or even to religious delusions about trespasses interpreted as having committed the unforgivable sin. This

Table 8.1: Theoretical Matrix of Possible Relationships Between Religiousness and Depression According to the Adapted Vulnerability-Stress Model of Depression.

	history		onset		presentation	course	
	vulnerability	main effect protective	provoking	stress buffer	symptom formation	depression maintaining	recovery-promoting
Behavior							
- organized (community)							
- private (prayer)							
Cognitive							
- personal beliefs							
- belief traditions							
Motivation							
- intrinsic							
- extrinsic							
Affective							
- God object relation							
e.g. supportive							
e.g. dominating							
e.g. neglect							

would imply a symptom-formation effect on the row for the cognitive dimension. As a second example, religious coping is not included as one of the main dimensions of religiousness, because it represents an application within this framework: If in times of adversity people intensify their prayer and thus prevent depression, stress-buffering effects can be located on the rows for private religious behavior and in the column of stress-buffering effects. Not all the positions on this chessboard are relevant to understanding the relationship between religiousness and depression. Questions arise as to which positions prove to be solid in the literature and which relevant clinical points can be derived from this approach.

3. RELIGION AND DEPRESSION: MAIN LINES AND PROTOTYPICAL FINDINGS

3.1. Meta-analyses

Two recent meta-analyses identified the main patterns of findings in the available empirical studies, including a focus on the distinctions between dimensions of religiousness. Hackney and Sanders (10) distinguished three dimensions: institutional religion (for example, church attendance), ideological religion (for example, belief salience or fundamentalism), and personal devotion (for example, intrinsic religious motivation). They performed a meta-analysis and showed that institutional religiousness was associated with slightly higher levels of mental distress (46 studies) and personal devotion with lower levels of mental distress (35 studies). Following a different strategy with 147 studies and focusing on depressive symptoms, Smith, McCullough, and Poll (11) report slightly more detailed findings. Again, intrinsic religious motivation was associated with lower levels of depressive symptoms, but the association between the measures of religious behavior and depressive symptoms were not significant. Moreover, Smith and colleagues identified both a weak main effect and a slightly more pronounced stress-buffer effect for people facing problems in old age. Furthermore, post-hoc analyses revealed that aspects reflecting a critical attitude toward religion, extrinsic religious motivation, and negative religious coping (for example, blaming God for difficulties) were associated with higher levels of depressive symptoms. The results of the meta-analyses suggest a main protective as well as a stress-buffer effect, but it should be emphasized that causal interpretations are not warranted.

3.2. Prayer

In meta-analyses and reviews, prayer is often categorized as religious behavior, but private prayer should not be confused with public religious participation. Prayer does not only involve the private aspect of contemplation, but the frequency of private prayer by far exceeds that of religious behavior in the context of attending services. Although prayer is viewed as an essential element of religiousness, only a limited number of studies have been conducted on prayer or other private religious behavior and depression, and the results are mixed. One possible reason for the conflicting results may have to do with the process of coping itself. People intensify their praying in times of adversity, which is when depressive symptoms and other signs of distress develop as well. If prayer is successful as a coping strategy, it can facilitate the recovery from depressive symptoms over time. Ai and colleagues illustrated this principle (12) with their observation that, retrospectively, prayer related to higher levels of depressive

symptoms in the period immediately following coronary bypass surgery, but this association was reversed after one year of follow-up.

Another perspective on prayer has to do with its perceived importance among patients admitted to a mental hospital. In a small sample (N = 50) of psychiatric inpatients in the United States, Fitchett and colleagues (13) described that prayer remained important for 80 percent of the patients, almost two-thirds of whom suffered from mood disorders. The percentage was similar in a comparison sample of medical and surgical patients. It is uncertain whether prayer is a successful strategy for coping religiously with depression, but the fact that people pray very often suggests that they strongly adhere to it. In a U.S. sample studied in North Carolina, the frequency of prayer among older adults with major depression was 80 percent weekly or more (14) compared to 46 percent in an Australian sample.(15) Despite these differences, the rates of prayer are substantial. Prayer did not relate to depressive symptoms in these studies.

3.3. Recovery from Depression

Several studies describe associations between aspects of religiousness and the outcome of depression. In three studies among (older) subjects with depression, intrinsic religious motivation,(16) salience of religion,(17) and positive religious coping (14) were associated with a better depression outcome. Church attendance had no significant association with the depression outcome in either of the above studies. However, in a large study among 1,000 hospitalized adults with pulmonary or cardiovascular disease and concurrent major depression, Koenig (18) did not observe a significant association between intrinsic religiousness and remission of depression. Church attendance, however, predicted a shorter recovery time, after multivariate adjustment for health and social support. Higher levels of religiousness can thus be assumed to predict a better depression outcome among older patients or subjects with a serious physical condition. The question remains as to whether the severity of the depression was similar between people still able to express high levels of religiousness and those unable to do so. It is not completely certain whether a history of previous depressive episodes or other markers of vulnerability could be sufficiently accounted for in these studies.

3.4. Type of Symptoms (and Syndromes)

Moral issues play an important role in the Judeo-Christian belief tradition, with its adherence to moral codes, emphasis on conscience, and keen awareness of guilt. People involved in religion may therefore more often report feelings of guilt, even though this may reflect more about their perceived moral standards and religious upbringing than about pathological guilt. Indeed, in a community-based study among older adults with a major depression in the Netherlands, depressed Roman Catholics and depressed Protestants more often reported feelings of guilt than depressed nonchurch members.(19) Stompe and colleagues (20) focused on the symptom of guilt in a cross-national comparison between depressive patients from Austria (Vienna) and Pakistan (Lahore). The authors stated that feelings of guilt may be prominent in non-Christian societies as well, for example, in Islamic cultures. In their empirical approach, they draw a distinction between ethical guilt representing more or less normal expressions of guilt and delusionlike ideas representing more exaggerated conceptions of guilt or false judgments about guilt. Ethical feelings were observed in both countries to the same extent, with Pakistanis generally only expressing mild self-reproach and Austrians tending to express feelings of guilt. Delusionlike ideas about guilt were less prevalent and only reported by Austrians.

The issue of symptom formation can also be addressed at a higher level, no longer regarding specific symptoms within the depressive syndrome but ascending to groups of symptoms. A relevant distinction here is drawn between internalizing and externalizing mental disorders. Internalizing disorders mainly correspond to depression and anxiety, whereas externalizing disorders manifest themselves in altered behavior

such as substance abuse or antisocial conduct. This type of categorization has been applied by Kendler and colleagues,(21) who assessed a wide range of aspects of religiousness in a population-based sample of twins in Virginia. They analyzed the associations between these aspects and the lifetime history of nine psychiatric and substance use disorders, internalizing as well as externalizing. In their study, the social dimensions of religiousness, such as church attendance, were associated with lower rates of all types of disorders under study. A positive God image (*Involved God*) was only associated with a lower prevalence of externalizing disorders. It might be useful to follow the approach taken by Kendler and colleagues, using different samples with respect to age, region, culture, or religious affiliation. With respect to religious affiliation, the last aspect, Levav and colleagues (22) showed that the rate of major depression was significantly higher among male Jews than among Roman Catholics and Protestants, but the rate of alcoholism among Jews was lower.

3.5. Pietistic Orthodox Calvinism

A particular aspect of the relationship between religiousness and depression can be found in one tradition, of a modest size, in the Netherlands. Strict adherence to Reformed, Calvinist doctrines is thought to give rise to a mind-set characterized by depressed mood, a tendency to refrain from pleasure, a sense of insufficiency, and guilt feelings. These aspects are in keeping with a more orthodox application of the doctrines of John Calvin and the Heidelberg Catechism. This catechism formulates three articles, one on misery, one on salvation (*How I may be delivered from all my sins and miseries),* and one on gratitude as requirements for knowing whether one will be saved. The emphasis on misery and powerlessness in Calvinist doctrine might have certain implications for mental well-being. In their small and relatively closed communities, pietistic orthodox Calvinists characterize their attitude as *heavy*, with positive social sanctions for behavior in line with the Catechism. There is ongoing interest in the Netherlands in this pietistic orthodox Calvinist tradition, and there are empirical indications that the rates of depression in these communities are twice as high compared to other rural communities.(23)

3.6. Pentecostals

The possible adverse effects of religious beliefs are not exclusive to pietistic orthodox Calvinists and may also pertain to a certain extent to Pentecostals. In a population-based study in North Carolina, Meador and colleagues (24) reported three times as high a risk for major depression among members of Pentecostal congregations as among members of other churches, after adjustment for several possible confounders such as life events and social support. One possible explanation the authors suggested was that especially depressed people may be particularly apt to affiliate themselves with the Pentecostals. A similarity between orthodox Calvinists and Pentecostals may be that their communities often combine a pietistic way of believing and strong, possibly over-regulating social networks.

3.7. Religious Discontent

In the literature on depression, a highly relevant type of relationship is the one between *religious discontent*, also referred to as *religious struggle* or *negative religious coping*, and depression. There is a reported link between criticism of God or a sense of being abandoned by God and higher levels of depressive symptoms.(25, 26) This research was carried out among samples of somatically ill hospitalized patients or older adults. The link between religious discontent and depressive symptoms is generally twice as strong as the one between intrinsic religious motivation or church attendance and depressive symptoms. Most studies nonetheless only included positive aspects of religiousness. Smith and colleagues (11) conclude in their extensive meta-analysis that researchers should devote more attention to negative forms of religiousness. Prospective research could for example shed light on whether feelings of religious discontent decrease or even disappear if

a depression ends, or if they represent, in fact, a risk factor for recurrent depression.

4. LIFE COURSE PERSPECTIVES

So far there exists considerable scientific evidence for a multifaceted relationship between religiousness and depression. The findings should be understood in their context, as is apparent from the very different samples, ranging from the community studies, samples of older people, hospitalized somatically ill patients, or psychiatric inpatients. Of course, knowledge of the religious tradition in the geographical region where studies have been performed is crucial to understand the types of relationships. A related perspective pertains to the age of the participants under study, the cohort in which they grew up, and their current stage of life. Is religion equally important throughout one's course of life? What can we learn from the few studies carried out among children and adolescents?

4.1. The Varieties of Religious Development

Individualization and secularization have permeated the Western world in the past century. Greater freedom has evolved to make choices to which extent a religious way of life fits to one's course of life, which will also relate to and depend on one's social roles and family ties, personal inclinations, character traits, and spheres of interest. It would be good to have greater insight into the choices people make with respect to spirituality and religion. In their study on *The Varieties of Religious Development in Adulthood*,(27) McCullough and colleagues suggest that religiousness does not follow one general trajectory throughout life, as seems to be suggested by higher levels of religiousness in later age. They conducted an empirical analysis, focusing on the importance of religion, in a sample of more than a thousand young Californians under study since 1940 with follow-up assessments for up to fifty years later. The results revealed three trajectories of religiousness: (1) about 40 percent of the sample followed a pattern starting with intermediate levels of religiousness that increase around age 54 and return to the initial level by age 80 (*parabolic class*), (2) about 40 percent of the sample exhibited a pattern with very low religiousness throughout their lifetime (*low/declining class*), and (3) less than 20 percent had high levels of religiousness that even increased throughout their lifetime (*high/increasing class*). In this study, the distribution of 40 percent parabolic, 40 percent low, and 20 percent high is fascinating, because similar distributions might well occur in other populations. This research suggests that, for a minority (perhaps a large minority), religion is very relevant throughout life; for others, there are stages when religion becomes relevant; and for another, substantial number, religion seems to remain entirely irrelevant. An exception to this last point is that people with an active resistance against religion sometimes will not be indifferent to religion at all and may have suffered from a too-strict religious upbringing in some cases.

In the course of a lifetime, some aspects of religiousness may become less important or less relevant to one's mental well-being and be replaced by other aspects. In adolescence, church attendance may affect moral directives, coping skills, and social functioning.(28) In adult life, an intrinsic religious motivation emerges as an aspect relevant to self-realization and self-determination, which are important for goal-directed behavior in the context of career development and family building.(27) In later life, both church attendance and intrinsic religiousness can play an important role as resources for coping with adversity. It is uncertain whether affective aspects of religiousness such as a perceived relationship with God or spiritual aspects such as an openness to transcendental experiences develop throughout the life cycle. Moreover, the social context, especially the degree of secularization, plays a decisive role in the extent to which people have a verbal repertoire to communicate about their religious or spiritual inclinations.

4.2. Children and Adolescents

One study performed by Rew and colleagues (29) in a pre-adolescent sample (8–12 years) in Austin,

Texas, focused on prayer. Prayer frequency was associated with social connectedness and sense of humor, but not with levels of perceived stress, possibly because the levels of stress in this population were generally low.

A review by Wong and colleagues (30) included twenty studies on the association between religiosity, spirituality, or both and mental health in adolescents in the 10 to 20 age range. They devoted specific attention to the various measures of religiosity and spirituality. The most pervasive finding produced by this strict and systematic approach was that church attendance (and other measures of institutional religiosity) in particular exhibited positive associations with mental health. This finding is quite different from the results of meta-analyses on religion and depression in samples of adults,(10, 11) where institutional measures exhibit the weakest correlations with mental health and devotional measures the strongest. Wong and colleagues suggest that the social and behavioral impacts of religiosity might be more beneficial to adolescents than to older adults because they provide adolescents with a sense of order and belonging during a potentially turbulent period in their development.

5. RELIGION AND BEREAVEMENT

Losing a spouse or lifelong companion is something that generally occurs in later life and confronts the individual with a difficult task. Although there is no need to comprehend the response of mourning as a mental disorder, it does require a thorough adaptation process generally accompanied by transient or longer lasting depressive moods or other depressive symptoms. In the stages of grief formulated by Kübler Ross,(31) the bereaved are apt to go through the normal psychological stages of *denial, anger, bargainin*g, *depression,* and *acceptance.* Although there is insufficient empirical evidence that all mourners go through all these stages in this sequence,(32) the stages provide a frame of reference for understanding some of the dynamic responses to bereavement and their interplay with religion.

In its myths and beliefs, religion has a great potential for helping people cope with the end of life, bereavement, and dying. It is possible to speculate on how religiousness relates to each of the five stages of grief. In the opinion of atheists, for example, the belief in an afterlife may be a form of denial. Anger might evoke problematic feelings among religious people, such as guilt about rebelling against the Creator or trouble expressing anger at God. Bargaining can be done in an effort to influence one's fate by altruistic behavior or adherence to rituals, as is observed among Roman Catholics. Calvinists might have compelling questions about whether or not they are predestined for salvation. Depression may follow any of the various religiousness and depression patterns outlined above. As to acceptance, the role of religiousness may relate to the outcomes of the previous stages. In any of the stages of grief, the religious community can often provide a certain degree of consolation, moral support, human contact, and sharing in ceremonies of mourning.

An intriguing hypothesis about the psychology of religion and bereavement derives from attachment theory. Kirkpatrick (33) stated that a personal relationship with God resembles a secure attachment to a primary caregiver. Along these lines, the emotional compensation hypothesis notes that the relationship with God provides comfort if a loved one dies and helps compensate for the lack of a love relationship.

Becker and colleagues (34) evaluated thirty-two studies on the relationship between religious and spiritual beliefs and bereavement. About half the studies reported a positive association. Nevertheless, the approaches exhibited considerable variation as regards the measures and outcomes. The vast majority of the studies examined samples consisting of white American Protestant females. One exception was a British study on the fourteen-month outcome of bereavement among 135 relatives of patients admitted to a center for palliative care.(35) Spiritual beliefs, as assessed with the Royal Free interview on religious and spiritual beliefs, (36) had a modest but robust association with a better grief outcome, even after adjustment for baseline depression scores. Because of the mixed and modest effects, Becker and colleagues concluded that the issue of whether religion is related to the grief outcome has not been resolved.(34) They comment that religious and spiritual beliefs can be expected to affect many other aspects besides depressive symptoms, such as autonomy, personal growth, or engagement in social activities.

6. RELIGION AND BIPOLAR DISORDER

By definition, the question of how religion relates to bipolar disorder requires an approach that addresses both poles. First, an approach to the depressive pole would need to fit into the vulnerability-stress model described above. Other, complementary principles might have to do with the relationship between religiousness and the manic phase. This simple suggestion does not consider the fact that the depressive and manic phases occur in succession and often depend on each other. Furthermore, the vulnerability-stress model also applies to the manic pole, at least in the first episodes of bipolar disorder. (37) In view of the sensitization phenomenon, the provoking effect of environmental stressors increases over time with successive recurrent episodes of mania. This means that, over time, minor stressors or even minimal stress may be sufficient to provoke a new episode. A related feature of bipolar disorder over time is the *kindling phenomenon*,(37) where the frequency of the recurrent episodes gradually increases and symptom-free intervals tend to shorten. Bipolar disorder medical treatment regimes not only aim to minimize the affective disturbances during the episodes, but also to prevent recurrent episodes and at least prevent the bipolar cycle from accelerating. Besides prolonging the symptom-free intervals, another task in the treatment of bipolar disorder is to help patients accept that they have a chronic mental disease, assist with social rehabilitation, and prevent demoralization.

The relationship between religiousness and the two poles of bipolar disorder spectrum may thus follow the vulnerability-stress model, with an emphasis on factors relating to the (cyclic) course. Moreover, becoming aware of one's chronic vulnerability will not be easy for most patients. An acceptance of this unfortunate condition is conceptualized as a loss situation, a loss of career possibilities and social roles, relational losses, and a loss of mental stability itself. Any loss evokes grief reactions and complicated losses, in turn, complicate the grief process itself. The basic stages of grief according to Kübler Ross are outlined above.

Regarding the relationship between facets of religiousness and bipolar disorder, four aspects deserve special mention.

1 *Symptom formation.* Symptom formation factors play a role in the stress-vulnerability model, but in the case of mania, religiousness cannot be regarded as a peripheral factor. During mania, many patients experience states of enlightenment and increased religious motivation, which easily shift to the level of religious delusions. Although religious delusions are discussed in chapter 7, the question remains as regards the extent to which aspects of religiousness such as the religious tradition influence the emergence of increased religious insights and emotions during the manic state.

2 *Religious experiences during mania.* Bipolar patients sometimes tend to conceal the experiences they have during the mania from mental health professionals, but still ponder about them or even cherish the memory of their enlightened state or spiritual insights, irrespective of the negative consequences of the manic episode. How should these religious insights be viewed? Would they undermine the grief process? Or would they serve to help to maintain self-esteem?

3 *Religious preoccupations as early signs.* When bipolar patients intensify their religious involvement, this may in turn lead to religious and spiritual preoccupations. Mental health professionals often recognize religious preoccupations as early signs of a new manic episode. This provides an opportunity to prevent a recurrent episode, but patients discover that their religious life leads to distrust from their clinicians, who feel the urge and responsibility to focus on the biological treatment regime. So the element of religiousness is not only a special domain in the contact between the patient and the clinician, it is also laden with suspicion.

4 *Disillusionment with religion.* There is a fourth aspect that may be relevant to the depressive episode as well as the symptom-free interval. After the mania, enlightened spiritual experiences often lose their charm once the euphoria has faded away. In the depressive state and the symptom-free interval, disillusionment with religion and spirituality may be experienced. This may obstruct the grief about having to cope with a chronic mental disorder and represent an additional loss in life, the loss of trust in one's religion. Religiousness and bipolar disorder may thus be deeply intertwined in the dramatic euphoric manifestation as well as in the component of loss. Religion may become the subject of cycling itself.

So far, very few studies have been conducted on religiousness or spirituality and bipolar disorder. In 1969, Gallemore and colleagues described that conversion experiences were more than twice as prevalent in patients with mood disorders.(38) However, patients with bipolar disorder did not differ from a control group with respect to other aspects of religiousness. Similarly, the above-mentioned study by Levav and colleagues did not reveal any differences in the prevalence of manic episodes in people of various religious affiliations. (21) In a small sample of psychiatric inpatients, Kroll and Sheehan (39) noted that manic patients reported higher personal religious experience rates (55 percent) than depressed patients (25 percent) or a national sample (35 percent). Two other studies on patients with psychosis (40, 41) showed that the prevalence of religious delusions was about equal among manic patients and patients with schizophrenic psychosis and about twice as high as among patients with a psychotic depression.

Findings of this type show how religion emerges in the phenomenology of the mania. A hypothesis can be formulated about symptom-formation effects in that people with a religious background may express manic symptoms in a more religious way than others.

In a study on bipolar patients in Texas, African-Americans report higher levels of spiritual and religious coping than Caucasians.(42) In a New Zealand study on eighty-one bipolar outpatients in a stable phase, a majority of the patients reported having found support in their religious and spiritual beliefs,(43) but 40% said the bipolar disorder led to a decrease in their religious faith. Patients hospitalized in the past five years report a higher frequency of church attendance. Regarding the special relationship between religiousness and bipolar disorder, many other elements still need to be examined over time in empirical studies on patients in manic states, symptom-free intervals, and depressed states, and on the interaction between patients and clinicians.

7. RELIGION AND SUICIDE

Ever since Durkheim's *Le Suicide* was published in 1897, there has been considerable awareness that religion may affect and attenuate suicide rates. Durkheim hypothesized that suicide rates would be higher in societies with lower levels of social integration (*egoistic* suicide) or with rapid changes and decreases in social regulation (*anomic* suicide).(44) Because predominantly Protestant societies are more likely to have developed modern economies with less social integration and regulation, there is a sociological explanation for the higher suicide rates in Protestant countries. According to Durkheim, Roman Catholicism has adopted an antimodernist stance, which in turn might have led to lower suicide rates. Roman Catholicism thus holds a more traditional position, but the levels of social integration and regulation are generally not as extreme as to produce other risks (*altruistic* and *fatalistic* suicides). Although this brief summary does not do justice to the highly original and influential work by Durkheim, the role of religious traditions has changed in the course of the past century. Moreover, in applying Durkheim's theory, the methodological caveat of research at an aggregate level (for example, of regions or countries) implies that no inferences can be made about minorities within these aggregated entities (*ecological fallacy*). Suicide, as an event, is relatively rare, and extremely large samples with a longitudinal design are required to obtain the best evidence pertaining to individual processes. Furthermore, the reliability of official suicide records might vary with the prevailing religious and ethical views in, for example, Roman Catholic regions.

The sociologists Pescosolido and Georgianna have granted considerable insight into how religious affiliations related to suicide rates in a sophisticated analysis of suicide data from 1970 in the United States.(45) They showed that suicide rates were lower in regions with more Roman Catholics and higher in regions with more liberal Protestants. In regions with high church attendance and low interfaith marriage rates, suicide was strikingly rare. Pescosolido and Georgianna postulated that the risk of suicide increases if social networks generate poor integration (for example, among atheists) or overly tight regulation (for example, with members subjected to a strong religious regulative authority, as in religious sects). They suggested a U-shaped curvilinear relationship between suicide rates and the degree of social integration and regulation, as is generated by the religious climate.

A valuable cross-cultural insight is provided by Simpson and Conklin, who summarized their cross-national findings based on suicide statistics from seventy-one countries: the percentage of Muslims is inversely related to the suicide rate.(46) Controlling for economic, social, and demographic characteristics did not eliminate the effect of Islam, and Simpson and Conklin also tried to discount the reliability level of the suicide statistics. As a possible explanation, the authors referred to Durkheim's theory on social integration and regulation, because Islam fosters a close religious community that orders the daily life of the adherents.

There are other explanations besides social integration for the lower suicide rates in regions with higher levels of religious affiliation. Neeleman and colleagues demonstrated in a cross-national analysis that religious beliefs were strongly associated with limited tolerance of suicide, and that, in turn, limited tolerance of suicide was more relevant to the association with suicide rates than religious involvement as such.(47) In an extensive sociological overview, Stack contended that only a few core religious beliefs (for example, in an afterlife) and prayer help prevent suicide.(48)

In a recent overview of the literature, Colucci and Martin described the main patterns in the empirical findings about religion and suicide.(49) They conclude that religious factors are generally associated with lower suicide ideation, more negative attitudes toward suicide, and lower suicide attempt rates. They feel, however, that many of the studies need to be replicated in other samples and cultures. Far more research has been conducted about religion and suicide statistics, and most of it indicates that various aspects of religiousness offer some protection against suicide.

In short, religion does seem to provide some protection against suicidal thoughts and behavior via better social integration (for example, embeddedness in a religious group), the contents of religious beliefs, or adherence to social norms such as the nonapproval of suicide. One of the few studies with individual data on religion and suicide should be cited here because of its revealing results.(50) Sorri and colleagues presented retrospective clinical data and interviews with the relatives of 1,348 individuals who committed suicide in Finland in 1988. They noted that a history of inpatient psychiatric treatment and a diagnosis of psychotic or depressive disorder were more common among religious people (18 percent). Sorri and colleagues concluded that their findings tended to imply that a higher level of mental suffering was necessary among the religious before suicide occurred.

8. A SUMMARY OF EMPIRICAL FINDINGS PERTAINING TO MOOD DISORDERS

In the following brief overview, eight statements are made that relate to the empirical findings.

1 [extensive evidence] Religiousness relates to some degree to better mental health in the community and represents a source of adaptive coping in times of adversity.
2 [some evidence] The recovery rate from depression is substantially better for patients who attach intrinsic value to their religious faith and patients involved in a religious community.
3 [good evidence] During depressive episodes, negative feelings such as discontent toward God or feeling abandoned by God are highly prevalent.
4 [some evidence] Religious beliefs and practices are equally common among psychiatric inpatients, including the depressed; the frequency of prayer may be even higher, irrespective of whether it leads to recovery from depression.
5 [some evidence] Depressed patients with a Christian background may be more likely to present with feelings of guilt.
6 [no evidence] During manic episodes, religious beliefs may transform, either via delusional inflation or via possibly more meaningful spiritual enlightenment, but tend to become the subject of cycling itself and to be surrounded by suspicion and disillusionment.
7 [mixed evidence] Religiousness may help people cope with bereavement and may lead to a better grief outcome, although it is uncertain whether this means less depression.
8 [sociological evidence] Religion may have a small protective effect against suicidal thoughts and behaviors, but should not be overestimated in the context of other risk factors.

9. APPLICATIONS TO CLINICAL PRACTICE

9.1. Why Raise the Subject of Religion and Spirituality in Clinical Contacts?

It might seem only logical to some clinicians, nurses, or therapists that religion and spirituality should be included as a regular theme, although this notion may meet with hesitation and even reluctance in others. Because the subject has multifarious aspects such as strict morality and adherence to literal beliefs and intolerance toward people of other faiths, feelings of embarrassment or annoyance are lurking or can provoke the conviction that the clinician does not have sufficient knowledge about religion and spirituality. Although some awareness of one's limitations often makes sense in mental health care, there can be advantages to discussing religiousness in clinical contacts. It might be worth considering and may outweigh the uneasiness described above.

The first assumption here is that mental problems in general and mood disorders in particular often raise questions about the meaning of life. This can either pertain to loss of meaning, or the revelation that one's life can be experienced at summits of meaning itself. Avoiding the matter of the meaning of life, whether accompanied by presumptions of a transcendent reality or not, may hide a relevant domain of the patient's life.

Without going into the field of pastoral care and theology, there are two practical ways to include religion and spirituality in clinical contacts with patients with mood disorders. The first is by examining in the diagnostic phase whether religious or spiritual ideas manifest themselves as psychiatric symptoms or seem to color the expression of symptoms. The second is by establishing a mutual understanding regarding how spirituality and religiousness represent a relevant domain in life. This can be an investment in the therapeutic relationship, and at some time in the treatment phase, it can lead to a referral to a pastoral counselor.

9.2. Diagnostic Phase

9.2.1. Depression

Patients with depressive disorders do not often spontaneously share their religious and spiritual views, questions, or experiences with their clinician or therapist. Particularly in the case of depressed patients, due to their tendency toward inhibition or poverty of speech, many elements in the diagnostic interview need to be raised actively by the interviewer. This requires additional efforts by the interviewer to get an impression of the patient's inner conflicts and private concerns, including remnants of hope. An open inquiry should avoid rapid conclusions about which problems might bother the patient the most. The investigation of mood, anxiety, substance use, psychotic experiences, physical state, and suicidal ideation all deserve equal attention. In the initial contact, the subject of spirituality and religiousness may be only briefly cited to show the patient that the subject will not necessarily be ignored in the future.

Several signs of depression can be experienced in a way relating to religion. With respect to depressive mood and anxiety, cognitions such as attributions of the currently depressed state to moral punishment may arise and connect to feelings of guilt or worthlessness. Anhedonia, energy loss, concentration problems, and fatigue may connect to a lack of purpose in everyday life and be related to a sense of abandonment by God or loss of an inner spiritual spark. As the evidence of discontent with God in times of depression proves to be fairly solid, one might inform the patient that many depressed patients experience these feelings and ask whether the patient recognizes this theme. A lack of perspective, loss of hope, and loss of self-esteem may turn into thoughts about death or activate latent cognitive schemes about self-annihilation as a last resort. A neutral inquiry about possible belief in an afterlife, heaven or hell, or reincarnation for adherents to Hinduism or some contemporary spiritual movements can often be added in the discussion about pondering death.

9.2.2. Mania

When a patient is in a manic state, the clinician frequently has to try to regulate the contact and avoid conflicts that would ruin the chance of a working alliance with the patient. Furthermore, manic patients tend to be talkative and force the interviewer to listen to facts, achievements, and associations about which the relevance is uncertain. It can thus frequently take some time for the clinician to conclude to which extent there is disorder in the structure of thought. Once that clinical conclusion is arrived at, the contents of thoughts seem to escape further consideration. It may nevertheless be fascinating to continue and to record what manic patients reveal about their religious and spiritual insights. Patients frequently report feeling in contact with cosmic energies and having religious experiences. Whether these experiences are classified as spiritual, religious, or delusional does not always receive sufficient attention. An important caveat is that, during the mania, mixed emotions may be hidden: the religious perspective, once the clinician asks about it, may reveal thoughts about humility toward God, shame about their current state of overconfidence, unfortunate expectations about the future, or even suicidal thoughts.

9.2.3. Grief

Although not a regular reason for consulting mental health services, encounters with individuals who have lost a spouse or someone they were close to are not exceptional and often require the best skills of tactful and empathic communication. An early inquiry about whether religion may in some way be a source of consolation or relief may reflect the clinician's personal reaction to manage a difficult and emotionally demanding subject. Emotional reactions to unanticipated situations tend to come in waves. Empathic listening and a focus on primary needs such as contact with relatives or friends may be more relevant in the first phase than inquiring about religion. A brief allusion to the subject of religion or spirituality can let the patient know that the subject will be open for discussion when the time comes. The mental health care professional can ask whether there are any religious rituals that can or should take place.

9.2.4. Suicidal Thoughts

Professional guidelines in several Western countries recommend a systematic suicide risk assessment. A rigid systematic approach should, however, be more than counterbalanced by an empathic approach to facilitate an alliance with the patient, which can serve as a life-saving bridge in moments of crisis. Two elements in the risk assessment may relate to religion or spirituality. First, the estimate of remaining hope: hopelessness occupies a central position in the development of suicidal thoughts. What sources of hope remain? For those with religious or spiritual faith, a perspective of hope may still be attainable. Second, to a certain extent religion itself has been shown to prevent suicide. However, this effect, examined in suicide statistics at aggregated levels, should not be estimated as more than modest. As a rule, the risk of suicide in situations of loss, severe depression, or psychosis and in people who experience hopelessness cannot completely be compensated by religiousness or spirituality.

9.3. Connect: Abridging Personal Styles

Discussing the patient's religious and spiritual history and experiences may provide an opportunity to examine the expression of psychopathology in religious terms, as well as to address existential questions and the potential of hope. Nevertheless, knowledge about what we can conclude from empirical research may not be sufficient. Patients may inquire about the religious preferences of the clinician, nurse, or therapist. Moreover, they may express their beliefs in a way that evokes uneasy feelings. Individual religious convictions will almost always differ between two individuals (clinician and patient) and tend to be very personal. Small differences might be noticed with even greater sensitivity than huge differences that are simply there because someone was raised in a different culture.

Another reason for feelings of uneasiness might be more relevant in that it is not the contents of the religious or spiritual beliefs that differ but the cognitive, emotional, and moral style. James Fowler, as a scholar of the psychology of religion, provides some organizing principles in this connection.(51) In his monograph *Stages*

Table 8.2: Brief Summary of Fowler's Stages of Faith. (51) Stages Printed in Bold Appear to be Prevalent in Adult Samples (Wulff, 1991, pp. 399–402).(52)

Stage		Period
1. Intuitive-projective faith	Imagination and imitation	Ages 3 – 7
2. Mythic-literal faith	Story, drama and myth; concrete reciprocity	School age
3. Synthetic-conventional faith	Shaping of the personal myth; staying close to expectations by others	Adolescence
4. Individuative-reflective faith	Relativism, critical, demythologizing; own responsibility for one's faith	Adolescence
5. Conjunctive faith	Revaluation of early imagination, narratives and symbols; dialectical and paradoxical	Midlife
6. Universalizing faith	Inclusive of all being; unifying and transforming; contagious; decentration from self	Rare

of Faith, Fowler theorizes about levels of faith development that run more or less parallel to cognitive, intellectual, and moral development. Table 8.2 summarizes the stages with keynotes as short characterizations.

The stages of faith can be helpful in estimating one's own preferred level of apprehending religion and spirituality and that of others. Recognizing that others tend to communicate at a different stage may neutralize feelings of uneasiness to some degree, because it is apparent that others adhere to different themes and thematic expressions and have different expectations concerning how to interact about these themes. Many mental health care workers may recognize their own stage of faith as *individuative-reflective*, allowing for a critical and sometimes skeptical attitude toward religion and spirituality. Pious church members may feel more comfortable with *synthetic-conventional faith*. Awareness of different ways to experience beliefs according to a categorization like Fowler's may make it easier to communicate with the patient. Using Fowler's stages, however, entails the

risk of a higher stage being equated with higher spiritual achievements or moral qualifications. In principle, a neutral assumption might be that, at each level, people can experience their spiritual life in optima forma.

No research has been conducted yet on whether patients with mood disorders experience changes in their stage of faith. One might imagine how certain cognitions during depression could tend to demythologize religious beliefs and lead to disillusionment. Manic patients, on the other hand, may be convinced of their supreme insights at the level of universalizing faith, although this may be at odds with inflated self-esteem.

10. CONCLUSION

As a main principle in the application of religious and spiritual themes in clinical practice, one should not divert from regular treatment strategies. Excessive enthusiasm on the part of mental health workers with respect to religion should be examined as a sign of counter-transference. However, including religion and spirituality sometimes leads to a better understanding, patients who see religion or spirituality as relevant. The therapeutic relationship may become more personal, which enhances some of the nonspecific therapeutic factors as formulated by Rogers (53): genuineness, empathy, and unconditional positive regard. Here, finding and maintaining hope in times of despair or disillusion represent an ongoing matter of clinical care and sensitivity.

REFERENCES

1. Kessler RC, Berglund P, Demler O, Jin R, Merikangas KR, Walters EE. Lifetime prevalence and age-of-onset distributions of DSM-IV disorders in the National Comorbidity Survey Replication. *Arch Gen Psychiatry.* 2005;62:593–602.

2. Kessler RC, Chiu WT, Demler O, Walters EE. Prevalence, severity, and comorbidity of 12-month DSM-IV Disorders in the National Comorbidity Survey Replication. *Arch Gen Psych.* 2005;62:617–627.

3. World Health Organization. *The World Health Report 2001.* Burden of mental and behavioural disorders. Chap. 2. Geneva, Switzerland: WHO; 2001.

4. Brown GW, Harris TO. *Social Origins of Depression; A Study of Psychiatric Disorder in Women.* London: Tavistock; 1978.

5. Cohen S, Wills, TA. Stress, social support, and the buffering hypothesis. *Psychol Bull.* 1985;98:310–357.

6. Glock CY. On the study of religious commitment. *Relig Edu Res Suppl.* 1962;57:98–110.

7. Rizzuto AM. *The Birth of the Living God. A Psychoanalytic Study.* Chicago: University of Chicago Press; 1979.

8. Lans, JV. Empirical research into the human images of God. A review and some considerations. In: Ziebertz, H-G, Schweitzer F, Häring H, Browning D, eds. *The Human Image of God.* Leiden, Netherlands: Brill Academic Publishers; 2001:347–360.

9. Pargament KI. *The Psychology of Religion and Coping; Theory, Research, Practice.* New York; London: The Guilford Press; 1997.

10. Hackney CH, Sanders GS. Religiosity and mental health: a meta-analysis of recent studies. *J Sci Study Relig* 2003;42:43–55.

11. Smith TB, McCullough ME, Poll J. Religiousness and depression: evidence for a main effect and the moderating influence of stressful life events. *Psychol Bull.* 2003;129:614–636.

12. Ai AL, Dunkle RE, Peterson C, Bolling, SF. The role of private prayer in psychological recovery among midlife and aged patients following cardiac surgery. *Gerontologist.* 1998; 38:591–601.

13. Fitchett G, Burton LA, Sivan AB. The religious needs and resources of psychiatric inpatients. *J Nerv Ment Dis.* 1997;185:320–326.

14. Bosworth HB, Park H-S, McQuoid DR, Hays JC, Steffens DC. The impact of religious practice and religious coping on geriatric depression. *Int J Geriatr Psychiatry.* 2003;18:905–914.

15. Payman V, George K, Ryburn, B. Religiosity of depressed elderly inpatients. *Int J Geriatr Psychiatry.* 2008;23:16–21.

16. Koenig HG, Pargament KI, Nielsen J. Religious coping and health status in medically ill hospitalized older adults. *J Nerv Ment Dis.* 1998;186:513–521.

17. Braam AW, Beekman ATF, Deeg DJH, Smit JH, Tilburg WV. Religiosity as a protective or prognostic factor of depression in later life; results from a community survey in the Netherlands. *Acta Psychiatr Scand.* 1997;96:199–205.

18. Koenig HG. Religion and remission of depression in medical inpatients with heart failure/pulmonary disease. *J Nerv Ment Dis.* 2007;195:389–395.

19. Braam AW, Sonnenberg CM, Beekman ATF, Deeg DJH, Tilburg WV. Religious denomination as a symptom-formation factor of depression in older Dutch citizens. *Int J Geriatr Psychiatry.* 2000;15:458–466.

20. Stompe T, Ortwein-Swoboda G, Chaudhry HR, Friedmann A, Wenzel T, Schanda H. Guilt and depression: a cross-cultural comparative study. *Psychopathology.* 2001;34:289–298.

21. Kendler KS, Liu X-Q, Gardner CO, McCullough ME, Larson D, Prescott CA. Dimensions of religiosity and their relationship to lifetime psychiatric and substance use disorders. *Am J Psychiatry.* 2003;160:496–503.

22. Levav I, Kohn R, Golding JM, Weissman MM. Vulnerability of Jews to affective disorders. *Am J Psychiatry.* 1997;154:941–947.

23. Braam AW, Beekman ATF, Eeden PV, Deeg DJH, Knipscheer CPM, Tilburg WV. Religious climate and geographical distribution of depressive symptoms in older Dutch citizens. *J Affect Disord.* 1999;54:149–159.

24. Meador KG, Koenig HG, Hughes DC, Blazer DG, Turnbull J, George LK. Religious affiliation and major depression. *Hosp Community Psychiatry.* 1992;43:1204–1208.

25. Fitchett G, Murphy PE, Kim J, Gibbons JL, Cameron JR, Davis JA. Religious struggle: prevalence, correlates and mental health risks in diabetic, congestive heart failure, and oncology patients. *Int J Psychiatr Med.* 2004;34:179–196.

26. Braam AW, Schaap-Jonker H, Mooi B, Ritter D, Beekman ATF, Deeg Djh. God image and mood in old age; results from a community-based pilot study in the Netherlands. *Mental Health Relig Cult.* 2007;11:221–237.

27. McCullough ME, Enders CK, Brion SL, Jain AR. The varieties of religious development in adulthood: a longitudinal investigation of religion and rational choice. *J Pers Soc Psychol.* 2005;89:78–89.

28. Smith C. Theorizing religious effects among American adolescents. *J Sci Study Relig.* 2003;42:17–30.

29. Rew L, Wong YJ, Sternglanz RW. The relationship between prayer, health behaviors, and protective resources in school-age children. *Issues Compr Pediatr Nurs.* 2004;27:245–255.

30. Wong YJ, Rew L, Slaikeu KD. A systematic review of recent research on adolescent religiosity/spirituality and mental health. *Issues Ment Health Nurs.* 2006;27:161–183.

31. Kübler Ross E. *On Death and Dying.* London, UK: Tavistock Publications; 1969.

32. Kastenbaum R. *The Psychology of Death.* 3d ed. London, UK: Free Association Books; 2000:222.

33. Kirkpatrick LA. An attachment-theory approach to the psychology of religion. *Int J Psychol Relig.* 1992;2:3–28.

34. Becker G, Xander CJ, Blum HE, Lutterbach J, Momm F, Gysels M, Higginson IJ. Do religious or spiritual beliefs influence bereavement? A systematic review. *Palliat Med.* 2007;21:207–217.

35. Walsh K, King M, Jones L, Tookman A, Blizard R. Spiritual beliefs may affect outcome of bereavement: prospective study. *Br Med J.* 2002;324:1551–1555.

36. King M, Speck P, Thomas A. The Royal Free interview for religious and spiritual beliefs: development and standardization. *Psychol Med.* 1995;25:1125–1134.

37. Kupka RW, Post R. Kindling as a model for recurrent affective disorders. In: Trimble MR, Schmitz B, eds. *Seizures Affective Disorders and Anticonvulsant Drugs.* Guildford, UK: Clarius Press; 2002.

38. Gallemore JL, Wilson W, Rhoads J. The religious life of patients with affective disorders. *Dis Nerv Syst.* 1969;30:483–487.

39. Kroll J, Sheehan W. Religious beliefs and practices among 52 psychiatric inpatients in Minnesota. *Am J Psychiatry.* 1989;146:67–72.

40. Brewerton TD. Hyperreligiosity in psychotic disorders. *J Nerv Ment Dis.* 1994;182:302–304.

41. Appelbaum PS, Clark Robins P, Roth LH. Dimensional approach to delusions: comparison across types and diagnoses. *Am J Psychiatry.* 1999;156, 1938–1943.

42. Pollack LE, Harvin S, Cramer RD. Coping resources of African-American and white patients hospitalized for bipolar disorder. *Psychiatr Serv.* 2000;51:1310–1312.

43. Mitchell L, Romans S. Spiritual beliefs in bipolar affective disorder: their relevance for illness management. *J Affect Disord.* 2003;75:247–257.

44. Durkheim E. *Le Suicide* [Suicide]. Paris: Presses Universitaires de France; [1897] 1960.

45. Pescosolido BA, Georgianna S. Durkheim, suicide, and religion: toward a network theory of suicide. *Am Sociol Rev.* 1989;54:33–48.

46. Simpson ME, Conklin GH. Socioeconomic development, suicide and religion: a test of Durkheim's theory of religion and suicide. *Soc Forces.* 1989;67:945–964.

47. Neeleman J, Halpern D, Leon D, Lewis G. Tolerance of suicide, religion and suicide rates: an ecological and individual study in 19 Western countries. *Psychol Med.* 1997;27:1165–1171.

48. Stack S. Suicide: a 15-year review of the sociological literature; Part II: modernisation and social integration perspectives. *Suicide Life Threat Beh.* 2000;30:163–176.

49. Colucci E, Martin G. Religion and spirituality along the suicidal path. *Suicide Life Threat Beh.* 2008;38:229–244.

50. Sorri H, Henriksson M, Lönnqvist J. Religiosity and suicide: findings from a nation-wide psychological autopsy study. *Crisis.* 1996;17:123–127.

51. Fowler JW. *Stages of Faith.* San Francisco: Harper & Row; 1981.

52. Wulff DM. *Psychology of Religion: Classic and Contemporary Views.* New York: John Wiley & Sons; 1991.

53. Rogers CR. The necessary and sufficient conditions of therapeutic personality change. *J Consul Psychol.* 1957;21:95–103.

9 Spirituality and Substance Use Disorders

ALYSSA A. FORCEHIMES AND J. SCOTT TONIGAN

SUMMARY

Spiritual values and meanings are important determinants and regulators of behavior, and a treatment model that recognizes this component offers a more integrated view of how to best treat addiction. The authors of this chapter approach the interface of spirituality and addiction from the premise that individuals possess a fundamental desire for meaning and purpose – components central to spirituality – and that the difficulty in fulfilling these needs sometimes results in destructive methods of coping, including the problematic use of substances. The authors propose a model of how spirituality is involved in the development and recovery of addiction. We then review relevant research literature and current methodological questions that consider spirituality as an independent, dependent, moderating, or mediating variable. Finally, clinical and practical implementations will be discussed and augmented with case studies.

I. INTRODUCTION

Conceptions of spirituality and addiction are intimately tied together in the United States. Twelve-step programs, founded on the doctrine and prescribed spiritual practices of Alcoholics Anonymous (AA), are the dominant models for recovery from addiction. Therefore, it is hard to speak about addiction without speaking about spirituality.

Spirituality is also addiction's Tower of Babel. There is little consensus among both professionals and laypersons as to what spirituality is, how it relates to religion, how it should be measured, how it relates to recovery from substance use disorders, where it belongs in formal treatment, and how relevant it is for recovery. Strong opinions have been voiced both for and against the inclusion of spirituality in addiction treatment. Some argue that it is one of the most important resources by which people achieve and maintain sobriety, while others argue that including spirituality within formal treatment or mandating patients to twelve-step programs is unconstitutional and challenges the separation of church and state. Overall, then, spirituality has been a significant source of conflict within the treatment of substance use disorders, and consequently, clinicians fall along the spectrum in deciding to either emphasize or avoid discussing this subject with patients.

This is an evidence-based chapter intended to help guide clinical practice. The authors begin with a definition of spirituality. We then propose a model for understanding the role of spirituality in the development and recovery from addiction as one way practitioners might understand this interface. We present the roots of the long-standing interface between spirituality and addiction as stemming from the twelve-step model, rooted in spiritual practice and beliefs. Included in the overview of the twelve-step model is a discussion of the frequency and magnitude of spiritual transformations that are often experienced by individuals during the process of recovery from addiction. We also present studies that have attempted to move outside of the twelve-step model and systematically incorporate spiritual disciplines as an intervention for addiction. We then engage the reader in some of the current debates concerning the interface of spirituality and religion, including a discussion of how spirituality can be classified as an independent, dependent, moderating, or mediating variable. Finally, the authors highlight clinical implementations of why, who, how, and when clinicians should discuss spirituality with patients in addiction treatment. The empirical and theoretical findings are augmented with case studies.

2. DEFINING SPIRITUALITY

The topic of spirituality is receiving increased attention in addiction research, evidenced by a steady escalation in publications and funded research since 1980.(1) Within the research literature, however, there is lack of clarity in the definition of spirituality. It is often confused with religion even though spirituality and religion are distinct constructs.(2)

In a review of the literature on addiction and spirituality, Cook examined 265 publications to identify the definition of spirituality by different authors.(1) Cook found that only 12 percent of the papers explicitly defined the term *spirituality*, 32 percent offered a description of the concept of spirituality, 12 percent defined a related concept (such as "the spiritually healthy person"), and 44 percent of the papers left the term *spirituality* undefined. Breaking the conceptual content of the definitions into component parts, Cook classified the content of the various definitions into thirteen conceptual components.(1) Cook found that the four components that were encountered most frequently and were most central to the definition of spirituality were transcendence, relatedness, core/force/soul, and meaning/purpose.(1) On the basis of Cook's descriptive analyses, a working hypothesis definition was proposed. Cook's definition (1) highlights the main components of how spirituality is understood within the addiction literature:

Spirituality is a distinctive, potentially creative and universal dimension of human experience arising both within the inner subjective awareness of individuals and within communities, social groups, and

traditions. It may be experienced as relationship with that which is intimately "inner," immanent and personal, within the self and others, and/or as relationship with that which is wholly "other," transcendent and beyond the self. It is experienced as being of fundamental or ultimate importance and is thus concerned with matters of meaning and purpose in life, truth and values (pp. 548–549).

3. THEORETICAL RATIONALE FOR THE RELATIONSHIP BETWEEN SPIRITUALITY AND ADDICTION

3.1. The Role of Spirituality in the Development of Addiction

There is, in human nature, a desire to connect with that which is beyond the self; that which gives life meaning. Despite this yearning, individuals are distracted from spiritual seeking as they are pulled toward the material world and offered alternative ways to silence this spiritual longing. Ram Dass (3) wrote:

It's not difficult to recognize how deep are the ways our mind has been conditioned to deal with unpleasant situations by resisting them. Throughout our whole lives we have been encouraged to do anything we can to escape from rather than to explore and investigate unpleasantness. ... It's not just physical pain we try to avoid, but all kinds of unpleasant conditions: boredom, restlessness, self-doubt, anger, loneliness, loss, feelings of unworthiness. In our culture we do all we can to push these experiences aside, or keep them at a distance. We choose to be entertained. (1985, p. 79)

Enticed by the temporary comfort that is offered through the use of a substance, an individual begins to see substance use as the shortcut to wellbeing. Gerald May (4) wrote, "If God indeed creates us in love, of love, and for love, then we are meant for a life of joy and freedom, not endless suffering and pain. But if God also creates us with an inborn longing for God, then human life is also meant to contain yearning, incompleteness, and lack of fulfillment" (p. 179). Absolving the state of yearning with a placating substance is an enticing alternative to the quest for spiritual fulfillment.

The writings of Alcoholics Anonymous echo this innate sense of awareness that a God concept resides "deep down in every man" (p. 55).(5) One of the founding moments of AA was a letter Bill Wilson, the co-founder of AA, received from Carl Jung. Bill W. had written to Jung telling him about the conversion experience and subsequent sobriety of Roland, a former patient of Jung's who had been told he was a hopeless alcoholic whose only possibility of recovery was through a spiritual experience. Jung's letter stated that he believed that Roland's "craving for alcohol was the equivalent, on a low level, of the spiritual thirst of our being for wholeness; expressed in the medieval language: the union with God" (p. 69).(6) Jung continued, "You see, 'alcohol' in Latin is spiritus, and you use the same word for the highest religious experience as well as for the most depraving poison. The helpful formula therefore is: *spiritus contra spiritum*" (p. 70).(6) Alcohol serves as a substitute for spirituality: without effort, the use of a substance offers a sensation that brings one nearer to the divine.

Gerald May (7) wrote, "Chemical abuse and dependency constitute for me the sacred illness of our time. In few other conditions does one come up so definitely against the fierce line between grace and personal willpower" (1992, pp. 160–161). Addiction characterizes an effort to control; it is an attempt to fill a spiritual void with chemical reality. As a consequence, rather than cultivating a stronger inner self and reinforcing one's inner strength, addiction moves individuals away from the core of their being. In the search for a simple solution, the use of a substance offers an instantaneous way to quiet restless thoughts, suppress discomforting feelings, and soothe the inside with something from the outside.

Sanderson and Linehan (8) describe attachment as "the mind's habitual clinging to feelings, thoughts, and behaviors that are ineffective or not reality based" (p. 205). Attachment to a substance is a futile attempt to impose direction in one's life; a direction that displaces one's prior values, meaning structures, and goals. Instead, individuals become concerned with purposeful action toward their next drink or their next high. In Tillich's (9) terminology, the substance becomes the individual's ultimate concern. The topic of attachment is apparent in the diagnosis of substance use disorders – part of the criteria for substance use disorders is that a great deal of time is spent in activities necessary to obtain the substance (American Psychiatric Association, 1994). May (4) describes the spiritual nature of addiction as "a deep-seated form of idolatry. The objects of our addictions become our false gods. These are what we worship, what we attend to, where we give our time and energy" (1991, p. 13).

Addiction also involves a setting apart from one's self, others, and the world – a direct opposition to spirituality's emphasis of oneness with all of humanity. The use of substances offers a way to "avoid being present to oneself" (p. 44).(4) Isolation from one's self is made possible through the distancing of self-awareness. Hull (10) proposed that alcohol reduces the user's level of self-awareness, thereby decreasing sensitivity to information about present and past behavior. If behavior "is, or has been, inappropriate and liable to self and other criticism, then a reduction in self-awareness may provide a source of psychological relief" (p. 138).(11) It is common for individuals with substance use problems to report that they feel disconnected from others, and as attachment to the substance increases there is a tendency to isolate from important relationships. In AA, a common term is "terminal uniqueness," describing the alcoholic's perception of extreme uniqueness and alienation from his or her peers. In Buber's (12) terms, isolation implies an I-It relationship, where others are viewed as a means to an end, echoing this idea of detachment from others.

From this perspective, substance use represents an attempt to fill a spiritual vacuum. The spiritual components of transcendence, relatedness, meaning and purpose, and core/force/soul are, using Jung's aphorism *spiritus contra spiritum*, displaced by the use of psychoactive substances. In an attempt to take the easier path to spiritual enlightenment, substance use moves the individual toward attachment and isolation and farther away from what they actually seek: purpose in life and connection to others. In this conceptualization, a path out of addiction is to increase one's spirituality as a way to find meaning and purpose.

3.2. The Role of Spirituality in Recovery from Addiction

The choice then, to continue to rely on self or to turn to something higher, is a risk of faith and is a source of ambivalence for many seeking treatment for substance use disorders. Recovery requires giving up the demand to control one's experience. Within Alcoholics Anonymous, the term *powerlessness* embodies the paradox of surrender: gaining more control by giving up control to something greater. Cole and Pargament (13) describe this process as one in which "the individual begins to see the self in relationship to a higher purpose or transcendent reality rather than the center of the world" (p. 185). In other words, "Our deep desire for this is not simply a spineless need to be without responsibility; rather it is a heartfelt longing to give ourselves, in love and honesty, to someone or something truly worthy" (p. 302).(14)

May (14) describes willingness as a "surrendering of one's self-separateness, an entering-into, an immersion in the deepest processes of life itself" (p. 6). The spiritual practices of prayer, meditation, and fasting are practices that require increased self-control and foster increased self-awareness. These practices require an acceptance of mystery, powerlessness, and an increase in self-awareness. Willingness implies humility and represents "spirituality's concern to preserve the sense of awe in the presence of mystery and an awareness of the strengths tapped by

an admission of powerlessness" (p. 40).(15) The reliance on a higher power is an act of willingness. The individual must exercise the willingness to accept acceptance, which, in Tillich's (9) terms is an act of faith. The acceptance of one's finitude represents a significant gain in spiritual maturity.

Hope is found in the discovery of a power greater than one's self and an openness to that which is beyond the realm of human understanding. In the spiritual sense, hope emerges after one turns toward meaningful existence with humility. Hope implies an effort to search for, find, and cling to something significant in living, and the willingness to accept the mystery of life. As Frankl (16) wrote, "Existence falters unless there is a strong ideal to hold on to" (p. 50). One way that hope is elicited is through the process of identifying one's personal values in a way that offers inner structure.(17) This increase in value-behavior consistency stems from an ability to see beyond and accept one's circumstance rather than dull one's feelings through the use of a substance. A hopeful attitude allows an individual to relate to oneself and others with a new outlook.

Frankl (16) highlighted humans' most fundamental similarities when he wrote, "There is no human being who may say that he has not failed, that he does not suffer, and that he will not die" (p. 73). Spirituality increases by focusing on similarities rather than differences and by opening one's self in a trusting relationship. As one shares personal experiences, trust and closeness inevitably develop, which enrich both individuals' appreciation of their humanity. It is a realization that allows an individual to feel cohesion and structure, knowing there is a transcendent core to which everything is connected. Here, the self and others are viewed as ends in themselves, reflecting Buber's I-Thou (12) relationship that involves an open, sharing, and complete relationship with another. In the culmination of spiritual gain, an individual reestablishes a connection to life and others.

From the perspective of a spiritual model of recovery from addiction, individuals engage in the process of moving toward increased meaning with a different perspective toward others and self. Reconnection is established to others and individuals are no longer in need of a substance to fill the innate desire for spiritual longing.

4. EMPIRICAL FINDINGS

4.1. Categorizing Research on Spirituality and Addiction

Geppert, Bogenschutz, and Miller (18) developed a comprehensive annotated bibliography on spirituality and addictions. A total of 1,353 papers met search criteria and were subsequently classified into ten categories, including spiritual practices and development and recovery, measurement of spirituality and addiction, and religious and spiritual interventions. Inverse relationships between religiousness and spiritual practices and substance use were consistently observed. Of the empirical studies reporting results of spiritual interventions for substance users, transcendental meditation and other forms of meditation were found to produce significantly reduced substance use. Finally, although there appears to be a consistently positive relationship between twelve-step attendance and involvement and various measures of spirituality or religiosity, a causal role of spiritual or religious change resulting from twelve-step participation has received mixed support, at best. The authors note that a majority of the research in spirituality and addiction has been concentrated in a few areas and point to a need for longitudinal and prospective studies that begin to explore the mechanisms of action of spirituality.

4.2. Twelve-Step Programs: A Spiritual Approach to Recovery from Addiction

In the recovery from substance use, researchers are beginning to address spirituality and religion as important factors, a long overdue realization the recovery program of Alcoholics Anonymous has promoted since 1935.(19) In the words of Bill W., the co-founder of Alcoholics Anonymous, those with substance abuse problems "have been not only mentally and physically ill, [they] have been spiritually sick" (p. 64).(5) In twelve-step programs such as Alcoholics Anonymous, members engage in specific prescribed behaviors to facilitate spiritual growth.

From the perspective of twelve-step programs, individuals must embrace the simplicity and submission of spiritual surrender and give up the need for heroic mastery of their own life.(5) Submission is apparent in the first step, as the process of surrender requires individuals to give up independence for proper dependence on God. Confession is also a part of the twelve-step tradition, when a member admits to himself or herself and others that he or she is an alcoholic. This theme is echoed again in the fifth step, when an individual admits to God, himself or herself, and another human being the exact nature of his or her wrongs.(5) Brenda Miller (20) argued that spiritual modeling, which she defined as "observing other persons who are exemplary in modeling spiritual practices," is a mechanism for the transmission of spirituality in AA (p. 233).(5) In AA, learning through modeling occurs as members share their experiences of "strength and hope" and work with a sponsor who has an understanding of the spiritual nature of the program.

4.3. Spiritual Transformations in Recovery from Addiction

Evidence of the importance of spirituality within an addiction population was supported in a study conducted by Robinson, Brower, and Kurtz.(21) Results of this study included the significant finding that 54.4 percent of patients entering treatment for alcohol problems had, at some time in their lives, had a life-changing spiritual or religious experience, compared to 39.1 percent in a large national survey. Alcoholics Anonymous holds that spiritual transformations are the mechanism for change and therefore transformational experiences are an important component of the AA program. The twelfth step assures "having [had] a spiritual awakening as a result of these steps" (p. 60).(5) Within Alcoholics Anonymous, the spiritual transformation is understood as the means to move from destructive independence to proper dependence on God and others.(22) The experience of a spiritual transformation in AA is defined by its ability to hold great personal significance, change self-perception, and enhance one's relationship to God and the world (Alcoholics Anonymous, 2001). These experiences are discrete and often occur in the absence of any significant external event and result in profound lasting changes, including stable sobriety. AA argues, however, that gradual processes, such as the kind described by James (23) in *The Varieties of Religious Experience*, are equally valid to the instantaneous variety.

In a study of Alcoholics Anonymous members who experienced transformational spiritual change,(24) findings indicated that prior to the transformational experience, most participants reported low levels of happiness, desire to live, feeling of being in control, having close and loving relationships with others, satisfaction with their life, a sense of meaning in their life, or a close relationship with God. After the transformational experience, participants reported an increase in happiness, the desire to live, satisfaction with their life, a sense of meaning in their life, and a closer relationship with God.

4.4. Moving Beyond Twelve-Step Programs: Research on Spirituality as a Protective Factor

The benefit of considering spirituality in the treatment of addiction has been advocated outside twelve-step treatment modalities, although a systematic integration has yet to be proposed.(22, 25) Spirituality and religiosity are well-known protective factors that consistently predict lowered risk of alcohol and drug abuse.(26, 27) According to Stewart,(28) who studied college students' spiritual and religious beliefs and their use of alcohol and drugs, spirituality was a protective factor in the decision of whether to use substances. The inverse relationship between spirituality and substance use is further supported by research on the role of spirituality in recovery. In a study of forty individuals in recovery from alcohol dependence, Jarusiewicz (29) reported that individuals maintaining sobriety indicated more evidence of spirituality than those who returned to problematic drinking.

What remains unknown, however, is whether it is spirituality that protects or whether it is the community or some other factor associated with spirituality that accounts for the lower substance use.

4.5. Research on Spiritual Disciplines in the Treatment of Addiction

Spiritual disciplines offer a way for individuals to increase their overall spiritual health through the use of specific practices. Practices such as meditation, service, and celebration promote lifestyle changes that foster spiritual development. Research evidence has supported the role of some of these disciplines as an intervention in the treatment of addiction. Inward disciplines, such as meditation, offer avenues of personal reflection and change. Outward disciplines, such as service, promote outward actions and lifestyle changes. The corporate disciplines, such as confession and celebration, bring us nearer to one another and to God.

In a review of the literature, three spiritual practices have received research attention. These practices are rooted in religious traditions, clearly indicating that religious resources have been brought to bear in addiction treatment.

Meditation. The practice of silent centering. The term *contemplation* is also reserved here for practices of silent centering, and thus is interchangeable with meditation. Marlatt and Kristeller (30) described the clinical effectiveness of meditation as a treatment for substance use disorders, and Witkiewitz, Marlatt, and Walker (31) offered preliminary data in support of mindfulness meditation as a treatment for addictive behavior.

Prayer. Prayer differs from but overlaps with meditation, with its primary purpose being encounter, communication, and communion with the Divine. Johnsen (32) found that individuals who used prayer and meditation following a twenty-eight-day inpatient treatment showed better treatment outcomes at a six-month follow-up.

Acceptance. There is a dialectic tension between accepting what is and seeking to change it, that is captured in the famous "serenity prayer" that has been adapted and widely used within Alcoholics Anonymous: "God grant us grace to accept with serenity the things that cannot be changed, Courage to change the things which should be changed, And the wisdom to distinguish the one from the other." Also included in the discipline of acceptance is the forgiveness of the self and others and the act of submission, giving up independence for a proper dependence on God. According to Lin and colleagues,(33) individuals randomized to an adjunct forgiveness intervention reported lower depression, anxiety, and substance use at a four-month follow-up.

Other than these studies that have examined the role of specific spiritual disciplines in the treatment of addictions, many other specific spiritual practices have not been studied empirically. Research is still in the early stages in determining which spiritual disciplines may predict positive outcomes better than others.

5. WHAT ROLE DOES SPIRITUALITY PLAY IN SUBSTANCE USE REDUCTION?

Spirituality has been studied from distinct perspectives, and it is extremely important to distinguish these perspectives when describing the role of spirituality in recovery. Spirituality has, for example, been investigated as it directly affects substance use (independent variable). In contrast, spirituality has also been investigated as an outcome arising from prescribed practices intended to reduce substance use (dependent variable). Third, spirituality has also been studied as a moderating variable in which people with some faith characteristic are more (or less) likely to accept spiritual interventions. And, finally, spirituality has been investigated as a mediator or mechanism variable that explains why particular behaviors are predictive of substance use reductions.

5.1. Spirituality as an Independent Variable

Spirituality has received mixed support as having a direct effect on later substance use. In a

recent book, *Sober for Good* (2001), Fletcher (34) discussed pathways to sobriety and noted, "Comments related to spirituality were among the five most frequent responses to open-ended questions about key things … used to get sober and stay sober" (p. 239). Additionally, Flynn, Joe, Broome, Simpson, and Brown (35) reported that 63 percent of their sample indicated that strength from spirituality was reported as an important factor in the recovery from cocaine dependence, and Koski-Jannes and Turner (36) found that spirituality was a factor associated with better maintenance of treatment gains.

Evidence of the importance of spirituality within an addiction population was also supported in a study conducted by Robinson, Brower, and Kurtz.(21) Results of this study included the background finding that 54.4% of patients entering treatment for alcohol problems had experienced, at some time in their lives, a life-changing spiritual or religious experience, compared to 39.1 percent in a large national survey. Participants in the Robinson et al.(21) study also rated their spirituality higher than their religiosity, and higher than did the national sample. Most important, after statistically controlling for self-reported frequency of AA attendance, positive gains in spiritual beliefs and practices significantly predicted reduced substance use.

It is important to note that, although patients' endorsement of the importance of spirituality tends to be high in case studies and the empirical literature, there is a larger body of work to the contrary. For example, the magnitude of the relationship between spirituality/religiosity scores measured at intake among an alcohol dependent sample (N = 1,726) and abstinence from alcohol (at a twelve-month follow-up) in an examination of Project MATCH participants was small and not clinically meaningful (37) albeit statistically significant. Finally, Miller, Forcehimes, et al.(38) conducted the first two systematic evaluations of the impact of a manual-driven intervention designed to explore and foster the practice of spiritual disciplines on addiction treatment outcomes. The authors anticipated that spiritual guidance would enhance spiritual experience and increase personal spiritual practices during follow-up, which, in turn, would affect substance use outcomes. In both trials, however, contrary to prediction, spiritual guidance had no effect on spiritual practices or substance use outcomes at any follow-up point.

5.2. Spirituality as a Dependent Variable

Robinson, Cranford, Webb, and Brower (39) reported significant six-month changes in spiritual and religious practices, daily spiritual experiences and forgiveness, positive religious coping, and purpose in life among their sample of substance abusers attending AA. Likewise, in Project MATCH, for example, 27.6 percent (n = 108) of the outpatient clients who attended AA during the twelve weeks of treatment (N = 391) also reported having had a spiritual awakening as a result of their AA attendance. In the aftercare sample, 569 clients reported attending some AA during treatment of which 29.3 percent (n = 167) reported a spiritual awakening in connection with AA attendance.(37) *Strong* evidence, across diverse measures of religiousness and spirituality, documents spiritual increases among AA members.

5.3. Spirituality as a Moderator Variable

A number of studies have investigated whether individual spiritual/religious beliefs and practices predispose a person to use spiritual-based interventions and, if so, whether they receive differential and improved benefit by attending such programs. Schermer and colleagues,(40) for example, reported that self-reported atheists were significantly less likely to attend AA relative to self-reported agnostics, spiritual, and religious persons. Interestingly, however, atheists who did attend AA reported equal benefit as religious and spiritual alcoholics. Likewise, Connors et al.(37) theorized that more spiritual/religious alcoholics would fare better when they received twelve-step facilitation therapy relative to cognitive behavioral or motivational enhancement therapy. Here, they reasoned that enhanced comfort with the therapeutic orientation of the spiritual-based

twelve-step therapy would produce improved outcomes. Contrary to predictions, neither compliance with therapy nor drinking outcomes differed for matched and mismatched alcoholics. More recently, Kelly et al.(41) reported that spiritual and religious beliefs of a sample of 160 adolescent inpatient substance abusers was unrelated to frequency of AA meeting attendance over an eight-year follow-up.

5.4. Spirituality as a Mediator Variable

It is possible that spirituality influences the causal pathway through a reduction of behavioral risks brought about by the promotion of a healthier lifestyle.(42) Spiritual disciplines, particularly those offering complex beliefs about human relationships, ethics, and life and death, are directly relevant to health, and spiritual feelings and thoughts might enhance coping skills. For instance, Krause (43) found that spiritual beliefs and practices were associated with higher self-esteem and feelings of self-worth, particularly among older adults. Ellison (44) reported a similar finding, indicating that individuals with a strong faith report feeling happier and more satisfied with their lives. Idler et al.(45) reported "spiritual interpretations of difficult circumstances may have the power to bring individuals to a state of peace of acceptance of a situation that cannot be altered and give them the ability to live with it" (p. 333).

Research support has also been found for physiological mechanisms that are altered through spiritual practices. Benson (46) found that certain spiritual practices (that is, prayer and meditation) elicited a "relaxation response," an integrated physiological reaction in opposition to the "stress response." This response resulted in a lowering of individuals' blood pressure, heart rate, and changes in brain wave activity.

Another possible mechanism is a social function that is altered through spiritual practices. Perhaps spirituality operates through an expansion of one's social support network by providing a sense of friendship and emotional support, such as that provided in a setting such as Alcoholics

Anonymous. The context of a spiritual community may be the protective factor, or it may be the community that is supportive of spirituality that accounts for the lower substance use. For instance, Kaskutas, Bond, and Humphreys (47) examined one-year outcomes in relation to AA participation and found that, although general support from others was associated with improvement in functioning, only specific support from AA members mediated abstinence. Additionally, having a greater number of sober individuals in one's social network was predictive of abstinence among alcohol-dependent persons.(48, 49)

6. SPIRITUALITY IN THE CLINICAL CONTEXT

6.1. Why Should Spirituality Be Discussed with Patients with Substance Use Disorders?

Within the larger framework of cultural sensitivity, spirituality is an issue that should not be compartmentalized as outside the psychotherapy domain. The separation between psychology and religion/spirituality stems from a long-standing antagonism between these fields.(50) Paralleling the recent increased attention spirituality is receiving in substance use research, it is also fairly recent in the clinical context that spirituality has been emphasized in the inclusive model of treating all the aspects of a person's experience. This complementary relationship is viewed as both helpful and respectful to the patients with whom practitioners work.

The word *religion* (re-ligare) is Latin for "to connect again," and this broadened definition expands the boundaries of organized religion to encompass a broader definition of spirituality and the emphasis on connection and meaning. Also, returning to the model described above, if addiction leads to disconnection (American Psychiatric Association, 1994) (7) following Jung's aphorism *spiritus contra spiritum*, spirituality is the natural path toward reconnection and is a particularly important consideration in the treatment of addictions.

6.2. Who Should Discuss Spirituality?

Although most clinicians regard their spirituality as important and regard religion as beneficial to psychological well-being, mental health practitioners remain much less religious than the general population.(50) Although patients often will regard spiritual and religious issues as directly relevant to their substance abuse problem, the therapist often will *not* be an expert in the spiritual/religious tradition of the patient and hence may not be qualified to offer advice within that tradition.

Many believe that leaders or experts in religion or spirituality are chosen or ordained to these positions after lengthy training and prayerful consideration. Research on the treatment of addiction suggests that practitioners delivering treatment do not need to have personal experience of addiction; rather the practitioner can use empathy in an attempt to understand the patient's situation.(51) Client-centered approaches, in particular, support the use of empathy as a way to create a collaborative relationship between the patient and practitioner. Thus, the skillful use of client-centered methods to draw out the patients' own meanings and understanding is perhaps more critical regarding patients' spiritual or religious journey than many other aspects of their psychological experience.

One consideration in determining who is qualified to discuss spiritual and religious issues with the patient concerns the difference between within-faith and between-faith interventions. Client-centered approaches are suitable for between-faith interventions, in which the therapist and patient's spiritual and religious beliefs are not necessarily convergent. When, however, a patient is seeking within-faith advice, it is then important for the therapist to recognize the need for expertise in this area and discern whether consultation is necessary or whether it is appropriate to refer the patient to someone more experienced and knowledgeable in this area. It is important to determine whether the patient's issue concerns a theological question that would be best addressed through a within-faith provider or a psychological issue that can be addressed using client-centered methods appropriate for between-faith interventions. It is also important for providers to be aware of referral sources and knowledgeable of local religious or spiritual leaders for consultation or referral purposes.

Given the lack of empirical data on the effectiveness of addiction counselors delivering spiritual guidance, it is important to consider how much expertise and knowledge the patient is seeking and or expecting from the practitioner. Practitioners must consider the possibility that a spiritual intervention may require the practitioner to be in more of an expert role and that providers need to have a sufficient level of expertise in the area of spirituality before addressing this issue with patients.

6.3. How to Raise the Issue of Spirituality

The question of how to raise the issue of spirituality with patients is a primary difficulty for practitioners and patients in addiction treatment. Some patients may not frame their dilemma as a spiritual one, others may have grown up without a spiritual vocabulary, and others may bear still-painful scars of exposure to toxic religion. Whatever the reason, many patients who wish to discuss spiritual issues may not know where to begin. Similarly, many providers struggle with how to raise this issue during assessment and treatment.

Open questions are a good place to start, because these questions challenge patients to reflect and to explore. Answering an open question requires not only content, but also some processing and organization of information. The provider therefore learns not only facts, but also something of how the person organizes meaning. These questions are appropriate during the clinical interview part of an assessment or during an intake or followup session as the provider begins to piece together the patient's narrative. Some examples of open questions to begin exploration of this area are

- What is your view of spirituality?
- To what/whom are you most committed in life?
- How do you understand the relationship between spirituality and addiction?

- How do you understand your purpose in life?
- What would you like to be different in your spiritual life a year from now?

6.4. When to Raise the Issue of Spirituality

Aside from mutual-help recovery programs, formal treatment programs rooted in a twelve-step model and specific treatments linking patients with twelve-step programs (for example, Twelve Step Facilitation), there is not an empirically based systematic approach for integrating spirituality in treatment. Therefore, there is little research regarding the timing of when a discussion of spirituality should be initiated or when spiritual growth should be encouraged.

The severity of the patient's substance use disorder may play a role in determining the most appropriate time to begin a discussion of spiritual issues. Findings from two recent clinical trials of a spiritual intervention delivered in an inpatient addiction treatment setting (Miller, Forcehimes, et al., in press) suggest that introducing spiritual exploration too early in treatment may be counterproductive. According to Maslow's (52) theory, people tend to fulfill needs in the hierarchical order of survival, safety, love and belongingness, esteem, self-actualization, and finally spiritual or transcendence needs. Perhaps, for individuals who are early in the recovery process, other needs are prioritized above spiritual ones, and the timing was not appropriate to attempt to facilitate spiritual growth. Severely substance-dependent individuals seeking treatment are often unemployed, lacking adequate social networks, struggling with housing and financial stressors, experiencing significant relationship conflicts, and often having complicated concurrent medical issues secondary to their substance use disorder. For these reasons, the authors suggested that patients' basic needs of safety, love, and survival were of greater necessity than working toward spiritual growth and that the intervention might have been better suited to aftercare.

This is not to suggest that it is definitely harmful to explore spirituality early on in treatment. This was a population with severe drug dependence, and alternative explanations for why the treatment effect was null are also plausible. Perhaps a discussion of spirituality is helpful early on in treatment, but encouragement to begin practicing specific spiritual disciplines was too burdensome during the early stages of recovery.

6.5. Case Studies

As we move into case studies of spirituality in addiction treatment, we offer three examples of how spirituality may play a part in treatment. The first is an example of how assessing a patient's spirituality can actually be considered treatment in and of itself. A second example is a vivid description of a spiritual transformation, which clinicians are likely to encounter and thus should be aware of the nature and magnitude of such a profound change.(21) Finally, the third case study describes a scenario in which it is appropriate for the clinician to refer the patient out for additional spiritual guidance.

Assessment as Treatment. In a recent clinical trial (53) designed to increase patients' practice of spiritual disciplines, an unexpected finding was that those assigned to the control condition still reported spiritual growth stemming only from the baseline assessment. The baseline assessment included several instruments designed to assess the patients' spiritual and religious background and beliefs. Unexpectedly, during the follow-up assessment, patients would often report things such as the following:

> I really started thinking about things after I did this first batch of paperwork. You know, since then, I realized how much I used to pray and how I'd really gotten away from that and I've started doing that again, you know, just praying to say thanks that I made it through another day, and asking God to watch over my kids, and stuff like that.

It seems then, that even though therapists may not directly explore issues of spirituality with a patient, the act of completing an assessment that included questions about the frequency of spiritual practices and religious attendance and involvement can increase levels of spiritual practice.

Understanding Profound Spiritual Transformations. Up to 54 percent of treatment-seeking individuals experience a profound spiritual experience that results in a magnitude of change.(21) Transformations are manifested dramatically, usually in a vivid, surprising manner without a salient external event. These events are highly significant for the individual experiencing them, and there is often a desire combined with a fear in discussing them with a professional. Understanding the nature of these experiences can assist in clinical work. Here is one such story:

> Jack had a troubled background, including sexual and physical abuse, exposure to gang violence, heavy drug and alcohol use, and financial struggles. He was a frequent drunk driver, but had never been given a DUI (driving under the influence of alcohol or an illicit substance). His transformational experience was a dream, which to him was more real than any dream he had ever experienced. In his mind's eye, he saw himself driving on the freeway after a long night of drinking. He hit the rail, the car spun, and he was involved in a head-on collision with another car. He could see himself getting out of the car, uninjured, to examine the damages. In the car, he saw the bloody wreckage of a family of four: the mother, in the passenger seat, was the only one breathing. The two small children had been thrown from the car, their small bodies distorted on the pavement, surrounded by pools of blood. The father had not been wearing his seatbelt and his head had gone through the windshield. Immediately sobered by the realization of

what he had done, he watched in horror as the mother got out of the car to examine the remains of her family. His dream flashed forward, and he saw himself in court, tortured by the agony of watching the mother sobbing. Then he saw himself in prison, unable to handle the misery he had imparted on this family. He awoke to reality just as he was losing consciousness in his dream as a result of hanging from the ceiling of his jail cell.

From the depths of despair, Jack woke up in a cold sweat and vowed to never drink or use again. And ten years later, he continues to keep that promise to himself.

In this case study, the issue is not so much how to evoke change or spiritual growth, but rather that the clinician should be aware of the nature of such experiences and be prepared to help the patients understand and integrate the experience within their spiritual framework.

Referring Out. Although we are encouraging the inclusion of spirituality, it is also important to note that there are times when referring the patient to someone within a particular religious tradition is acceptable and even advisable. Consider the following example:

Jon is a 52-year-old man seeking treatment for alcohol dependence. He was diagnosed with alcoholic cardiomyopathy and recently informed that the heart damage and heart failure was irreversible and that it is unlikely he will survive a heart transplant. During the intake session, Jon tells the therapist that he is a devout Catholic and that he has questions about whether or not he has lived a good enough life to go to heaven and whether God will forgive him. The therapist realizes that Jon is wanting specific answers related to a particular religious tradition, so arranges for Jon to meet with a priest once a week.

In this example, the therapist is aware that the patient is seeking theological rather than psychological questions regarding his religious background and the nature of sin and salvation. For this within-faith intervention that the patient is seeking, the therapist is correct to refer these questions to a clergy member. It may be appropriate for the practitioner to continue to see the patient for substance abuse treatment in adjunct to seeing the priest for end-of-life questions, and this should be discussed between patient and therapist to determine the patient's needs.

7. CONCLUSION

The traditions of Alcoholics Anonymous emphasize the vital importance of spiritual growth and transformation in recovery from substance dependence. Outside of the twelve-step model of recovery, spirituality is receiving increased attention, evidenced in both funded research and etiological and treatment models of addiction. Clinicians and researchers continue to be challenged by the complexity of defining what spirituality is (and is not), the perspectives by which it is classified, and how to systematically integrate it into addiction treatment. The authors have proposed one way of examining the development of addiction as related to spiritual deficit and recovery from addiction as related to spiritual growth. Clinicians are encouraged to explore, encourage, and support patients' spiritual background and desire for spiritual growth and are offered suggestions for how to integrate spirituality into the treatment of addictions.

REFERENCES

1. Cook CH. Addiction and spirituality. *Addiction.* 2004;99:539–551.
2. Miller WR, Thoresen CE. Spirituality, health, and the discipline of psychology. *Am Psychol.* 2004;59.1:54–55.
3. Dass R, Gorman P. *How Can I Help: Stories and Reflections on Service.* New York: Alfred A. Knopf; 1985.
4. May G. *Care of Mind/Care of Spirit.* San Francisco: Harper Collins; 1992.
5. AA World Services: *Alcoholics Anonymous: The Story of How Many Thousands of Men and Women*

Have Recovered from Alcoholism, 4th ed. New York: 2001.

6. Wilson BW, Jung CG. Spiritus Contra Spiritum. The Bill Wilson/C.G. Jung Letters, *The roots of the society of alcoholics anonymous. Parabola.* 1987;12:68–71.

7. May G. *Addiction and Grace.* San Francisco: Harper Collins; 1991.

8. Sanderson C, Linehan MM. Acceptance and forgiveness. In: Miller WR, ed. *Integrating Spirituality into Treatment: Resources for Practitioners.* Washington, DC: American Psychological Association; 1999:199–216.

9. Tillich P. *Dynamics of Faith.* New York: HarperCollins; 2001. (Original work published in 1957).

10. Hull JG, Toung RD, Jouriles E. Applications of the self-awareness model of alcohol consumption: predicting patterns of use and abuse. *J Pers Soc Psychol.* 1986;51:790–796.

11. Orford J. *Excessive Appetites: A Psychological View of Addictions,* 2nd ed. New York: John Wiley & Sons; 1985.

12. Buber M. *I and Thou.* New York: Simon & Schuster; 1970.

13. Cole B, Pargament K. Spiritual surrender: a paradoxical path to control. In: Miller WR, ed. *Integrating Spirituality into Treatment: Resources for Practitioners.* Washington, DC: American Psychological Association; 1999:179–198.

14. May G. *Will and Spirit.* San Francisco: Harper Collins; 1982.

15. Kurtz E. *Not-God: A History of Alcoholics Anonymous.* Hazelden: Center City, MN; 1999.

16. Frankl VE. *Man's Search for Meaning.* New York: Pocket Books; 1963.

17. Yahne CE, Miller WR. Evoking hope. In: Miller WR, ed. *Integrating Spirituality into Treatment: Resources for Practitioners.* Washington, DC: American Psychological Association; 1999:217–234.

18. Geppert C, Bogenschutz MP, Miller WR. Development of a bibliography on religion, spirituality and addictions. *Drug Alcohol Rev.* 2007;26.4:389–395.

19. Tonigan JS, Toscova RT, Connors GJ. Spirituality and the 12-step programs: a guide for clinicians. In: Miller WR, ed. *Integrating Spirituality into Treatment: Resources for Practitioners.* Washington, DC: American Psychological Association; 1999:111–132.

20. Miller B. Intergenerational transmission of religiousness and spirituality. In: Delaney H, Miller WR, eds. *Judeo-Christian Perspectives on Psychology: Human Nature, Motivation, and Change.* Washington, DC: American Psychological Association; 2005:227–244.

21. Robinson EA, Brower KJ, Kurtz E. Life-changing experiences, spirituality and religiousness of persons entering treatment for alcohol problems. *Alcoholism Treat Quart.* 2003;21.4:3–16.

22. Kurtz E. The historical context. In: Miller WR, ed. *Integrating Spirituality into Treatment: Resources for Practitioners.* Washington, DC: American Psychological Association; 1982:19–46.

23. James W. *Varieties of Religious Experience.* Mass Market Paperback; 1902.

24. Forcehimes AA, Feldstein SW, Miller WR. Glatt's curve revisited: the development of transformational change in Alcoholics Anonymous. *Alcoholism Treat Quart.* 2008;26:241–258.

25. Tonigan JS, Toscova RT, Connors GJ. Spirituality and the 12-Step programs: a guide for clinicians. In: Miller WR, ed. *Integrating Spirituality into Treatment: Resources for Practitioners.* Washington, DC: American Psychological Association; 1999:111–132.

26. Miller WR. Researching the spiritual dimensions of alcohol and other drug problems. *Addiction.* 1998;93:979–990.

27. Zimmerman MA, Maton KI. Life-style and substance use among male African-American urban adolescents: a cluster analytic approach. *Am J Comm Psychol.* 1992;20:121–138.

28. Stewart C. The influence of spirituality on substance use of college students. *J Drug Educ.* 2001;31:343–351.

29. Jarusiewicz B. Spirituality and addiction: relationship to recovery and relapse. *Alcoholism Treat Quart* 2000;18:99–109.

30. Marlatt GA, Kristeller JL. Mindfulness and meditation. In: Miller WR, ed. *Integrating Spirituality into Treatment: Resources for Practitioners.* Washington, DC: American Psychological Association; 1999:67–84.

31. Witkiewitz K, Marlatt AG, Walker D. Mindfulness-based relapse prevention for alcohol and substance use disorders. *J Cogn Psychother.* 2005;19:211–228.

32. Johnsen E. The role of spirituality in recovery from chemical dependency. *J Addict Offender Couns.* 1993;13:58–61.

33. Lin W, Mack D, Enright R, Krahn D, Baskin T. Effects of forgiveness therapy on anger, mood, and vulnerability to substance use among inpatient substance-dependent clients. *J Consul Clin Psychol.* 2004;72:1114–1121.

34. Fletcher A. *Sober for Good: New Solutions for Drinking Problems – Advice from Those Who Have Succeeded.* New York: Houghton Mifflin; 2001.

35. Flynn PM, Joe GW, Broome KM, Simpson DD, Brown BS. Looking back on cocaine dependence: reasons for recovery. *Amn J Addict.* 2003;12:398–411.

36. Koski-Jannes A, Turner N. Factors influencing recovery from different addictions. *Addict Res.* 1999;7:469–492.

37. Connors GJ, Tonigan JS, Miller WR. Religiosity and responsiveness to alcoholism treatments: matching findings and causal chain analyses. In: Longabaugh RH, Wirth PW, eds. *Project*

MATCH: A Priori Matching Hypotheses, Results and Mediating Mechanisms. Rockville, MD: US Government Printing Office; 2001.

38. Miller WR, Forcehimes A, O'Leary M, LaNoue M. Spiritual direction in addiction treatment: two clinical trials. *J Subst Abuse Treat*, 2008;35:434–442.

39. Robinson EA, Cranford JA, Webb JR, Brower KJ. Six-month changes in spirituality, religiousness, and heavy drinking in a treatment-seeking sample. *J Stud Alcohol Drugs.* 2007;68:282–290.

40. Schermer C, Tonigan JS, Miller WR. Atheists, agnostics and alcoholics anonymous. *J Stud Alcohol.* 2002;63.5:534–541.

41. Kelly JF, Brown SA, Abrantes A, Kahler CW, Myers, M. Social recovery model: An 8-Year investigation of adolescent 12-step group involvement following inpatient treatment. *Alcohol Clin Exp Res.* 2008;32:1468–1478.

42. Gorsuch RL. Religious aspects of substance abuse and recovery. *J Soc Issues.* 1995;51:65–83.

43. Krause N. Religiosity and self-esteem among older adults. *J Gerontol Psychol Sci.* 1995;50B:236–246.

44. Ellison CG. Religious involvement and subjective well-being. *J Health Soc Beh.* 1991;32:80–99.

45. Idler EL, Musick MA, Ellison CG, et al. Measuring multiple dimensions of religion and spirituality for health research: conceptual background and findings from the 1998 General Social Survey. *Res Aging.* 2003;25:327–365.

46. Benson H. *The Relaxation Response.* New York: Avon; 1975.

47. Kaskutas LA, Bond J, Humphreys K. Social networks as mediators of the effect of alcoholics anonymous. *Addiction.* 2002;97:891–900.

48. Witbrodt J, Kaskutas LA. Does diagnosis matter? Differential effects of 12-step participation and social networks on abstinence. *Am J Drug Alcohol Abuse.* 2005;31:685–707.

49. Bond J, Kaskutas LA, Weisner C. The persistent influence of social networks and alcoholics anonymous on abstinence. *J Stud Alcohol.* 2003;64:579–588. In: Delaney H, Miller WR, eds. *Judeo-Christian Perspectives on Psychology: Human Nature, Motivation, and Change.* Washington DC: American Psychological Association; 2003:227–244.

50. Delaney HD, Miller WR, Bisonó AM. Religiosity and spirituality among psychologists: a survey of clinician members of the American Psychological Association. *Prof Psychol Res Pr.* 2007;38.5:538–546.

51. Miller WR, Rollnick S. *Motivational Interviewing,* 2nd ed. New York: Guilford Press; 2002.

52. Maslow AH. *Toward a Psychology of Being.* New York: Van Nostrand; 1968.

53. Forcehimes A. InSITE: Integrating spirituality into the inpatient treatment experience (Doctoral dissertation, University of New Mexico, 2007). Dissertation Abstracts International 2008;68:4822.

10 Religion, Spirituality, and Anxiety Disorders

HAROLD G. KOENIG

SUMMARY

Anxiety disorders are widely prevalent in the United States and around the world. Religious beliefs and activities are likewise prevalent and are often inversely correlated with anxiety symptoms. Furthermore, clinical trials show that religious therapies from a variety of religious traditions appear to improve anxiety disorder symptoms to a degree that is equal to or greater than traditional secular therapies. Religious involvement may also exacerbate anxiety in certain individuals, and anxious individuals may sometimes distort or manipulate religion to serve neurotic ends. Anxiety can also be a powerful motivation for religious activity as persons turn to religion to cope with the distress that anxiety causes. In this chapter, I

1 discuss whether religion is the cause or the consequence of anxiety disorder.
2 examine research on the relationship between religion and anxiety in specific disorders (generalized anxiety disorder, panic disorder, post-traumatic stress disorder, obsessive-compulsive disorder, and phobia).
3 illustrate how religion may improve or exacerbate anxiety with specific case examples.
4 examine implications for clinicians in the assessment and treatment of anxiety disorders (including specific ways that religion can be used in the management of anxiety disorder).
5 discuss how to untangle the complex interaction between religion and anxiety by consultation, referral, or co-therapy with pastoral counselors.

Anxiety, worry, and nervousness are common in today's society where the average person has numerous roles to play and must encounter stressors from many different sources as part of normal daily life. There is a difference, however, between this "normal" anxiety and the anxiety experienced by those with anxiety disorders. When worry and tension continue over time and symptoms become so intense that they interfere with a person's ability to function at work or in social relationships, then an anxiety disorder is said to be present. Anxiety disorders are among the most prevalent of psychiatric conditions diagnosed in epidemiologic surveys of the general population. According to the National Comorbidity Survey Replication, the lifetime prevalence of anxiety disorders in the United States is 28.8 percent (1) and the twelve-month prevalence rate is 18.1 percent.(2) This means that almost one in every three Americans has had an anxiety disorder at some time in the past, and one in five met criteria for an anxiety disorder within the past year. This makes anxiety disorder the most common psychiatric problem in the general U.S. population, more common than either depression or alcoholism. The lifetime prevalence for anxiety disorders around the world is about 17 percent, although methods of measurement vary and may not be directly comparable with U.S. figures cited above.(3)

This chapter examines the role of religion/spirituality in the development, course, and treatment of anxiety disorders. It is sometimes said that religion "comforts the afflicted and afflicts the comforted." However, religion may also afflict the afflicted in some circumstances, particularly individuals already vulnerable to depression or anxiety. Conventional wisdom would argue that religious teachings about hellfire, punishment, and damnation could worsen psychiatric symptoms in the individual predisposed to anxiety. Freud described religion as the "obsessional neurosis of humanity" and believed that most people would be better off without it.(4)

These negative aspects of religion, however, may have been overemphasized by mental health professionals in the past, and the benefits of religion underemphasized. There is little doubt that throughout history, many of the anxieties and worries that humans faced as they encountered the immense and threatening universe around them were dealt with through religious belief, which provided peace, security, and a sense of control.(5)

The chapter will also focus on the role that religious beliefs and practices play in the assessment and management of anxiety disorders. Anxiety disorders addressed in this chapter include generalized anxiety disorder, panic disorder, posttraumatic stress disorder, obsessive-compulsive disorder, and phobia. I examine the relationship of these disorders to religion, rather than spirituality, because religion can be more easily measured, and there is more agreement on what religion actually is (versus spirituality).(6) Before proceeding in that regard, however, I first examine how religion and anxiety may affect one another.

1. RELIGION AS A CAUSE

Some studies show a positive cross-sectional relationship between religious involvement and anxiety.(7) In other words, the greater the religious involvement, the greater the anxiety. This is particularly true when religion is measured as either extrinsic religiousness,(8–10) (where religious involvement is motivated by external concerns other than religion, such as economic or social goals) or negative religious coping (where God is seen as punishing, distant, abandoning, or powerless).(11) In contrast to extrinsic religiosity is *intrinsic* religiosity, which describes religious involvement motivated by religion itself, where religious concerns are the ultimate goal and

end of the religious activity. Intrinsic religiosity is often inversely related to anxiety (that is, the intrinsically religious person is less anxious than others).(8, 12–14)

Furthermore, there is uncertainty about what the positive associations reported between religion and anxiety in cross-sectional studies really mean. Do they exist because religion causes people to become more anxious or because anxiety motivates people to become more religious (like the soldier who prays for safety or turns to God while being shot at by the enemy)?

As noted earlier, certain religious teachings about the afterlife and possible retributions there for less-than-devout behavior could indeed foster anxiety in vulnerable persons. Anxiety may appear in religious persons who are not living up to the high expectations of their faith with regard to spiritual progress. These individuals may worry about not being "good enough" to please God (for Christians, Jews, or Muslims) or to improve their karma for the next rebirth (for Hindus or Buddhists). Such concerns could create psychological strains that increase anxiety. Although systematic longitudinal research documenting such phenomena is lacking, simple logic make such clinical scenarios quite plausible (even if they are not widespread, as suggested by the research below).

2. RELIGION AS A COMFORT

Although religion can potentially arouse anxiety, much data from cross-sectional and longitudinal studies also suggest a protective effect for religion. Indeed, these epidemiological associations are buttressed by a handful of randomized clinical trials showing that religious interventions decrease anxiety and other symptoms of distress. For example, Hughes and colleagues (15) examined the cross-sectional relationships between social support, religiosity, and anxiety in 282 hospitalized patients with heart disease. This patient population is of particular importance given the negative effect that anxiety has on cardiac outcomes. In the Hughes study, greater religiosity was related to lower state anxiety and also lower trait anxiety. Although those who were more religious also had greater social support, which helped to explain the relationship between religiosity and trait anxiety, this could not account for the relationship with state anxiety. In a second cross-sectional study, Wollin and colleagues examined children just prior undergoing general anesthesia. They found that children with the greatest anxiety were those whose mothers did not practice a religion.(16) At least two prospective studies have found that anxiety symptoms decreased in persons following religious conversion or rededication to religion,(17, 18) and one recent study found that patients with panic disorder who reported religion as very important to them recovered more quickly in response to traditional cognitive-behavioral therapy.(19) Finally, two randomized clinical trials in patients with generalized anxiety disorder (GAD) reported that religious interventions added to secular treatments resulted in faster improvement of symptoms compared to secular interventions alone.(20, 21)

3. RELIGION AND SPECIFIC ANXIETY DISORDERS

I now review these studies in greater detail so that psychiatrists can have a better sense of what exactly was examined and what was found.

3.1. Generalized Anxiety Disorder

Patients are diagnosed with a generalized anxiety disorder (GAD) when they have a long history of worrying about many things, both minor and major, and these worries cause dysfunction in their daily lives. Religious interventions appear to be effective in this type of anxiety disorder based on the following three randomized controlled trials.

First, Azhar and colleagues randomized sixty-two Muslim subjects to traditional treatment (supportive psychotherapy plus anti-anxiety drugs) or traditional treatment plus religious practices, such as prayer and reading verses from the Holy Koran.(20) Those who received therapy supplemented with religious practices improved significantly faster than those receiving traditional therapy.

Second, Razali and colleagues examined the effects of Muslim-based cognitive-behavioral therapy (CBT) on anxiety symptoms in a study in which they randomized eighty-five religious and eighty nonreligious Muslims with GAD to either standard treatment (benzodiazepines, supportive psychotherapy, and simple relaxation exercises) or standard treatment plus use of the Koran and Hadith (sayings of Mohammed) to alter negative thoughts and behaviors and increase religiousness.(21) Religious subjects receiving the religious CBT recovered significantly faster than religious subjects receiving standard treatment alone; however, religious CBT had no impact in nonreligious subjects.

Finally, Zhang and colleagues examined the effects of Chinese Taoist cognitive therapy (CT) in 143 Chinese patients with GAD who were randomized to Taoist CT, benzodiazepines (BDZ) only, or combined Taoist CT and BDZ treatment.(22) Subjects receiving BDZ treatment alone experienced a rapid reduction in GAD symptoms by one month, but these benefits were gone by six months of follow-up. Those receiving Taoist CT alone had little improvement in symptoms at one-month follow-up, but showed significant symptom reduction by six months. Those in the group receiving both Taoist CT and BDZ experienced significant symptom reduction at both one- and six-month follow-ups. However, there was no way to determine whether there was anything therapeutic about the religious aspects (Taoist) of CT or whether improvements were simply due to the nonreligious aspects of CT.

3.2. Panic Disorder

Panic disorder (PD) involves brief but recurrent feelings of extreme fear associated with physical symptoms such as rapid heart rate, difficulty breathing, and fear of dying. In some cases, panic disorder may be associated with agoraphobia or fear of the "market place" (open spaces or crowds). Such patients may be literally imprisoned in their homes, fearful that if they go out into the open where others congregate, they will experience panic and not be able to escape. This disorder is very disabling both because of the psychological anguish that it causes during an attack and because people restrict their lives to avoid recurrence of symptoms.

Religious involvement may help to relieve panic symptoms, particularly when accompanied by traditional psychotherapy. For example, Bowen and colleagues in Saskatchewan, Canada, explored coping and motivation factors related to treatment response in fifty-six patients with PD participating in a psychotherapy clinical trial.(19) Subjects were treated with group CBT, and then were followed for up to twelve months after the baseline evaluation. Self-rated importance of religion was a significant predictor of improvement in panic symptoms and reduced perceived stress at the twelve-month follow-up. Investigators concluded that high importance of religion reduced PD symptoms by decreasing levels of perceived stress.

3.3. Post-Traumatic Stress Disorder

Religion is a source of coping for many persons suffering from severe trauma. Post-traumatic stress disorder (PTSD) results when people cannot psychologically integrate a traumatic experience, allowing it to continue to overwhelm them. These persons' worldviews have been so shaken by the traumatic event that the world no longer appears predictable or controllable. This results in a paralyzing type of anxiety whenever anything reminds them of the traumatic event. When religious worldview is affected and faith is weakened or lost (that is, spiritual injury), PTSD symptoms may be particularly persistent and unresponsive to therapy. For example, consider a study of 1,385 veterans from Vietnam (95 percent), World War II and/or Korea (5 percent) involved in outpatient or inpatient PTSD programs. (23) In this study, conducted by the Veterans Administration (VA) National Center for PTSD and Yale University School of Medicine, investigators found that a weakened religious faith was an independent predictor of use of VA mental health services. This effect was independent of (and stronger than) severity of PTSD symptoms

or level of social functioning. Investigators concluded that the use of mental health services was driven more by a weakened religious faith than by clinical symptoms or by social factors.

3.4. Obsessive-Compulsive Disorder

Steketee and colleagues examined the relationship between religiosity and obsessive-compulsive disorder (OCD) symptoms in thirty-three patients with OCD and twenty-four patients with other anxiety disorders.(24) Although they reported that religiosity was significantly correlated with severity of OCD symptoms, they found no relationship between religiosity and general anxiety, social anxiety, or depressive symptoms, suggesting specificity for the relationship between religion and severity of OCD symptoms within patients with OCD. They did not, however, find a difference in degree of religiosity between the patients with OCD and the patients with other anxiety disorders. All associations were cross sectional, so it is not possible to say whether religiosity led to greater OCD symptoms in OCD patients or whether OCD symptoms led to greater religiosity. Furthermore, again no relationship was found between OCD (as a disorder) and religiosity.

More recent research has also failed to find evidence to link religiousness to OCD as a disorder. For example, investigators in Tel Aviv, Israel, compared religiosity between twenty-two OCD patients, twenty-two panic disorder patients, and twenty-two normal controls undergoing surgery, matching these groups by age and gender.(25) No difference in religiosity was found between these groups on any of the five measures used to assess religiosity, except that patients with panic disorder scored significantly lower on religiosity than did surgery controls. Other studies of OCD patients from a variety of religious backgrounds have likewise found no relationship between religiousness and OCD as a disorder.(26–28)

In fact, there may be a bias that favors the detection of OCD symptoms in religious persons.(29) OCD symptoms scales appear to be contaminated with questions that traditionally religious persons tend to answer in the affirmative, which could bias these scales toward detection of OCD symptoms in religious persons. This could help to explain why religiosity and severity of OCD symptoms are associated in OCD patients, but that there is no difference in religiosity between subjects with OCD and those with other psychiatric disorders or those without any psychiatric disorder.

There may also be a difference between religious patients with OCD and patients with OCD who have religious obsessions. When religious obsessions and compulsions are present, these patients may have a worse prognosis. For example, a study of sixty outpatients with OCD in Spain that followed subjects for one to five years found that those with sexual or religious obsessions had poorer long-term outcomes despite traditional treatment.(30) Another study of 153 outpatients with OCD in London, England, enrolled in a randomized clinical trial of behavioral therapy found that the presence of sexual and religious obsessions again predicted poorer outcomes.(31) Although a form of faith-based cognitive therapy has been developed to help treat religious patients with OCD, it is not clear that this treatment is as effective in OCD patients with religious obsessions.(32)

3.5. Phobia

Phobias are fears that relate to specific situations, such as fear of heights, fear of spiders, fear of open spaces, and so forth. When a phobic person is exposed to the feared stimulus, anxiety increases to distressing levels. The person then seeks to escape the stimulus – which, if successful, results in a reduction of anxiety – and avoid it in the future. Phobias are the most common of all anxiety disorders in the general U.S. population and can be quite disabling, depending on the type of phobia.

Although not much research has been done on religious involvement and phobia, a few studies are relevant. Morse and Wisocki surveyed 156 persons aged 60 to 90 years whom they recruited from senior centers throughout western Massachusetts.(33) Religious characteristics

measured were membership in church/temple, religious attendance, and religion as a source of comfort. Scores on these questions were then summed to create a religiosity index, and subjects were dichotomized into those with high and low religiosity. Subjects with high religiosity reported significantly fewer phobia symptoms as measured using the Symptom Check List-90 (SCL-90).

In another study, we examined the relationship between religious involvement and phobias in a random sample of 2,969 community-dwelling persons of all ages living in the piedmont area of North Carolina (Wave II of the National Institutes of Health Epidemiologic Catchment Area study).(34) Participants were divided into three groups by age: 18 to 39 years (young), 40 to 59 years (middle aged), and 60 to 97 years (elderly). Diagnoses of phobia and other anxiety disorders were made using *Diagnostic and Statistical Manual of Mental Disorders, Third Edition* (*DSM-III*) criteria; recent (past six months) and lifetime rates were determined. Young subjects who attended religious services at least weekly experienced significantly lower six-month rates of agoraphobia (2 percent versus 5 percent). Middle-aged persons attending services at least weekly had significantly lower six-month rates of social phobia (0.2 percent versus 3 percent), and those claiming to be "born again" had both lower six-month and lower lifetime rates of social phobia. However, in the young group, subjects for whom religion was "very important" had significantly higher six-month rates of simple phobia (10 percent versus 5 percent). No significant associations were found in the elderly group.

In the most recent study, an Internet survey of 1,402 adults, investigators examined the association between psychiatric disorders and religious characteristics.(35) A subscale of the Symptom Assessment-45 Questionnaire was used to identify psychiatric disorders, including phobia. Religious characteristics assessed were religious fundamentalism, religious attendance, frequency of prayer, and belief in an afterlife. Results indicated that there was no relationship between phobia and either religious fundamentalism or religious attendance. However, frequency of prayer was related to significantly higher phobia scores, while belief in an afterlife was related to significantly lower phobia scores. In fact, of the twelve characteristics measured, age was the only characteristic that predicted fewer phobia symptoms more strongly than did belief in an afterlife.

Thus, the particular way that religion is measured, the age of the person, and the specific type of phobia are all important in determining associations between religion and phobia.

4. CASE EXAMPLES

The research above suggests that religious involvement is generally related to fewer anxiety symptoms and less anxiety disorder. However, it is useful to examine individual cases that illustrate the use of religion in either alleviating or exacerbating anxiety. The names below are fictitious to protect patient confidentiality.

4.1. The Worrier

Jane is a 40-year-old mother of three children ranging in age from 4 to 10. She has a lifelong history of being a "worrier." Just about everything seems to make her anxious. As soon as one problem is solved, she quickly begins to worry and ruminate about other issues. When under a lot of stress, her worrying gets much worse – to the point that she is unable to function. Prior to seeking psychiatric help, she often had to ask her eldest child to watch the younger children and even cook supper for the family. Jane simply didn't have the energy or the patience to do this. Her constant worrying also interfered with her marital relationship. She felt an intense need to control all decisions related to family matters and would not listen to her husband or allow him a role in these decisions. This resulted in frequent and heated arguments.

Frustrated with her anxieties and fearful that her husband would leave her, Jane saw a psychiatrist who diagnosed her with generalized anxiety disorder. He gave her a prescription of the medication buipirone, which she was to take three times per day. Although this medicine was

partially effective, it left her with considerable residual anxiety. Always a religious person, Jane turned to this source for help with her anxiety. In addition to taking the buspirone, she now copes with her many worries through prayer, reading the Bible, and help from her faith community. Prayer enables her to give up some of her need for control to God and consequently makes her feel more peaceful. When she is in deep, serious prayer, she finds herself relaxed both emotionally and physically. Reading positive religious scriptures also helps to counteract her negative, anxiety-provoking thoughts. Reading stories about Biblical figures overcoming their fears gives her hope, and the promises in scripture of God's continual presence makes her feel calmer.

As she began to feel better, Jane also became more active in her religious community. This increased her social contacts, which provided her with more emotional support outside her family and gave her ways to reach out to others in need of help. This, in turn, reduced her worrying (or at least got her mind off of herself and her problems). Praying with other church members and singing hymns during the church service also gave her a sense of peace and reduced her sense of isolation. Thus, the combination of the medicine prescribed by her psychiatrist and greater involvement in religious activities has improved Jane's quality of life and reduced her GAD symptoms.

4.2. Panic at Night

Tom, a 28-year-old salesman, sees a psychiatrist for the treatment of panic disorder. Tom originally began having panic symptoms at night, when he would awake early in the morning with his heart racing, short of breath, and feeling like he was dying. His doctor initially treated him with a combination of paroxetine 40 mg per day and clonazepam 1.0 mg twice daily, with fairly good results. Nevertheless, he continued to occasionally awake with panic-like symptoms. Although they didn't escalate into a full-blown panic attack, they disturbed him enough that he could often not go back to sleep. Switching the clonazepam to 2.0 mg at bedtime helped to control these episodes, but they did not go away. Whenever he was stressed out over a big sales deal, the panic-like symptoms at night would return, overriding even the medication.

Knowing that Tom was a religious man from taking a spiritual history, the psychiatrist suggested that he try meditation. The psychiatrist described several different kinds of meditation: Hindu-based transcendental meditation, Buddhist-based mindfulness meditation, and Christian-based centering prayer. Tom said he would try the Christian-based centering prayer, but as a devout Catholic, he was not interested in Eastern religious practices. His psychiatrist suggested he try centering prayer for twenty minutes before going to bed at night and then again for twenty minutes on arising in the morning. If he awoke with panic-like feelings, he was instructed to go through his centering prayer routine for twenty minutes. After about four weeks of this practice, Tom noticed that the frequency of his panic feelings at night began to decrease. Even when they appeared, the centering prayer caused them to quickly subside. Tom eventually combined centering prayer with repetition of the Lord's Prayer, which continues to work for him and is more consistent with his faith tradition.

4.3. Lost Faith

John, a 23-year-old soldier, was on his third tour of duty in Baghdad, Iraq, when his best friend Joe, riding next to him in a jeep, was killed by a roadside explosive device. The two men were very close. Joe had saved John's life, once pulling him out of a burning building after he had lost consciousness from smoke inhalation and another time dragging him to safety out of the line of fire after he had been wounded. John couldn't believe that his friend was now dead. "Why hadn't the bomb killed me instead?" thought John. It just wasn't fair. For nearly three years, he and his friend had been inseparable partners. Both had strong religious faith and prayed regularly together for protection over each other and their families. Why would a loving God have allowed

this? It didn't make sense. If God allowed this, thought John, then he didn't want anything to do with God. He would simply make it on his own. Doing that, however, would prove to be more difficult then he imagined.

After he returned home from Iraq, he discovered that his wife had fallen in love with someone else and asked him for a divorce. On top of that, he couldn't find work anywhere, particularly since he had only partial use of his left arm where he had been wounded during his last tour of duty. He was able to drive an army jeep, but that was about all, and this skill now was hardly something that someone would hire him for. Shortly after returning home, John began having nightmares and flashbacks of his war experiences, found himself avoiding news programs reporting on war events and action-type TV shows, and noticed that he startled easily whenever someone came up behind him or surprised him. Life had become painful and was losing meaning for him. What reason did he have to continue living? Over time, the emotional burden that he was carrying became heavier and heavier. He sought help at the Veterans Administration (VA) hospital in the psychiatric outpatient clinic. The psychiatrist he saw diagnosed him with depression and PTSD from his war experiences and started him on medication. The psychiatrist also scheduled him to see a social worker for counseling. John stabilized after about three to six months of this treatment, but he did not return to his usual self. For the past several years, he has continued to seek help at the VA for his emotional problems. Although the medicine has been helpful and the counseling useful, no one has asked him how his wartime experiences affected his religious faith.

4.4. Devout and Prayerful

Roberta is a 60-year-old accountant. Two years ago her husband suffered a fatal injury at his workplace. She now lives alone and, other than driving back and forth to work, lives a pretty quiet life. Members of her congregation, family, and friends have long known Roberta for her religious devotion. She attended religious services before work every morning at 7:00 a.m. at the local Catholic church and prayed the rosary at least five times per day. She rose up early each morning because it took her several hours to get dressed and get ready for work and church. When she attended religious services, she would always light a candle for her two sons, which she believed would protect them physically and help them to lead good lives. Praying the rosary was also for her sons, but also for her ailing mother and for protection against the dangers of living alone.

Whenever circumstances prevented her from either attending daily Mass or saying the rosary on time, Roberta became very upset and angry at whoever interfered with her routine; she also became extremely anxious and had to call each son and her mother to assure herself that they were OK. When anything disturbed her religious routine, she would call her sons and mother exactly three times each. Although they tried to understand, this upset her sons who had busy lives themselves. Although such behaviors were not new for Roberta, they had increased in frequency and intensity since her husband died.

Roberta also had some other strange behaviors that members of her church simply explained as, "that's Roberta." She would walk from her house to the church every morning at the exact same time and using the same route and could be seen walking from square to square on the sidewalk, being careful not to step on the lines. She also avoided opening the door of the church (and her home) without first taking out her handkerchief and cleaning off the doorknob (or wrapping it with the handkerchief as she turned the knob). If she touched any part of the doorknob with her hands, then she would immediately go wash her hands.

One day Roberta was hospitalized for a short period following a small stroke. She was unable to attend Mass during this time. She became very upset in the hospital and demanded that the nurse allow her to leave so that she could attend Mass. As a result, a psychiatric consultation was obtained, and Roberta was diagnosed with obsessive-compulsive disorder (after the psychiatrist obtained a full history from her sons). She was placed on medication, and arrangements were made for follow-up after hospital discharge with a behavioral therapist. Although medication reduced her intense need for attending Mass daily and praying the rosary, she refused to see the behavioral therapist and continued to have active symptoms, especially when her routine was disrupted.

4.5. Trouble Crossing Streets

Phil is 52 years old, divorced, and lives in a large city where he moved about six months ago after losing his job in the small town where he had lived and worked most of his life. Since moving to the city, Phil obtained work as a nurse's assistant (orderly) on the evening shift of a large hospital. Although he liked his job, Phil had one particular problem that made his life difficult: crossing streets. Because he lived fairly close to his workplace, Phil was able to make it almost all the way to work without crossing any major streets. This took considerable effort and time. If he walked directly to work from his apartment, he could get there in about two minutes. The circuitous route that he took to avoid crossing streets, however, took him about twenty minutes. Despite this route, however, he had to cross one large street to get to the hospital. This was not a new problem for Phil. He had had trouble crossing large streets even in the small town where he had lived. Prior to and during a street crossing, his heart would race and he would experience extreme anxiety. That anxiety quickly abated whenever he was able to either avoid crossing or after he had crossed over. His fear of crossing streets, however, had gotten much worse since taking this new job in the city, which had much larger and busier streets. Phil had actually missed a couple of shifts at work because he had become so anxious trying to cross the street in front of the hospital that he had to return home and call in sick for the day.

Phil was reluctant to seek help from a psychiatrist, because the cost of living in the city was high, and his medical insurance paid only half of the cost of mental health visits. However, if this continued, he might lose his job. So Phil obtained an appointment with a psychiatrist who prescribed a small dose of lorazepam, which he was to take forty-five minutes before leaving home. The psychiatrist also gave him a referral to a therapist. Although the medication helped, it sedated him and made him feel sleepy at work, so he stopped the medication. Concerned about the cost of seeing a therapist, he instead sought help from the rabbi at the synagogue he was attending.

The rabbi listened carefully to Phil and then came up with a suggestion. He encouraged him to say quietly (but out loud) to himself the Twenty-third Psalm as he came closer and closer to the feared street. He was to recite the entire psalm before reaching the street, and then, just before crossing, he was to start over and repeat the entire psalm as he was crossing the street. After being sure that the light was green, the signal to cross was present, and no cars were coming (or had stopped), he was to step out into the crosswalk and walk across while saying the psalm and thinking about the meaning of each verse.

The first time he tried this, it didn't work well. His anxiety level continued to rise as he got closer and closer to the street, and by the time he actually got there, he was so anxious that he forgot the words to the psalm. His mind raced with fear, he got discouraged, and he went back home, calling in sick for the day. Nevertheless, he tried it again the next day as his rabbi had instructed. The second time wasn't quite as bad as the first time, and at least he remembered the words of the psalm and got across the street (more, however, because he was afraid of losing his job if he missed two days in a row). Over the next week, he carried out this ritual every day going to and returning from work. Although his anxiety level fluctuated from day to day, his fear gradually began to decrease. After three weeks of this practice, he was able to cross the street with only minor anxiety and from then on did not miss work again for that reason.

5. APPLICATIONS TO CLINICAL PRACTICE

Research findings and case reports such as those described above have many potential clinical applications that have to do with both the assessment and treatment of patients with anxiety disorders.

5.1. Assessment

The most important application involves the psychiatrist taking a thorough and detailed spiritual history from the patient and perhaps from other sources as the patient gives permission (family, friends, and/or clergy). How detailed that spiritual assessment is depends to some extent on whether the psychiatrist is only prescribing medication, prescribing medication and doing therapy, or doing therapy alone. Even if only medication is being prescribed, the spiritual assessment can provide information on whether the patient has religious beliefs that might conflict with the taking of medication.

Does the patient feel that taking medication is consistent with his or her religious beliefs? How does the patient's family and faith community feel in this regard? Is this acceptable, or is taking medication seen as counter to religious beliefs emphasizing a complete dependence on God? Anything less than complete dependence on God (such as taking medication or relying on therapy from a mental health professional) may be viewed by some as unfaithful. The religious patient's compliance with the prescribed treatment, especially over the long term, will depend heavily on the answers to such questions. If the psychiatrist brings up these concerns right from the start and allows the patient to discuss them in a supportive, accepting, and understanding atmosphere, then the patient will feel free to discuss these issues with the psychiatrist at a later date should they become relevant.

If psychotherapy is contemplated, or even simple psychological support, then a more detailed spiritual assessment will be needed to more fully understand the role that religious beliefs play in the patient's coping and in the dynamics of his or her psyche. This should initially be done in a positive and supportive manner. Does the patient have any religious or spiritual beliefs? Are these beliefs important to the patient? If so, when did they become important and why? Has the patient had any key religious transformations or other experiences with religion that changed him or her in some significant way? What are the specific religious beliefs and practices of the patient, and how does the patient see these as now affecting his or her life? What benefits does the patient obtain from religious beliefs/practices? What are some of the negative aspects of religious involvement as the patient perceives? Do religious/spiritual beliefs provide comfort, or alternatively, have they ever been a cause for stress and distress? Does the patient think there is a relationship between religious or spiritual beliefs and his or her symptoms? How might such beliefs influence decisions regarding medications or psychotherapy? How does the patient's religious community view psychiatric care, and are they likely to be supportive or discouraging in this regard?

Some areas may need to be explored in greater depth. First, to what extent are religious beliefs being used in a healthy way to cope with emotional problems? Usually, there is a component of healthy, positive religious coping that is present. This component is supportive, encouraging, and brings hope and meaning to the patient's life, despite painful struggles. Religious community involvement may be a key component of the patient's social support system, even more important than family members. The religious patient's primary friendships may come from the religious community, and those supportive relationships may influence the success of his or her coping efforts.

There may also be a negative component to the religious coping, particularly among those who are less religious or no longer religious. To what extent is there a component of unhealthy religious coping present that reflects anger at and disappointment with God, a clergy person, or faith community? The patient may phrase this in terms of feeling punished by God, deserted by God, or seeing God as distant, uncaring, and impotent. There may be anger at clergy or at other members of the faith community because they have not called or shown interest in the patient's problems. As noted, the original emotion driving such negative religious coping responses is

usually anger. While not always, sometimes that anger is present because of an unhealthy, distorted understanding of God or the faith community. The patient's relationship with God and expectations from clergy may be influenced by poor relationships with parental figures who were experienced as uncaring, deserting, or abusive, which is then projected onto God or other religious figures.

Second, to what extent is the patient using religious beliefs and activities to block constructive changes that need to be made to live a freer and more fulfilling life? Religion can be either a motivating force for change and healing, or the patient can use religion as a defense to avoid making necessary changes in ways of thinking and relating to others. Usually, both are going on to some extent. The psychiatrist's job in therapy is to determine to what extent each of these dynamics is present. If a force for positive change, then religious involvement should be supported; if a defense against positive change, then the pathological use of religion may need to be gently confronted.

6. TREATMENT

6.1. Inquire

The spiritual assessment itself is a powerful intervention. Simply asking questions about this area of patients' lives will cause them to think more about these issues and will help them to realize their potential for either good or harm. Given the important role that religion can play in holding together the patient's psyche, it is important to show genuine respect for religious beliefs during both assessment and treatment and communicate appreciation of their value to the patient. Of course, this applies to patients who are religious and value religion, not to the person who has no interest in religion. Care, however, must be taken before concluding that the patient has no interest in religion and that religion has no relevance, even for the most fervent agnostic or atheist (and possibly even more so for these patients than for others, because they have taken a stance against religion, which may conflict with cultural norms).

6.2. Support

During initial inquiry and throughout most of the treatment (certainly treatment with medications and in situations where therapy is purely supportive), the psychiatrist should support the patient's religious beliefs. Such support depends on whether the patient's religious beliefs are generally healthy, appear to be anxiety relieving, and especially if there is a situational stressor that is driving anxiety. Support should be shown in the way that the therapist makes inquiries about the religious beliefs of the patient. Facial expression, tone of voice, body posture, head nodding, and verbal expressions of support should all be used. Being sincere is crucial, because the patient will quickly sense if sincerity is absent. The psychiatrist's realization that much objective research and logical sense dictates that religion can be a tremendous resource should help him or her convey that sincerity to the patient.

6.3. Using Beliefs in Therapy

If the patient is religious, if religious beliefs are generally healthy and nonobstructive to therapy, if the therapist is well informed about the patient's religious belief system, and if the therapist has had training on how to address religious or spiritual issues (that is, some kind of clinical pastoral education), then he or she may consider using the patient's religious beliefs in the therapy itself. This is particularly true when doing supportive, cognitive-behavioral, or interpersonal psychotherapy with patients who have anxiety disorders. This will be discussed below within a Judeo-Christian framework, about which the present author is familiar.

6.4. Supportive

The purpose of supportive therapy is to provide emotional and social support to persons who are dealing with overwhelming real-life stressors.

Anxiety symptoms themselves can be stressors (as the old saying goes, "There is nothing to fear but fear itself"). Although there is much within Judeo-Christian beliefs that appears nonsupportive, such as teachings about hell, damnation, and devils, there are also many teachings that are positive, uplifting, confidence building, and hope conveying. Take for example the book of Psalms, which contains many scriptures that emphasize God's love and nearness (Ps. 139), protection (Ps. 91), power to make a difference (Ps. 68), and reliability (Ps. 31). These may be used to help the anxious patient to feel reassured and more confident. Many scriptures emphasize the peace that religious beliefs provide (Isa. 59:19; John 14:27; Col. 3:15; Rom. 5:1; 2 Thess. 3:16), and describe ways to achieve that peace (2 Cor. 13:11; 1 John 4:18). If the patient has strong religious beliefs, then he or she may believe that the words of scripture are words directly from God and may, therefore, receive those words as the ultimate authority. The therapist may provide the patient with a list of scriptures to meditate on or to repeat when facing situations that might arouse anxiety or fear.

6.5. Cognitive-Behavioral

Maladaptive cognitions that involve catastrophizing are common among persons with anxiety disorders. These negative thoughts, and the behaviors associated with them, create fear and anxiety. Cognitive-behavioral therapy (CBT) seeks to challenge these exaggerated negative cognitions and behaviors and replace them with more positive ways of thinking and behaving that are optimistic and realistic. For that reason, CBT is one of the most common treatments for anxiety disorders. A form of religious CBT has been developed that relies on Biblical scriptures to challenge negative self-talk,(36, 37) and this therapy has been shown in at least one randomized clinical trial to achieve benefits equal to or superior to traditional CBT in religious patients.(38) Positive supportive scriptures are used to counter negative thoughts about the self and the situations or surroundings that generate anxiety. For example, if the patient routinely thinks that he or she is in danger, out of control, or dwells on disasters that might happen, then this patient would be instructed to modify his or her thinking so it will be more consistent with what Biblical scriptures are saying.

In fact, scriptures instruct people to dwell on the positive, not the negative: "Finally, brethren, whatsoever things are true, whatsoever things are honorable, whatsoever things are just, whatsoever things are pure, whatsoever things are lovely, whatsoever things are of good report; if there be any virtue, and if there be any praise, *think on these things* [emphasis added]" (Phil. 4:8).* For religious patients with anxiety disorders, then, the following scriptures may be used to alter negative thinking. These represent promises by God to his people:

- "Do not be anxious about anything, but in everything, by prayer and petition, with thanksgiving, present your requests to God" (Phil. 4:6).
- "Do not be afraid; you will not suffer shame. Do not fear disgrace; you will not be humiliated. You will forget the shame of your youth and remember no more the reproach of your widowhood" (Isa. 54:4).
- "You will not fear the terror of night, nor the arrow that flies by day, nor the pestilence that stalks in the darkness, nor the plague that destroys at midday. A thousand may fall at your side, ten thousand at your right hand, but it will not come near you" (Ps. 91:6–7).
- "I will not fear the tens of thousands drawn up against me on every side" (Ps. 3:6).
- "God is our refuge and strength, an ever-present help in trouble. Therefore we will not fear, though the earth give way and the mountains fall into the heart of the sea, though its waters roar and foam and the mountains quake with their surging" (Ps. 46:1–3).
- "Do not fear, O Jacob my servant; do not be dismayed, O Israel. I will surely save you out

---

* Scripture verses taken from the Holy Bible, New International Version. Copyright © 1973, 1978, 1984, International Bible Society.

of a distant place, your descendants from the land of their exile. Jacob will again have peace and security, and no one will make him afraid" (Jer. 46:27).

- "So do not fear, for I am with you; do not be dismayed, for I am your God. I will strengthen you and help you; I will uphold you with my righteous right hand" (Isa. 41:10).
- "For I am the Lord, your God, who takes hold of your right hand and says to you, Do not fear; I will help you" (Isa. 41:13).

Although the scriptures above are from the Judeo-Christian Bible, other world religions have similar teachings that build confidence and may calm the anxious person. Recall that both Muslim and Buddhist (Tao) forms of CBT for anxiety disorders exist and have been studied in clinical trials.(21, 22) The type of religious CBT chosen, of course, should match the religion of the patient.

Furthermore, the particular cultural environment may influence whether or not the psychiatrist uses religious scriptures to combat dysfunctional cognitions. For example, while religious CBT may be perfectly acceptable in the United States, South America, the Middle East, Africa, and other religious areas of the world, in more secular areas (such as found in some countries of Europe), it may meet with resistance from patients and peers. Regardless of cultural context, as mentioned earlier, a spiritual history is always required to determine whether patients might be receptive to such an approach.

6.6. Interpersonal

Some experts view the experience of interpersonal loss and disordered attachment as the underlying causes for much of human psychopathology. Interpersonal psychotherapy (IPT) is a method of addressing these issues within a therapeutic framework.(39) Patients with anxiety disorders often have problems with attachment rooted in their early developmental experiences and relationships with parents. Religious IPT may facilitate healing of these early relationships by focusing on the person's image of God and substituting a relationship with God for missing or disordered parental attachments. Theophostic therapy is a Christian counseling method used to help patients recall suppressed or hurtful memories (often involving relationships with parental figures) so they can be healed in the present.(40)

7. ENCOURAGING/PRESCRIBING RELIGION

In rare instances, the psychiatrist may gently encourage religious beliefs or activities that patients may not be currently engaged in, but have been involved in previously. Such encouragement should focus on the patient's faith tradition. Considerable care needs to be taken, however, because encouragement or prescription is a much more aggressive approach. It is quite possible that the patient will see this as coercive (which is not acceptable). Most psychiatrists will not feel comfortable encouraging religion, and it is questionable as to whether this activity is even ethically permissible. However, if the anxious patient is socially isolated and in need of support, was once involved in religious practices, and there are potentially removable barriers to resumption of religious involvement, then the psychiatrist may bring this up in therapy and consider encouraging the patient to re-engage in such activity. Before doing so, the psychiatrist would be wise to check with an expert in pastoral care and counseling. Nevertheless the problems that can result from mental health professionals trying to evangelize patients of no religion or a different religion from their own are legion, given the personal nature of religious belief and the power differential in the relationship between patient and psychiatrist.(41) Furthermore, the focus of therapy should always be on the patient, not on the therapist or the therapist's need to share his or her faith.

8. CHALLENGING UNHEALTHY RELIGION

As noted above, religious beliefs may not always be helpful for patients with anxiety disorder, or the patient may be using religion in a harmful or unhealthy way. For example, the patient with generalized anxiety disorder may be focusing on religious scriptures that warn about the dangers and agonies of hell. Anxious patients may fear that their failure to live up to religious ideals has destined them for an eternity of pain and suffering in the afterlife, and their anxious temperament may cause them to dwell on such fears.

William is a 56-year-old teacher who has suffered from generalized anxiety for most of his life. He has found great comfort in his religious beliefs, in attending his Baptist church and spending time with the friends he has made there, and in reading the Bible that gives him hope and courage. However, he sometimes worries about whether he is really "saved," and whether he has lived a good enough life to make it to heaven. He had a dream the other night that he was in hell, and he woke up in a cold sweat. He could not get this off his mind all day. When he went in to see his psychiatrist for his usual appointment, he told the psychiatrist about the dream. The psychiatrist listened carefully and helped the patient explore his feelings about the dream.

In other cases, the anxious patient may cope with anxious feelings by taking on an air of superiority or self-righteousness, and then condemn others whom he or she views as not living right or believing correctly. Such attitudes may interfere with social relationships, lead to isolation, or even result in paranoid thoughts about others.

Stephanie is a 35-year-old wife and mother of three. She is the member of a fundamentalist religious group, which she encouraged her family to join. She is a perfectionist in her expectations of herself and others. Stephanie believes that only those in her religious group possess the truth, and others are wrong and going to hell, even those within her own congregation who are not living up to her high religious standards. She is often critical of others, especially members of her family but also others outside the family as well. This has interfered with her relationships, causing rifts within the family and also isolation from others in her community and congregation. By feeling better than others, Stephanie covers up a deep-seated insecurity and poor self-image. She is scrupulous and controlling, fearful that if she is not in control, then bad things will happen – as they have happened before. As a child she was quite sensitive and needy, and she was criticized mercilessly by a judgmental mother with similar emotional problems. She wonders whether her husband is having an affair, and at times can't understand why he would love her.

Patients may also misinterpret or misapply religious teachings, using them in a rigid and inflexible way that leads to excessive guilt and compulsive behaviors. Religious teachings encourage persons to regularly perform religious rituals, pray without ceasing, practice self-sacrifice, and focus on others' needs. Each of these, while healthy if done in moderation, can also be unhealthy if taken to an extreme.

Bob is a married 32-year-old computer science teacher with two young children. He is active in his church, where he is a deacon. He attends every social event at church and spends many hours cleaning up and putting things back in order at the end of church functions. Bob has to put everything back in exactly the same place or he feels anxious. He must check the locks on the church several times after locking up, and sometimes has driven back to the church fearing he has left it unlocked. He has similar fears about locking up his own home at night. Bob's wife has complained to him on more than one occasion that he hardly ever spends time with his two children, and she would like to do other things

with him besides going to church. Bob, however, explains that he is serving God and is committed to the church, and that if he doesn't do it then no one else will do it right. Because his wife has now threatened to leave him, and he cannot seem to alter his behavior, Bob has come to see a psychiatrist for help.

As noted earlier, patients may also use religion defensively to avoid addressing issues in therapy. Here, the patient uses religious justifications for ways of thinking or behaving that really have nothing to do with religion, but everything to do with the patient's desire to resist needed change.

Sarah is a divorced 42-year-old sales clerk. Sarah has as history of being raped and brutally beaten about twenty years ago when someone broke into her home during a robbery. She continues to suffer nightmares of the attack, cannot watch violent movies, and suffers from chronic depression and anxiety. She is quite religious and uses much religious jargon in talking about her past and present life. She has attended many religious revivals and healing services and reports having demons exorcised from her on more than one occasion. Since her divorce, she has had many male boyfriends in brief relationships but is unable to establish a lasting, intimate relationship because of the fear that comes over her whenever the relationship deepens. A psychiatrist diagnosed her with PTSD. In addition to treating her with medication, the psychiatrist referred her for therapy to help in her relationships with men. Whenever the therapist talks to her about the rape event, she immediately begins using religious explanations to minimize the event, claiming that the Lord healed her of all that when she underwent exorcism. She then tries to change the subject. She has been in therapy for almost a year but is not making much progress.

If religious beliefs are being used neurotically to obstruct needed changes or psychological insights, then after a therapeutic relationship
has been established the psychiatrist may need to
gently challenge those beliefs (as noted above).
However, unless the therapist has pastoral counseling training and is quite familiar with the religious tradition of the patient, it may be best to
seek consultation or referral to someone with
pastoral counseling experience.

9. PASTORAL REFERRAL OR CONSULTATION

Whenever complex religious issues or conflicts
are present, the psychiatrist should always consider consultation, referral, or co-therapy with a
pastoral counselor. Under certain circumstances,
such referral should come sooner rather than
later if religious issues are present and appear to
be related to the anxiety disorder. These circumstances include those when the clinician is not
very knowledgeable about religious issues, when
the particular religious background of the patient
is different than the clinician's, or when the patient
requests such referral. In religious patients with
anxiety disorders, particularly if the disorder has
been present for many years, psychological and
religious issues are almost always deeply intertwined. This may even be true for nonreligious
patients and is the reason why a spiritual history
is necessary for all patients.

Effective pastoral consultation or referral
requires that the psychiatrist identify a pastoral
counselor whom the psychiatrist can work with
and who has the skills to help patients in these
situations. Pastoral counselors typically have four
years of college, three years of postgraduate theological education, and either a master's degree or
doctorate in counseling. If trained pastoral counselors are not available, then clinicians should get
to know the clergy in their area who do counseling and are open to consultation and referral
(especially the clergy of patients that they may
be seeing, although that will depend on patients'
preferences). It may be helpful to have a meeting
or lunch with clergy before referring anyone to
them to get a sense of their experience, skills, and
approach to counseling. Community clergy vary
widely in the type and extent of training, from no
training to modest exposure to counseling techniques in seminary. Some clergy may seek additional training, although that is not always true.
Regardless of their level of training, clergy on
average spend about 15 percent of their time in
marital, family, or individual counseling and are
often the first persons that religious persons go to
for help with their emotional problems.(42)

Clergy should not be brought in, however, until
the clinician has a thorough understanding of the
patient's problems and a therapeutic relationship
has been established. The clinician will also need
to prepare the patient for pastoral involvement by
emphasizing the importance of religious issues
and admitting his or her lack of expertise in this
area, requiring consultation. Of course, before
involving clergy or pastoral counselors (other
than when obtaining informal consultation),
explicit permission from the patient is needed.

10. CONCLUSIONS

Religious beliefs and practices are often inversely
correlated with anxiety symptoms or disorders,
but not always so. Religion helps many patients
with anxiety disorders to cope with their symptoms, and religious therapies are effective in
reducing symptoms of anxiety. Religion may
also exacerbate anxiety disorder; patients with
anxiety disorder may manipulate or distort religion; and patients may use religion defensively to
avoid healthy change. Clinicians with appropriate
training can use the religious beliefs of patients
to help treat anxiety disorder by supporting,
encouraging, or directly using those beliefs in
therapy. Trained pastoral counselors and clergy
can be helpful when religious beliefs need to be
challenged or when religious beliefs are deeply
interwoven with psychopathology.

REFERENCES

1. Kessler RC, Berglund P, Demler O, Jin R,
   Merikangas KR, Walters EE. Lifetime prevalence and age-of-onset distributions of DSM-IV

disorders in the national comorbidity survey replication. *Arch Gen Psychiatry*. 2005;62:593–602.

2. Kessler RC, Chiu WT, Demler O, Walters EE. Prevalence, severity, and comorbidity of 12-Month DSM-IV disorders in the national comorbidity survey replication. *Arch Gen Psychiatry*. 2005;62:617–627.

3. Starcevic V. Review: worldwide lifetime prevalence of anxiety disorders is 16.6%, with considerable heterogeneity between studies. *Evid Based Ment Health*. 2006;9:115.

4. Freud S. Future of an Illusion. In: Strachey J, trans. and ed. *Standard Ediction of the Complete Psychological Works of Sigmund Freud*. London: Hogarth Press (published in 1962); 1927:43.

5. Koenig HG. *Faith and Mental Health: Religious Resources for Healing*. Philadelphia: Templeton Foundation Press; 2005.

6. Koenig HG. Religion, spirituality and medicine in Australia: Research and clinical practice. *Med J Aust*. 2007;186(10):S45–S46.

7. Wilson W, Miller HL. Fear, anxiety, and religiousness. *J Sci Stud Relig*. 1968;7:1.

8. Baker M, Gorsuch R. Trait anxiety and intrinsic–extrinsic religiousness. *J Sci Stud Relig*. 1982;21:119–122.

9. Bergin AE, Masters KS, Richards PS. Religiousness and mental health reconsidered: a study of an intrinsically religious sample. *J Couns Psychol*. 1987;34:197–204.

10. Tapanya S, Nicki R, Jarusawad O. Worry and intrinsic/extrinsic religious orientation among Buddhist (Thai) and Christian (Canadian) elderly persons. *Aging Hum Dev*. 1997;44:75–83.

11. Boscaglia N, Clarke DM, Jobling TW, Quinn MA. The contribution of spirituality and spiritual coping to anxiety and depression in women with a recent diagnosis of gynecological cancer. *Int J Gynecol Cancer*. 2005;15(5):755–761.

12. Bivens AJ, Neumeyer RA, Kirchberg TM, Moore MK. Death concern and religious beliefs among gays and bisexuals of variable proximity to AIDS. *Omega*. 1994–1995;30:105–120.

13. Kraft WA, Litwin WJ, Barber SE. Religious orientation and assertiveness: relationship to death anxiety. *J Soc Psychol*. 1986;127:93–95.

14. Ryan RM, Rigby S, King K. Two types of religious internalization and their relations to religious orientations and mental health. *J Pers Soc Psychol*. 1993;65:586–596.

15. Hughes JW, Tomlinson A, Blumenthal JA, et al. Social support and religiosity as coping strategies for anxiety in hospitalized cardiac patients. *Ann Beh Med*. 2004;28(3):179–185.

16. Wollin SR, Plummer JL, Owen H, Hawkins RM, Materazzo F. Predictors of preoperative anxiety in children. *Anaesth Intensive Care*. 2003;31(1):69–74.

17. Cooley CE, Hutton JB. Adolescent response to religious appeal as related to IPAT anxiety. *J Soc Psychol* 1965;56:325–327.

18. Paloutzian RF. Purpose in life and value changes following conversion. *J Pers Soc Psychol*. 1981;41:1153–1160.

19. Bowen R, Baetz M, D'Arcy C. Self-rated importance of religion predicts one-year outcome of patients with panic disorder. *Depress Anxiety*. 2006;23(5):266–273.

20. Azhar MZ, Varma SL, Dharap AS. Religious psychotherapy in anxiety disorder patients. *Acta Psychiatr Scand*. 1994;90:1–3.

21. Razali SM, Hasanah CI, Aminah K, Subramaniam M. Religious – sociocultural psychotherapy in patients with anxiety and depression. *Aust N Z J Psychiatry*. 1998;32:867–872.

22. Zhang Y, Young D, Lee S, et al. Chinese Taoist cognitive psychotherapy in the treatment of generalized anxiety disorder in contemporary China. *Transcult Psychiatry*. 2002;39(1):115–129.

23. Fontana A, Rosenheck R. Trauma, change in strength of religious faith, and mental health service use among veterans treated for PTSD. *J Nerv Ment Dis*. 2004;192:579–584.

24. Steketee G, Quay S, White K. Religion and guilt in OCD patients. *J Anxiety Disord*. 1991;5:359–367.

25. Hermesh H, Masser-Kavitzky R, Gross-Isseroff R. Obsessive–compulsive disorder and Jewish religiosity. *J Nerv Ment Dis*. 2003;191(3):201–203.

26. Greenberg D, Shefler G. Obsessive compulsive disorder in ultra-orthodox Jewish patients: a comparison of religious and non-religious symptoms. *Psychol Psychother*. 2002;75(2):123–130.

27. Tek C, Ulug B. Religiosity and religious obsessions in obsessive–compulsive disorder. *Psychiatry Res*. 2001;104(2):99–108.

28. Okasha A, Lotaief F, Ashour AM, El Mahalawy N, Seif El Dawla A, El-Kholy GH. The prevalence of obsessive compulsive symptoms in a sample of Egyptian psychiatric patients. *Encephale*. 2000;26(4):1–10.

29. Yossifova M, Loewenthal KM. Religion and the judgement of obsessionality. *Ment Health Relig Cult*. 1999;2(2):145–151.

30. Alonso P, Menchon JM, Pifarre J, et al. Long-term follow-up and predictors of clinical outcome in obsessive–compulsive patients treated with serotonin reuptake inhibitors and behavioral therapy. *J Clin Psychiatry*. 2001;62(7):535–540.

31. Mataix-Cols D, Marks IM, Greist JH, Kobak KA, Baer L. Obsessive–compulsive symptom dimensions as predictors of compliance with and response to behaviour therapy: results from a controlled trial. *Psychother Psychosom*. 2002;71(5):255–262.

32. Gangdev PS. Faith-assisted cognitive therapy of obsessive-compulsive disorder. *Aust N Z J Psychiatry*. 1998;32:575–578.

33. Morse CK, Wisocki PA. Importance of religiosity to elderly adjustment. *J Relig Aging*. 1987;4:15–25.

34. Koenig HG, Ford S, George LK, Blazer DG, Meador KG. Religion and anxiety disorder: an examination and comparison of associations in

young, middle-aged, and elderly adults. *J Anxiety Disor.* 1993;7:321–342.

35. Flannelly KJ, Koenig HG, Ellison CG, Galek K, Krause N. Belief in life after death and mental health: findings from a national survey. *J Nerv Ment Dis.* 2006;194(7):524–529.

36. Propst LR. *Psychotherapy in a Religious Framework: Spirituality in the Emotional Healing Process.* New York: Human Sciences Press; 1987.

37. Backus W, Chapin M. *Telling Yourself the Truth.* Minneapolis, MN: Bethany House Publishers; 2000.

38. Propst LR, Ostrom R, Watkins P, Dean T, Mashburn D. Comparative efficacy of religious and nonreligious cognitive-behavior therapy for the treatment of clinical depression in religious individuals. *J Cons Clin Psychol.* 1992;60:94–103.

39. International Society for Interpersonal Psychotherapy. Interpersonal psychotherapy: an overview. http://www.interpersonalpsychotherapy.org/. Accessed August 9, 2007.

40. Theophostic.http://en.wikipedia.org/wiki/Theophostic. Accessed August 10, 2007.

41. Spero MH. Countertransference in religious therapists of religious patients. *Am J Psychother.* 1981;35:565–575.

42. Weaver AJ. Has there been a failure to prepare and support Parish-based clergy in their role as front-line community mental health workers? A review. *J Pastoral Care.* 1995;49:129–149.

11 Religion/Spirituality and Dissociative Disorders

PIERRE-YVES BRANDT AND LAURENCE BORRAS

SUMMARY

The connection between religion/spirituality and dissociative disorders is complex. Possession states cannot always be interpreted as a kind of dissociative disorder. The chapter begins with the famous case of Achille being "exorcised" by Pierre Janet and reminds us of how the healing task of medical doctors is distinct from that of priests. It then continues by discussing how the *Diagnostic and Statistical Manual of Mental Disorders, Fourth Edition, (DSM-IV)* approaches complaints of possession (Code F 44.9). During the twentieth century, the multiple personality diagnosis was renamed "dissociative identity disorder" and constitutes only one subcategory of dissociative disorder. The prevalence of dissociative disorders is difficult to establish. It depends on cultural aspects (the Ross-Spanos controversy). Descriptions of cases show the variety of relationships between religion and dissociative disorders: identity disorder with religious content but without possession (case 1), divine possession (case 2), and demonic possession (case 3). Anthropological criticism applied to the assimilation of possession with dissociative disorders brought about the introduction of the concept of "associative disorder." The chapter concludes with the discussion of the possible collaboration between psychiatrists and clergy, exorcists or shamans when a person is said to be possessed. This chapter attempts to show under which conditions an ethno-psychiatric consultation may be helpful.

I. CHAPTER OVERVIEW

According to epidemiologic studies, dissociative disorders have a lifetime prevalence of about 10 percent.(1) Dissociative symptoms may occur in acute stress disorder, posttraumatic stress disorder, somatization disorder, substance abuse, mood disorders, psychoses, dissociative identity disorder, trance, and possession trance. Although dissociative trance disorders, especially possession disorder, are probably more common than is usually thought, little systematic research into this phenomenon has been done in psychiatry. Moreover, encounters with these disorders are increasingly likely for mental health professionals, who may be unaware of the phenomenon.

The experience of being "possessed" by another entity holds different meanings in different cultures. Possession states are often interpreted as being nonpathological: affected individuals can even achieve higher status when they are viewed as having supernatural powers of healing and understanding. Alternatively, when individuals become so distressed and dysfunctional that they seek assistance from healers and mental health professionals, the interpretation of their suffering as the consequence of a possession by entities like bad spirits depends on the cultural background of the healer. In other words, such cases are challenging to diagnose and treat: viewing the diagnosis of possession as abnormal constitutes a culturally oriented decision.

The first issue to discuss, then, is the question of diagnosis. In the international classifications of mental disorders, dissociative or possession trance is not considered to be a normal part of a broadly accepted, collective cultural or religious practice. A short historical perspective on possession phenomena and exorcism will be followed by a brief reminder of what the *DSM-IV* and the *International Statistical Classification of Diseases and Related Health Problems 10th Revision* (*ICD-10*) say about dissociative disorders. The place of possession in these classification systems will open the discussion of cross-cultural variations. How do members of different cultures differ and agree in their experience of and response to the phenomenon of possession? What is this phenomenon like in different cultural settings? The different approaches will be presented here.

This discussion will then allow us to consider the diagnosis and the treatment of dissociative disorders from a differential diagnosis point of view. Once again, cultural factors play an important role: Dissociative disorders are not diagnosed with the same frequency in Europe and North America.

The discussion will be illustrated by descriptions of modern cases of psychiatric patients who believed they were possessed and how they were managed from both religious and medical perspectives. An anthropological analysis will then lead up to the conclusion, which is dedicated to the question of how religious authorities, ethnopsychiatrists, and clinicians could collaborate.

2. A HISTORICAL PERSPECTIVE

Historically, the diagnostic category of dissociative disorders developed in several stages. According to Spanos,(2) the history of dissociation began in the nineteenth century with the diagnosis of traumatic hysteria. Charcot believed that the "nervous shock" following a traumatic accident could produce a frightening idea, which was then unconsciously transformed into hysterical symptoms. Janet (3) used the concept of dissociation to describe the process of splitting and automatism of ideas. According to his theory, these dissociative ideas are organized into a state of consciousness that is different from normal consciousness. To illustrate this model he presented the case of

Achilles, a 33-year-old man who believed he was possessed by the devil, which developed due to his remorse at having been unfaithful to his wife on a business trip.(4) This thought, which tormented him unconsciously, was experienced by Achilles as a secondary demonic personality. Janet unhesitatingly qualified the treatment, which consisted of modifying the traumatic memory through hypnosis, as a modern exorcism. Later, this specific clinical case was reinterpreted according to the theory of multiple personalities. Multiple personality disorder later became a diagnostic category of its own in the *DSM-III*.

Janet's explanation of the phenomenon of possession as a dissociative symptom with religious content contrasts with the religious interpretation, which describes possession as the expression of an invasion of the body by spiritual forces. The conflict between these different interpretations of the phenomenon of possession originally began several centuries earlier. The conflict came to a head in 1707, when King Louis XIV promulgated the law under which priests, monks, and nuns who practiced medicine in France had to pay a fine of 200 French livres (p. 15).(5) This decision was a result of the concerted efforts of medical professionals to legitimize the practice of medicine. It allowed them to obtain social recognition and even gave them the supreme authority over health. With the establishment of medical schools in different universities and steadily increasing political support, physicians (doctors), who were considered as mere artisans in the Middle Ages, gained the status of recognized scientists. This evolution was accompanied by a new definition of the line separating religious and medical treatments. From that point on, everything belonging to the domain of the spirit was answerable to the authority of the church or of philosophy, whereas the human body, considered as an animal or a machine, fell under the authority of medicine. Therefore, a priest, for example, who practiced the laying on of hands on a sick person suffering from a fever and who prayed for that person's health, could be accused by doctors of practicing illegal medicine as an act of unlawful competition unless the priest could prove that the origins of the fever were exclusively spiritual.

The distinction between illness and the phenomenon of possession appeared in the Roman ritual that Pope Paul V promulgated in 1614. Through a differential approach, this ritual ascribed three signs to the demon possessed: (1) pronouncing or understanding words in a language unknown by the possessed person, (2) revealing hidden knowledge, and (3) the exhibition of a force that transcends the natural human condition.

In practice, priests who performed exorcisms were more likely to express aversion toward religious things as the determining criterion. For this reason, Gassner (1727–1779), a priest who practiced exorcism in the regions of Constance and Ratisbonne, took the precaution of starting with what he called a *trial exorcism* (p. 85).(6) To ensure that he did not cross over into the sphere of the medical doctor, he began the ritual by presenting a crucifix and asking the individual to kiss it. He also sprinkled holy water, and so on. If the individual remained quiet and peacefully submitted to the veneration of holy objects, then their suffering was caused by a natural illness and they had to be seen by a medical doctor. But if the person began to blaspheme and/or have convulsions, then their suffering was caused by a supernatural illness requiring treatment by an exorcist.

This specific division of tasks is not exclusively reserved to Catholicism. The way of expressing our symptoms has been strongly influenced by this division of tasks, which partly explains why patients who consult a doctor whose practice corresponds to the Western medical paradigm prefer not to formulate their suffering in religious language in front of the doctor. Instead, it is to their religious authorities that they address their metaphysical fears or, if they feel the need, their requests for prayers or rituals. For this reason, individuals who believe that they are possessed and that they need the help of an exorcist rarely discuss this within the context of a psychiatric consultation.

3. DISSOCIATIVE DISORDERS AND POSSESSION IN DSM-IV AND ICD-10

In the American Psychiatric Association's *DSM-IV, Text Revision* (*DSM-IV-TR*), the multiple personality diagnosis has been renamed the "dissociative identity disorder (DID)." It now constitutes only one of the five subcategories of dissociative disorder, along with dissociative amnesia (DA), dissociative fugue, depersonalization disorder, and dissociative disorder not otherwise specified (DDNOS). Complaints of possession are considered a kind of dissociative disorder because the individual presents a state of mind that appears to be under the control of two or more entities that organize the individual's psychic life. But possession is no longer considered a form of multiple personality disorder as it was in the *DSM-III*. The *DSM-IV* places pathological possession in the category of possession trances under the diagnosis of dissociative disorder not otherwise specified (Code F 44.9). This shows that a clear distinction has been made between the phenomenon of possession and DID.

The criteria for the differential diagnosis clarify this distinction. While the DID is described as a "mental state where separate and distinct different personalities can cohabit (criterion A), and where one after another can take control of the person's behaviour (criterion B)," in mental states of trance or possession (DDNOS), "subjects typically say that spirits or entities coming from the outside have entered their body and have taken control of it." The cultural dimension is important here. The *DSM-III* continued to associate possession with a multiple personality disorder, whereas the *DSM-IV* specifies that dissociative states of trance are disturbances "related to certain places or cultures" and are not necessarily of a pathological nature. The *ICD-10* also has a category for trance and possession disorder.

The *ICD-10* provides a special category for dissociative disorder called trance disorder and possession states. In this group of disorders, there is a temporary loss of identity and awareness, and the individual may appear to be taken over by another personality, a spirit, or a deity.

These disorders are limited to occurrences that are involuntary, unwanted, and occur outside of accepted religious or cultural experiences. Psychoses, multiple personality disorders, substance-induced disorders, and temporal lobe epilepsy are excluded. This classification takes into consideration the sizable number of dissociative disorder diagnoses that occur in nonindustrialized nations and were previously diagnosed as atypical dissociative disorder or dissociative disorder not otherwise specified.(7)

4. POSSESSION IN VARIOUS CULTURAL CONTEXTS

The concept of possession exists in all parts of the world. A review based on 488 societies showed that 74 percent had one or more forms of possession belief (p. 249).(8) Possession beliefs may or may not be linked to trance behavior. In some cultures, when someone becomes the new king, the soul of his predecessor enters him. During the enthronement ritual, a brief possession trance can accompany the entrance of the soul. Afterwards, the new king will be considered as permanently possessed by the soul of his predecessor. Similarly, when Christians say they are inspired by the Holy Spirit, this kind of "divine possession" may be expressed by trance behavior. These two examples, the king possessed by the soul of his predecessor and Christians possessed by the Holy Spirit, represent positive conceptualizations of possession.

Possession can also refer to negative experiences. Bourguignon considers trances as a kind of altered state of consciousness. She noticed that trances were not necessarily associated with the concept of possession, and when examining geographic distribution, she observed that trances were highly correlated with America. She described hunter-gatherer societies in which trances were actively sought out, especially by men, and sometimes with the help of drugs (South America). In contrast to this type of trance with positive connotations, the possession trance is significantly correlated with agricultural societies in sub-Saharan Africa and with the circum-Mediterranean region.

This type of trance, which mostly affects women, has more negative connotations.

Two main modes of traditional intervention can be undertaken when a person complains of being possessed by bad spirits or demons, whether a state of trance is observed or not: exorcism or manipulation. Exorcism denotes rituals that aim to expel negative forces. Manipulation involves rituals that seek to integrate negative forces. In many cultures, the coordination of such rituals is entrusted to a person who has special knowledge about altered states of consciousness and possesses special healing powers. This person is thought to have a kind of authority over negative forces, either to chase them away or negotiate an alliance with them. Exorcism can be understood as religious coping, with God, gods, or good spirits *against* demons, whereas manipulation can be understood as religious coping *with* demons.

In a study focused on traditions in Morocco, Hell (9) shows that the treatment of possession includes a differential diagnosis. When the misfortune is caused by a spirit (*djinn*) of lesser importance, the exorcism is performed by a learned and lettered man (a *fiqh* or *taleb*) reciting verses from the Koran and carrying out purification rituals. But if the spirit (*djinn*) is more powerful, the only solution may be to seek the help of a traditional brotherhood that practices a possession ritual. The brotherhood of the Gnawa is the most renowned for its practice of rituals of possession. By working with the spirits over extended periods during these rituals of possession, the possessed person learns how to establish an alliance with the hostile forces. The idea that exorcists deal with different levels of negative forces is common in different cultures.

5. THE DISTRIBUTION OF DISSOCIATIVE DISORDERS

Epidemiologic studies find a prevalence of dissociative disorders of around 10 percent in the general population and of around 16 percent in psychiatric inpatients, with a female predominance.(1)

The higher rate of dissociative disorder diagnoses in the United States compared to other regions of the world, notably in Europe, has given rise to different interpretations. Some believe the reason is a better capacity to diagnose a complicated disorder. For others, the reason is a social movement that encourages physicians to diagnose very sensitive patients with this disorder. It is a fact that only a limited number of psychiatrists are responsible for the vast majority of dissociative disorder diagnoses. These different points of view have prolonged the Ross-Spanos controversy about multiple personality disorder. Spanos believed this disorder was an artifact of the doctor-patient relationship, whereas Ross thought that it was simply a disorder that was very complex to diagnose.(10) The *DSM-IV* shows a great deal of precaution by stating that this disorder could be specific to certain cultures. Could this be an indication that the cultural dimension of personality should not be underestimated?

Possession cannot always be interpreted as a kind of dissociative disorder. From a cross-cultural perspective, we have seen that it is not necessarily considered pathological. When the individuals who complain of being possessed require medical treatment, their psychological organization is not always of a dissociative nature (that is, exclusively falling within the dissociative disorder category). In fact, as the expression of a belief, possession can be combined with different forms of disorders. According to Janet, possession was considered a form of hysteria. However, it can also appear in association with schizophrenia or dissociative symptoms, as the following cases will illustrate.

6. DESCRIPTIONS OF CASES

None of the cases described below of patients suffering from DID manifested an identity of a religious nature. Patients who believe that they are God, Jesus, or a religious leader to whom a higher mission has been addressed are usually considered to be suffering from delusions of grandeur. These delusions are classed within the category of positive symptoms of psychotic disorders, which are more severe than dissociative disorders. The first case presented below

has similarities with this diagnosis. The description of the second case provides an example of divine possession. The predominant trait of the "presence" inhabiting the sufferer contrasts with demonic possession, of which an example will be described in the third case.

6.1. Case 1

At the age of around 20, Mr. H. decompensated after a frightening experience when he was attacked with a knife. He began to have regular auditory hallucinations. He heard voices, either of Jesus talking to him or maybe his future self. Later on, he realized that he had heard voices when he was about 13 or 14 years old. These voices sometimes seemed to belong to dissociated personalities who controlled his body. He said, "Because if I connect myself to my core personality, I feel like I am paralyzed" and "Someone else has controlled my muscles for the past two years." He then explained that it was either his future personality (self) or Jesus who controlled his body, and that they were very careful to closely imitate his core personality. He recounted that the dissociative symptoms were at first associated with posttraumatic stress disorder, because they appeared after he was attacked. The diagnosis of schizophrenia with dissociative symptoms was only established later. He himself believed that he was suffering from a dissociative disorder (multiple personality disorder). If a psychiatrist had confirmed the diagnosis of multiple personality disorder, would his suffering have more clearly taken on that form? At one point, he attempted to commit suicide. He discussed this event in these words: "At that time, another personality controlled my body …; it was the other personality who swallowed the pills; it was not my current personality." However, he did not identify that personality. His religious beliefs did not help him to cope with his suffering; on the contrary, they seemed to intensify it. Voices told him that he would become the greatest saint in human history, but examples of the saints before him, such as Jesus, show that sanctification cannot be attained without experiencing severe suffering. However, he thought that the voices were kind because they encouraged him by promising a better future. He prayed often, validating his prayers with self-inflicted suffering even though he realized that God wasn't doing anything. This didn't prevent him from devotedly practicing his religion on an individual basis, nor did it keep him from calling himself a Catholic. His religiosity allowed him to have interesting discussions with his brother who was a priest. Religion principally provided him with a framework to interpret the meaning of life and suffering. It also helped him to maintain a rational stance toward his ideas of grandeur and toward his unfulfilled expectations that he would be healed and his suffering would be gone.

6.2. Case 2

One evening, at the age of 17, Elise had a strange experience on the beach.(11) Colors transformed into a rainbow; she felt a strange sense of well-being and suddenly heard voices that told her to throw herself into the water: "Chase away the good; chase away the evil; fly away into the duct." She then threw herself fully dressed into the sea. Her parents found her much later on the beach having an imaginary conversation with a group of people. According to Dumet and Ménéchal, who originally described the case, when she talked about the subject of her conversion, she was trying to "convince them [her parents] of her divine possession" (p. 159). Her family and friends had doubts about the truth of her experience, and she started to doubt the reality of the experience herself. "She had firmly believed in it for years, and her life had been transformed afterwards. This inspired her to write, and it also made her feel that she wasn't alone in life anymore, that someone was with her and in her who would always follow her. It was comforting and alarming at the same time" (p. 159). In their description of this clinical situation, Dumet and Ménéchal mention the dissociation of the being, the absence of unity of the self and the feeling of being inhabited by someone else. They do not hesitate to note that the feeling of having someone inside you is linked to the concept of possession, but

they hasten to add that the appearance of this presence in Elise "is just an unconscious way of occulting the void or rather the feeling of being sucked into nonexistence that she had felt since the loss of the maternal object" (p. 165). Her symptomology led them to believe that she had a schizophrenic pathology. However, Elise's experience on the beach in Normandy at the age of 17 had permanently changed her perception of the external world and of herself. While she is now 24 years old, the feeling of not being alone anymore, of being inhabited by someone else, does not alarm her. This unique experience, which she still refers to, is also a source of creative energy. Since then, she has written a novel and poetry. Two years ago, she went to Paris to take theater lessons. It is difficult for her to make sense of her disturbing experience and to accomplish her artistic projects. Of course, she is also troubled by a feeling of persecution. But when a teenager experiences a feeling of possession, is the cause always to be found in a form of psychic dissociation? Wouldn't it be more appropriate to talk about the difficulties experienced in incorporating conflicting psychic aspects in a case like Elise's? Wouldn't it make more sense to think of these difficulties as being the result of an incapacity to make the distinction between the inside and the outside, to define the limit between what constitutes "me" and what belongs to the "other"? Every culture furnishes landmarks for the constitution of psychic containers (or "psychic envelopes," using an expression introduced by Anzieu).(12, 13) Perhaps these landmarks were unclear in Elise's case.

6.3. Case 3

In 1994, Father Schindelholz published the narrative of the case of Barbara, a 19-year-old girl who lived in a city in Switzerland.(14) He recounts that a Zurich psychiatrist diagnosed Barbara with diabolic possession. The physician believed that what the young girl was suffering from was not a matter of medical science. As a result, the Catholic family began to look for a priest who would be able to help her. In the narrative, Father

Schindelholz provides a description of Barbara's symptoms. At the end of August 1971, "Besides various unexplainable afflictions, scratches suddenly appeared all over her legs and red spots covered her face. At that time, she had to quit her job. Coughing, suffocating, rigid fingers, and back pain became more and more common. She also had the feeling that somebody was pushing needles into her head, neck, lungs, and stomach. Whenever she entered a Catholic church (she belonged to this faith), she was immediately able to fold her rigid fingers and the coughing stopped instantaneously" (p. 10). Her health problems forced her to quit her job in a children's home. Barbara recounts that some time earlier, during a lunch break, she had been reading about the life of a saint, and she had told herself that she'd like to have a little of that saint's sanctity. When she laid the book down, she suddenly heard a lugubrious voice. At the end of October 1971, she began to develop tremendous physical strength: During a crisis, four men were required to keep her lying on her bed. On October 29, she started hearing voices and talking to them. The appearance of her face changed. She grimaced full of hatred, becoming unrecognizable during that time – always between 11 p.m. and 1:30 or 2 a.m. There were seven different masculine voices who refused to tell her their names, but who introduced themselves with numbers. They talked a great deal and answered questions. Number 1 was a bit boorish and number 2 seemed to be the spokesperson for the others. Number 2 was the one who talked the most and was present at each session. Number 3 appeared only rarely and was extremely violent. His voice was coarse and raucous. He violently threw Barbara against the walls and threw objects across the room. Sometimes Barbara had to put her head under the cold water faucet for fifteen minutes in the winter time. Her physical health remained unaffected although she was a frail girl weighing no more than forty kilograms at that time. Number 4 was haughty and arrogant and appeared only rarely. Number 5 was genteel, and the language he used was very refined. Number 6 was more serious and did not often participate. Number 7 revealed his identity

only at the end of the ordeal, "saying that he was a prince of hell" (p. 11). All of this went on for six and a half years, occurring about 80 percent of the time. However, the voices did not disturb her at three different times of the year: Christmas, Easter, and during the summer holidays. Father Schindelholz carried out many exorcism rituals during these years, always at the girl's home (she still lived with her parents). He only performed these rituals between 11 p.m. and 2 a.m. when the voices manifested themselves, and someone else always attended these sessions. These witnesses, her family and close friends, met to help support Barbara during her crises. After awhile, her parents were the only ones who continued to attend.

Father Schindelholz describes his first meeting with Barbara, when he arrived at 9:30 p.m. at the family home. "She came up to me immediately when the door was opened. She greeted me with a smile and a cheerful 'Good evening father.' But I perceived an expectation in her; she had the look of someone who asks: 'Is this one capable of more than the others'" (p. 13). Afterwards, everybody sat down and chatted about everyday things. Barbara listened closely to the conversation and laughed heartily when somebody told a joke. Nothing seemed to distinguish her from other girls her age. Father Schindelholz noticed that there were no watches or clocks in the room and that Barbara wasn't wearing one either. Suddenly she stood up very straight and went quickly to her room. The priest looked at his watch; it was 11 p.m. Everybody followed her. "The young girl had thrown herself on the couch and was writhing in a strange way. I watched her attentively, but she didn't seem to pay any attention to the people around her. She was short of breath, gasping, and her face was slightly redder than before. Her mother sat down beside her. The rest of us were standing above her. I took the risk of asking the ritual question: 'Who are you?' A sudden spurt of saliva in my direction was the answer. I stepped back and asked the same question, which triggered a litany of irate curses in response. I was able to catch a few words like: 'pork of a dog, dirty pig, head of a monkey, balls of a sheep,

and so on. ...' Each insult was followed by snarl-
ing, grimaces of hate and bulging eyes filled with
blood. It was already another, unrecognizable living being which was lying there. This being was
the opposite of the girl I had seen before who
had been so quiet, sweet, relaxed, gentle and gay"
(p. 14). He then offered to perform an exorcism.
After the parents agreed, he took out his prayer
book. He recounts that the demons tried to rip
it away from him. The book flew into the air.
"We immediately attached Barbara onto her bed,
where she struggled violently, trying to break
away. Four strong men had to hold her, while she
spit at them and scratched them. I thought that
the moment was right to start the exorcism, and
I made the sign of the cross while throwing some
holy water on the poor creature. The reaction
was immediate. She tried vainly to break free,
crying and hurling curses at us. She belched out
a series of extremely violent curse words, but I
went on with the prayer. I wanted to observe during this first exorcism session whether the four
characteristic signs of possession would manifest
themselves" (p. 15). The priest then noted that
all of these signs were soon observed. A long
monitoring process then began. The priest went
to see Barbara regularly at her home to perform
exorcisms. Between his visits, her mother called
him nearly every evening after 11 p.m. so that
the numbered voices could speak to him on the
phone, usually for fifteen to thirty minutes.

No immediate improvement was visible. On
the contrary, no progression was seen at all. At
the beginning of November 1972, after performing several exorcisms, the priest wrote to the
family that he was not sure that he could still
oversee the case. On November 16, the mother
replied that the night before she had cleaned the
kitchen three times between 12:30 and 1:15 a.m.
because "the numbers" had covered it with sugar.
The priest advised her to go on a pilgrimage to
Lourdes or Lisieux, places that were known for
their beneficial effects on visitors. A pilgrimage
was organized for Easter of 1973. During the mass
in the basilica of Lisieux, one of Barbara's hands
closed and she could no longer open it. She had
to go home with her hand in this position.

After the summer holidays, "the numbers"
started to appear again. To help her begin working again, she was given typewriting tasks to
perform at home. In the evening, "the numbers"
destroyed the work done during the day. On
July 9, 1974, when the numbers left Barbara as
they did every year for the summer holidays, they
announced that they would be back on August 5.
A second pilgrimage to Lourdes was undertaken on July 25. Everything seemed normal. On
August 5, at 11 p.m., the numbers were back. A
turning point occurred at the end of October 1975
when the numbers announced that they would
leave Barbara one day when their "leader" told
them to do so. But before that, they specified that
they wanted a prey. In fact, it took several more
years. On March 3, 1978, the numbers dictated an
important text, of which an excerpt reads: "The
bitch was left at our disposal. We could harass her
because the one at the top allowed us to. We tried
to use the strategy of illness, but we failed to bring
her to our side. 'Mister W.' also helped us a lot in
our work, but it has been a lost cause since the
beginning. Why did we really come? A very long
time ago, someone cursed Barbara's grandfather,
a curse related to a certain 'book.'... Mr. W. called
us and asked us to help him through our work;
that's why so many of us came. Mr. W. belongs to
us .... We are seven numbers. We cannot reveal
our names; it would be too dangerous, too dangerous for us. The solution is called 1/2 + 1/2 = 1.
That means that when the bitch gets married, we
will have to leave forever. Without conquering!
We are damned, damned! cursed! damned!"

Barbara's grandfather had died in 1977.
Mister W. was an acquaintance of the family.
Barbara's mother was convinced that this man had
been practicing black magic against them. In April
of 1978, Barbara was "released." At that point,
number 7 spoke for the first time and revealed his
name: "I am Astaroth." The priest identified him
with a pagan divinity in the Bible and said that
this divinity was the symbol of a powerful demon.
(He said, this divinity is mentioned in the Bible;
Astaroth is a plural. See Judg. 2.13, 1 Sam. 7.3 and
12.10, and 1 Chron. 6.56). A few months before
Barbara was "freed," she had become involved in

a romantic relationship with a friend. Her boyfriend never found out what happened to her after 11 p.m. They got married in the autumn of 1978. In 1994, when the story was published, the couple already had two children.

From a psychodynamic point of view, it seems important to emphasize that Barbara didn't have a romantic relationship until after her grandfather's death and that when her anticipated marriage, which meant leaving her parent's home, was announced in March of 1978, it was followed by the end of her ordeal. What effect did the curse that lay on her grandfather's shoulders have on Barbara's incapacity to start her own life? What was the nature of the relationship between Barbara and her grandfather? Was it necessary for him to die for a man to occupy a place in Barbara's life? Was he the prey the numbers asked for before their departure?

A psychoanalytic approach would certainly look for an unresolved intrapsychic conflict, perhaps stemming from incest, that caused the neurosis. In fact, several of Barbara's symptoms correspond to the classical description of hysteria. Father Schindelholz was convinced that Barbara was not suffering from hysteria, schizophrenia, or a paranoid disorder. He believed that the fact that Barbara remembered what the numbers had said after the episodes was proof that they were not psychiatric phenomena. This allowed her to write down most of what happened (p. 16). In fact, this criterion is insufficient.

Ellenberger documented all the cases of multiple personalities while trying to classify all the clinical varieties of the phenomenon. There are cases of multiple personalities who are simultaneous or successive, mutually conscious of each other or mutually unaware of each other, and even cases where only one of the personalities is aware of the other.(6) The remark that Barbara was aware of what happened while she was possessed after the episodes is Father Schindelholz's attempt to find a criterion that would make it possible to clearly distinguish possession from a psychiatric disorder. His attempt must be considered within the larger context of the different interpretational conflicts that have characterized the debates between

medical doctors and priests since the eighteenth century.

Did Barbara suffer from hysteria or possession? Answering that question would lead us to reproduce the same distribution of tasks established between clerics and physicians in the eighteenth century. A different approach might be more fertile. This approach admits the possibility that diverse interpretational levels coexist, with Barbara's suffering in a central position. From a psychopathological point of view, Barbara's psychological manifestations would undoubtedly have been interpreted as a phenomenon of hysteria. Diverse forms of somatization (coughing, suddenly paralyzed members, convulsions, and so forth) are considered to be distinctive features of hysteria. The problems were solved when Barbara became involved in a durable relationship with a man of her age, making us think that an intrapsychic conflict was the source of her suffering. Barbara's case was not considered from that point of view. The phenomenon was interpreted from the point of view of her family's system of beliefs: a demonic possession. It is interesting, however, to note the fact that, after six years of treatment, Barbara was freed from her suffering without resorting to psychiatry.

Should we compare the efficacy of the two different systems of treatment? In this specific case, limiting the phenomenon to a psychiatric diagnosis of hysteria without taking into consideration its spiritual meaning would probably have made Barbara and her family feel misunderstood, which could have led them to refuse the treatment. By listening to Barbara and her family over an extended period and letting them guide his interventions, Father Schindelholz was able to offer Barbara the therapeutic support that helped her to get through a difficult chapter in her life and achieve independence. We should mention that the priest felt on several occasions that he could not understand the reality he was confronted with. When reading his narration, it seems that the positive outcome was brought about despite his expectations. His merit consists in his endurance; he did not abandon Barbara when he could have considered the case hopeless. Too often, spiritual authorities are unaware of the relationship that is established between themselves and the person in need of help when they begin an exorcism. A lack of professionalism in the management of the therapeutic bond and the environment that is established through the practice of exorcism can have very damaging effects. Instead of considering that spiritual and psychic suffering are mutually exclusive and necessitate two different modes of treatment, it seems wiser, in certain cases, to try to integrate both approaches.

7. ANTHROPOLOGICAL CRITICISM

There is a principal criterion given in the *DSM-IV* to differentiate a possessed person from a person suffering from a DID, meaning someone who has several identities whether they are conscious of each other or not. In cases of possession, the identity that takes the control of the person is felt to be coming from the outside. The difference is essentially a question of how the person identifies with the different entities: a possessed person would at least sometimes identify himself or herself with the spirit he or she feels possessed by. In other words, in a case of possession, when the spirit or the entity speaks through a human being using "I," the spirit or entity is not thought to have its origin in the subject it talks through. In the list of examples of dissociative trances that are not considered as pathological, the *DSM-IV* tends to use the term *possession* with cultural differences. However, the case of Barbara, the presence of exorcist priests in each diocese of the Roman Catholic Church all over the world, and the practice of exorcism in Pentecostal evangelic churches in North America as well as in Europe show that the phenomenon of possession should not be exclusively associated with or limited to the non-Western world. This concept is part of the modern Western world as well. Certainly some would say that anthropological pre-modern conceptions are still present in the Western world and that religious environments support their conservation. But we believe that the opposition between what comes from the "inside" and what comes from the "outside" goes beyond culture. This opposition makes it possible

to describe the multiplicity of the human psyche and identity and makes us question whether the term *dissociation* is appropriate to describe this phenomenon. When an individual describes himself as being confronted with or having to face a spirit or an entity that comes from the outside and lives within him, why should we only talk about "dissociation" and not about "association" also? Systematically using the term *dissociative* reveals that, although we recognize that subjects can feel that external entities have penetrated their bodies, only one diagnosis is acceptable to us: their psychic cohesion is fragmented. This brings us to question an implicit assumption in this categorization; a fragmented identity or a multiple identity can only be the result of dissociation. Thus, before such a fragmentation, the human psyche was necessarily a coherent whole, complete and unified. From this point of view, every kind of psychic evolution that leads toward a certain multiplicity can only be the result of a loss of cohesion. The Western world is influenced by what Clifford Geertz calls "the occidental notion of the person"(15) which

1 tends to use the terms *individual* and *person* as if their meaning were equivalent; in other words, individual identity and personal identity are thought of as synonyms.
2 qualifies identity, in particular individual identity, according to two criteria: unity and uniqueness.

Accordingly, the person is seen in the Western world "as a cognitive universe that more or less determines behaviour, like a dynamic centre of consciousness, emotion, judgement and organized action integrated into a distinctive whole, and that, at the same time, is opposed to other wholes and to the natural and social environment." However, Geertz notes that in a broader global context of different cultures, this conception of a person is quite unusual. Several studies of intercultural psychology (16) or studies concerning the personality in the ancient world (17–19) (p. 55) (note 17) and (pp. 72–73) (note 18) have shown that, in most cultures, identity in the sense of uniqueness is assigned to a social group such as a family or a clan rather than to an individual. In other words, the *individual identity* is thought to be determined by the social group of origin.

The modern Western world conveys the project to mold distinctive individual identities with a high level of self-awareness and a high level of autonomy. We cannot contest the legitimacy of such a cultural project. Nevertheless, it does seem valid to question the actual degree to which this project has been accomplished in Western populations. What proportion of the population has actually achieved such maturity? The question can be considered from a sociological point of view and also from the point of view of developmental psychology. At what point in development is this psychic maturity attained? We would like to examine the following problem: Because the integration of psychic functions and the differentiation of identity are not innate, dissociation can only jeopardize that which has already been integrated. When a unified, differentiated identity has not (yet) been constructed, what paradigm can be used to examine the disturbances stemming from multiplicity?

Two hypotheses underlie our line of reasoning. First of all, the hypothesis of the incomplete asserts that a being is in a constant process of growth (becoming). A being is never a whole, nor a finished entity. This statement is nothing original; it is amply affirmed in psychotherapy: The confrontation with what lacks (failings, absence, project not yet achieved) is decisive for the elaboration of desire. But this aspect has been systematically forgotten in the exploration of the phenomenon of possession – the notion that a subject can be confronted with situations for which he is unprepared and which he is psychically unable to elaborate on a psychological level seems to be inconceivable. The second hypothesis is that of the possibility of intrusions, of a break-in. The trauma theory (20) examines psychic contents that break into a psyche that is not ready to assimilate them (for example, soldiers who witness traumatic scenes of violence during the war, persons present when a bomb explodes in a subway). Such contents can become obsessing: Although the scene took place a long time

ago, every time it is evoked it seems to be as vivid as it was the first time (for example, a soldier who was suddenly attacked during the night; many years later, he is woken up with a start every night by this scene). In that case, it means that these contents are not developed, not fantasized, not symbolized. If such contents trigger a dissociation, this would only be a secondary effect; it would be a disorder resulting from a weakened psyche trying to integrate these contents (compare the crypt concept introduced by Abraham and Torok).(21)

When the subject is not undergoing a psychic disorganization of what has already been constructed, but suffers from the presence of psychic contents that he is unable to deal with, wouldn't it be wiser to designate this as an "associative disorder" rather than a "dissociative disorder"? This might help to show that the subject has taken elements inside himself (for example, fantasies and fears) that do not belong to him (for example, proxy traumas). The same can be said of victims of torture. Some disorders result from the assimilation of the torturers by persons tortured.(22) In other words, the disorder appears because the person was trying to integrate a psychic content that he shouldn't.

8. COLLABORATION BETWEEN PSYCHIATRISTS AND RELIGIOUS PROFESSIONALS

When a person is said to be possessed, a question comes to the fore: What should the clergyman or religious authority (priest, pastor, exorcist, or shaman) be responsible for and what should the psychiatrist be responsible for? Both parties, based on their systems of reference, are concerned about the person's autonomy. For the clergyman, the exorcist, or the shaman, the person who complains of being possessed is thought to have lost his autonomy to think or act. The person is dominated by forces that he cannot control. To be liberated, the possessed person counts on the authority of the expert on spiritual matters. The spiritual authority assumes that benevolent spiritual forces (gods, protecting ancestors, spirits, among others) will intervene and serve as allies to the exorcist or shaman. The efficacy of the intervention under-taken largely depends on the extent to which the possessed person, his family, and friends accept it.

For the psychiatrist, the goal is the patient's psychic autonomy. The complaint of possession will be interpreted as a paranoid delusion or as the expression of the patient's dependence on thoughts of persecution. A therapeutic strategy could con-sist of reinforcing the "self" by helping the patient develop a rational stance toward the entities he feels possessed by. The analysis could consist of demon-strating that some of the patient's ideas are incoher-ent or, in a more radical way, arguing against the existence of the spiritual entities mentioned by the patient and suggesting that he ignore these entities to show him that they only have the power that he gives them. This strategy can be effective, but it can also be a complete failure because of the violent confrontation involved between the demons or evil spirits and the authority of the psychiatrist. Even worse, this strategy can lead to a conflict in the patient's loyalties that he cannot deal with, when medical compliance involves the humiliation of his native culture or religious faith.

To avoid provoking a confrontation between antagonistic systems, the psychiatrist can choose to occupy the position of someone who would like to establish links between the two worlds of mean-ings. The aim is not for the psychiatrist to give up his own system of reference. The challenge is to include the patient's cultural perspective, the spiri-tual counselor's cultural perspective, and the clini-cian's psychological viewpoint in the discussion. At the least, the patient must realize that the psychia-trist is willing to take cognizance of the patient's per-sonal system of reference. Collaboration between the psychiatrist and the patient's religious system is not always possible. For example, the patient may seek the help of an exorcist who considers that his intervention is incompatible with any psychiatric intervention. The aim would then be to help the patient position himself so that he can accept the support of the medical system without necessarily betraying his own system of reference. In any case, the psychiatrist should be aware that his domain of competence is based on a Western definition of illness and suffering. Despite the difficulty he

may have in accepting that the patient attributes a different meaning to illness and suffering, the psy-chiatrist will benefit from taking a different point of view into account. Understanding the role the patient assigns him in his own system of reference can only be helpful to the psychiatrist. To help the patient view the therapeutic interventions of the healers that belong to his system of reference from a critical angle, he must also develop an analytical point of view toward the psychiatric interventions recommended within the context of the medical system. Within the care setting, the aim is to pro-vide therapeutic possibilities that help the patient make choices leading to a higher level of psychic autonomy.

9. ETHNOPSYCHIATRIC CONSULTATIONS

An "ethnopsychiatric consultation" (a term coined by Georges Devereux who introduced the concept) can be helpful in this approach.(23) During such a session, a psychiatrist and co-therapists from differ-ent cultural backgrounds meet with the patient to discuss his symptoms and specific problems. Each co-therapist can explain how these problems would be interpreted by the system of reference that he represents. In other words, the co-therapists play the role of cultural mediator to facilitate the inter-pretation of one reference system through another. Possession can take on different meanings depend-ing on the patient's system of reference. This spe-cial session can help him to more clearly formulate the meaning of possession in his own system of reference. As we saw in Barbara's case, possession is not always the result of cultural interpretations originating outside the Western world. Thus, an ethnopsychiatric consultation could also be useful to patients coming from families with deep Western roots. In this case, the participation of co-therapists who can describe how the Catholic Church or dif-ferent protestant and evangelical groups interpret possession and exorcism would be important. Such a session can help develop better communication between the patient and the psychiatrist and facili-tate the construction of a common system of ref-erence incorporating the meanings of the patient's system of reference as well as the meanings of the medical system. This can allow both participants, the psychiatrist as well as the patient, to continue the treatment without each being locked into his own system of reference. The ethnopsychiatric setting helps construct a sphere that contains enough space for both of them, but that also forces them to change. This does not mean that the ethnopsychiatric consultation becomes a session for deliverance prayers, exorcism, or possession rituals. Because Devereux has constructed the concept of ethnopsychiatric consultation as a possible component of a medical treatment, the consultation is supposed to be under the responsibility of a doctor. So, even if one of the co-therapists had the status of a religious authority in the patient's system of reference, the ethnopsychiatric consultation is conducted by a doctor and takes place within the framework of the medical system of care. As a unique psychiatric setting, this consultation enriches traditional medical treatment and provides the opportunity for individuals from different cultures to construct a common frame of reference. Although this frame is medical and not religious and belongs to the Western system of care, this doesn't prevent a debate about whether religious rituals are appropriate. The topic can be discussed, but the final decision should be left to the patient and his family and friends. The purpose of the discussion should be to help provide a meaning for the decision to make use of religious rituals or not.

ACKNOWLEDGMENTS

With our grateful acknowledgments to Dr. Franceline James, ethnopsychiatrist in Geneva, for her remarks.

REFERENCES

1. Ross CA, Duffy CMM, Ellason JW. Prevalence, reliability and validity of dissociative disorders in an inpatient setting. *J Trauma Dissociation*. 2002;3: 7–17.
2. Spanos NP. *Multiple Identities and False Memories: A Sociocognitive Perspective.* Washington: American Psychological Association; 1996.
3. Janet P. *Major Symptoms of Hysteria.* New York: Macmillan; 1925.
4. Janet P. *The Major Symptoms of Hysteria: Fifteen Lectures Given in the Medical School of Harvard University.* New York: Macmillan; 1907.
5. Rausky F. *Mesmer ou la révolution thérapeutique.* Paris: Payot; 1977.
6. Ellenberger HF. *The Discovery of the Unconscious.* New-York: Basic Books Inc., Publishers; second printing; 1970.
7. Coons PM, Bowman ES, Kluft RP, Milstein V. The cross-cultural occurrence of multiple personality disorder: additional cases from a recent survey. *Dissociation.* 1991;4(4):124–128.
8. Bourguignon E. *Psychological Anthropology: An Introduction to Human Nature and Cultural Differences.* New York: Holt, Rinehart and Winston; 1979.
9. Hell B. *Possession et chamanisme: Les maîtres du désordre.* Paris: Flammarion; 1999.
10. Ross CA. *Multiple Personality Disorder: Diagnosis, Clinical Features and Treatment.* New York: John Wiley; 1989.
11. Dumet N, Ménéchal J. *15 cas cliniques en psychopathologie de l'adulte.* Paris: Dunod; 2005.
12. Anzieu D. *Le Moi-peau.* Paris: Dunod; 1995.
13. Anzieu D, Briggs D. *Psychic Envelopes.* London: Karnac; 1990.
14. Schindelholz G. *Exorcisme, un prêtre parle.* Porrentruy: Editions Le Pays; 1994.
15. Geertz C. "From the natives point of view": on the nature of anthropological understanding. In: Basso KH, Selby HA, eds. *Meaning in Anthropology.* Albuquerque: University of New Mexico Press; 1976:221–237.
16. Triandis HC, Bontempo R, Villareal MJ, Asai M, Lucca N. Individualism and collectivism: cross-cultural perspectives on self-ingroup relationships. *J Pers Soc Psychol.* 1988;54(2):323–338.
17. Malina BJ. *The New Testament World.* Atlanta: John Knox; 1981.
18. Malina BJ, Neyrey JH. First-century personality: dyadic, not individual. In: Neyrey JH, ed. *The Social World of Luke-Acts.* Peabody, MA: Hendrickson; 1991:67–96.
19. Brandt P-Y. *L'identité de Jésus et l'identité de son disciple: le récit de la transfiguration comme clef de lecture de l'évangile de Marc (NTOA 50).* Fribourg: Editions Universitaires, Göttingen: Vandenhoeck & Ruprecht; 2002.
20. Lebigot, F. *Traiter les traumatismes psychiques. Clinique et prise en charge.* Paris: Dunod; 2005.
21. Abraham N, Torok M. *L'écorce et le noyau.* Paris: Flammarion; 1987.
22. Sironi F. *Bourreaux et victimes: Psychopathologie de la torture.* Paris: Odile Jacob; 1999.
23. Devereux G. *Essais d'ethnopsychiatrie générale.* Paris: Gallimard; 1970.

12 Self-Identity and Religion/Spirituality

PIERRE-YVES BRANDT, CLAUDE-ALEXANDRE FOURNIER, AND SYLVIA MOHR

SUMMARY

Self-identity results from construction. Self-consciousness is achieved in several steps. Based on the attachment bond, the infant's self is constructed within the framework of the first dyadic relationships, particularly the relationship with the mother. It successively enriches itself with new self senses (Stern). By language and by the access to the symbolic function, infants get more directly in contact with cultural constructs, reference points they can identify with. Thus, religious figures replace attachment figures and play the role of substitute of the parental figures. Based largely on a definition of self-identity by Ricoeur, this chapter shows how the religious dimension of the self stems from the interaction between processes one can identify with, present ever since infancy, and the cultural environment the individual comes into contact with. Religious traditions carry reference points one can identify with especially via accounts, rites, and roles. Highlighting the aspects one must take into consideration when providing therapeutic treatment, we illustrate these processes of identification by three case studies. Religion can help restore identity but it can also weaken it. When the patient and the therapist come from very different cultural contexts, it is important for the therapist to try to integrate the patient's reference system to support the therapeutic alliance.

I. INTRODUCTION

Since the beginning of the twenty-first century, narcissistic issues have become quite meaningful in the clinical picture. The increased fluidity of reference points has rendered identities more unstable, more blurred. For a certain number of our contemporaries, this context weakens the construction of the relationship with the self. When this situation is experienced in a painful manner, it results in a feeling of identity loss with a depressive component, or even in identity disorders with psychotic characteristics (identity confusion in the manic form of a grandiose self or schizoid organization, for instance). The need to relieve this suffering manifests as a quest for landmarks, in the hope of reassurance or even confirmation of one's true self (for example, in the fields of sexual orientation, intergenerational relations, professional, or vocational choices). This expectation applies to all systems that provide a sense of purpose, among which religions play a special role.

2. THE ROLE OF RELIGION/SPIRITUALITY IN THE CONSTRUCTION OF SELF-IDENTITY

How can a religious system or spiritual framework address this need? Let us note from the start that individual identity is not an automatic given. It results from development during which psychological processes are at work. Based on initial figures of attachment, the infant's and then the child's self is constructed according to parental models. Afterwards, by progressive socialization, the child gets in contact with an increasingly vast circle of figures to identify with (potentially). In adolescence, some of these figures (peers, adult role models, or idealized historical or fictional characters) will play a decisive part in finding the strength to break away from the family environment. All these processes at work from birth until adolescence remain active throughout adult life. The interactions between religion/spirituality and identification models are circular. Religious behavior and spiritual values are transmitted by means of an identity model of the child or adult. From an early age via the adults in their lives, individuals come into contact with religious or spiritual figures that help them shape their identities. The models lauded by religions and the religious or spiritual figures taken as role models are created partly based on identity bearings discovered during development. The terms *father, mother, brother, sister, friend, lover, companion,* and so forth are often applied to religious models. The transmission of religious aspects of identity, however, is not limited to interpersonal relations. Socialization assumes the ability to find one's place in a group. Children very rapidly become familiar with customs and learn to assume roles, not only in contact with their parents, but also in larger social groups.

3. CHAPTER ORGANIZATION

After providing a definition of self-identity, this chapter will begin by presenting the developmental aspects that condition the construction of the self. We will then discuss the construction of a core self, the constitution of the first psychic envelope. Then we will approach the role of identification processes in the construction of a differentiated self-identity. These aspects will be articulated by means of attachment theory. After that, we will go into detail on the interactions between religion/spirituality and identity construction. Toward this aim, we will examine religious figures as figures of attachment, the role of the parental figures, and then its extension to the relationship between the individual and the group. This will allow an emphasis on various forms of collective symbols provided by the cultural environment: the identification figures presented in parables, the identification models conveyed in rites, and the social roles. We will then present and analyze a few cases, some of which were followed up with psychiatric treatment or psychotherapy. The conclusion will provide a multicultural perspective

on these issues. In summation, we will first examine how a religious or spiritual experience can threaten the cohesion of the self and then explore under what circumstances religion/spirituality can contribute to reestablishing identity. Second, we will discuss the provisions involved in considering the patient's reference system in the treatment process. The goal is to determine, for each case, what in the patient's religious and spiritual referents will permit the establishment of a secure, defined self-relationship and lead to accepted social roles.

4. DEFINITION OF SELF-IDENTITY

The philosopher Paul Ricoeur distinguished between the *idem-identity* and the *ipse-identity*.(1) The *idem*-identity designates what is not altered by time. In relation to the individual, it traces back to one's genetic code as would be true for fingerprints, for example. On a psychological level, it defines the character in the sense of the personality traits that individuals preserve throughout their lives. This is a static definition of identity. On the contrary, the *ipse*-identity designates the continuity of the relationship with the self through the inevitable alterations and discontinuities over a lifetime. This definition is a dynamic one; it takes into consideration the formation of the individual. Of course, individual identity is supported by one's genetic foundation. Nevertheless, knowing only somebody's genetic code is surely not enough for assessing an individual's identity. One's psychological being is constantly developing through interaction with the environment. The feeling of identity, the feeling of "being oneself," and the individual's self-image are the result of an ongoing process of construction that is a continual quest for balance. In this regard, the self is an entity situated at the interface of the intrapsychic and the social constructs of the personality.

This entity must be distinguished from other entities used to refer to the subject. The self is neither the *ego* nor the *id*. The self designates self-representation; how individuals think of themselves in the long term. This representation is inevitably culturally dependent: it contains a certain concept of self-identity that can vary in function of age, sex, and social position. It is "how the subject is advised to think of himself or herself."

So that this self does not remain an auxiliary, peripheral being (a false self?), it has to be taken charge of by the *ego* (according to Freudian terminology here), which adjusts the degree of centrality it grants to the identifications offered by the (representation of the) self conveyed by culture. Furthermore, preferences in this field are more or less influenced by the family environment.

At each stage of their existence, individuals construct the self their ego is able to undertake, by means of identity representations provided by their environment. A transformation of the self can result from reorganization caused by endogenous factors (new cognitive abilities, new impulsive expressions), or by exogenous factors (access to a new social position, confronting situations that are not easily assimilated by the already constructed self). Transformation of the self means: access to a new identity (pp. 56–57).(2)

This definition of the self should not be mistaken with the Self defined by Carl Gustav Jung as an archetype whose function is the union of opposites and that is perceived by the ego as transcendent as it is able to integrate the ego and what the ego is not able to integrate, or shadow. For Jung, the relationship between the Self and the ego is situated at the level of the intrapsychic. What we mean here by self is, on the contrary, located where the ego meets with its environment. It is an effect of symbolism that language construction and self-representation are necessary in communicational exchange.

5. DEVELOPMENTAL ASPECTS OF IDENTITY CONSTRUCTION

In his works on the interpersonal world of the infant,(3) Daniel Stern pinpoints the emergence of a sense of self to a very young age. Already at two to six months, an infant begins to have the sense of a core self. The permanence of the contact with his own body allows him to recognize himself as a physical entity with its own cohesion and continuity. He experiences the permanent availability of the sensory and proprioceptive feedback coming from his own body, as opposed to the exterior signals coming from outside his self. This description connects what Didier Anzieu called the "Moi-peau,"(4) or "skin-ego". The feelings of identity and self-representation are based on the construction of a psychic envelope, which develops using the bodily envelope for support. The bodily envelope is a border between the body and the outside world and an internalization of this first experience of creating an inner vessel within oneself. This sense of a "core self as a separate, cohesive, delimited physical entity with its own awareness of activity, affection, and temporal continuity" (p. 21),(5) will deepen at the age of seven months with *the sense of a subjective self*, when the baby is able to attribute to others the capability of having a mental state similar to its own. Then, during the second year of life, this sense is further enriched by *the sense of a verbal self*, which forms with the beginnings of verbal language.

The emergence of these different definitions of the self is achieved in and by interpersonal relationships, particularly with the mother (or with any other person in charge of mothering). This relationship, integral to identity, is first of all an affective one. Daniel Stern referred to it as "affective attunement." The attunement can be seen as the mother's response to the child's spontaneous activity and particularities. This response is both a validation of and a support to their activity. There are of course different levels of attunement, ranging from a pure and simple rebuff to modeling appropriate behavior (*the good-enough mother*, according to Winnicott).

The affective attunement is present from the emergence of the *sense of a core self* (in holding, handling, and presenting objects). Infants will internalize "schemas-of-being-with," which will serve as a model for future interactions. Thus, the "tickle the tummy" game is learned from the mother, but it is recognized when played with other people. In other words, the identity is constructed in the relationship with the mother but is maintained in a prototype recalled by a cue. Identity is not part of the actual goal. By the range of affective attunements that she provides, the mother will validate or repudiate certain experiences. Together with the creation of *the sense of a core self*, this initiates differentiation between the social self and the disavowed self. The *social self* is created by the experiences of the self that are selected and attributed value because they satisfy somebody else's needs and desires. The *disavowed self* consists of a conglomerate of disavowed self-experiences that are not easily expressed using language. During development, the social self will be perceived as a *false self* in personal experiences further determined by the "internal conception," to which being one's *true self* will be attributed. This is because the social self satisfies the desires of others before its own.

With the emergence of *the sense of a subjective self* and of the infant's newly acquired ability to recognize in others a mental state similar to its own, the domains of privacy and intimacy become possible. A third domain of the self is established, the *private self*, composed of experiences one does not share, but that are not disavowed. The emergence of *the sense of a verbal self* creates a new way of being-with between mother and child by resorting to verbal symbols in sharing meaning. In this sense, language acquisition is not only regarded as an access to individuation, but also as a powerful means of maintaining union. Indeed, learning language strengthens the psychological bond first with relatives and then with other members of the language's culture. This developmental vision of early childhood (0–2 years old) conceives of a forging of the identity within the crucible of the relationship. Infants establish themselves by

internalizing types of intersubjective relationships, that is, various forms of "being-with." They are regarded from the start as differentiated beings. Another perspective on the construction of identity emphasizes the *object* of the relationship; the person in the relationship rather than the manner of relating to him or her. This distinction matters from the moment we want to follow Freud's reasoning and associate partial identification with only certain traits of a person, as opposed to a global identification with him or her.

6. THE PROCESS OF IDENTIFICATION

According to a Freudian interpretation, identification is "the act by which an individual becomes identical to another, or by which two human beings become identical" (p. 187).(6) Freud distinguishes three identification modes: a primary identification, a secondary identification, and a partial identification.

Primary identification is born in the first relationship with the mother. It is the original form of connection to another person, marked from the outset by affective ambivalence. Contrary to Stern, Freud did not consider infants to be differentiated from the very beginning. Rather, he assumes that as long as both sexual and generational lack of differentiation predominate in the first relationship with the mother, the ego and the alter-ego are not clearly differentiated and that, strictly speaking, an object relation cannot be established. The difference between Stern's and Freud's points of view results from a difference in criteria when talking about differentiation. From his research on babies, Stern was able to highlight an infant's sense of self that implies the ability to differentiate between self and others long before the other is constructed as a love object different from the self, according to Freud's criteria. Characterized by primitive orality, the primary identification is thus an identification with the relative, the mother figure. It is experienced and symbolized as a bodily operation: incorporation. Freud believes that, in the same way, during mourning the lost object is incorporated and empowered at the same time with a loss of interest in the individual's social life.

Secondary identifications overlay this chronologically preceding primary identification. This process is no longer achieved by incorporation, but rather by introjection. This process conveys people and with them their inherent qualities from the inside to the outside in a fantastical mode. Contrary to incorporation, it does not necessarily imply reference to bodily limitations.

Contrary to the first two identification modes, the third one, partial identification, can be achieved without any relationship of love or hatred. On the basis of ability, or will, subjects can identify themselves, or put themselves in the same situation (community) as a person. Moreover, identification can concern a person's unique trait.

According to Freudian theory, identity can (from the view of the second stage) be traced back to the construction of the self, of the ego. In the end, it stems from the product of the three identification modes. The construction of the individual's identity is thus initially marked by the dyadic relationship (more or less undifferentiated according to the authors' required criteria) with the mother.

As mentioned previously, primary identification is the basis of the identifications that follow. Individual identity will develop based on this relationship with the mother. This dyadic relationship takes the lead, provides protection, and assuages anguish. From the point of view of its object, the relationship can be projected at a higher level onto a divine figure. It is therefore the maternal function (the qualities special to mothering) that is projected on divinity (which is, in this sense, sexually undifferentiated) (Freud, 1927).

The triangular relationship including a third party succeeds this dyadic relation. The third role is that of the father. Freud theorizes on the establishment of this three-way relationship by means of the Oedipus complex. He estimates it emerging at around 3 to 5 years of age, but it begins even sooner. This relational switch is simultaneous with the beginnings of sexual differentiation. Young children learn that they are a boy or a girl. The father interrupts the privileged relationship between mother and child. He necessitates a sort of forsaking, a necessary separation from the mother. For the young boy, this break leads to a relationship of rivalry and love with the father. The young boy will thus identify himself with the father while simultaneously being his rival (for access to the mother). Through this experience of duality, trying to keep two parental images together (the good and the bad father, according to Mélanie Klein), the child integrates two structural taboos, just as much individual as collective, which are the taboo on incest and the taboo on murder. As much as in the introjection of the parental images, what will survive in the formation of the personality is what has been internalized from the relationships among the members of the triad. From a religious point of view, the father's arrival marks the arrival of law, of separation, and of judgment. In representation of the divinity, the paternal characteristics projected onto the divine figure do not erase the maternal traits, but rather join them. In adolescence, becoming a man or a woman (a sexually differentiated adult) allows access to reproduction and therefore to identifications with paternal or maternal qualities and with the qualities of parents and adults in general. These partial identifications go together with an attack on the parental imagos, a confrontation that is necessary for differentiation. Adolescents must be able to assert themselves through rebellion to escape identification with a role model. Each integration of differentiation (subject/object, pleasure-ego/reality-ego, differences in sex or generation) can be traumatic if there are no anticipatory representations. "The cleavage of the Ego is a denial of these differences when they catch by surprise an unprepared by anticipatory representations Ego" (p. 98).(7) It is therefore a lack of sufficient representative introductions that make identity crises traumatic for the child.

As demonstrated by Freud, religious figures can be empowered via the unresolved oedipal conflict to escape such a growth process and to lead to what he calls neurotic religion. However, religious figures can also serve as a support in facing a growth crisis, either by offering counter-models allowing teenagers to assert themselves before the parental figures, or else by helping them surpass a deficiency or a loss by accepting the limits of the human condition. (8) Following the mode of partial identification, children will pursue the construction of their identity through the selection of attitudes, choice of behaviors, and integration of value systems. This construction clearly stems from the constant interaction with the educational environment. It can thus include an emphasis, marked by the educational environment, on a religious or spiritual dimension.

7. ATTACHMENT AND IDENTIFICATION

Parental figures are the first identifying figures. However, before orienting the construction of the identity by encouraging certain attitudes or dependencies, the parental figures are responsible for establishing a bond for the infant that serves as a foundation for identification. This basic function has been more thoroughly described by attachment theories. The attachment bond especially has been researched in the context of the relationship between trauma and resilience. Studies on attachment are responsible for the greatest and best contributions to understanding the capacity for coping with trauma. Attachment theories have truly expanded through the work of John Bowlby.(9) According to Bowlby, "Psychological development exists in newborns' ability to establish a secure mode of connection with a close adult. It is this mode of connection that allows them to progressively distance themselves from their mothers and to explore the world while still being sure of their mothers providing the security and affection they need." Two important ideas emerge from these works. First of all, the importance of early care becomes evident. According to Donald Winnicott's terminology, a "good enough mother" is the one who gives the child basic psychological security, allowing him or her to deal with later trauma. Second, and what the attachment theorists are currently developing, children must be able

to benefit from at least one secure attachment bond, from a stable landmark, to support them in the various difficult situations they must overcome. Boris Cyrulnik was primarily responsible for the promotion in France of the idea of "development tutors" or "resilience tutors."(10) These "resilience tutors," who are not medical care professionals, are suitable for ensuring a secure attachment, strengthening a person's self-esteem in a delicate situation, and helping to make sense of life's events. According to Serge Tisseron, "The idea is to allow psychologically fragile people to create self-images, as well as images of others, that are able to think, feel, and distinguish between representations and emotions that are shared and those that are personal. In the end, these persons must arrive at a self-image that is capable of creating and breaking bonds, both in a self-to-self dialogue – deep down inside – and in exchanges with others" (p.24).(11) In this way, they bear the history and thus the child's identity during periods of great fragility. "Resilience tutors" are co-authors of the child's history, allowing him or her to recreate self-images and images of others.

At this stage, it becomes possible to see how impulse theory and attachment theories complement each other. It is relationship, such as defined by Daniel Stern in affective attunement or by John Bowlby in internal operating models, that contributes to the internalization of parental figures. These parental figures are stable and formative in a secure attachment that introduces the pleasure of a relationship; they are much less formative when the forms of attachment are insecure and are built on anxiety. Stable and structuring attachment figures favor introjection. They support the child or adult in the processes of symbolization and liaison (according to the language of metapsychology). For Serge Tisseron, "the capacity for introjection … is part of an intersubjective process between the child – or the adult – and a third person who fulfils maternal functions" (p.116).(11) Attachment figures that are not very formative will favor what Nicolas Abraham and Maria Torok refer to as "inclusions," a kind of pocket containing psychological elements that can produce strange manifestations in which subjects do not recognize themselves.(12)

In summary, the attachment relationship is a foundation and a vector for the internalization of the parental figures. It responds to a primary need. It is on the basis of this maternal function, later replaced by others, that the secondary and the partial identifications develop, allowing access to the symbolization processes (communication codes, access to language). In this way, the internalization of the relationship with stable and structuring parental figures depends on attachment and, therefore, on the subject's capacities of symbolization such as employment, learning of ritual practices, and construction of social roles.

8. RELIGIOUS FIGURES AND ATTACHMENT

Mary Ainsworth has shown how, on the path to adulthood, the first attachment figures are replaced by sexual partners, family members (grandparents, brothers, sisters, or other kin), and members of peer groups.(13) Therapists also are assigned the role of an attachment figure. To fully benefit from psychotherapy, it is imperative that the patient lean on a secure base.(9) From a developmental point of view, religious figures play the role of attachment figures, because they offer a secure relational frame. Ainsworth notes that priests or pastors are also potential attachment figures. In the religious field, divinities or saints can be used as reassuring figures. It is worth considering up to what point we can speak of attachment figures when perceptible contact is not possible.

In the psychology of religion, Granqvist and Kirkpatrick have developed the idea that religious figures would fill a lack of attachment bonds and play the role of "resilience tutors" by incarnating the parental function. In most Western religious traditions and in attachment research, the religious individual's close relationship with a personal God is central.(14) In Bowlby's normative attachment conceptualization, the term *attachment relationship* does not refer to any type of close relationship but exclusively to those that

meet four criteria: proximity maintenance, safe haven, secure base, and separation distress.(15) Granqvist's and Kirkpatrick's studies are based on the assumption that these four criteria are reasonably met as concerns the relationship of the believer with a spiritual object/figure. Hence, it is suggested that some aspects of attachment are similar for the believer in relation to his or her spiritual object/figure and for the child in relation to her parents, that is, they serve the function of obtaining/maintaining a sense of perceived security when in distress.(16) There are several means available for the religious individual to establish a sense of proximity or closeness to a spiritual figure/object, such as using symbols, engaging in rituals, and prayer.(14) Regarding the safe haven aspect of attachment, one of the best documented findings in psychology of religion is that believers turn to God in situations of distress. Such situations are diverse and include loss through death and divorce,(17) emotional crises,(18, 19) and relationship problems,(20) all of which are likely to activate the individual's attachment system. Two different modes of psychological coherence related to spiritual/religious coping have been described. The correspondence hypothesis suggests that there is a correspondence between early child-parent interactions on the one hand and a person's ability to cope in relation to a spiritual object/figure on the other. According to this hypothesis, a secure attachment history would enable a person to use a spiritual/religious object/figure as an attachment figure, which proximity would help regulate affects. The compensation hypothesis suggests that an insecure attachment history would lead to a strong religiousness/spirituality as a compensation of the lack of perceived security.(21)

9. RELIGIOUS FIGURES PLAYING THE ROLES OF PARENTAL FIGURES

Referential religious figures can bridge the gaps between identification figures. In certain religious traditions, people practicing a religious function are called *father* or *mother*. These same denominations can be applied to saints or to divine figures. In other words, believers are invited to situate themselves in a child-parent relationship. Antoine Vergote and Alvaro Tamayo have collected studies that have highlighted the way in which a divine figure, in the Christian context but also outside this context, combines paternal and maternal aspects.(22) Compared with the father's image or to the mother's image, God's image joins paternal traits such as maintaining order and providing protection with maternal traits such as unconditional love and kindness. These results, although based on a population of Belgian children, could be generalized to other cultural environments.

In the same vein, on a basis of case studies on a psychiatric population, Rizzuto (23, 24) shows how much God's figure builds on the foundation of a given individual's parental figures. This gives way to contemplation of two types of therapeutic intervention while dealing with patients to whom God or a divine figure plays an important role. In one scenario, the therapist can try working on the perception of divine figures to alter the bond to the paternal or to the maternal figure. This involves inviting the patients to explore their representation of God or other divine figure by asking whether it corresponds to their system of beliefs and whether this figure is influenced by the figures of their own parents. A second possibility is investigating whether this divine figure plays the role of an attachment figure or of an identification figure and whether it is possible for the patient to draw support from the figure to face her difficulties and build her own identity.

10. THE INDIVIDUAL AND THE GROUP

The collective dimension is an essential element for the construction of the religious/spiritual identity of the individual. The need for protection and affective proximity can also be filled in a religious community, as a way station for the family environment. Attachment theory is not exactly an adequate framework for describing this function fulfilled by a group, because it applies in theory to the relationship between two individuals. The

function of the receiving and protective group will be better described in terms of a substitute of the maternal envelope (Winnicott, 1968).(25) The source of religious or spiritual references mobilized by the subject to interpret the world is not initially inherent to the individual, but is rather found in cultural constructions. The subject turns to her culture to find the words and the conceptual and behavior categories for interpreting her experiences. Thus, there are special rites of passage that accompany the important transformations of a major life event, such as birth, coming of age, marriage, or death. Nevertheless, in Western or Westernized societies, there is a clear tendency to individualize the rites. It is in this context that David Le Breton (26) interprets adolescents' risky behaviors as attempts to fill the void of the rite of passage from childhood to adult life in these societies. By putting their life in danger, adolescents try to test their limits. This should be understood as a sort of cry for help, an attempt to provide oneself with an understanding of the path to adult status. However, without clear signals coming from the outside, young people are in danger of taking risks unaware. Extreme sports without sufficient training, car racing, overdose, and excessive dieting are all attempts to ensure that one is in control of one's own life and of the world. Adults know that such control can only be relative and limited. Their task is to protect the children, who are still incapable of recognizing their limits, and to help them get to know themselves so that they can become autonomous. In other words, the construction of the individual identity is achieved through recognition from others. It is in the confrontation between the representation I have of myself and the representation that others convey to me that I learn who I am. Nonetheless, this confrontation is not only focused on the construction of the specific identity. Surely, if everything goes well, individuals will learn to know themselves thanks to an image sent to them by their environment. However, a society's educational system is also an expression of expectation the society has of the individual: that she adjust to fit the environment. The construction of the self is not only contained in the representation of what constitutes the individual on the basis of independent choices. The self is also shaped by the environment that guides the choices. The self-image an individual projects thus results from a compromise between what the individual emanates and what the society expects. The quality of an individual's integration in her life environment will depend on the extent of this compromise of combining individual and collective expectations.

II. COLLECTIVE SYMBOLIZATION OF THE INDIVIDUAL IDENTITY

Any given society proposes a culturally shared conception of self-identity. The cultural representations that convey it vary. It can be expressed through artistic productions. Self-awareness, attitudes, and behaviors that can be lent to an individual are defined in novels, children's stories, documentary films, and fiction movies. Advertisements, interviews, news stories, social roles dictated by professional activities, law, education, and health systems are all vectors that shape the conception of a given society's self-identity. Religious institutions or the circumstances responsible for the relationship with the unpredictable, transcendence, and the afterlife also contribute to the conception of the self. Hence, tales displaying mythological, divine, ancestral, or exceptional historical figures serve as a support to identification. Christian tradition heavily emphasizes the *imitation of Christ*. To cite only a few examples, Moses is the classic example for a Jew, Buddha for a Buddhist, and a Sufi master for certain Islamic groups. Thus, in various religious traditions, exemplary figures contribute to the foundations of identity. Accounts of these figures' lives are told, and episodes from these lives are taken as examples to follow. By reading or listening to these accounts, the reader or listener sets up the processes of identification necessary to understand the story. The identity can then be built by complete or partial appropriation of the figure brought out in the story, or, on the contrary, by antagonistic reaction to this figure. In this case, the account can waken experiences

of the self to which the subject had not previously had access. In other words, at certain moments of their lives, individuals can manage to make sense of the situation they are in by identifying similarities to a situation experienced by a central figure of the religious tradition they have chosen. It is then an already-experienced situation that is retold through a story about a figure from the past. In all these cases, the cohesion of the identity is found following the narration mode. The transformation of identity, threatening the continuity of the self, is supported by the narrative plot: By telling the story of this transformation, individuals reestablish continuity beyond the rupture. Herein lies the identity, in the sense of the *ipse*-identity, such as suggested by Paul Ricoeur.(1) The staging of identity construction in stories shows the narrative character of the individual identity. The stories are the collective symbolization.

Another form of symbolization of self-identity is its *mise-en-scene* during rites. Rites are cultural devices built to shape the identity of those taking part in them. Thus, there are rites of passage to mark coming of age, marriage, or death. The words, the concepts, or the behaviors established by these rites often contain an important religious or spiritual dimension. Although each rite of passage is generally experienced only once by an individual, other rites, such as collective or individual prayers, taking part in the Eucharist, confession, family or community celebrations, or pilgrimages, are reiterative. Whichever form they take, these rites provide bearings that can be used for identification shared by those adhering to the tradition that conveys them. Their function is one of facilitating integration into society and social roles.

As for rites of passage, they could be thought to only spur a transformation in the intended individuals. However, every person present at the event reflects on his or her own path. Participation means putting oneself in a position of identification. For some of them, it means preparing for what they will one day be called on to experience; for others, reliving a past rite. In a narrative or ritual manner, stories and rites symbolize a process of construction of this identity. They direct the roles to be played.(27) In anticipation of experiences that patients could perceive as threatening the cohesion of the self, rites and stories propose interpretation models of these experiences as social roles one must assume. Psychotherapy operates in the same way. In a therapeutic setting marked by a certain rituality, it allows playing various roles through interactive sequences integrating narrative aspects.

12. CASES WITH RELIGIOUS/SPIRITUAL ASPECTS

The case descriptions provided here have been chosen to show how various aspects of what constitutes a religious tradition can be invoked by an individual during the process of constructing his or her identity. The first case refers to a person of Christian tradition, while the second and the third cases concern individuals of Muslim tradition. What these case studies highlight is not restricted to these particular traditions. The first case illustrates how a girl's difficult time in distancing herself from her mother is accomplished in late adolescence and then in young adulthood with the help of a community structure and of attachment and identification figures of religious nature. The second case highlights the nature of identification potentially contained in the practice of a rite, but also the extent of the contact that can be established with a secure foundation relationship. The third case demonstrates how religious traditions furnish social roles.

12.1. Case 1

Sister B. is a nun in a Benedictine monastery. She says she has been suffering from asthma ever since she was a child. She thus describes the relationship between her and her mother as stifling. Her parents were bakers and she was allergic to flour. In adolescence, she managed to distance herself by going abroad for her professional training. She reports that her asthma attacks stopped after a prayer with a charismatic group, where she experienced the Spirit of Peace. From

a charismatic perspective, the Spirit of Peace is considered to be a divine gift. The body collapses. If the person is standing, she falls without being hurt and remains like this for a while. Those who have experienced this describe it as a deep relaxation in which all internal tension disappears. A feeling of well-being takes its place, providing reassurance of being accompanied by a kindly presence. Sister B. was 23 when she had this experience. She attributes it as the result of a journey of several years, made after several successive steps. At the age of 33, she entered the monastery. A few months later, while still a novice, she was sent with a group of nuns to a field to collect stones and throw them into a tractor. They were supposed to clear the field of stones before plowing. This was dusty work, which set off an asthma attack. Reinterpreting what happened at this specific moment, Sister B. believes that the attack was triggered by fear. "It plunged me back into a situation in which I could only suffocate and I was in complete crisis." Ten years before, she had been healed in a miraculous way, she recounts, and then wonders if she ought to doubt this healing. Her superior again sent her to gather stones, thus confronting Sister B. with an impossible task, as she describes it. She recounts, "I prayed a lot and then asked the Virgin Mary to accompany me, as I realized I had experienced a lot and could do a lot of impossible things without suffering an asthma attack. I thought this was a step I had to take." During this new shift of stone collecting, she didn't have an asthma attack. "I came back with a stone; I took the most beautiful one, I didn't throw it in the tractor, but put it in my garden apron; I took it with me to the monastery and put it in a small sanctuary in the garden, where there is a statue of Saint Mary, and said: here, this is the stone of victory." She laughs and continues, "So, through an Impossible Task, as Saint Benedict describes it, I had really overcome something." This account illustrates well how attachment coordinates with identification.

First, charismatic prayer, with its lullaby-like songs, built a maternal setting in which Sister B. experienced profound security. The account was not detailed enough to tell if a specific member of the charismatic group played an intermediary role as an attachment figure, or if the secure bond was directly established with God within the protective framework of the praying group. At the monastery, however, the attachment relationship was established with the Virgin Mary through prayer. This was how she developed a secure relationship through which she was able to identify herself with Saint Benedict, founder of the Benedictine order she wanted to join. The construction of her monastic identity was shored exclusively upon exemplary figures from the past. There was also a human religious figure, present at her side: the novices' superior. She represented both an identification figure for Sister B., because she entered the convent before her, and a possible attachment figure, because she was dedicated to helping the novices as a guide. At the convent, Sister B. built her identity by depending not only on saints' figures, but also on the nuns around her, especially the novices' superior, called "Mother Superior." In this role, the superior served as a mother, an intermediary for attachment, and simultaneously, as a sister, an intermediary for identification.

12.2. Case 2

Ms. T. is 27 years old. She is a university student. She has been diagnosed as suffering from schizophrenia following a social breakdown and hospitalization. Her parents are both nonpracticing Muslims. Her mother comes from an Arabic country and her father is English. The patient reports that she prays many times a day, alone at home, but that she never goes to the mosque. She also says that her beliefs help her find comfort, although she says she is not sure of her creed. "They are MY beliefs; I find it difficult to answer your questions." One of the present difficulties she identifies is failing her university exams. When in an exam setting, panic and anxiety prevented her from performing satisfactorily. After a period of treatment, she returned to her studies and succeeded in passing the exams two years in a row. She says that prayer helped her to overcome her panic and anxiety. During a control

session, questions were asked about the form and the content of this prayer to identify the coping process employed. It was obvious that the patient was talking about her own act of prayer, and not about others praying for her. It was also obvious that she was talking about the act of prayer that she reports practicing many times a day. It was nevertheless impossible to determine conclusively what kind of prayer she was practicing: the ritual Muslim one, five times a day, or a more personal one. This case allows us to highlight two approaches to coordinating religion/spirituality with the self and with individual identity.

First possibility: She draws her strength from ritual practice of Muslim prayer. In this case, it is the identification with a reference group that strengthens her personal identity. In stressful situations, the feeling of being a good Muslim makes her feel secure. While not sure of herself when articulating her beliefs, she could have found a means of leaning on a firm point of reference: all Muslims recite prayers five times a day. Because her parents are not practicing followers, she doesn't have the opportunity of being taken to the mosque. Social breakdown is one of the characteristic symptoms of schizophrenia. Reciting the five prayers at home could be a means of establishing a link with a reference group and therefore reducing the feeling of isolation. From this point of view, the coping process can be described as a support found in the possibility of being like everybody else. The indications for treatment would therefore consist in extending this process onto other ways of "being like everybody else." Knowing that psychological illness has a tendency of being experienced as a loss of commonality with the other humans ("Am I normal?"), and knowing as well that the paranoia in certain ideas attack the consistency of the subject's identity, knowing that one is "like everybody else" can be reassuring. Of course, in a Western country, practicing the daily five prayers does not permit identification with the entire society. The subjects will identify themselves with the group they feel they belong to. By reciting the daily prayers, Ms. T. can feel she belongs to the Muslim community. Regarding her recovery, it could be useful to attempt to extend this process to other areas such as hobbies or clothing, for example. It remains to be seen whether the goal of having the same hobbies as other young people her age (Muslims or not Muslims), or dressing like other young girls her age would help the patient fight against social breakdown and find more confidence in public and in interpersonal relations.

Second possibility: Praying helps Ms. T. to maintain contact with a reassuring figure, that is, God. In this case, the content of the prayer does not necessarily consist in recited formulas but perhaps rather in a private conversation with God, or even a silent certainty of being in contact with the divine presence. Praying could be a means of recalling the security of previous experiences, or it could be a kind of psychological envelope created to finally achieve a secure self. From this point of view, the coping process would result from the activation of the attachment bond where the divine figure replaces the previous attachment figures. Indications for treatment would consist in encouraging the patient to pray every time she feels nervous and begins to panic, especially when she is confronted with a feeling of emptiness.

Being able to distinguish between these two forms of praying is very important because they call for distinct coping strategies. Of course, these strategies can be combined. During ritual prayer, the Muslim believer can both strengthen her feeling of belonging to a community of believers and her relationship with Allah. It is also possible that praying combines the recitation of the five daily prayers with other more personal instances of praying. It is also possible, however, that they practice only one kind of praying, which essentially entails only one of the processes described. Therefore, if Ms. T.'s praying consists exclusively of reciting the five daily prayers, and she does not rely on them to experience a secure relationship with God, but rather to experience the reassurance of praying properly and being a good Muslim, there are strong chances that the suggestion to pray whenever she starts to panic will not help. As a matter of fact, reciting the daily prayers means reciting them at precise hours.

As for the feeling of panic, it can surface at any time of day. If, on the contrary, her praying is not centered around the five daily prayers but rather around establishing contact with God at various moments throughout the day, especially during times of panic, a "be like everybody else" coping strategy would not apply. The suggestion to try to strengthen her feeling of belonging with young people her age by trying to be like them risks not having any effect because it is not directly linked to the coping mechanism she has created through prayer to face the panic of exams. This is why it would be more judicious to suggest that she find strength in prayer every time that she feels helpless during the day and not only when dealing with exams. (Later, it was found that this option was the correct one.)

12.3. Case 3

Mr. Z. is an immigrant worker of Muslim origin from a nonpracticing family environment. When he left his country, he started using cocaine and LSD. He also lost contact with all religious Muslim influences. He stopped taking drugs four years ago when he married a woman who came to join him from his country of origin. Since then, two children have been born. He claims to have returned to religious practice at the same time and has become very devoted to it. He goes to the mosque every Friday and recites his prayers five times a day. He declares, "Thanks to religion, I don't do anything foolish and I don't sin." He complains of auditory hallucinations, mainly insults, and of recurrent headaches. When he prays, he is attacked by a strong desire to insult God. He stopped working a few months ago, but is supported by social services. He spends a lot of time in bed and says that his wife complains about him not taking care of the children. Regarding his recovery, the issue at hand is to help him take action. The most important area in which an improvement would be desirable for both the patient and his family environment is the patient's involvement in raising his children. We examined the role religion plays among the different resources at the patient's disposal. Indeed, when questioned on what helps him confront the illness, the patient himself confirms that his religious tradition helps him in this regard. On the other hand, when it comes to his role as a father, he is helpless and very detached from his children. He does not have a role model from his own experience as a child, because his father died when he was 2 years old. During a session with his doctor, it clearly appears that his renewed involvement in Islam has allowed this man to recreate his cultural environment. He stays at home most of the time with his wife and children. His wife goes out very rarely. This environment gave his essential identity the necessary support to help him overcome the crises of quitting drugs and being unemployed. This coping strategy, however, risks enabling a breakdown, which could in time further damage his ability to support himself. The challenge lies in how he will assume his parental responsibility. It was suggested to his doctor that Mr. Z. be brought back to the religious imperative "I want to be a good Muslim," an approach that has helped him confront his difficulties for four years. This involves asking Mr. Z. how his choice of being a practicing Muslim connects to being a good father. One must remember that Islam is passed on through the father and therefore the father's role in maintaining and perpetuating the religious tradition is important. In other words, this means that being a father and raising children is linked to religious membership. If, as Mr. Z. confirms, getting back in touch with Islam helped him face his difficulties, it is plausible that his difficulty in fulfilling his role as a father could also be remedied with the help of the religious references he relied on for other issues. It could even be suggested to him that trying to be a good father is not an optional activity, but a necessary consequence of his choice to practice Islam. It could then be suggested that he reflect on what his religious tradition has to say on this subject. Through the construction of the paternal role, Mr. Z. was confronted with a transformation of identity. Owing to his personal history, he struggled to find a role model to whom he could refer. During the therapy session,

there was a discussion on whether the return to Islam for guidance on the paternal role was truly religious in nature, or whether it was more about seeking reference to the cultural environment of the country of origin. This would be an appropriate time to highlight that religion does not only involve intimate beliefs such as "God exists," "God loves me," "God punishes me," and so forth. On the contrary, religion also encompasses the symbolic systems that humans have devised to explain the meaning of life in relation to events in human existence. Such systems offer guidelines for all aspects of life and bring together beliefs and practices that are regulated within various religious institutions.

13. RELIGION CAN ALSO WEAKEN IDENTITY

As we have already seen, religion/spirituality can help restore identity when facing threatening conditions such as those experienced by patients with severe mental symptoms (that is, patients with long-term disorders like schizophrenia). However, religious experiences can also disturb and destabilize. For example, reproaches heard in a sermon could be understood as persecution, a missionary appeal read in a sacred book could nourish delusions of grandeur, or the experience of a ritual or meeting where all members start to adopt the same behavior could lead to the anguishing feeling of losing contact with oneself. Experiences of losing awareness of the distinction between the self and the nonself, regarded by some as mystic experiences, could for others be very distressing and disturbing.(28) Even when the religious dimension does not disturb an individual, it does not necessarily favor the individual's autonomy. Hence, an attachment relationship experienced with religious figures can be reduced to a mere displacement of the primary relationship. Such a relationship thus has the effect of reinforcing a regressive attitude. From a therapeutic point of view, keeping a critical eye on the role played by the religious dimension in identity construction is thus important. When the religious dimension is a part of the patient's reference system, one must make sure that it favors the integration of all aspects of identity.

14. MULTICULTURAL PERSPECTIVE

From a multicultural perspective, the patient's reference system – especially the conception of the self unique to this system – does not necessarily coordinate well with the therapist's model of medical care and psychological health. Is there a risk of a conflict between two conceptions of individual identity? Under which circumstances would it be possible to establish a therapeutic alliance between the therapist and the patient's religious/spiritual (cultural) reference system? It is the therapist's responsibility to build this therapeutic alliance. In terms of roles, the therapeutic relationship, in its basic structure, assigns the mother's role to the therapist. The therapist has to offer the patient a protective vessel for his or her suffering. This vessel refers back to a third party: the medical model of interpretation of psychological disorders. When this medical model seems incompatible with the patient's reference system, it is up to the therapist to adjust the therapeutic relationship to the patient's reference system. The first effort will be one of translation: an attempt to interpret the functions, categories of a particular element in the patient's belief system, in terms of the medical system. First of all, this involves establishing the foundation for the subject's identity cohesion. Contrary to what seems evident to the modern Westerner and thus to Western medicine, individual identity does not rely on the construction of a psychological core-self in every culture. In many cultures, the cohesion of the individual identity, what protects the individual against intrusions or mental breakdown, is collectively guaranteed by belonging to a group. The treatment then requires the therapist to take into consideration this way of perceiving one's relationship with oneself and to adapt the treatment by integrating, according to the specific case, the family and cross-generational dimensions – sometimes including even relationships with ancestors and gods. It is not that the success of the therapeutic

intervention depends on the therapist's adherence to the patient's system of meaning. However, it is in the caregiver's best interest to understand how the patient interprets his or her actions and, if necessary, to suggest other interpretations. Medical treatment in a multicultural context requires the construction of a therapeutic framework based on a conception of the self that is valid for the patient. A proposal of therapeutic intervention that compels the patient to completely forsake his culture has little chance of success. Hence, it is more about building an intervention framework that draws support from the conception of the self adhered to by the patients and that translates the potential therapeutic course of action into terms of the patient's identity construction. Such an approach requires a lot of creativity. In the end, if successfully achieved, it will have brought about a reorganization of the patient's identity, integrating elements belonging to the patient's culture of origin and those originating in the therapist's medical system.

REFERENCES

1. Ricoeur P. *Soi-même comme un autre*. Paris: Seuil; 1990.
2. Brandt PY. Se trouver d'ailleurs comme par surprise. In: Mancini S, ed. *La fabrication de psychisme: Pratiques rituelles au carrefour des sciencs humaines et des sciences de la vie*. Paris: La Découverte; 2006:55–78.
3. Stern D. *The Interpersonal World of the Infant: A View from Psychoanalysis and Developmental Psychology*. New York: Basic Books; 1985.
4. Anzieu D. *Le Moi-peau*. Paris: Dunod; 1995.
5. Stern D. *Le monde interpersonnel du nourisson: une perspective psychanalytique et développementale*. Paris: PUF;1989:21.
6. Laplanche J, Pontalis JB. *Vocabulaire de la psychanalyse*. Paris; PUF: 2002 (original ed. 1967).
7. Cosnier J. Les vicissitudes de l'identité. In: Alleon AM, Morvan O, Lebovici S, eds. *Devenir « adulte » ?*. Paris: PUF; 1990:95–111.
8. Grom B. *Religionspsychologie*. München/Göttingen: Kösel/Vandenhoeck & Ruprecht; 1992.
9. Bowlby J. *Attachment and Loss (3 vol.)*. Harmondsworth/ Ringswood: Penguin Books; 1991.
10. Cyrulnik B. *Un merveilleux malheur*. Paris: Odile Jacob; 1999.
11. Tisseron S. *La résilience*. Paris: PUF; 2007.
12. Abraham N, Torok M. *L'écorce et le noyau*. Paris: Flammarion; 1987.

13. Ainsworth MDS. Attachments beyond infancy. *Am Psychol.* 1989;44:709–716.

14. Kirkpatrick LA. Attachment and religious representations and behavior. In: Cassidy J, Shaver PR, eds. *Handbook of Attachment: Theory, Research, and Clinical Applications.* New-York: Guilford; 1999:803–822.

15. Hazan C, Zeifman D. Pair bonds as attachments: evaluating the evidence. In: Cassidy J, Shaver PR, eds. *Handbook of Attachment: Theory, Research, and Clinical Applications.* New-York: Guilford; 1999:336–355.

16. Sroufe LA, Waters E. Attachment as an organizational construct. *Child Dev.* 1977;48: 1184–1199.

17. Granqvist P, Hagekull, B. Religiosity, adult attachment, and why "singles" are more religious. *Int J Psychol Relig.* 2000;10:111–123.

18. James W. *Varieties of Religious Experiences.* New-York: Longman Green; 1902.

19. Starbuck ED. *The Psychology of Religion.* New-York: Charles Scribner's Son; 1899.

20. Ulman C. Cognitive and emotional antecedents of religious conversion. *J Pers Soc Psychol.* 1982;43:183–192.

21. Granqvist P, Hagekull B. Religiousness and perceived childhood attachment: profiling socialized correspondence and emotional compensation. *J Sci Stud Relig.* 1999;38:254–273.

22. Vergote A, Tamayo A, eds. *The Parental Figures and the Representation of God.* The Hague [etc.]: Mouton; 1981.

23. Rizzuto AM. *The Birth of the Living God: A Psychoanalytic Study.* Chicago: University of Chicago; 1979 (Trotta, 1999).

24. Rizzuto AM. Object relations and the formation of the image of God. *Br J Med Psychol.* 1974;47: 83–99.

25. Winnicott DL. *Holding and Interpretation: Fragment of an Analysis.* New York: Grove; 1968 (1987).

26. Le Breton D. *Conduites à risques: des jeux de mort au jeu de vivre.* Paris: PUF; 2002.

27. Sundén H. *Die Religion und die Rollen: Eine psychologische Untersuchung der Frömmigkeit.* Berlin: Töpelmann; 1966.

28. Hulin M. *La mystique sauvage.* Paris: PUF; 1993.

13 Personality, Spirituality, Religiousness, and the Personality Disorders: Predictive Relations and Treatment Implications

RALPH L. PIEDMONT

SUMMARY

The purpose of this chapter is to demonstrate the conceptual and empirical value of religious and spiritual constructs for understanding and treating individuals with a personality disorder. Using the Five-Factor Model of Personality (FFM) as the organizing framework, it was shown that spirituality and religiousness (collectively referred to as numinous constructs) represent qualities not redundant with the FFM domains and are universal aspects of functioning. These numinous constructs have a causal impact on psychosocial functioning. The value of spirituality and religiousness in treating those with a personality disorder lies in the anti-narcissistic aspects of the numinous. Spirituality calls us to see larger patterns and relationships that bring forth greater honesty and intimacy with others. The therapeutic value of spirituality is overviewed in the treatment of borderline, narcissistic, anti-social, and schizotypal disorders. Other potential clinical values for spirituality in treating the remaining disorders are discussed.

I. INTRODUCTION

According to the *Diagnostic and Statistical Manual of Mental Health Disorders, Fourth Edition* (*DSM-IV*),(1) a personality disorder (PD) represents a rigid and ongoing pattern of thoughts and behaviors that deviate markedly from the expectations of the culture of the individual who exhibits them. These patterns are inflexible, nonadaptive, and consistent across many situations and represent disturbances in at least two of the following:

cognitions, affect, interpersonal functioning, and impulse control. Although these dysfunctions represent deviations from expected norms, individuals with a PD do not see their eccentricities as problem inducing, despite the fact that they may experience significant distress or impairment in social, occupational, or intrapsychic functioning. Overall prevalence rates vary for the PDs in general and for each specific PD depending on the nation examined, the region of the country (that is, urban vs. rural), and gender. Samuels et al.(2) noted in a U.S. community sample an overall prevalence of 9 percent. Unmarried men with a high school education or less were most vulnerable. Similar findings were noted by Torgersen, Kringlen, and Cramer (3) using a representative sample of Norwegians. They found a 13.4 percent prevalence rate, again with single, unmarried individuals being most at risk. Torgersen et al. also provided a review of ten other studies conducted in the United States and Europe that found rates for PDs ranging from 5.7 percent to 22.5 percent (median prevalence of 11.1 percent). Finally, Maier, Lichtermann, Klingler, and Heun (4) found with a German sample a 10 percent prevalence rate. Overall, it seems reasonable to conclude that approximately 10 percent of the general population may suffer from a PD.

This is a rather large percentage of individuals, and such human volume carries with it significant costs not only in terms of pain, suffering, and impaired functioning, but also economically, in dollars and cents. A number of studies have examined the actual social and economic costs of the treatment of individuals with PDs, and values can range into the tens of thousands of dollars in lost work productivity, health care, and treatment costs.(5, 6) Fortunately, however, psychotherapy does offer an option to help individuals with PDs to cope better with their circumstances and to reintegrate back into society. Bartak, Soeteman, Verheul, and Busschback (7) found in their literature review that psychotherapy can be quite effective in treating PDs, evidencing a large statistical effect in comparison to control groups. Gabbard, Lazar, Hornberger, and Spiegel (8) found that psychotherapy has a beneficial economic effect when used in the treatment of severe PDs by reducing long-term costs for inpatient care and work impairment.

Although help for characterological impairment is available, improvements in psychotherapy can be made and efficacy rates can be increased. To advance, treatment requires a greater understanding of the PDs, the factors that contribute to their development, and identification of new personological resources that can be exploited in treatment. The purpose of this chapter is to provide a new perspective on PDs from the vantage point of the Five-Factor Model of Personality (FFM). The origins and development of this model will be presented, and its relationship to the personality disorders will be outlined. Readers will then be introduced to the realm of the numinous. The term *numinous* refers to the general dimension of psychological constructs assessing that which is considered hallowed, sacred, and awe-inspiring, such as spirituality and religiousness. The relationship of these types of variables to the FFM will be outlined, and their value as empirically viable constructs reviewed, especially as they relate to PDs . The role of these numinous constructs for understanding the PDs and implications for treatment will be discussed. To understand personality dysfunction, one needs to understand those motivational qualities that constitute the personality.

2. DEVELOPMENT OF THE FIVE-FACTOR MODEL OF PERSONALITY

Literally thousands of personality trait variables are available today in hundreds of different inventories and scales. Such a cornucopia of constructs can easily lead to confusion when

deciding which traits to use. Fortunately, recent research has discovered that the majority of these traits cluster themselves around five broader dimensions known as the *Five Factor Model of Personality* (FFM).(9) These "Big Five" factors are: *neuroticism*, the tendency to experience negative affect; *extraversion*, which reflects the quantity and intensity of one's interpersonal interactions; *openness to experience*, the proactive seeking and appreciation of new experiences; *agreeableness*, the quality of one's interpersonal interactions along a continuum from compassion to antagonism; and *conscientiousness*, the persistence, organization, and motivation exhibited in goal-directed behaviors.(10) Research has shown that these five dimensions do provide a useful language for talking about trait variables and that these factors do predict a wide range of important psychosocial outcomes, including mental and physical health, occupational, academic, and intrapersonal criteria.(11)

These five dimensions have shown themselves to represent a rather comprehensive taxonomy of personality traits. A taxonomy is simply a framework for classifying things on the basis of their similarity. To accomplish this, one needs to identify all the necessary qualities that distinguish the entities that are to be classified, and these distinguishing characteristics must be mutually exclusive. In the FFM, each of the domains is independent of the others, and research has shown that these dimensions appear to represent the majority of variance found in most personality measures. Table 13.1 provides a short overview of this work.

A number of studies have evaluated the degree to which these five personality dimensions overlap with psychological constructs from different theoretical models. Simply put, these studies asked the question, "Are the qualities represented by the dimensions of the FFM the same as those found in other scales, or do they represent something different?" As can be seen in Table 13.1, whether using a measure of Murray's needs, Gough's folk concepts, Jungian typologies, interpersonal behaviors, or vocational interests, the dimensions of the FFM are present among these theoretically diverse

Table 13.1: Bibliography of Joint Analyses Using the Dimensions of the FFM.

Instrument	Construct Measured	Findings
Adjective Check List	Murray's needs, Folk constructs	All five factors found
Basic Personality Inventory	Normal personality domains	All five factors found
California Psychological Inventory	Folk constructs, normal personality	Agreeableness under-represented
Edwards Personal Preference Schedule	Murray's needs	All five factors found
Eysenck Personality Profiler	Biologically based personality constructs	No openness found
Guilford-Zimmerman Temperament Survey	Trait personality constructs	All five factors found
MCMI I & II	Axis II constructs	All five factors found
MMPI	Axis I constructs	Openness not well represented
Myers-Briggs Type Indicator	Jungian personality constructs	Neuroticism not found
Personality Research Form	Trait personality constructs	All five factors found
Self-Directed Search 3	Vocational interests	Neuroticism not well represented
16PF	Trait personality constructs	All five factors found

Adapted from Piedmont RL. *The Revised NEO Personality Inventory: Clinical and Research Applications.* New York: Plenum Press; 1998. With kind permission of Springer Science and Business Media.

instruments. A large literature has developed showing that the dimensions of the FFM are quite comprehensive and represent the essence of what is traditionally considered "personality."

Research has shown that the FFM dimensions are linked to one's genetic makeup, about one-half the variance observed in traits is inherited from our parents. Traits also have been shown to generalize cross culturally, so the same patterns in behaviors, attitudes, and actions we see in Western culture are also found to occur in other cultural contexts, such as in Asia and Africa. Traits represent human universals for understanding behavior.(12) Perhaps the most intriguing aspect of research on traits has been the discovery that one's trait profile does *not* change in adulthood. After age 30, all things being equal (for example, no psychotherapy or religious conversions), personality seems to be pretty much set; our trait dispositions will remain stable over our adult lives. The value of this finding is that once someone's trait standing is known, accurate predictions about his or her behavior can be made well into the future. However, until age 30, personality is still in flux and capable of modification. But after 30, an adaptive orientation to the world emerges that leads us to pursue personal goals that are the most satisfying to our needs (for example, the achievement-oriented person will seek out competitive situations, the extravert will seek out the company of others). Thus,

the dimensions of the FFM represent genotypic aspects of the individual, biologically based entities that govern the course of adult strivings.

The value of the FFM is twofold. First, the FFM provides an efficient framework for organizing personality-related issues around these five dimensions. The personological qualities associated with these dimensions have been nicely outlined for both normal and clinical samples. (11, 13) For example, neuroticism has been linked with risk for a psychiatric disorder and burnout; extraversion and agreeableness define interpersonal styles; openness to experience relates to curiosity, empathy, and dogmatism; and conscientiousness is related to achievement outcomes in school, work, and athletic environments. Thus, to obtain a comprehensive assessment of an individual, a clinician would want to make sure that any measure contains information from all these domains.

The second value of the FFM is that it provides straightforward, clear language for describing and discussing personality-related information. The dimensions of the FFM provide a sort of latitude and longitude for understanding personality constructs. By mapping scales from different measures onto these five factors, one can understand similarities and differences among the constructs. Correlations with the FFM dimensions can be the personological fingerprint for a scale; an indication of those qualities reflected in its score. This parsing ability is perhaps the most important feature of the FFM. It enables one to avoid what Block (14) has referred to as the "jingle and jangle fallacies." These terms refer to, respectively, the tendency to see scales as being similar, or different, on the basis of their label rather than on any empirical evidence. The former term sees convergence where none may exist, and the latter term allows useless redundancy to develop. Perhaps the least useful place to look for a scale's meaning is its name. Unfortunately, these "fallacies" too often characterize the field of assessment.

One case in point relates to research that examined the relationship between Type A personality styles and coronary heart disease (CAD). The Type A Behavior Pattern (TABP) was an identified aspect of personality that was related to actual physical illness.(15) The time-pressured, high-achieving, hyper-alert mental condition that characterized the TABP seemed to lead men to develop fatal heart problems. Although early research was supportive of the link between TABP and CAD, later studies failed to find consistent relationships between the personality style and health. What was identified as the "toxic component" to CAD was anger and hostility. Individuals having problems with expressing anger in healthy ways seemed most at-risk. But even here, the relationship was not always observed; some measures of anger seemed to predict CAD, but others did not. It was not until various measures of anger were examined within the context of the FFM that the puzzle was finally solved.

It turned out that there are two types of anger. One type, characterized by emotional outbursts of screaming, yelling, and emotional upset is frequently seen when someone gets frustrated or is provoked by another. The other type of anger does not show any type of negative emotional arousal but rather reflects the malevolent attitude, "You hurt me and I will hurt you more." One type of anger is affective in nature and the other more interpersonal and attitudinal. When correlated with the FFM measures, the first type related strongly with neuroticism (reflecting the

presence of negative affect), while the second type correlated with low agreeableness (reflecting a very cynical, self-centered, mistrustful orientation). Surprisingly, it is the second type of anger, related to low agreeableness that is related to CAD.(16) By mapping these measures of anger onto the dimensions of the FFM, we were able to develop a more sophisticated and nuanced understanding of what is meant by *anger*. Although there are many scales that carry the label *anger*, they are not all measuring the same constructs. There are different types of anger, each with their own very different psychological and health-related implications. The FFM helps us to clarify what our constructs measure and gives us a language for thinking more precisely about personality.

3. THE FFM AND THE PERSONALITY DISORDERS

Because PDs represent enduring patterns that characterize an individual's long-term functioning, it seems reasonable to conclude that such maladaptive patterns would be related to one's underlying personality structure. Much has been written concerning the linkages between the FFM and the PDs and the numerous conceptual issues associated with these comparisons (see Costa & Widiger (17) for an overview). Suffice it for our purposes to note that associations between the FFM and the PDs provide two points of interest. First, associations between these two sets of constructs demonstrate that personality disorders represent more extreme variants of the normal personality dimensions. The FFM dimensions represent a robust and economical set of personological qualities that are useful for understanding adaptive and nonadaptive aspects of functioning. Second, the pattern of correlations between the FFM domains and the PD dimensions can, as noted above with anger, help to elaborate the kinds of temperaments underlying these disorders. Such information can facilitate differential diagnosis and enhance therapy by identifying relevant etiological factors and anticipating treatment issues.

Table 13.2: Partial Correlations Between SCID-IIP Screener Scales and FFM Personality Domains Controlling for Acquiescence.

SCID-IV PD Scale	FFM Personality Domain				
	N	E	O	A	C
Avoidant	.50***	−.52***	−.19***	−.08	−.17**
Dependent	.43***	−.12	−.17**	−.03	−.32***
Obsessive-Compulsive	.32***	−.09	−.08	−.30***	.24***
Passive-Aggressive	.60***	−.23***	−.06	−.47***	−.33***
Depressive	.64***	−.41***	.04	−.36***	−.23***
Paranoid	.52***	−.31***	.00	−.55***	−.21***
Schizotypal	.29***	−.19***	.21***	−.31***	−.20***
Schizoid	.10	−.36***	−.11	−.22***	−.15**
Histrionic	.19***	.37***	.14	−.22***	−.17**
Narcissistic	.33***	.00	.06	−.56***	−.16**
Borderline	.66***	−.22***	.07	−.48***	−.38***
Antisocial 1 (Adult Behavior)	.32***	−.01	.10	−.51***	−.42***
Antisocial 2 (Youth Behavior)	.21***	−.05	.15**	−.39***	−.23***

$N = 302$

Note: N = Neuroticism, E = Extraversion, O = Openness, A = Agreeableness, C = Conscientiousness.
*** $p < .001$, ** $p < .01$, $p < .05$, two-tailed

Adapted from Piedmont RL, Sherman MF, Sherman NC, Williams JEG. A first look at the DSM-IV structured clinical interview for personality disorder screening questionnaire: more than just a screener? *Meas Eval Couns Dev.* 2003;36:150–160.

Table 13.2 provides the results of one study that correlated scores from the *Structured Clinical Interview for DSM-IV Personality Disorders Screening Questionnaire* (SCID-IIP) (18) and the FFM personality domains.(19) (Data are provided to show heuristic support for the arguments being made here. However, familiarity with interpreting partial correlations is not essential for understanding the points being made in the text. Readers so inclined can skip any review of the tabled data.) The SCID-IIP is a self-report questionnaire that contains the diagnostic items for each of the PDs. Individuals rate on a 1 to 5 scale the extent to which each behavior is self-descriptive (for example, Do you often feel nervous when you are with other people?). These data were based on a student sample of 302 individuals and are representative of findings from other studies using other instruments. (Saulsman and Page (20) provide a meta-analysis of these relationships.) Two points of interest emerge from Table 13.2. First, all the PD scales correlate with at least one of the FFM domains. Thus, characterological dysfunctioning

can be seen as a more extreme variant of the normal dimensions of personality. Particularly (high) neuroticism and (low) extraversion are most strongly related to the PD scales, indicating that affective dysphoria and social withdrawal are key components to impairment regardless of how it is categorized. Agreeableness and conscientiousness are also related, indicating a selfish, impulsive orientation behind many of the PDs. Interestingly, openness has only a few points of overlap, indicating that qualities associated with permeability and rigidity are less strongly reflected in the current set of nosological definitions.

A careful examination of each PD scale's relationship to the FFM domains also provides important insights into the personological dynamics of each disorder. For example, consider the FFM correlations for the avoidant PD scale. Notice, those who score high on this scale also score high on neuroticism and low on extraversion. The low extraversion (that is, introversion) makes sense for this group. They tend to avoid contact with others and prefer a more solitary orientation. The positive correlation with neuroticism indicates that these individuals are also anxious and distressed; they avoid groups because they may fear negative evaluations by others or making social blunders. Those with an avoidant PD possess a clear social phobia that may underlie their withdrawal. Next, consider the correlations found with the schizoid PD scale. Here is another disorder that is characterized by social withdrawal and isolation. Like the avoidant PD, the schizoid PD also scores low on extraversion, reflecting the desire for privacy and seclusion. However, the schizoid scale does not correlate with neuroticism, indicating that those with a schizoid PD, *unlike* the avoidant PD, do not systematically experience social phobia as a cause of their withdrawal. Those diagnosed as a schizoid are not necessarily threatened by groups nor do they fear social contact in the ways that those with an avoidant PD do. Given that these two types of disorders may present in similar ways, knowing individuals' scores on these FFM domains can be quite helpful in making a differential diagnosis.

The FFM provides a useful empirical and interpretive framework for understanding a wide range of psychological functioning and can be useful in highlighting motivational qualities relevant in diagnosis and treatment. Miller,(13) drawing on information from his own clients, provided useful clinical information into how individuals high and low on each of the five personality domains would present themselves in therapy. He also outlined some of the key problems these clients were likely to experience along with potential treatment opportunities and pitfalls. For example, individuals high on neuroticism present themselves with a variety of negative affects. Their presenting problems span the full spectrum of neurotic pains. Such individuals may always experience personal pain regardless of how much therapy they receive, although such emotional distress can certainly motivate patient compliance with treatment. Miller also noted that those low on neuroticism and high on conscientiousness had better ratings of treatment outcome. In a study of outpatient substance abusers, I noted

that those high on neuroticism benefited from client-centered therapy and systematic desensitization, while problem-solving advice was not seen as effective with these types of clients. Those high on agreeableness responded well to the AA and NA programs, while those low on agreeableness responded well to relaxation sessions, art therapy, and journaling.(11) The FFM has much to offer our understanding of Axis II functioning (i.e., PD clinical presentations).

The question that we come to now concerns how spirituality and religiousness fit into this model. A number of important issues will be raised in the following sections that concern what added value these constructs bring to our understanding of Axis II functioning over the FFM. But first, these constructs need to be defined in ways that are amenable to scientific analysis.

4. DEFINING AND MEASURING SPIRITUALITY AND RELIGIOUSNESS

Because spirituality and religiousness are seen by many as being conceptually overlapping, in that both involve a search for the sacred,(21) some researchers prefer to interpret these two dimensions as being redundant.(22) Musick, Traphagan, Koenig, and Larson (23) have noted that in samples of adults, these two terms are highly related to one another. They questioned whether there is a meaningful distinction between these two constructs or if any disparities are simply an artifact of the wishes of researchers hoping to find such differences (p. 80). Nonetheless, there are those who emphasize the distinctiveness between these two constructs.(24, 25) Here, spirituality is viewed as an attribute of an individual (much like a personality trait) while religiosity is understood as encompassing more of the beliefs, rituals, and practices associated with an institution.(26) Religiosity is concerned with how one's experience of a transcendent being is shaped by, and expressed through, a community or social organization. Spirituality, on the other hand, is most concerned with one's personal relationships to larger, transcendent realities, such as God or the universe. In an effort to operationalize these two constructs in a manner that would solidly ground them in mainstream psychological theory and measurement, I created the *Assessment of Spirituality and Religious Sentiments* (ASPIRES)(27) scale. In this measure, there is a single broad dimension that captures the spirituality domain and two scales that assess the religiousness domain. Each will be discussed in turn.

In the ASPIRES, spirituality was defined as an intrinsic motivation of individuals to create a broad sense of personal meaning within an eschatological context. In other words, knowing that we are going to die, spirituality represents our efforts to create meaning and purpose for our lives. This need for meaning is seen as an intrinsic, universal human capacity.(25) The scale assessing spirituality is named the *Spiritual Transcendence Scale* (STS). The STS was developed to capture those aspects of spirituality that cut across all religious traditions (see Piedmont (27) for how this scale was developed). This unidimensional scale contains three correlated facets: *Universality*, a belief in the unity and purpose of life; *Prayer Fulfillment,* an experienced feeling of joy and contentment that results from prayer and/or meditation; and *Connectedness* a sense of personal responsibility and connection to others.

In contrast to spirituality, religiousness is not considered to be an intrinsic, motivational construct. Rather, it is considered to represent a *sentiment*. Sentiment is an old term in psychology and reflects emotional tendencies that develop out of social traditions and educational experiences.(28) Sentiments can exert a powerful influence over thoughts and behaviors, but they do not represent innate, genotypic qualities like spirituality. That is why the expression of sentiments (for example, religious practices) can and does vary over time and across cultures. There are two measures of religious sentiments on the ASPIRES. The first is the *Religiosity Index* (RI). The RI examines the frequency of involvement in religious rituals and practices (for example, how often does one pray, how often does one attend religious services). It also queries the extent to which religious practices and involvements are important. *Religious*

Crisis (RC) is the second measure and examines the extent to which an individual feels alienated, punished, or abandoned by God (for example, I feel that God is punishing me). What is of interest about these items is that they address the negative side of religiousness, when faith and belief become sources of personal and social distress. This scale enables an examination of the extent to which disturbances in one's relationship to God can affect one's broader sense of psychological stability.

The five ASPIRES scales (the three facet scales of the STS plus the two religious sentiments scales) provide a relatively comprehensive assessment of the numinous dimension. Compared to most measures in this field, the ASPIRES has a rather large and comprehensive body of validity evidence. The increasing popularity of the ASPIRES can be attributed to its ability to address critical empirical questions about the utility of any measure of spirituality or religiousness. The next section will outline the four key validity issues and why the ASPIRES is an important measure for understanding normal and clinical aspects of psychological functioning.

5. FOUR KEY VALIDITY ISSUES FOR THE ASPIRES

Perhaps the single most important question to be asked of any measure of spirituality and religiousness is whether the construct represents something unique about the individual. Critics of spiritual research are concerned that numinous constructs are only the "parasitization" of already existing personality variables.(29) To be of value, measures of the numinous need to demonstrate that they capture nonredundant aspects of the individual and therefore provide insights into functioning that are missed by current psychological constructs. A number of studies have jointly factor-analyzed the ASPIRES scales along with measures of the FFM and have consistently shown that the two sets of constructs are mutually independent.(24, 30) Thus, spirituality can be argued to represent the *sixth* major personality domain.(24)

Knowing that spirituality and religiousness represent unique personological qualities, the second key issue is to demonstrate that these numinous constructs are related to important psychosocial criteria *over and above* the predictive power of established personality constructs. In short, to what extent do spiritual scales evidence incremental validity over the FFM domains? A growing literature continues to document that the ASPIRES scales do indeed predict a wide range of outcomes over and above the FFM personality domains in both normal (24, 27) and clinical samples.(31) The data further demonstrated that while both the spiritual and religious sentiments scales predict some outcomes in common (for example, Satisfaction with Life, Self-Actualization, and Purpose in Life), these constructs also evidenced incremental validity over each other. In some instances, the STS was the sole predictor of outcomes (for example, Positive Affect, Individualism, and Social Support), while in other instances the religious sentiments scales were the only predictors (for example, Attitudes toward Sexuality, Negative Affect, and Pro-social Behavior). Thus, although these two types of constructs are highly correlated, they do have sufficient unique predictive power to warrant their use as separate scales. These data suggest that different psychological systems mediate the expression of spirituality and religiousness.

The third major validity issue addresses whether spirituality is indeed a universal aspect of human functioning. It has long been known that the majority of measures designed to assess spirituality are rooted in Christian-based perspectives,(32) reflecting mostly a mainline Protestant orientation.(33) Is the STS simply a measure of this ideology or would non-Christian individuals and those from other cultures find these concepts relevant? Research using the ASPIRES with non-Christian groups (for example, Jewish, Hindu, and Muslim) and across cultures (for example, India, Korea, Philippines, and Mexico) continues to find the scales and their related constructs to be reliable and valid with these diverse groups.(25, 34–36) The fact that the spiritual concepts in the ASPIRES can be readily translated into languages sharing no common root history with English strongly supports the universal salience of these ideas. Only genotypic qualities can evidence such cross-cultural generalizability.

The final, and perhaps most essential, issue concerns the ultimate nature of the relationship between spirituality, religiousness, and psychological functioning. As Emmons and Paloutzian (37) (pp. 392–393) noted, "We do not yet know whether personality influences the development of religiousness…, whether religiousness influences personality…, or whether personality and religiousness share common genetic or environmental causes." If one's orientation to the numinous develops out of one's sense of personhood, then it is the level of psychological adjustment that forms the experiences of the numinous. Like any other behavior, relationships with some ultimate reality are reflections of more basic psychological dynamics. However, if spirituality and religiosity have a causal impact on our psychological system, then these variables become important conduits through which growth and maturity can be focused. In this scenario, the quality of one's relationship to the transcendent has important implications for our own psychological sense of stability. Disturbances in our relationship to the transcendent can have serious repercussions for the rest of our system. Demonstrating that numinous constructs serve as causal inputs into our psychic systems would have far reaching implications for how the social sciences conceptualize individuals and would open the possibility for a whole new class of potential therapeutic strategies.(38)

Employing structural equation modeling (SEM), a growing number of studies are examining which of these two options is more likely correct.(39) Piedmont (40) showed in both U.S. and Filipino samples, and with self- and observer ratings, that spirituality (as measured by the STS) was best described as a *causal input* into our psychological sense of emotional well-being. Our relationship with a perceived transcendent reality has important implications for our inner sense of emotional stability. It has also been demonstrated that spirituality was a causal predictor of psychological growth and maturity.(39) Further, spirituality was shown to be a predictor of religious involvement. Certainly these findings have far-reaching implications for how the social sciences conceptualize individuals and open the possibility for the development of a whole new class of potential therapeutic strategies that involve numinous-related motivations.

Given the empirical robustness of the ASPIRES scales and their relatedness to emotional stability, it is a reasonable next step to examine how these constructs relate to Axis II functioning. Are they significant causal predictors of characterological dysfunctioning? Can disturbances in our relationship with the transcendent create intrapsychic conflicts? Or, does the development of mental illness undermine spiritual and religious strivings?

6. SPIRITUALITY, RELIGIOUSNESS, AND PSYCHOPATHOLOGY

As noted above, the majority of research with numinous constructs has focused on general factors of well-being and life satisfaction. When research includes clinical dimensions, they are mostly affective in nature (for example, depression, anxiety, and hopelessness).(41) Findings here show significant relationships between numinous constructs and affective dysphoria. An epidemiologic survey of Canadians showed that religious involvement was related negatively to depression.(42) MacDonald and Holland (43) examined the relationship between measures of spirituality and religious involvement with the Minnesota Multiphasic Personality Inventory-2 (MMPI-2) scales. In general, involvement in religious activities and higher levels of spirituality were associated with lower levels of pathology. Interestingly, both studies found that religious involvement was a better predictor than spirituality.

Very little research has been done examining how explicit psychopathologic variables (for example, symptom dimensions and diagnostic criteria) are related to spiritual and religious constructs. One study examined the relationship between symptom scores and spiritual well-being in a sample of African-American patients with a first-episode schizophrenic disorder. Consistent with the literature for nonclinical samples, there was a negative correlation between these two sets of constructs.(44) Carrico et al.(45) applied a path model to examine the role of spirituality on depressive symptoms in HIV-positive persons. They found that a model specifying spirituality as a causal input (albeit an indirect effect) into the experience of depressive symptoms fit the data well. In contrast to the above research, both of the studies found spirituality negatively related to symptom experiences. Lavin (46) employed a cross-lagged panel design to demonstrate in a sample of adults that negative images of God (that is, high on neuroticism and low on agreeableness) led to higher self-ratings of symptomological distress over time. Although these studies provide support for the causal precedence of numinous constructs, it remains yet to determine the power of religious involvement and spirituality relative to each other in predicting symptom experience.

Piedmont, Hassinger, Rhorer, Sherman, Sherman, and Williams (47) provided the only known data linking measures of spirituality and religiousness to Axis II constructs. The relationship between the five ASPIRES scales and two measures of Axis II functioning (the SCID-IIP PD Scales described above and the *Schedule for Nonadaptive and Adaptive Personality* [SNAP (48)]) were examined while controlling for the predictive effects of the FFM personality domains. SEM analyses were also conducted comparing different models that varied the causal relationship between the two sets of constructs. Because the findings were similar for both Axis II measures, only the results with the SCID-IIP PD scales will be discussed here. The data for these findings are based on the responses of 342 undergraduate volunteers from a midwestern state university.

Table 13.3 presents the partial correlations between each of the ASPIRES scales and the SCID-IIP PD scales, controlling for the predictive effects of personality. Thus, these coefficients

Table 13.3: Partial Correlations Between the SCID-IIP Axis II PD Scales and the ASPIRES Spirituality and Religious Sentiments Scales Controlling for FFM Personality Domains.

SCID-IV PD Scale	ASPIRES Scale					
	PF	*UN*	*CN*	*R*	*RC*	ΔR^2
Paranoid	−.05	−.07	.04	−.07	**.16****	.03*
Schizoid	−.01	−.03	**−.13***	.03	**.15****	.04**
Schizotypal	**.16****	**.15****	.04	.08	**.15****	.07***
Antisocial-Adult	**−.15****	**−.11***	−.02	**−.25*****	**.21*****	.08***
Antisocial-Youth	.10	.10	−.01	**.15****	−.03	.03*
Borderline	−.11	−.06	.02	**−.17****	**.26*****	.06***
Histrionic	.01	.07	.01	−.02	**.13***	.01
Narcissistic	−.07	−.01	−.04	−.09	**.16****	.06***
Avoidant	**−.14***	**−.12***	−.10	−.09	**.16****	.02*
Dependent	−.02	−.05	.00	−.02	.07	.01
Obsessive-Compulsive	**.18*****	**.11***	.03	**.24*****	.00	.06***
Passive-Aggressive	.01	−.01	.00	−.03	**.22*****	.05***
Depressive	−.10	**−.14***	−.09	−.12	**.23*****	.05***
ΔR^2	.14***	.12***	.07*	.17***	.11***	

$N = 342$. $p < .05$; ** $p < .01$; *** $p < .001$, two-tailed. PF = Prayer Fulfillment, UN = Universality, CN = Connectedness, R = Religiosity Index, RC = Religious Crisis.

Note: Correlations in bold indicate a significant predictor in the regression analysis.

Adapted from Piedmont RL, Hassinger CJ, Rhorer J, Sherman MF, Sherman NC, Williams JEG. The relations among spirituality and religiosity and Axis II functioning in two college samples. *Res Soc Sci Stud Relig.* 2007;18:53–74.

reflect the *unique* overlap between the numinous scales and Axis II functioning. There are four points of interest here. First, with the exception of the dependent scale, all the PD scales correlate with at least one of the ASPIRES scales. The numinous constructs relate to almost the entire spectrum of disorders. Second, the two religious sentiments scales appear to have more numerous associations, and of higher magnitude, than the STS facet scales. Thus, learned religious sentiments may be more salient for understanding Axis II issues than spiritual motivations. Third, two series of regression analyses were performed to obtain the amount of overlapping variance. The last row of Table 13.3 indicates the amount of unique variance that each of the ASPIRES scales has in common with all of the SCID-IIP PD scales once the influence of personality is removed. As can be seen, the PD scales explain from 7 percent to 17 percent of the variance in each ASPIRES scale. These would be considered very large effect sizes.(49) Finally, the last column in the table evaluates the amount of unique shared variance between each PD scale and the five ASPIRES scales, controlling for the predictive effects of personality. In all but two instances (the Histrionic and Dependent PD scales), the ASPIRES scales uniquely account for a significant amount of variance in each PD scale (from 2 percent to 8 percent). The magnitude of these effects would be considered moderate to strong. The bolded correlations indicate those scales that emerged significant in the regression. It is interesting to note that the religious sentiments scales were the consistent predictors while the STS facet scales tended to drop out of the analyses.(50)

The second phase of this study was to apply SEM to evaluate models that varied the causal relations between the ASPIRES scales and the PD scales. Model 1 examined the causal impact of both personality and spirituality on Axis II functioning. Model 2 examined the causal impact of both personality and religious sentiments on Axis II functioning. Model 3 reversed the causal sequence and evaluated the impact of personality and Axis II functioning on religious sentiments.

The results indicated that the data had modest fit with Model 1. Interestingly, the pathway from spirituality to Axis II functioning was nonsignificant. This indicated that Spiritual Transcendence does not have any substantive relationship with this outcome. Thus the observed correlations presented in Table 13.3 above can be attributed to method artifacts in the data (for example, the reliance on all self-report data and sample specific error). The results for Model 2 indicated much better fit of the data to the model. The pathway from religious sentiments to Axis II functioning was significant, indicating that one's religious involvements do have a significant, unique causal impact on characterological impairment. Model 3 had the worst fit of all, indicating that religious sentiments being a consequence of one's personality and temperamental dysfunctionality is not very likely. That this pattern of findings was also replicated with the SNAP PD scales provides strong support for the position that individuals who are not actively involved in the religious practices of their faith and also are experiencing distress in their relationship with a transcendent being are likely to develop psychological instability.(46) It is important to note that these relationship problems with the transcendent are not a function of one's innate interpersonal style (qualities of personality), nor a function of interpersonal impairment due to the personality disorder dynamics. The predictive power of the Religious Sentiments scales was not mediated by these other related constructs. There appears to be something unique about the relationship with the transcendent that affects one's affective and cognitive processes.

The independence of spirituality from Axis II functioning raises the possibility that spirituality may serve as an important personological resource for treatment of PDs. Spirituality's lack of involvement in the pathognomonic process suggests that these motivations may not be distorted or impaired among individuals with Axis II issues. In other words, individuals experiencing a personality disorder do not necessarily have an impaired spirituality. Although its expression may appear odd or unusual in relation to more traditional presentations, it nonetheless can provide the individual with an important adaptive resource. Thus, working with spirituality around issues of transcendence may be able to provide a more realistically based set of perceptions and beliefs that can be therapeutically useful.

7. THE ROLE OF SPIRITUALITY IN TREATING PERSONALITY DISORDERS

The emphasis of this section will be on how spiritually related constructs can be deployed therapeutically to provide adaptive skills and potential self-transformation. How this is accomplished varies widely, from using more broadly defined meditative and mindfulness techniques to promote self-awareness,(51) to applying techniques and activities that will directly access existential and spiritual questions (for example, past life regression, chanting, and bibliotherapy),(52) to incorporating specific scriptural passages that both guide the therapy and provide relevant reflections that speak to core issues of spirituality.(38, 53) Finding ways to spiritually intervene is a young area, and there are a growing number of treatment-related texts now appearing.(54), (55) Applications of spiritual and religious techniques to the PDs has so far been limited to just handful of the disorders (for example, borderline, narcissistic, schizotypal, and antisocial). The utility of the numinous for treating the others still needs to be researched. The remaining part of this chapter will overview some of the clinical issues related to select PDs.

7.1. Schizotypal PD

Perhaps one of the central issues in managing patients with apparent religious delusions or ideas of reference is to accurately discern whether these "disturbances" reflect cognitive distortions or real mystical/spiritual experiences. This is particularly critical when dealing with individuals from non-Western cultures, where more animistic religious beliefs and rituals that involve "spirits" and "demons" exist. To the untrained eye, valid mystical experiences may appear as psychotic-like episodes, and to treat them as such clinically would be inappropriate.

Only one study to date has empirically examined mystical experiences among psychotic inpatients, religious contemplatives, and normal adults. (56) Interestingly, it was found that psychotics and contemplatives could not be discriminated on the bases of their scores on a mystical experience scale. Both groups reported experiences that were phenotypically comparable. However, the two groups were differentiated on the basis of their scores on a narcissism scale; the psychotic group scoring significantly higher. Selfishness, self-involvement, and grandiosity are clear characteristics of a nonspiritual orientation.(50) However, positive signs of a real transcendent experience include a sense of wholeness, perfection, joy, and acquired insight. Psychotic experiences will have the effect of promoting psychological fragmentation, while true mystical experiences result in an enhanced sense of personal integration. Lukoff (57) provided a useful orientation for differentiating between a true "spiritual emergency" and a psychotic episode.

But spirituality can also be a useful therapeutic resource for those with a schizotypal PD, regardless of whether their "mystical experiences" are valid or not. Lukoff outlined a number of useful techniques for managing such clients, such as mindfulness and promoting a connection to the transcendent. Building a personal relationship to God can be helpful in building an identity, creating greater self-responsibility, and promoting hope. Keks and D'Souza (58) also believed that numinous constructs can help individuals gain a sense of self and develop a better sense of personal support for themselves. Involvement in supportive religious communities can help to melt stigmas associated with having a psychiatric label and provide increased personal meaning.

7.2. Borderline and Narcissistic PDs

Khalsa (51) believed that psychospiritual interventions can help clients with these PDs create for themselves an inner mental state that is dynamic, attractive, peaceful, and creative. Spiritual techniques help to promote more internally stable emotional states. This is accomplished by using a blend of Dialectical-Behavior Therapy (DBT) in conjunction with various yoga and meditative practices. The goal is to help individuals identify their core personality and to embrace it as a first step in making a personal transformation. The meditative practices help clients to sit with their thoughts and to see how they initiate emotions.

Lawrence (53) viewed the narcissistic PD as much of a spiritual issue as a psychological one. Using more Western religious techniques, she argued that a developing relationship with God can serve as a useful intrapsychic object that can provide personal security to the client enabling him or her to counter the inner vulnerabilities that compromise the narcissist from developing and maintaining healthy interpersonal relationships. Lawrence relies on an explicitly Christian framework for providing the basis to the intervention process. Spiritual growth is linked directly to psychological growth and maturity, with the client-God relationship being the core element to the treatment process. Of course, the generalizability of this model is limited to those who accept established views of Christian theology.

7.3. Antisocial PD

Martens (52) argued that spiritually oriented psychotherapy could be a powerful intervention for antisocial and psychopathic personalities. Spirituality can be useful in promoting authenticity, moral and social capacity, and a greater faith in life. Martens' approach uses more eclectic strategies than those outlined in the previous two sections. His "spiritual psychotherapy" is "intended for patients with spiritual interests and latent abilities to develop spiritual activities. During spiritual psychotherapy, spiritual themes like getting wisdom … coping with loneliness … authenticity … development of personal ethics will be discussed" (p. 207). The goal of this approach is twofold: (1) to help clients find a way out of their psychosocial problems and (2) to create a healthy attitude toward themselves and the world by examining the spiritual dimensions of life.

Piedmont (31) examined the predictive role of spiritual transcendence as a predictor of outcome from an outpatient substance abuse treatment program. Participants were long-term drug and alcohol users from an inner city, mostly homeless, population. The group's overall personality profile showed low levels of both agreeableness and conscientiousness, a pattern characteristic of the antisocial PD (see Table 13.2). The six-week intensive program was fundamentally a spiritually oriented intervention that included a number of other modules (for example, vocational training, AA/NA groups, health awareness, and group therapy). Participants attended the program five days week, for six hours a day. Individuals completed a number of psychosocial measures and the STS. Over the course of treatment, individuals experienced significant reductions in emotional distress, improvements in coping abilities, and increased levels of spirituality. Interestingly, the STS facet scales of Universality and Connectedness were the most robust predictors of self and therapist ratings of outcome. Both of the facet scales stress one's relationships to others. Universality reflects a recognition of life as being interconnected. Individuals are part of a larger social reality, a community of "oneness" that transcends the many differences we experience in this life. Connectedness stresses the importance of the individual and his or her responsibility in caring for, responding to, and being involved with the many social communities that a person is part of (for example, family, neighborhood, and community). Enabling individuals to emotionally invest in supporting communities may lead to generative beliefs that provide a motivation for change.

For those with an antisocial PD, creating an awareness of social responsibility works against the more manipulative, selfish orientation that characterizes this disorder. As Piedmont (31) (p. 220) noted, "Spirituality's therapeutic effect may be in its ability to reintroduce [individuals who have been socially marginalized] as meaningful players in the larger human polity. Spirituality stresses the value of people despite their brokenness; it emphasizes the importance of each person's life in maintaining the integrity of the fabric of human experience."

8. THE CURATIVE POWER OF SPIRITUALITY

Why does spirituality present as a useful therapeutic resource for treating personality disorders? There are certainly many answers to this question ranging from a belief in the healing power of God's grace to the perspective that spirituality represents a "master motive" that organizes the personality and brings coherence to its strivings. It is my opinion that the value of spirituality is that it serves as an antidote to narcissism. A materialistic, self-centered approach to life, where one is always concerned with obtaining gratification of personal needs and wishes, leads to an impulsive style that can be easily frustrated by the demands of life. Here, life goals are usually oriented to the short term and relationships are usually manipulative and emotionally superficial. Spirituality, on the other hand, represents a lifestyle that is transpersonal in nature, where one recognizes a transcendent reality that calls individuals to set personal goals along an eternal continuum. A spiritual perspective recognizes that birth and death are only developmental signposts along a much longer ontological process. Recognizing one's connections to all life and embracing one's responsibilities to care for others create relationships that are emotionally deep, generative, and mutually satisfying.

Being able to step outside of oneself and to put one's life into a larger interpretive context can be emotionally healing and liberating. Committing to this larger vision allows individuals to find personal stability and coherence, even during times of fluidity and disjuncture. For individuals locked into their own narrow worlds of emotional pain, personal ineptitude, and interpersonal inadequacy, this broader meaning may provide ways of coping with stressful events or creating buffers against negative feelings. It may also represent a higher level of personality maturity.

It is interesting to note that in reviewing the literature on spirituality and the Axis II PDs, the types of disorders that are discussed all involve narcissism as a fundamental characteristic. The antisocial, narcissistic, schizotypal, and even borderline represent disorders where selfishness and manipulativeness are salient. It now seems evident that spirituality should be an important curative factor with these types of disorders. However, the question still remains to be answered whether spirituality and religiousness would be relevant for treating other PDs that are less narcissistically oriented, like the avoidant, obsessive-compulsive, schizoid, and histrionic. Perhaps other aspects of spirituality may be relevant, such as prayer fulfillment.

Prayer fulfillment correlates significantly with positive affect. Individuals who are able to establish an emotional connection to a transcendent being are able to derive a sense of joy and contentment above and beyond what can be predicted by personality (that is, levels of extraversion). Prayer fulfillment has been shown to be a buffer to the experience of burnout, at least among clergy. Religious involvement (for example, frequency of prayer and attending religious services) has been shown to be negatively related to neuroticism; those who involve themselves in the rituals and practices of their faith seem to experience less negative affect. So perhaps concerning those PDs that are highly correlated with neuroticism (for example, avoidant, dependent, depressive, and paranoid; see Table 13.2), the dimensions of Prayer Fulfillment and Religiosity may be most relevant for treatment. It is up to future research to examine these issues.

9. THE DARK SIDE OF THE NUMINOUS

A colleague of mine would always say, "The brighter the light, the darker the shadow" when we would witness talented people making surprising personal blunders. This clever saying reminds us that all things in life carry with them assets and liabilities, and spirituality is no exception. Although the numinous mostly carries with it positive potentialities, one must also be aware of the potential adverse affects it may have. One aspect of this was noted earlier in describing the

impact of religious crisis and its very toxic impact on psychosocial functioning. Having a relationship with the transcendent can be uplifting and supportive, unless one is feeling victimized and/or abused. In working with individuals who may be religiously oriented or helping clients develop a deeper spirituality, one needs to be careful that the spirituality that arises is not a source of pain, guilt, or exclusion.(58)

Martens (52) cautions that some clients, especially those with an antisocial PD, may use spiritual information to manipulate others or to appear that they have grown to gain release from psychiatric facilities. Employing spiritual material in therapy with clients having a comorbid psychotic or delusional disorder may foster the development of delusional ideation that may strengthen their resistance to treatment. Of course in both scenarios, a trained clinical eye is important. Being able to discern between real spiritual growth and superficial accommodating is key. However, discernment between psychotic/delusional behavior of a religious nature and actual spiritual experiences requires a more developed clinical palate.

Working with religious-oriented clients or attempting to incorporate spiritual and religious techniques into treatment requires that therapists develop basic competencies in numinous-related issues. Understanding various religious faiths in terms of their practices and philosophies is an important first step. Such knowledge helps give insight into a client's worldview and outlines moral beliefs. However, as this chapter has shown, spirituality is more than a demographic variable. It is a significant psychological construct that also needs to be understood in its own right. Making effective spiritual interventions can be facilitated if the therapist has experience with the underlying numinous issues. With the inclusion in the *DSM-IV* of a new diagnostic category named *Religious or Spiritual Problem* (V62.89), therapists need to be alert to the influence of spiritual and religious dynamics and their impact on a client's larger clinical situation. Determining whether a spiritual crisis represents a real psychosocial decompensation or the precursor of enhanced transpersonal growth is critical to the accurate diagnosis and effective treatment of the client.

10. SUMMARY

These findings have considerable significance for clinicians who may be skeptical about numinous variables, perhaps viewing them as "fuzzy" constructs. Taken together, the information presented here should lend confidence to professionals regarding the empirical viability and conceptual soundness of numinous scales: They can meet the empirical criteria of scientific method and rigor. Spirituality and religiousness relate to how an individual creates a broad sense of personal meaning for his or her life. Creating meaning can have an important impact on the quality and stability of one's psychic life. As was demonstrated here, spirituality can have a buffering effect on life's stressors by creating a source of inner joy and contentment despite the distress. Further, disturbances in our relationship to a transcendent being can have a direct negative impact on our functioning. Feeling punished and shunned by the God of one's understanding can create much disruption in one's sense of self and emotional stability. In treating PDs, therapists need to include a consideration of the client's spiritual orientation and bring this information into treatment. Helping the client to work through perceived problems in their spiritual world can help restore a sense of calmness and stability. Working to improve a more spiritual sense of meaning can enable a client to develop other psycho-social connections that can help facilitate the ongoing treatment process. A wide variety of techniques are already available for moving clients in a more spiritual direction, and therapists should acquaint themselves with them.

REFERENCES

1. American Psychiatric Association. *Diagnostic and Statistical Manual of Mental Disorder*, 4th ed., text ed. Washington, DC: Author; 2000.

2. Samuels J, Eaton WW, Bienvenu OJ, Brown CH, Costa PT, Nestadt G. Prevalence and correlates of personality disorders in a community sample. *Br J Psychiatry*. 2002;180:536–542.

3. Torgersen S, Kringlen E, Cramer V. The prevalence of personality disorders in a community sample. *Arch Gen Psychiatry*. 2001;58:590–596.

4. Maier W, Lichtermann D, Klinger T, Heun R. Prevalences of personality disorders (DSM-III-R) in the community. *J Pers Disor*. 1992;6:187–196.

5. Rendu A, Moran P, Patel A, Knapp M, Mann A. Economic impact of personality disorders in UK primary care attenders. *Br J Psychiatry*. 2002;181:62–66.

6. Van Asselt ADI, Dirksen CD, Arntz A, Severens JL. The cost of borderline personality disorder: societal cost of illness in BPD-patients. *Eur Psychiatry*. 2007;22:354–361.

7. Bartak A, Soeteman DI, Verheul R, Busschbach JJV. Strengthening the status of psychotherapy for personality disorders: an integrated perspective on effects and costs. *Can J Psychiatry*. 2007;52:803–810.

8. Gabbard GO, Lazar SG, Hornberger J, Spiegel D. The economic impact of psychotherapy: a review. *Am J Psychiatry*. 1997;154:147–155.

9. Digman JM. Personality structure: emergence of the five-factor model. *Annu Rev Psychol*. 1990;41:417–440.

10. Costa PT, Jr, McCrae RR. Normal personality assessment in clinical practice: the NEO Personality Inventory. *Psychol Assess*. 1992;4:5–13.

11. Piedmont RL. *The Revised NEO Personality Inventory: Clinical and Research Applications*. New York: Plenum Press; 1998.

12. McCrae RR, Allik J. *The Five-Factor Model across Cultures*. Dodrecht, The Netherlands: Kluwer Academic Publishers; 2003.

13. Miller T. The psychotherapeutic utility of the five-factor model of personality: a clinician's experience. *J Pers Assess*. 1991;57:415–433.

14. Block J. A contrarian view of the five-factor approach to personality description. *Psychol Bull*. 1995;117:187–215.

15. Friedman M, Rosenman RH. Association of a specific overt behavior pattern with increases in blood cholesterol, blood clotting time, incidence of arcus senilis and clinical coronary artery disease. *J Am Med Assoc*. 1959;2208:828–836.

16. Barefoot JC, Dodge KA, Peterson BL, Dahlstrom WG, Williams RB, Jr. The Cook-Medley hostility scale: item content and ability to predict survival. *Psychosom Med*. 1989;51:46–57.

17. Costa PT, Jr, Widiger TA. *Personality Disorders and the Five-Factor Model of Personality*, 2nd ed. Washington, DC: American Psychological Association; 2002.

18. First MB, Gibbon M, Spitzer RL, Williams JBW, Benjamin LS. *User's Guide for the Structured Clinical Interview for DSM-IV Axis II Personality*

Disorders (SCID-II). Washington, DC: American Psychiatric Press; 1997.

19. Piedmont RL, Sherman MF, Sherman NC, Williams JEG. A first look at the DSM-IV structured clinical interview for personality disorder screening questionnaire: more than just a screener? *Meas Eval Couns Dev.* 2003;36:150–160.

20. Saulsman LM, Page AC. The five-factor model and personality disorder empirical literature: a meta-analytic review. *Clin Psychol Rev.* 2004;23(8):1055–1085.

21. Hill PC, Pargament KI. Advances in the conceptualization and measurement of religion and spirituality: implications for physical and mental health research. *Am Psychol.* 2003;58:64–74.

22. Zinnbauer BJ, Pargament KI, Scott AB. The emerging meanings of religiousness and spirituality: problems and prospects. *J Pers.* 1999;67:889–920.

23. Musick MA, Traphagan JW, Koenig HG, Larson DB. Spirituality in physical health and aging. *J Adult Dev.* 2000;7:73–86.

24. Piedmont RL. Spiritual transcendence and the scientific study of spirituality. *J Rehab.* 2001;67:4–14.

25. Piedmont RL, Leach MM. Cross-cultural generalizability of the Spiritual Transcendence Scale in India: spirituality as a universal aspect of human experience. *Am Behav Sci.* 2002;45:1888–1901.

26. Miller WR, Thoresen CE. Spirituality and health. In: Miller W, ed. *Integrating Spirituality into Treatment*. Washington, DC: American Psychological Association; 1999:3–18.

27. Piedmont RL. *Assessment of Spirituality and Religious Sentiments, Technical Manual*. Baltimore, MD: Author; 2004a.

28. Ruckmick CA. *The Brevity Book on Psychology*. Chicago, IL: Brevity Publishers; 1920.

29. Buss DM. Sex, marriage, and religion: what adaptive problems do religious phenomena solve? *Psychol Inquiry.* 2002;13:201–203.

30. Piedmont RL, Mapa AT, Williams JEG. A factor analysis of the Fetzer/NIA Brief Multidimensional Measure of Religiousness/Spirituality (MMRS). *Res Soc Sci Stud Relig.* 2006;17:177–196.

31. Piedmont RL. Spiritual transcendence as a predictor of psychosocial outcome from an outpatient substance abuse program. *Psychol Addict. Behav.* 2004b;18:223–232.

32. Hall TW, Tisdale C, Brokaw BF. Assessment of religious dimensions in Christian clients: a review of selected instruments for research and clinical use. *J Psychol Theol.* 1994;22:395–421.

33. Gorsuch RL, Miller WR. Assessing spirituality. In: Miller WR, ed. *Integrating Spirituality into Treatment*. Washington, DC: American Psychological Association; 1999:47–64.

34. Cho I. *An Effect of Spiritual Transcendence of Fear of Intimacy*. Unpublished masters thesis, Torch Trinity Graduate School of Theology, Seoul, Korea; 2004.

35. Goodman JM, Britton PJ, Shama-Davis D, Jencius MJ. An exploration of spirituality and

psychological well-being in a community of orthodox, conservative, and reform Jews. *Res Soc Sci Stud Relig.* 2005;16:63–82.

36. Piedmont RL. Cross-cultural generalizability of the Spiritual Transcendence Scale to the Philippines: spirituality as a human universal. *Ment Health Relig Cult.* 2007;10:89–107.

37. Emmons RA, Paloutzian RF. The psychology of religion. *Annu Rev Psychol.* 2003;54:377–402.

38. Murray-Swank N, Pargament KI. God, where are you? Evaluating a spiritually-integrated intervention for sexual abuse. *Ment Health Relig Cult.* 2005;8:191–203.

39. Dy-Liacco GS, Kennedy MC, Parker DJ, Piedmont RL. Spiritual Transcendence as an unmediated causal predictor of psychological growth and worldview among Filipinos. *Res Soc Sci Stud Relig.* 2005;16:261–286.

40. Piedmont RL. Spirituality as a robust empirical predictor of psychosocial outcomes: a cross-cultural analysis. In: Estes R, ed. *Advancing Quality of Life in a Turbulent World*. New York: Springer; 2006:117–134.

41. Wink P, Killon N, Larsen B. Religion as moderator of the depression-health connection: findings from a longitudinal study. *Res Aging.* 2005;27: 197–220.

42. Baetz M, Griffin R, Bowen R, Koenig HG, Marcoux E. The association between spiritual and religious involvement and depressive symptoms in a Canadian population. *J Nerv Ment Dis.* 2004;192:818–822.

43. MacDonald DA, Holland D. Spirituality and the MMPI-2. *J Clin Psychol.* 2003;59:399–410.

44. Compton MT, Furman AC. Inverse correlations between symptom scores and spiritual well-being among African-American patients with first-episode schizophrenia spectrum disorders. *J Nerv Ment Illness.* 2005;193:346–349.

45. Carrico AW, Ironson G, Antoni MH, Lechner SC, Duran RE, Kumar M, Schneiderman N. A path model of the effects of spirituality on depressive symptoms and 14-h urinary-free cortisone in HIV-positive persons. *J Psychosom Res.* 2006;61:51–58.

46. Lavin LP. *The effect of outpatient therapy on a client's image of God*. Unpublished doctoral dissertation, Loyola College in Maryland; 2001.

47. Piedmont RL, Hassinger CJ, Rhorer J, Sherman MF, Sherman NC, Williams JEG. The relations among spirituality and religiosity and Axis II functioning in two college samples. *Res Soc Sci Stud Relig.* 2007;18:53–74.

48. Clark LA. *Schedule for Nonadaptive and Adaptive Personality: Manual for Administering, Scoring, and Interpretation*. Minneapolis, MN: University of Minnesota Press; 1993.

49. Hunsley J, Meyer GJ. The incremental validity of psychological testing and assessment: conceptual, methodological, and statistical issues. *Psychol Assess.* 2003;15:446–455.

50. Maltby J, Garner I, Lewis CA, Day L. Religious orientation and schizotypal traits. *Pers Ind Diff.* 2000;28:143–151.

51. Khalsa MK. Alternative treatments for borderline and narcissistic personality disorders. In: Mijares S, Khalsa G, eds. *The Psychospiritual Clinician's Handbook.* New York: The Hayworth Reference Press; 2005:163–182.

52. Martens WHJ. Spiritual psychotherapy for antisocial and psychopathic personality: some theoretical building blocks. *J Contemp Psychother.* 2003;33:205–218.

53. Lawrence C. An integrated spiritual and psychological growth model in the treatment of narcissism. *J Psychol Theol.* 1987;15:205–213.

54. Aten JD, Leach MM. *Spirituality and the Therapeutic Process: A Comprehensive Resource from Intake to Termination.* Washington, DC: American Psychological Association; 2008.

55. Richards PS, Bergin AE. *A Spiritual Strategy for Counseling and Psychotherapy.* Washington, DC: American Psychological Association; 2003.

56. Stifler K, Greer J, Sneck W, Dovenmuehle R. An empirical investigation of the discriminability of reported mystical experiences among religious contemplatives, psychotic inpatients, and normal adults. *J Sci Stud Relig.* 1993;32:366–372.

57. Lukoff D. Spiritual and transpersonal approaches to psychotic disorders. In: Mijares S, Khalsa G, eds. *The Psychospiritual Clinician's Handbook: Alternative Methods for Understanding and Treating Mental Disorders.* New York: Haworth Press; 2005:233–257.

58. Keks N, D'Souza R. Spirituality and psychosis. *Aust Psychiatry.* 2003;11:170–171.

14 Religion, Spirituality, and Consultation-Liaison Psychiatry

HAROLD G. KOENIG

SUMMARY

Religious beliefs and practices play an important role in enabling medical patients to cope with disability, dependency, fear, loss of control, and unpleasant medical symptoms. Besides influencing the development and course of emotional disorders such as depression and anxiety, religion can play a role in a host of other psychiatric conditions that mental health professionals are likely to encounter in medical settings, including somatization, agitation, behavioral problems, and substance abuse. In each of these conditions, religion can serve as either a resource or a liability. Religious beliefs may facilitate psychiatric care, or alternatively, conflict and interfere with it. For these reasons, and to provide culturally sensitive care, psychiatrists and other mental health professionals need to understand how religion can influence the onset, course, and treatment of conditions for which medical physicians are likely to consult them. In this chapter, I describe research on and case examples of how religion can influence patients' mental health. I also provide recommendations on how to take a religious/spiritual history, what to do with this information, and when pastoral care collaboration or referral is necessary. Given the wide prevalence of religious beliefs and behaviors in medical patients, and their potential impact on both mental health and medical prognosis, it is essential that clinicians consulting on these patients be informed.

Consultation-liaison psychiatry is growing rapidly and will continue to do so as our populations age, chronic illness increases, and persons with acute medical problems are hospitalized or treated in outpatient settings. The need for a distinct psychiatric approach to patients with acute, chronic, or terminal medical illnesses is now fully recognized. This chapter focuses on the emotional challenges and psychiatric illnesses that medical patients experience. In particular, it explores the roles that religion/spirituality play in the presentation and management of these conditions. Research is reviewed, cases are presented, and clinical applications (spiritual interventions) are discussed from a multicultural perspective that includes collaboration with chaplains, pastoral counselors, and community clergy.

I. REASONS FOR PSYCHIATRIC CONSULTATION

The most common reasons why medical physicians are likely to consult psychiatrists in acute medical or surgical settings are the following: anxiety, depression, psychosis, somatoform disorders, pain, posttraumatic stress disorder (PTSD), substance abuse, delirium, agitation, psychosis, and dementia.(1) In one early study conducted in a general hospital setting, reasons for psychiatric consultation were 35 percent depression, 29 percent uncooperative/management problem, 23 percent bizarre behavior or affect, 22 percent delirium, 19 percent previous psychiatric history, 16 percent maladjustment to illness, and 14 percent suicidal behavior.(2) Depression, suicidal behavior, and maladjustment to illness, then, make up the vast majority of consultations. Similarly, psychiatric consultation for nursing home patients is heavily weighted toward depression or behavioral disturbances related to depression, anxiety, dementia, pain, and maladjustment to illness.(3) Many of these same conditions are related to or affected by religious beliefs and practices, as is their management.

2. COPING WITH MEDICAL ILLNESS

Psychiatrists need to understand psychological and social factors that underlie common emotional and other psychiatric problems found in medical patients. Unlike psychiatric patients, who often have prior personal and family histories of psychiatric illness, childhood trauma, and/or personality issues, medical patients have usually been psychologically stable until they developed medical illness. The onset of health problems, then, often underlies depression, anxiety, and other psychiatric disturbances.

Chronic medical conditions, and especially acute exacerbations of those illnesses, pose enormous challenges to the patient's ability to cope. If there is also a history of prior psychiatric illness, then coping with medical problems may be even more difficult. Challenges include adjustment to loss of health and vigor, loss of energy and sleep, acute or chronic pain, increases in disability, changes in roles played in family and society, difficulty maintaining social relationships, trouble making new friends, loss of ability to work, loss of ability to meet life goals, loss of the ability to make a positive difference in others' lives, and most difficult of all, loss of a sense of purpose and meaning in life. The result of these losses and changes: anxiety, humiliation, despair, and loss of hope.

2.1. Loss of Health and Vigor

Health and physical vigor are usually taken for granted until they are lost, but once lost their value suddenly becomes apparent. To be free of physical symptoms and able to work and play without restriction are perhaps the most precious abilities that humans possess. No matter how much financial resources, power, or influence one has, without physical health, independence, and energy, it is difficult to enjoy life. Physical health is that one commodity that cannot be bought, and when disease takes it away, there may be nothing that one can do to get it back.

2.2. Loss of Energy and Sleep

Health problems often drain the patient's vitality, as the body tries to fight off the illness. This may leave little energy for physical or emotional activities that bring pleasure and enjoyment. If the medical condition also interferes with sleep (as do illnesses such as congestive heart failure, restless leg syndrome, painful neurological conditions, and arthritis), then the fatigue of insomnia adds to and magnifies the physical and emotional exhaustion. Feeling tired all the time can itself lead to depression or other psychiatric problems, because this interferes with meaningful activities and relationships.

2.3. Acute or Chronic Pain

There is a heavy overlap between pain and depression, which reinforce one another. Pain forces one's attention to the body part affected, making it difficult to think about anything else except a desire to relieve or escape the pain. Pain, especially when chronic, can completely dominate the patient's life, affecting sleep, hobbies, work, and relationships with family and friends. The treatments for pain, in fact, may also have negative consequences because they interfere with level of alertness, ability to communicate, drive, and function effectively. This can result in anxiety and depression, which further magnify or worsen the physical pain experienced.

2.4. Increase in Disability

As chronic illness affects physical function and ability to care for the self, there is an increasing need to depend on others. There are few things that people value more than independence and ability to control the direction of their lives. No one wants to be a burden on others, especially in independent societies such as the United States and Europe. Dependency can be particularly disturbing in situations where caregivers become resentful over their extra burdens, and then communicate this resentment directly or indirectly to the dependent person. Is there any wonder why level of disability is one of the strongest predictors of depression in medical patients?

2.5. Change of Roles in Family and Society

When patients are no longer able to work, generate an income, or contribute to family responsibilities, their importance and leadership positions in family and community are affected. The sick or dependent person often loses value and respect in the eyes of family members and society. This loss of "position" can be very distressing, especially for those who derived a great deal of satisfaction in being independent and able to provide for themselves and others.

2.6. Loss of Social Relationships

Patients with chronic and/or serious medical illness have a difficult time both maintaining social relationships and making new ones. Hearing difficulties may interfere with communication, and chronic disability may impair mobility necessary to attend social events. Medical symptoms, especially loss of energy, can keep patients in their homes or rooms and may reduce motivation to get out for social interactions. Social isolation, then, becomes a huge problem for those with chronic illness and may lead to depression, which may increase social withdrawal and increase loneliness. A vicious cycle quickly develops with increasing social isolation and increasing depression, which feed on each other.

2.7. Loss of Ability to Work

Work not only structures how people spend their time during the day, but also is a major source of identity and self-esteem for many. Not being able to work or contribute meaningfully because of medical illness or disability can be devastating. Loss of work can also mean loss of ability to generate income and provide support for self and others. If depression is to be successfully treated

over time, then issues related to loss of work must be addressed.

2.8. Loss of Opportunities to Meet Life Goals

Medical illness may portend permanent changes in physical functioning or may limit cognitive abilities, which can result in the realization that lifetime goals in work, career, or family may never be achieved. These patients need to identify new goals that are within their remaining abilities given their physical limitations. Patients may need counseling to develop their abilities so that worthwhile life goals can be successfully pursued despite limitations. Keeping motivation, hope, and vision alive become crucial.

2.9. Loss of the Ability to Make a Difference

Until becoming sick, many patients may have taken pride in making a positive difference in people's lives. Providing for family, raising children, contributing to church or community, helping a neighbor, contributing to goals in the workplace, and so forth may have been important and meaningful. Illness can interfere with all that, particularly when illness is chronic. Inability to make a positive difference, or its opposite, seeing oneself as making a negative difference in family or friends' lives, can be devastating to self-esteem and self-image.

2.10. Loss of Purpose and Meaning in Life

Any one or a combination of the above losses can leave patients feeling as if their lives have lost meaning and purpose, and that they no longer have a reason for living. Such feelings lead to hopelessness, discouragement, loss of motivation for self-care, and can ultimately lead to the conviction that life is not worth living and that death is the only way out. Although antidepressants, anti-anxiety drugs, and other biological treatments can be extremely helpful in relieving painful symptoms, they do not address the core issues driving depression. Incomplete or only partial treatment response, which is so common in medical patients, may be due to lingering existential concerns that were not adequately addressed as part of the overall treatment plan.

Given the massive losses and life change that physical illness causes, it is not surprising that depressive disorders are so common in hospital settings. Eventually, patients' efforts to meet these multiple challenges become exhausted. Our studies show that rates of major or minor depression in older patients acutely hospitalized with medical illness approximate 50 percent,(4) and, rates are even higher among younger hospitalized patients where medical illness and disability are not "on time" as they are in older adults.(5) The majority of these depressive disorders are undiagnosed and untreated.(6) Even if depression is identified as a problem, primary care physicians often lack the training to manage such disorders appropriately.(7) Despite their lack of expertise in treating depression, medical physicians refer only about 10 percent of these patients to psychiatrists, even when the patient has a major depressive disorder.(7) Some physicians may rationalize that patients with chronic illness and multiple losses have a good reason to be depressed, and so there is no need for treatment of this "normal" reaction to illness. Such therapeutic nihilism can only be addressed by education and by the experience of positive results when these patients are treated or referred for psychiatric care.

Because emotional disorders in medical patients are often a direct result of inability to cope with massive life change and loss, mental health specialists should seek out resources that can help patients adjust successfully to illness. Identifying and supporting such coping resources can complement existing biological, psychological, and social therapies.

3. ROLE OF RELIGION/SPIRITUALITY

Consultation-liaison (CL) psychiatrists and other mental health professionals should be aware of the roles, both positive and negative, that religious beliefs and practices can play in the adjustment of patients to medical illness. On the one hand, religious beliefs may be a symptom or cause of psychiatric disorder. On the other hand, religion may be a powerful coping resource for some patients, prevent the development of emotional disorder, or reduce the time it takes for these disorders to remit. Let us consider each of these possibilities below.

3.1. Religious Belief as a Symptom

Religious beliefs may be a symptom of depression or other emotional illness. For example, the medical patient may attribute the extreme guilt and sadness from their depressive disorder to having committed the "unpardonable" sin that dooms him or her to eternal damnation and suffering. The patient may feel great remorse and sense of failure and explain these feelings as punishment for trespasses of some sort, either real or imagined. Religion may also be used to normalize weight loss or improper attention to nutrition. The religious patient may try to cover up anorexia or weight loss by claiming that he or she is fasting for religious reasons. In all these instances, the religious belief is used to justify symptoms whose underlying cause is depression, not religion. In this case, then, the depressive symptom does not result from religion, but from the underlying depressive disorder and is simply explained by the patient in religious terms because of his or her religious worldview.

3.2. Religious Belief as a Cause

In some instances, religious beliefs may actually lead to the development or worsening of emotional disorder in vulnerable individuals. Religious beliefs and teachings may promote feelings of excessive guilt or remorse. Here, religious belief is contributing to the worsening of symptoms. High religious standards and values may be difficult to live up to. Honesty, generosity, selflessness, kindness, and gratefulness are difficult to live out even by the most saintly among us. How often such guilt or shame occurs – and proof that it is the religion that is the origin of the negative emotional symptoms – is uncertain, given the lack of research in this area. Conventional wisdom and clinical experience, however, suggest that this does happen. Prospective studies are needed to help to sort out cause versus effect (that is, whether religion causes depressive symptoms, or whether depressed patients are more likely to gravitate toward religion because it offers comfort or healing).

3.3. Religious Belief as a Coping Behavior

Rather than being a cause for depression or a symptom of it, religious beliefs and practices may be used by patients to cope with the pain and suffering that depression causes. This may be particularly common in medical patients (versus psychiatric patients) where emotional disorder is more often the result of difficult circumstances (situational depression). Religious beliefs may help medical patients to reframe their losses in a more positive light, give a sense of purpose and meaning, and provide hope that something good can result from the situation.

4. RELIGION AND DEPRESSION

Because depression is so common and resistant to treatment in patients with medical illness and disability, CL psychiatrists will be frequently called on to manage these patients. Although antidepressant medication and psychotherapy have an important place in the treatment of medically ill patients with depression, they are often not sufficient. Treatment-resistant depression or partially treated depression is extremely common, even after all traditional psychiatric therapies have been tried. Thus, helping patients identify resources that can help them adapt to the disturbing symptoms of medical illness or to the psychological distress of chronic disability or dependency is an important task.

A number of cross-sectional and prospective studies in medical inpatients suggest that religious coping is common in such settings and is associated with more rapid adaptation to medical illness and disability. This is especially true for patients with the most severe illness and greatest

disability and those whose physical conditions are not responding to medical treatments.

In the early 1990s, we studied a consecutive sample of men admitted to the medical and neurological services of the Veterans Administration Medical Center in Durham, North Carolina.(8) Eight hundred and fifty men aged 65 or older were examined for depressive symptoms using the self-rated thirty-item Geriatric Depression Scale (GDS) and Brief Carroll Depression Scale (BCDS); patients over age 70 years were also assessed with the observer-rated seventeen-item Hamilton Depression Rating Scale (HDRS). Religious coping was measured using the three-item Religious Coping Index (RCI) whose scores range from 0 to 30. In that study, 21 percent of patients indicated that religion was the "most important factor" that enabled them to cope, and 56 percent indicated that they depended at least a large extent on religion to cope.

In the cross-sectional analysis that used a multivariate model to control for nine other patient characteristics relevant to depression, RCI scores were significantly and inversely related to both self-rated (GDS) and observer-rated (HDRS) scales. Particularly important, this association was strongest for men with the most severe disability. In the longitudinal phase of the study, all subjects readmitted within the sixteen-month study period and subsequent five months (average follow-up six months) (n = 202) were reassessed for depressive symptoms (combination of GDS and BCDS). The baseline RCI score was the only characteristic that predicted fewer depressive symptoms on follow-up, after controlling for baseline depression and other covariates.

Although religious beliefs and practices appear to protect against the development of depression, religious people do get depressed. Even when that happens, however, depressive disorder appears to remit more quickly in these patients (that is, adaptation occurs more quickly). At least two studies in medical inpatients are relevant in this regard. In the first study, eighty-seven hospitalized medically ill patients on general medicine, cardiology, and neurology services of Duke Hospital were diagnosed with depressive disorder using the

Diagnostic Interview Survey (which makes diagnoses using the *Diagnostic and Statistical Manual of Mental Disorders, Third Edition, DSM-III*, criteria).(9) Intrinsic religiosity (IR) at baseline was measured using an established ten-item intrinsic religiosity scale. Patients were followed for an average of forty-seven weeks, and baseline predictors of speed of depression remission were analyzed using Cox proportional hazards regression. After controlling for baseline physical, psychological, and social characteristics, for every ten-point increase on the IR scale (that ranged from ten to fifty), there was a 70 percent increase in the speed of remission (Hazard Ratio = 1.70, 95% Confidence Interval = 1.05–2.75). As in the earlier study, among a subgroup of patients whose physical illness was either not improving or was getting worse (n = 48), effects were particularly strong. For those patients, every ten-point increase on the IR scale predicted over a 100 percent increase in speed of depression remission (HR 2.06, 95% CI 1.02–4.15).

In a second much larger study, researchers systematically identified 1,000 medical inpatients with depressive disorder. All subjcet were over age 50 and had congestive heart failure and/or chronic pulmonary disease.(10) Depressive disorder was diagnosed using the Structured Clinical Interview for Depression (SCID). Detailed information was obtained on depression, psychiatric and social characteristics, physical health, and religious involvement. Patients were followed after discharge (over twelve weeks for those with minor depression; over twenty-four weeks for those with major depression). Again, Cox proportional hazards regression was used to examine the independent effects of religious involvement on time to depression remission, controlling for baseline characteristics. Of the 1,000 depressed patients identified at baseline, follow-up data on depression course was obtained on 87 percent.

Results indicated that patients who attended religious services and participated in other group-related religious activities remitted from their depressions significantly faster than did less religiously involved patients. This effect persisted after controlling for other baseline characteristics and could not be explained by social support.

More important, patients with a *combination* of frequent religious attendance, prayer, scripture reading, and high intrinsic religiosity (14 percent of the sample) went into remission 53 percent faster than other patients (HR = 1.53, 95% CI 1.20–1.94, p = 0.0005, n = 839) after controlling for multiple baseline demographic, psychological, social, and medical predictors. Social support explained only 15 percent of this effect. Based on these results, investigators concluded that depressed medical inpatients who were highly religious (as determined by multiple indicators of religious involvement), particularly those involved in religious community activities, remitted faster from depression than other patients.

5. SUICIDAL THOUGHTS AND BEHAVIOR

Chronic medical illness is associated with high rates of successful suicide, even though contact with medical providers may be frequent. These patients are often reluctant to share suicidal thoughts with their physicians because of the stigma that depression carries with it. Other patients may try to recruit their medical providers to assist them in committing suicide, which can prompt referral to a psychiatrist for evaluation and management.

In some cases, suicidal (or homicidal) thoughts may be prompted by religious delusions. For example, a mother developed the religious delusion that her two young children would be forever damned to hell if she did not kill them. She drowned both children in the bathtub. Another example is that of a young man who felt extreme religious guilt for not living up to his religious ideals. He reasoned that if he killed himself, then this would be sufficient punishment to prevent his eternal damnation for the sins he had committed. He hung himself in his garage. Certain radical fundamentalists (for example, extremist Muslim groups) may favor suicide and homicide as an act of service to God. Most religious doctrines and teachings in almost every major religion around the world, however, discourage suicide. This is particularly true for suicide as a solution to personal suffering.

In some Eastern cultures (Japan and some areas of China), suicide may be viewed as an honorable act in certain rare circumstances (after shameful deeds or in service to country), but it is not condoned to avoid or escape from pain and suffering. Within Judeo-Christian faith traditions, to kill oneself is equivalent to murder, for one of the Ten Commandments is "Thou shalt not kill," and there is no distinction made between killing one's self or killing others. Such prohibitions are powerful deterrents to the sequence of psychological events that eventually lead to successful suicide.

Religious and spiritual beliefs often help people to cope with the pain and suffering that lead to suicidal thinking, and thereby convey hope and meaning that can prevent suicide. Religious involvement can also surround the suicidal person with a community of people who can support the person and help him or her bear the emotional burden. "Am I my brother's keeper?" asked Cain in Genesis. God's answer, "You bet you are." At the heart of some faith communities (although not all) is the care that members demonstrate toward one another. This is the ideal that the Christian scriptures (and the scriptures of other world religions) emphasize. "Whoever does not love does not know God, because God is love" (1 John 4:8, NIV).

Plenty of research supports the claim that religious involvement can prevent suicide in those with or without medical illness. People with strong religious beliefs, particularly if involved in a supportive religious community, have fewer thoughts about suicide, have more negative attitudes toward suicide, and commit suicide less often than those who are not religious. In a review of sixty-eight studies that examined the relationship between suicide and religion, fifty-seven (84 percent) found that religious persons were more negative about suicide, had fewer thoughts about it, attempted it less, and were less likely to complete suicide. In these studies religiousness was measured in many different ways: from frequency of religious activities to degree of personal religiousness to regional rates of religious book publication. Countries of the world that publish fewer books on religion have higher suicide rates than countries that publish more religious books.(11)

Critics say that areas of the world that are more religious often have stronger cultural taboos about committing suicide, which then affect whether or not cases of suicide are reported. Muslims, for example, strongly condemn suicide, whereas members of Eastern religious traditions such as Buddhists, Hindus, Chinese, and Japanese religions are more tolerant (with Christians and Jews falling in between, depending on how conservative their beliefs are).(12, 13)

More recent studies on religion and suicide include subjects of different ages across the life span and from various ethnic groups. Because suicide rates are greatest at the age extremes (adolescents/teenagers and older adults), studies in these populations are particularly relevant. Greening and Stoppelbein examined religiousness and suicidal attitudes in 1,098 Caucasian and African-American adolescents, asking them to rate the likelihood that they would ever commit suicide. (14) Investigators controlled analyses for depression severity, hopelessness, social support, and style of causal attribution. Of all these characteristics, religious orthodoxy (commitment to core beliefs) was the single strongest predictor of negative attitudes toward suicide. Furthermore, while severity of depression predicted a greater self-reported future likelihood of committing suicide, greater religious orthodoxy reduced the likelihood of depressed adolescents saying that they would ever die by suicide (that is, religious orthodoxy moderated the effect of depression on suicide).

The same pattern appears to be true in older adults, where the suicide rate is higher than any other population group. In a study of 835 urban low-income African-Americans, with an average age of 73 years, Cook and colleagues examined predictors of active and passive suicidal ideation.(15) Passive suicidal ideation is a desire to die or wish to be dead, but no active plans or intentions to end life. Active suicidal ideation involves more serious plans on how to commit suicide and active desire to harm self. Of the multiple characteristics measured (anxiety, social dysfunction, somatic symptoms, low social support, absence of a confidante, older age, lower education, more depressive symptoms, and poorer cognitive functioning), only two characteristics independently predicted *passive* suicidal ideation: depressive symptoms and low religious coping. Low life satisfaction and low religious coping were also the only characteristics that independently predicted *active* suicidal ideation.

The inverse relationship between religiousness and suicidal ideation is also present in patients with severe medical illness, which brings this topic into the realm of CL psychiatry. For example, McClain and colleagues examined the relationship between spiritual well-being, depression, and desire for death in 160 terminally ill cancer patients with less than three months to live.(16) Scales measuring depressive symptoms, hopelessness, attitudes toward a hastened death, and the FACIT-Spiritual well-being (SWB) scale were administered to patients. A single item measured recurrent thoughts of death or suicide on a scale from absent to "high risk requiring suicide precautions." SWB was significantly and inversely related to a desire for hastened death, hopelessness, and suicidal thoughts, and of all variables, was the strongest predictor of these three outcomes – even stronger than severity of depression. In fact, while depression was strongly correlated with desire for a hastened death in those with low SWB, no correlation was found between depression and suicidal yearnings in those with high SWB. This study, published in *The Lancet*, concluded that SWB provided substantial protection against end-of-life despair.

Examining attitudes toward euthanasia and assisted suicide in an Australian outpatient cancer population,(17) Carter and colleagues studied the impact of mental health and other characteristics in predicting attitude toward these suicide-related practices. The sample consisted of 228 patients attending an oncology clinic in Newcastle, Australia. Possible predictors of suicidal attitude included demographic characteristics, disease status, mental health (depression, anxiety, and prior suicide attempts), and quality of life. Results indicated that the majority of respondents supported euthanasia (79 percent) and physician-assisted suicide (69 percent). Only 2 percent, however, had ever asked

their physician for either euthanasia or physician-assisted suicide. Active religious belief was the most important predictor of attitudes toward all three suicide-related behaviors (euthanasia, assisted-suicide, and personal support for euthanasia or assisted-suicide). Patients with an active religious belief were 79 percent less likely to have positive attitudes toward euthanasia, 65 percent less likely to have positive attitudes toward assisted suicide, and 74 percent less likely to personally support euthanasia or assisted-suicide (all highly statistically significant). Interestingly, depression, anxiety, recent suicidal ideation, and history of suicide attempt were unrelated to any of these three outcomes once active religious belief was take into account.

5.1. Timely Psychiatric Care

Religious beliefs and activities may also affect suicide rates in other ways besides simply prohibiting suicide. In particular, religious involvement may increase the likelihood that persons with suicidal thoughts will obtain timely psychiatric care. Members of the religious community often consider it an obligation to check on those who may be depressed or otherwise at risk for suicidal thoughts. This may be particularly true for those with medical illness or in other difficult life situations obvious to members of their faith community. First, as noted earlier, the support from members of the congregation may help to reduce the negative emotions responsible for the desire to commit suicide. Second, church members may encourage people to seek professional assistance for their problems before those problems get to a point that suicidal thoughts develop. Third, if suicidal thoughts are already present, then members of the religious community are likely to encourage the suicidal person to seek professional help to relieve their distress or discover alternative ways of dealing with the problem besides suicide.

I Want to Die

Richard is a 70-year-old retired businessman who lost his wife of forty-five years, Ethyl, to cancer two years ago. He has chronic lung disease from years of smoking cigarettes, and drinks about three shot-glasses of vodka every night to relax and help him get to sleep. Richard and his wife had few social activities during their adult years, focusing most of their time on their children and work, although they did attend religious services regularly together. For many years, he served as an usher in his Methodist congregation, although he had to stop this activity about a year ago because of health problems. Nevertheless, he continued to attend religious services, albeit on an irregular basis in recent days. Richard had not been doing well since his wife passed away. He missed her terribly, especially when he would retire to bed at night. She had slept there next to him for over four decades and now her side of the bed was empty. He also had a lot of shortness of breath due to his worsening lung disease and spent most of the day inside his home watching TV and sleeping on-and-off. Becoming more and more depressed, Richard started having suicidal thoughts. He had a shotgun in the garage and began thinking about using it to take his life.

Around this time, a member of his church, Sam, called Richard on the telephone to find out how he was doing. Sam hadn't seen him in church for the last two Sundays, and so had become concerned. Richard broke down on the phone. He confessed to Sam that things had been really difficult for him, and told him, "I just want to die and be with Ethyl again." Sensing Richard's distress, Sam told him that he was coming right over. When Sam arrived, he found Richard sitting on the couch with a blank expression on his face. When Richard saw Sam, he broke into tears. After listening to Richard for a while, Sam insisted that he take Richard to see his family physician. Richard reluctantly agreed. After talking with Richard and learning about his thoughts of dying, the family physician called a psychiatrist colleague and made an appointment for Richard that afternoon. Sam assured the physician that he would take Richard to the appointment.

Religious involvement, however, does not always increase the likelihood that persons at risk for suicide will seek timely psychiatric care. In fact, religious beliefs may delay necessary psychiatric care by encouraging treatments within the faith community, thereby allowing depression or other psychiatric illness to worsen and suicidal behavior to emerge. Lack of timely referral, or negative attitudes within a religious congregation toward psychiatric care, can be at fault for unnecessary suicides.

Depending on God

Sherry is a 37-year-old unmarried woman who was recently diagnosed with rheumatoid arthritis. Due to the pain and disability that this illness caused, she sought help from her pastor to cope. Her pastor encouraged her with scriptures from the Bible, prayed with her, and suggested she become involved in a women's group at church. After three months of counseling, however, Sherry felt no better. Her pain was worse and the depression had become more severe. In fact, she was so depressed that she didn't have the energy or the concentration to pray, read the Bible, or get involved in the women's group, which made her feel guilty and like a failure. In fact, the depression got so bad that she barely had enough desire to get up in the morning and drive to her job as a department store clerk, which she was depending on to pay her bills. She had been late to work several times now, and was fearful of losing her job.

When she asked her pastor if perhaps she should seek professional psychiatric care, he encouraged her to "depend entirely on God" for healing and suggested that her desire to seek psychiatric care was a sign of her weak faith. Soon, feeling trapped in a situation that seemed to be without escape, she developed suicidal thoughts and took an overdose of pain medications. Luckily, she was found in time by a neighbor and rushed to the hospital, where she was successfully treated for the overdose. There Sherry was referred to a psychiatrist who began her on antidepressant medication. In four weeks, she was back to work and feeling more like herself again. She found another church and became an active member there.

6. ANXIETY IN MEDICAL SETTINGS

Although this topic is covered more fully in Chapter 10, I address anxiety disorders here in the context of medical illness, where CL psychiatrists are likely to be called on for assistance. Patients may have a variety of worries and fears when they are hospitalized with medical illness. Loss of control and feelings of helplessness drive anxiety in this setting. Patients are fearful of what their medical illness may mean for their own future and the future of their families. They may be worried about the results of lab tests or procedures. Some patients may become anxious after being told about a disabling or terminal diagnosis. In some cases, the anxiety may become paralyzing, especially if patients have a history of anxiety problems in the past.

Religious beliefs may influence the type and the severity of anxiety that patients experience. On the one hand, religious worries may center on concerns about salvation, fear of hell, or guilt over becoming sick. Such patients may become preoccupied with religious worries or become involved in a frenzy of religious behaviors such as compulsive prayer activity or repeated confessions. These behaviors may extend beyond "normal" kinds of religious involvement and become pathological in nature.

On the other hand, religious beliefs may help medical patients cope with the anxiety due to medical illness, or if an anxiety disorder is present, help patients cope with the pain and suffering that the anxiety causes. Religious beliefs and practices can give patients a sense of control over what is happening to them. Prayer gives patients something they can do, which may help to make a real difference in their situations. Patients may believe that prayer will physically heal their illness or give them the strength to cope with illness. The effectiveness of prayer in relieving anxiety depends on the strength of the patient's religious belief, the specific kinds of religious beliefs as they relate to healing, and the use of prayer in the past as a coping behavior.

Meditation may also help to relieve anxiety, although through a different mechanism than the kind of personal prayer described above. Personal prayer depends on the patient's relationship with God and is heavily dependent on cognitive processes (for example, belief, commitment, and trust). Meditation in the Eastern religious traditions of Hinduism (transcendental meditation) or Buddhism (mindfulness meditation), however, involves more of a behavioral mechanism. The clearing of the mind and a repetition of a sound, word, or phrase while sitting in a certain position, causes reflex relaxation – almost like biofeedback or progressive muscle relaxation – and if done consistently, can reduce anxiety or tension. This kind of meditation does not depend on a strong belief in, personal relationship with, or communication with God, but rather on a practice that involves a specific spiritual behavior that through physical procedures results in a deep, relaxed state. Herbert Benson has called this bio-behavioral reflex the Relaxation Response.(18)

A number of randomized clinical trials have shown that religious-based psychotherapy or psychotherapy supplemented by religious practices, may increase the speed of remission of anxiety, especially generalized anxiety disorder (GAD), which is common in medical settings. For example, Azhar and colleagues (19) randomized sixty-two Muslim patients with GAD to either traditional treatment (supportive psychotherapy and anti-anxiety drugs) or traditional treatment plus religious psychotherapy. Religious psychotherapy involved use of prayer and reading verses of the Holy Koran specific to the person's situation. Patients receiving the religious psychotherapy improved significantly faster than those receiving traditional therapy.

Likewise, Razali and colleagues (20) tested the effects of a Muslim-based religious cognitive psychotherapy (RCP) as a treatment for GAD in eighty-five religious and eighty nonreligious Muslims. Religious and nonreligious subjects were randomized to either the intervention group or to a control group. All subjects received standard treatment for GAD including benzodiazepines (BZD), supportive psychotherapy, and/ or simple relaxation exercises. Patients in the intervention group received cognitive therapy that included use of the Koran and Hadith (sayings of Mohammed) to alter negative thoughts and behaviors and to increase religiousness. Each of the four groups (religious subjects receiving RCP, religious controls, nonreligious subjects receiving RCP, and nonreligious controls) was assessed at four, twelve, and twenty-six weeks after the start of the intervention. Results indicated that religious subjects who received RCP improved significantly faster than religious controls. However, no difference was found between nonreligious patients receiving RCP and nonreligious controls. This study suggests that religious therapies work best in religious patients.

Finally, Zhang and colleagues examined the effects of Chinese Taoist-based cognitive psychotherapy (CTCP) in 143 Chinese patients with GAD.(21) Subjects were randomized to CTCP only (n = 46), benzodiazepines only (BDZ) (n = 48), or combined CTCP and BDZ treatment (n = 49). CTCP combined cognitive therapy and Taoist philosophy (using the thirty-two character Taoist formula). Those in the CTCP and combined groups received one hour of CTCP weekly for four weeks and then twice monthly one–hour sessions for the remaining five months. Subjects receiving BDZ remained on the same dose of medication for the final five months of the study. Results indicated that patients receiving BDZ treatment alone experienced the most rapid reduction in GAD symptoms, but that these beneficial effects were gone by six months. CTCP alone had little effect on symptoms in the short-term (at one month) when compared to BDZ therapy, but showed significant symptom reduction by six months. Combined treatment with both CTCP and medication showed symptom reduction at both one and six months. The major problem with this study was that the design made it impossible to determine whether the religious aspect of the cognitive therapy had anything to do with the benefits observed (because a secular cognitive therapy group was not included in the study to compare with the CTCP group).

Finally, there is some evidence that cognitive therapy in patients with panic disorder works better if the patient is more religious (see Chapter 10). Patients with strong religious beliefs depend on religious scriptures for comfort, particularly those scriptures promising that they are loved and never alone, and that there is nothing to fear, even death itself. These are powerful cognitions that can counteract anxious thoughts that may contribute to panic or other severe anxiety symptoms.

I'm Afraid

Janet is a 27-year-old unmarried schoolteacher who lives with her parents. She has recently been diagnosed with a rare form of breast cancer and is undergoing chemotherapy. Janet was in the hospital getting her weekly chemotherapy when she woke up suddenly in a panic. Her sister Sally, who was sitting across the room reading, immediately came to her bedside and asked what was wrong. Janet frantically told her, "I'm afraid I'm going to die. I can't get my breath and my heart is jumping out of my chest. Am I dying? Please help me!" The patient's sister rang the patient's call bell to alert the nurse on duty and then reached over and gently took Janet's hand. Sally said, "Janet, let's pray." When Janet nodded consent, Sally said a short comforting prayer asking God to calm her sister's nerves, give her a deep sense of peace, and let her know that God loved her, was with her now, and would never leave her. Gradually, Janet began to calm down. Her breathing slowed, and she became less frantic. After about 10 minutes, the nurse on duty came into the room, apologizing profusely for her tardiness (there had been another emergency on the ward and the nurse was preoccupied with that situation). By the time she arrived, however, Janet was feeling better and in control. The prayer had helped.

7. SOMATOFORM DISORDERS

Somatoform disorders are physical complaints or signs for which no physical etiology can be identified and are therefore thought to be due to psychological causes (that is, are somatic manifestations of psychological pathology). Among the most common and well-known somatoform disorders are conversion disorder, somatization disorder, and hypochondriasis.

There is little systematic research on whether somatoform disorders are more or less frequent among religious persons compared with the nonreligious. Only four studies have examined the relationship between religion and somatization (two studies coming out of our research group). In the first of these, Chaturvedi and Bhandari reported religious differences in beliefs about the underlying cause of psychosomatic complaints. (22) In a small sample of thirty-one psychiatric outpatients (twenty-four Hindu, seven Muslims) in Bangalore, India, they found that Muslims were more likely than Hindus to report that their illnesses were the result of physical causes despite the fact that they were told they were of psychological origin.

Second, a study by Koenig and colleagues reported results from the North Carolina site of the National Institutes of Mental Health Epidemiologic Catchment Area survey (n = 2,969). (23) No difference was found in rates of somatization disorder based on any religious characteristic, including religious attendance, prayer/Bible study, religious TV/radio, importance of religion, religious affiliation, or "born again" status (the latter involves making a conscious commitment to

turn one's life over to God and live life in a way that reflects the life of Jesus Christ). This is the only study that examined a random sample of community-dwelling residents diagnosed with somatization disorder using a structured psychiatric interview (Diagnostic Interview Schedule) and using *DSM-III* criteria.

Third, in a study of 300 primary care patients in Greece, Androutsopoulou and colleagues found that Muslims scored significantly higher than Christians on the somatic complaints subscale of the General Health Questionnaire, a difference that persisted after controlling for other covariates including gender.(24) It is not clear, however, what this finding means because complaint of somatic symptoms by primary care patients does not necessarily indicate a somatization disorder.

In the most recent study, Flannelly and colleagues conducted an Internet survey of 1,403 readers of *Spirituality & Health* magazine using the Symptom Assessment-45 Questionnaire, with a subscale that measures somatization.(25) They found no relationship between somatization and frequency of religious attendance or religious fundamentalism. Although a weak *positive* association was found between frequency of prayer and somatization, there was also a weak *negative* association between belief in an afterlife and somatization. Overall, then, there is little evidence for a relationship between somatization disorder and religious involvement.

Although not associated in general, a connection between somatization disorder and religion may sometimes occur, even if not very frequently. Such cases received an unusual amount of attention during the late nineteenth century because of historical trends at the time they were reported. During this period, the French Revolution had succeeded in throwing off the last vestige of religious influence. This is when the famous French neurologist Jean-Martin Charcot claimed that there was a connection between religion, hysteria (a form of conversion disorder), and other neurological illnesses.(26) Charcot emphasized the physical positioning and posture of Catholic saints as depicted in famous religious paintings from the early Middle Ages through the seventeenth century. Using more than five dozen illustrations, he argued that the Catholic mystics in these paintings were actually examples of hysteria (St. Catherine of Sienna being the prototype). (27) Paintings of saints in positions of prayer and even those of the crucifixion were said to illustrate hysteria. In some cases, Charcot actually claimed that these saints were suffering from opisthotonus (a severe hyperextension of the head in which the head, neck, and spinal column enter into a bridging or arching position). Charcot believed that the ecstatic states of the religious in these great works of art were manifestations of psychopathology. A more detailed and fascinating discussion of this topic is provided elsewhere.(28) Charcot's writings and teachings are particularly relevant because Freud would later train under Charcot, and the development of Freud's negative views toward religion could have been due to Charcot's influence.

Might religious beliefs contribute to the development of some kinds of somatoform disorders as Charcot argued and Freud would later emphasize? Examples of physical manifestations of psychological conflicts related to religion include the phenomenon of stigmata, where a physical wound (or bleeding) appears spontaneously on the body of a religious person in the same location as the wounds suffered by Jesus. (29, 30) The Italian priest, Padre Pio, is reported to have had stigmata on his hands, feet, side, and chest.(31) Other more contemporary examples of physical manifestations of spiritual-psychological forces might include the "faint" that occurs when someone is "slain in the spirit" at a Pentecostal healing service (where the minister places his hand on the forehead of a member of the congregation, who then faints and falls to the ground) or perhaps even the manifestation of "speaking in tongues." While not examples of somatoform disorders, they do illustrate how physical manifestations may occur as a result of religious beliefs acting through psychological-physiological processes.

There have also been reports of more serious religion-related conversion disorders that interfere with functioning and cause great distress and suffering. According to *DSM-IV*, conditions that occur in a specific religious or cultural context are diagnosed as "culture-bound syndromes," and are often characterized by dissociation and seizure like manifestations.

Please Don't Kill Me

Sarah is a 24-year-old married, unemployed Puerto Rican woman, with two children ages two and four. She presented to a neurologist with the complaint of "seizures" that were completely incapacitating her. Sarah was diagnosed with tonic-clonic generalized seizures and treated with carbamazepine. Despite this treatment, she continued to have seizures two or three times per week. She would typically have a headache, and then soon afterward would become unconscious and begin tonic-clonic movements, which would last for about ten minutes. After arousing, she would not recognize family members and wanted to leave the home. After the seizures, she would sometimes hallucinate a threatening female figure and was observed by family members to be begging, "Please don't kill or harm me." Further history revealed that two years before the seizures began, at the age of 17 years old, Sarah witnessed the suicide of her grandmother, who burned to death when she set fire to her home. Sarah felt guilty over this because she thought that if she had alerted people sooner, they could have saved the grandmother's life. When asked to explain her behaviors, Sarah said that she and her family believed in espiritismo (Spiritist religion) and participated in séances. They believed that disturbed spirits could take possession of the living, especially spirits of persons who had died a violent death. Such spirits could linger indefinitely in space and attack people to extract revenge. After twenty-two treatment sessions in psychotherapy over several months and nearly a year of follow-up with less frequent sessions, her psychogenic seizures nearly completely subsided. This patient's story is based on a case reported in the literature.(32)

The resolution of this case depended on the therapist addressing the patient's symptoms from her religious viewpoint. The therapist only gradually introduced the notion that there were other possible explanations for her symptoms, including unresolved guilt over the death of her grandmother. The therapist also used rituals in line with espiritismo beliefs to help the patient assist the grandmother out of her trapped place in the spirit world and on to a more peaceful and restful existence.

8. PAIN

The topic of religion often comes up when talking about pain and suffering. In fact, many of the world's great religions may have arisen in response to the difficulties that self-conscious humans faced when struggling with difficult life and death situations. These religions all address suffering as a central part of their rituals and theological traditions. Religious beliefs may be a cause for, a response to, or a way of coping with painful medical conditions, and consultation-liaison psychiatrists need to be familiar with how religion and pain interact and are connected.

First, religious beliefs, particularly if rigid and inflexible, may worsen pain. Religious patients may feel guilty for having a painful condition and seek to understand why God is allowing them to suffer so. They may feel that God is punishing them for past sins, or doesn't care, or isn't able to make a difference in their pain. Such religious cognitions may worsen the patient's psychological state, which can exacerbate the pain, adding spiritual suffering to physical suffering. Although such "negative religious coping" in response to pain is not particularly common in medical settings,(33) it does occur, and patients need to be asked about it. Pastoral care referral is often necessary to help patients deal with such religious struggles.

Second, and much more common in medical patients, is that religion is turned to in an attempt to cope with the pain. Patients may pray, read religious scriptures, or engage in religious rituals to help them deal with pain, especially the emotional consequences of the pain, that is the anxiety, sense of helplessness, and hopelessness that chronic pain frequently causes. The following clinical case, which illustrates the positive role that religion can play in coping with pain, appeared a few years ago in the *Journal of the American Medical Association*. This is a real case, although the name has been changed to ensure confidentiality.

I Pray

Margaret is an 83-year-old widowed woman who sees a physician in Boston, Massachusetts. Her doctor is an attending physician at Beth Israel Deaconess Hospital and is a professor of medicine at Harvard Medical School. Margaret has multiple chronic medical problems, including advanced diabetes mellitus and hypertension. The diabetes is probably the cause for a diffuse polymotor and sensory neuropathy that has resulted in chronic, progressive pain. Margaret has had chronic pain for almost fifteen years now, and the pain has proven resistant to most traditional treatments, including gabapentin, topiramate, mexiletine, tramadol, rofecoxib, celecoxib, acetaminophen, codeine, oxycodone, and a fentanyl patch. The pain appears to be neuropathic in nature and is narcotic-resistant. Her neurologist has signed off the case, saying there is nothing more he can do for her. When she goes to see her internist, the doctor doesn't have much to offer her. Most of the time, Margaret and her doctor just sit and talk about her pain and the challenges she faces with functioning, because little else can be done. Despite her long-standing chronic pain, Margaret is doing well from a psychological standpoint. She is optimistic, hopeful, and positive in her outlook. When her doctor asks her how she maintains such a positive attitude, she says that religion helps. Here are her words:

I don't dwell on the pain, you know. Some people are sick and have pain, and it gets the best of them. Not me. Praying eases the pain, takes it away. Sometimes I pray when I am in deep, serious pain; I pray, and all at once the pain gets easy. Praying helps me a lot. I feel that has helped me more than the medication. A doctor is a doctor. Not everybody is bound to believe in God. It's your own mind, your thought, and your belief. The doctor gives you medicine. God works through the doctor. He is a great physician and He heals, but you have to believe. I believe in God. He's my guide and my protector. Whenever you pray, you will get healing from God. You will. But you must have that belief. Because if you don't believe in God and turn your life over to Him, it's nothing doing. You can't just pray, "God, I'm suffering, and I ask You to heal my body." It don't work like that. You have to really be a child of God.(34)

The role of religion in coping with pain is described above from a Judeo-Christian religious perspective. Religious coping, however, is not restricted only to this faith tradition. All the other major world religions – Islam, Buddhism, Hinduism, and the Chinese religions – address the problem of pain and suffering in their unique ways. Patients from Eastern religions may seek to detach themselves from the pain (or from the need to be free of the pain). In these traditions, pain may be given meaning and purpose by associating it with "karma." By suffering willingly and bravely, this will ensure a better, happier life in their next rebirth. Eastern meditative practices, such as "mindfulness" meditation in the Buddhist tradition or "transcendental" meditation in the Hindu tradition, may further help to relieve pain by focusing the mind elsewhere, thereby blocking pain pathways in the brain.

For example, Kabat-Zinn and colleagues (35) described the effects of mindfulness meditation as part of a Stress-Reduction and Relaxation Program

(SRRP) in ninety highly screened chronic pain patients. The intervention was carried out over ten weeks (there was no control group, so this was an observational study only). Comparison of measurements before and after the SRRP intervention showed a statistically significant reduction in pain, mood disturbance, and psychological symptoms. Furthermore, pain-related drug use decreased and self-esteem increased. Effects were independent of sex, source of referral, and type of pain. Although there was no true control group, the course of symptoms in patients receiving the SRRP intervention was compared to a parallel group of patients being seen in another pain clinic (n = 21). The comparison patients did not show similar improvement after treatment with traditional protocols. Improvements in pain in SRRP patients were maintained for fifteen months for all but one measure of pain.

Religious involvement may also help to reduce the secondary complications seen in chronic pain patients, including substance abuse (alcohol and illicit drug use) and pain medication addiction. By providing an alternative coping behavior that is under the patient's control, there is less of a need for these more self-destructive behaviors. Many, many studies show an inverse relationship between religious involvement and substance abuse. In our review of this literature, eighty-six studies examined the relationship between religious involvement and alcohol; seventy-six of those studies found significantly lower alcohol use, abuse, and addiction in those who were more religious.(36) The findings are even more striking for illicit drug addiction. Of the fifty-two studies that examined religiousness and drug use, forty-eight found that those who were more religious were less likely to use drugs. Although I'm not aware of any studies of religion and substance abuse in chronic pain patients, the general relationship is likely to hold true for these patients as well.

Religious beliefs and practices may either speed the resolution of pain or reduce the perception of pain. The Kabat-Zinn study above found that pain symptoms were improved after ten weeks of mindfulness meditation and relaxation. Eastern meditation, however, is not the only religious practice associated with pain reduction. For example, Christian prayer was examined as an intervention in the treatment of pain in patients with advanced rheumatoid arthritis. Matthews and colleagues conducted a randomized clinical trial designed to examine the effects of in-person intercessory prayer ministry (IPM) as an adjunct to standard medical care for patients with rheumatoid arthritis. (37) Forty patients (82 percent female, all-white, mean age 62) who had active rheumatoid arthritis were given a three-day IPM intervention that included six hours of instruction and six hours of direct-contact prayer ("laying-on-of-hands"). Subjects were assessed at three and twelve months post intervention. Before and after comparisons revealed significant overall improvement ($p < 0.0001$), with sustained reductions in tender joints (seventeen versus six), swollen joints (ten versus three) ($p < 0.001$), self-reported pain ($p < 0.004$), fatigue ($p = 0.007$), and functional impairment ($p = 0.007$). Number of tender joints was less in the prayed for group compared to subjects randomly assigned to a waitlist control group at six months ($p = 0.02$).

9. DEMENTIA, AGITATION, BEHAVIORAL DISTURBANCE

Psychiatrists are often called to acute care hospitals or long-term care facilities to see patients with delirium, agitation, and/or psychosis. These conditions can be due to dementia, side effects of medication, or an underlying undiagnosed medical or psychiatric illness. Assuming that medical or medication side effects are not the cause, what can be done? Usually, the psychiatrist will prescribe an antipsychotic or a sedative (benzodiazepine) to calm the patient down. Unfortunately, these medications all have major adverse side effects that interfere with quality of life and may cause direct injury to the patient because they reduce alertness and impair balance, and antipsychotics can have negative neurological, cardiovascular, and metabolic consequences. Is there anything else that can be done besides tranquilizing these patients with drugs? Might religion help out in this regard?

Although there has been no systematic research on this topic, there are a plethora of case reports from nurses and other clinicians in long-term care settings who report that religious interventions may be useful in such circumstances, particularly if the patient is religious. These interventions include holding religious services, singing religious hymns, praying with, or reading religious scriptures to patients (the Psalms, for example).

I'm Scared

Hilda is an 86-year-old patient in a nursing home. She was diagnosed with Alzheimer's disease about five years ago. After a couple years, she became unable to care for herself, forcing her family to put her in a nursing home. Hilda is often agitated, especially when the nurses try to give her a bath in the morning. She is also paranoid and believes that the nurses are stealing from her and may even be poisoning her food. When she gets agitated, she sometimes strikes out at the nursing staff and may even assault other residents on a rare occasion (slapping them). During agitation spells, she refuses all of her medication, including the low dose antipsychotic that the psychiatrist prescribed for her agitation and paranoia. When asked why she would not cooperate with the nursing staff, Hilda's only response was, "I'm scared."

One day when Hilda was having one of her fits during the morning bath, the nurse's aide caring for her began to quietly sing a religious song ("Amazing Grace"). To her surprise, Hilda began to sing along with her. As she sang, she calmed down and became much more cooperative. Further history from the family revealed that Hilda had been a devout church member when she was younger and served as a member of the church choir for many years. Once the nursing staff learned about the aide's experience, whenever they wanted Hilda to calm down or cooperate with care, they would quietly sing "Amazing Grace" with her.

When patients with dementia have a religious background that includes a heavy emphasis on rituals (if Catholic, for example, saying the rosary or receiving communion), then engaging the patient in such rituals or prayers may help to reduce agitation and increase cooperation. Repeating the Twenty-Third Psalm or the Lord's Prayer with the patient may have the same effect. Again, however, a thorough religious history is necessary from the patient (or from the family, if the patient cannot remember or communicate). Several types of religious interventions may need to be tried, although finding out which religious behaviors, rituals, prayers or hymns, were particularly meaningful to the patient will probably be most successful. If the patient has never been particularly religious, however, such interventions are unlikely to help.

Religion can also assist patients cope with the stress involved in the development of dementia, especially the early stages when patients still have insight into what is happening to them. This is a time when emotional distress (depression or anxiety) is common. If religion has been of value to patients in the past, then it may be used to help calm them as they recognize that they are losing control. Praying with patients, reading religious scriptures to them, or singing favorite religious hymns may all serve to calm their emotions, just as described above for patients with more advanced dementia with agitation.

There is even some evidence suggesting that religious involvement may forestall the development of cognitive impairment in older adults (38) or may slow its progression in Alzheimer's disease.(39) Because depression and high stress may increase levels of serum cortisol, and because cortisol has adverse effects on the brain (particularly on the large pyramidal cells in the temporal lobes),(40) a mechanism does exist by which religious involvement could help to preserve memory functions. By reducing depression or speeding its remission, and/or decreasing stress levels, religion could prevent the increase in serum cortisol that adversely affects brain

cells. Lower cortisol or healthier cortisol rhythms among those who are more religious have already been demonstrated in several studies.(41–43)

Whether or not religious involvement helps to prevent cognitive decline in normal aging or dementia, we know that such involvement can be helpful to those caring for patients with dementia. It is often the caregiver who brings the patient with dementia to see the psychiatrist, and level of caregiver burden is a strong predictor of whether patients with dementia can be cared for at home (versus placement in a nursing home). Caregiver stress also affects both the mental and physical health of the caregiver. A number of studies have demonstrated that religious beliefs and practices are associated with lower caregiver stress.(44–46) Religious belief often gives the caregiver a sense of meaning and purpose in their caregiver duties and provides a community of support that can help counteract the isolation and loneliness of the caregiver role.

10. SUBSTANCE ABUSE

Psychiatrists are often called in when medical patients are withdrawing from alcohol or illicit drug use. Co-morbid substance abuse is widespread among patients with chronic physical health problems, as self-medication with these substances promises at least temporary relief of their suffering. What is the role of religion in substance abuse disorders, and how might religious factors influence the management of these patients?

First, as noted earlier, there is a large research literature showing that religious persons are less likely to abuse alcohol and drugs. The result is that these conditions are less likely to be a problem in patients who are more religiously involved. Religious involvement from an early age helps to prevent the onset of alcohol/drug abuse and addiction. Furthermore, it provides an alternative coping behavior (prayer, scripture reading, rituals, and community support) that can counter the stress that may drive people to use these substances. In addition, religious experiences and spiritual interventions have been shown to be effective in helping persons recover from substance abuse and addiction. In a study published in the *American Journal of Psychiatry* in 1953, Lamere reported, "In the generations covered by this survey, religion was often a powerful force in promoting abstinence [from alcohol] and 13, or 24% of these 53 who quit [outside of a terminal illness], did so in response to spiritual conversion."(47) In his classic study of the life history of alcoholics, Harvard psychiatrist George Vaillant likewise notes, "In the treatment of addiction, Karl Marx's aphorism 'religion is the opiate of the masses' masks an enormously important therapeutic principal. Religion may actually provide a relief that drug [and alcohol] abuse only promises."(48)

Spiritual principles of recovery have been operationalized in AA and NA. These programs, run by recovered substance abusers, have been enormously successful worldwide. The key to that success have been the following factors:

1 Admission of powerlessness (that the addicted person does not have within them the power to overcome their problem alone; that is, "I have sinned and cannot beat this problem on my own")
2 Surrender to a Higher Power (for many, this is God, and such surrender involves religious conversion; however, this is not always the case)
3 Commitment to help other brothers or sisters with alcohol addiction by supporting them and helping them to remain sober (that is, "love thy neighbor")

Thus, from a religious view, the process is confession, surrender, and loving others – often considered the key and most essential doctrines of the religious faith (at least in the Judeo-Christian tradition).

Thus, in managing patients with substance abuse problems, the psychiatrist may consider referring these patients to an AA or NA group. If those groups are not readily available, then similar resources should be identified and the addicted person connected to them. The faith community often provides supportive relationships not centered on drinking alcohol or use of drugs as the addicted person's prior community

of support was. Getting away from relationships with other active substance abusers may be key to maintaining sobriety.

11. RELIGION AS A DETERRENT TO PSYCHIATRIC CARE

Although religious beliefs and practices may help medically ill patients and their families to cope with the stress of medical illness, they can sometimes lead to the avoidance of mental health care. Although I have already discussed this above in the example concerning suicidal risk, I will elaborate further here because the potential for conflict is so serious. Given the long and generally antagonistic relationship between religion and mental health professionals, beginning with Freud in the early 1900s, devoutly religious patients may avoid psychiatric treatments with medication or psychotherapy. They may argue that praying, trusting in God, reading the Bible or other religious scriptures, and going to religious services is all that is necessary to cope with the stress of medical illness, and the need to seek professional mental health care may be viewed as having insufficient faith or religious commitment. Although today this is becoming less common and occurs primarily in small fundamentalist religious groups, such negative views of psychiatry and mental health care may be subtle and prevent or delay psychiatric care. For example, clergy may provide counseling to persons with chronic medical illness without recognizing the development of severe depression or suicidal thoughts, resulting in a delay in referral for antidepressant treatment. Although no systematic research exists on how frequently this occurs, anecdotal cases and news reports illustrate the disastrous consequences that can result.

Just Pray More

Catherine is a 36-year-old housewife and mother. She has three children, all under the age of 5 years. Catherine first noticed that she was becoming depressed after the birth of their third child when she began experiencing extreme fatigue, lack of motivation, and a voracious appetite. It got to the point that when the baby cried at night, she was unable to get up to change the baby's diapers and feed him. Instead, she begged her husband to do so. She also stopped making meals for the family and spent most of the day either in bed or sitting in front of the television set. Catherine and her husband are members of a fundamentalist Christian community in Houston, Texas. Her husband, getting more and more upset over Catherine's condition, took her to see their pastor. The pastor began counseling with Catherine, encouraging her to just pray more, read the Bible regularly, and attend religious services every week. He also asked her about any sin in her life and emphasized her need to confess the sin before she would feel better. Despite the visits with her pastor, she became more and more depressed. Catherine's husband asked the pastor if he should take her to see psychiatrist, given that she was doing worse. The pastor discouraged him, saying that all Catherine needed to do was put her entire faith in God, confess her sin, and pray and that seeing a psychiatrist was equivalent to putting her faith in man instead of in God.

12. RELIGION AS A FACILITATOR OF PSYCHIATRIC CARE

On the other hand, involvement in most mainstream religious groups can also increase the likelihood of early detection of mental illness and facilitate psychiatric referral. Increased levels of support and contact with other members of a faith community can result in early detection and encouragement to seek care. Religious people, because they have relationships with others within their community, are less able to avoid seeking help because others are more likely to be checking on them, calling them, visiting them, or seeing them during religious activities.

Religious involvement may also encourage compliance because religious people are taught to respect authority and to be responsible. Biblical scriptures encourage the faithful to do as those in authority tell them:

> Obey your leaders and submit to their authority. They keep watch over you as men who must give an account. Obey them so that their work will be a joy, not a burden, for that would be of no advantage to you. (Heb. 13:17)[1]

> Everyone must submit himself to the governing authorities, for there is no authority except that which God has established. The authorities that exist have been established by God. (Rom. 13:1)

Psychiatrists and other mental health professionals may be seen as authority figures whose instructions must be followed, increasing patients' likelihood of compliance with medication and psychotherapy. Furthermore, if psychiatric illness is viewed as a biological illness that requires treatment, then scriptures that advocate respect for the body (which the brain is obviously part of) may enhance compliance with medical treatments:

> Don't you know that you yourselves are God's temple and that God's Spirit lives in you? If anyone destroys God's temple, God will destroy him; for God's temple is sacred, and you are that temple. (1 Cor. 3:16–17)

Finally, religious values promote a responsible lifestyle. Religious persons may see themselves as having been given the gift of life and special talents that they must use to serve God and their fellow humans, rather than bury those talents. (See Matthew 25:15–28.) Because good mental health is necessary to fully use one's talents, religious persons may be more willing to seek and comply with treatment when their mental health is compromised.

[1] All citations from the Holy Bible are from the New International Version (NIV).

I Need Help

George is a 46 year-old electrician who attends a local Baptist church with his wife. George is a deacon in the church and makes regular mission trips to Guatemala to help build houses for poor families. One day at work when fixing a transformer on an electrical pole, he tripped on a loose wire and fell about thirty feet to the ground, landing on his side. George was hospitalized with five broken ribs, a crushed pelvis, a fractured femur (upper leg) and radius (wrist). After surgical stabilization of his fractures, he was transferred to the rehabilitation section of the hospital. Recovery was slow, and after about six weeks of little improvement, George got discouraged and start to give up hope that he was ever going to recover enough to go home and resume his work and ministry. Actually, his physical recovery was right on schedule, and now it was his emotional state that was holding him back. One day, he told his physical therapist, "I need help. I'm so discouraged that I don't want to try any more. But I know that God has a plan for my life, and I won't be able to live out that plan unless I started to feel better." The therapist asked George if he would mind if the therapist spoke with his physician and ask him to obtain psychiatric consultation. George replied, "If a psychiatrist can do something to make me feel like praying again, reading the Bible, and getting back on the mission field, then I want to see him."

Systematic research has examined the relationship between religious activity and use of mental health services. For example, investigators analyzed data from the 2001–2003 National Survey on Drug Use and Health to examine the relationship between religion and use of mental health services.(49) Two large subgroups were identified: those with moderate (n = 49,902) and with serious mental illness/emotional distress (n = 14,548). Sophisticated probit models were used to examine past twelve-month use of outpatient mental health care and prescription medications. Religious measures were frequency of religious attendance, strength of religious beliefs, and influence of religious beliefs on decisions. Other variables controlled in the analyses were *DSM-IV* disorders, symptoms, substance use and related disorders, self-rated health status, and sociodemographic characteristics.

Researchers found that in those with moderate mental illness/emotional distress, there was a positive relationship between religious attendance and increased outpatient mental health care use; however, importance of religious beliefs was inversely related to outpatient use. In the group with serious mental illness/emotional distress, religious attendance and importance of religious beliefs were both positively related to outpatient mental health service use and medication use; however, influence of religious beliefs on decisions was inversely related to outpatient mental health services. The authors concluded that these findings argued against the widespread notion that religious involvement discouraged use of mental health services, especially among those with serious mental illness.

Other research that has examined the relationship between religion and use of mental health services is the NIMH Epidemiologic Catchment Area Survey (the first large community study to determine rates of psychiatric illness in the community based on criteria established in the *DSM*).(50) This study reported that Pentecostals (fundamentalist Christians) in North Carolina were less likely to use psychiatric services than mainline Protestants. However, when analyses were stratified by frequency of religious attendance, the low rate of mental health services use was almost completely confined to Pentecostals who attended religious services infrequently. In fact, despite a 30 percent prevalence of mental illness in this subgroup of Pentecostals, not a single person had seen a mental health professional in the previous six months. In contrast, Pentecostals who attended religious services at least weekly used mental health services at two to six times the rate of other Protestants. In fact, Pentecostals who attended church frequently used these services more appropriately (that is, those with diagnosed mental illness sought mental health services, while those without mental illness were unlikely to seek such services). Thus, even among fundamentalist religious groups, those who are active in their faith community use mental health services as much or even more frequently than those from more mainline or liberal religious traditions (and use those services more appropriately).

13. WHAT SHOULD PSYCHIATRISTS DO?

What should the CL psychiatrist do with this information? How might it change his or her assessment and management of the patient? In my discussion above, I inferred numerous ways that psychiatrists could take advantage of the information presented in this chapter. However, I succinctly summarize here some common assessment and management strategies.

13.1. Take a Spiritual History

The initial assessment of the medical patient should always include a spiritual history as part of the social assessment. The following questions should be asked:

- What is the patient's religious or spiritual background (denomination, faith tradition)?
- Is religion/spirituality used to cope with stress?
- Is religion/spirituality a source of support or a cause of stress and conflict?
- Are there religious/spirituality beliefs that might influence psychiatric care or conflict with psychiatric treatments (psychotherapy or medication)?
- Is the patient a member of a religious/spiritual community, and is that community supportive or nonsupportive (and how)?
- Are there any spiritual needs that someone with expertise in pastoral care could help address?

The psychiatrist may also wish to expand the spiritual history to obtain a deeper understanding of the role of the patient's religious/spiritual beliefs in health or pathology. (See *Spirituality in Patient Care* for a more in-depth spiritual history for the mental health patient.(51)) If any issues come up that the psychiatrist is not familiar with or competent to address, then referral to a chaplain (in the hospital) or a trained pastoral counselor (in the community) is indicated.

13.2. Take a Spiritual History from Other Sources

If the patient is unable to give a spiritual history because of altered mental status or dementia, then take the spiritual history from family, friends, or the patient's minister. Note, however, if obtaining the history from anyone but a competent patient, it is necessary to obtain approval from the patient's power of attorney (POA) for healthcare decisions or guardian. If this person knows the patient well (such as a family member), the POA/guardian would be the recommended person to obtain the spiritual history from. Because this is a delicate and personal area, special care needs to be taken when exploring spiritual issues with anyone but the patient.

13.3. Anticipate Religious Resistances

Some patients will use religious beliefs as a defense against making needed life changes for health and growth or as a defense against taking medication with unpleasant side effects. For example, bipolar or schizophrenic patients may refuse mood stabilizers or antipsychotics on religious grounds, when in reality they simply don't like the side effects of these medications. This also applies to treatments for medical disorders. The hypertensive patient may refuse blood pressure medications for similar reasons, claiming that God will heal him or her (or that God's will be done). Religious teachings may also be used to avoid changing behaviors that are adversely affecting mental or social health. For example, the patient with an obsessive or compulsive personality is involved in so much religious activity in church that he or she neglects dependent family members, causing social strife. Another example might be the refusal of psychotherapy because of a desire to rely entirely on religious therapies.

13.4. Acquire Psychodynamic Insights

Taking a detailed and thorough spiritual history can provide psychodynamic insights that may be useful in psychotherapy. Although less of an issue for the medical patient than for the psychiatric patient, in medical patients with a history of psychiatric problems, this will be relevant. The stress of medical illness may trigger deep-seated psychological conflicts, especially those regarding dependency, which could cause agitation and irritability sufficient to interfere with medical care (or may even precipitate suicide).

Religious issues related to image of God, derived from unhealthy parental relationships, may need to be addressed. Religious guilt over past lapses in judgment may surface at this time, as patients fear retribution in the next life. Childhood abuse may give rise to shame and feelings that patients are not "good enough" to receive God's love, mercy, and blessings. Some religious patients may be distressed over thoughts that God is punishing them, has deserted them, or is powerless to make a difference in their situation. Research shows that religious conflicts of this nature may affect the medical condition of the patient and even lead to premature mortality.(52)

13.5. Respect Religious Beliefs

The psychiatrist should always and at all times show respect for patients' religious beliefs. This is even true for patients whose religious beliefs are conflicting with medical or psychiatric care. Bear in mind that these beliefs are usually intensely held and serve a variety of psychological functions, some healthy and some unhealthy. Even if unhealthy, however, the psychiatrist must establish a therapeutic alliance with the patient before attempting to change or alter those beliefs. Showing respect for patients' religious beliefs will facilitate the develop-

ment of that alliance and allow the psychiatrist to later challenge unhealthy beliefs if necessary.

13.6. Support Religious Beliefs

If the patient's religious beliefs are generally healthy (and the vast majority of nonpsychiatric medical patients' religious beliefs will be healthy and adaptive), then the psychiatrist should consider supporting those beliefs. Bear in mind that the psychiatrist is being asked here to support the patient's religious beliefs, not introduce new beliefs or proselytize his or her own beliefs. Support for patients' religious beliefs can be conveyed in many ways, both verbally and nonverbally. Efforts to ensure that patients' spiritual needs are being met and that religious resources are made available are important ways of demonstrating support.

13.7. Use Religious Beliefs in Counseling

Some psychiatrists with pastoral training may decide to use the patient's religious beliefs as part of therapy. This is particularly true with medical patients who are dealing with overwhelming situational stressors related to illness, disability, pain, and other medical symptoms (and the patient's psyche is relatively healthy). Integrating religious beliefs into psychotherapy should only be done with religious patients and would not be useful for nonreligious patients in most circumstances. Research shows that such integration (as in religious cognitive-behavioral therapy) is most effective for religious patients,(53) and may not be effective in the nonreligious.(20) The religious patient will likely be quite responsive and appreciative to such integration, whereas the nonreligious patient may be offended. On the other hand, integrating religion into psychotherapy can be done whether the *therapist* is religious or not. In fact, some research shows that religious cognitive therapy is more effective if delivered by *nonreligious* therapists than by religious therapists.(53) The reasons for this are not entirely clear. Perhap nonreligious therapists in this study were more objective, more accepting and less judgmental, or more rigorously applied the religious therapy according to protocol because it was less familiar to them.

13.8. Prescribe Religious Beliefs/Activities

Prescribing religious beliefs or practices for non-religious patients is not recommended. This can be viewed as coercive and should be avoided. If the patient is religious and is using religious beliefs to cope, then pointing out the benefits of religious practice as demonstrated repeatedly in the research literature as described here, would be supportive and encouraging to the patient. Doing so with nonreligious patients, however, would not be supportive in most cases and confusing and upsetting, particularly in patients struggling with medical stressors.

13.9. Collaboration with Chaplains, Pastoral Counselors, and Community Clergy

There will be many instances when the psychiatrist will wish to seek assistance or counsel from a chaplain or pastoral counselor in the management of religious patients. This would be particularly true when religious conflicts are present or when religion is important to the patient and the psychiatrist is unfamiliar with the patient's religion or uncomfortable dealing with it. In hospital settings, chaplains are readily available to assist in this way and are trained to address religious/spiritual issues from a multifaith perspective.

Of course, the psychiatrist must obtain approval from the patient before bringing in a religious professional. Many patients, however, may not understand what chaplains or pastoral counselors do or the type of training that they receive to address emotional and spiritual issues. Thus, the psychiatrist should explain this to the patient, and if the psychiatrist doesn't know the competencies of a chaplain/pastoral counselor, then further information should be sought (see *Spirituality in Patient Care*).(51) In some instances, the mental health professional will want to include the patient's clergy, especially if (1) chaplains or pastoral counselors are

unavailable, (2) the patient prefers, and/or (3) the religious tradition of the patient is not well known.

14. CONCLUSIONS

Psychiatrists will often be called on to see medical patients with psychiatric disturbances, especially as our population ages and the number of persons with chronic, disabling medical conditions expands. Medical physicians without special training and expertise in these matters will call on psychiatrists to assist them in the management of patients with emotional disorders such as depression and anxiety related to difficulties coping with medical illness. Psychiatrists will also be consulted on issues related to somatoform disorders, chronic pain syndromes, agitation, behavioral disturbances, and substance abuse. Religious beliefs and practices play a key role in enabling many medical patients to cope with overwhelming circumstances. They may also play a role in other psychiatric disorders as well, either as a resource or as a liability. Religious beliefs may facilitate psychiatric care and compliance with treatment, or they may conflict with and impede psychiatric care. CL psychiatrists and other mental health professionals working in medical settings need to learn about the religious/spiritual beliefs of patients by conducting a thorough and detailed spiritual history, findout what to do with this information, and recognizing when pastoral care collaboration or referral is necessary.

REFERENCES

1. Leigh H, Streltzer J. Handbook of Consultation-Liaison Psychiatry. New York, NY: Springer; 2007.
2. Karasu TB, Plutchik R, Steinmuller RI, Conte H, Siegel B. Patterns of psychiatric consultation in a general hospital. Hosp Community Psychiatry. 1977;28:291–294.
3. Callegari CM, Menchetti M, Croci G, Beraldo S, Costantini C, Baranzini F. Two years of psychogeriatric consultations in a nursing home: reasons for referral compared to psychiatrists' assessment. BMC Health Serv Res. 2006;6:73.
4. Koenig HG, George LK, Peterson BL, Pieper CF. Depression in medically ill hospitalized older

adults: prevalence, correlates, and course of symptoms based on six diagnostic schemes. Am J Psychiatry. 1997;154:1376–1383.

5. Koenig HG, Meador KG, Shelp F, Goli V, Cohen HJ, Blazer DG. Depressive disorders in hospitalized medically ill patients: a comparison of young and elderly men. J Am Geriatri Soc. 1991;39:881–890.

6. Koenig HG, George LK, Meador KG. Use of antidepressants by non-psychiatrists in the treatment of hospitalized medically ill depressed elderly patients. Am J Psychiatry. 1997;154:1369–1375.

7. Koenig HG. Physician attitudes toward treatment of depression in older medical inpatients. Aging Ment Health. 2007;11(2):197–204.

8. Koenig HG, Cohen HJ, Blazer DG, et al. Religious coping and depression in elderly hospitalized medically ill men. Am J Psychiatry. 1992;149:1693–1700.

9. Koenig HG, George LK, Peterson BL. Religiosity and remission from depression in medically ill older patients. Am J Psychiatry. 1998;155:536–542.

10. Koenig HG. Religion and remission of depression in medical inpatients with heart failure/pulmonary disease. J Nerv Ment Dis. 2007;195:389–395.

11. Stack S. Religiosity, depression, and suicide. In: Schumaker JF, ed. Religion and Mental Health. New York: Oxford University Press; 1992:87–97.

12. Kok L-P. Race, religion and female suicide attempters in Singapore. Soc Psychiatry Psychiatric Epidem. 1988;23(4):236–239.

13. Wikan U. Bereavement and loss in two Muslim communities: Egypt and Bali compared. Soc Sci Med 1988;27(5):451–460.

14. Greening L, Stoppelbein L. Religiosity, attributional style, and social support as psychosocial buffers for African American and White adolescents' perceived risk for suicide. Suicide Life Threat Behav. 2002;32(4):404–417.

15. Cook JM, Pearson JL, Thompson R, Black BS, Rabins PV. Suicidality in older African Americans: findings from the EPOCH study. Am J Geriatr Psychiatry. 2002;10(4):437–446.

16. McClain CS, Rosenfeld B, Breitbart W. Effect of spiritual well-being on end-of-life despair in terminally-ill cancer patients. Lancet. 2003;361(9369):1603–1607.

17. Carter GL, Clover KA, Parkinson L, et al. Mental health and other clinical correlates of euthanasia attitudes in an Australian outpatient cancer population. Psycho-Oncology. 2007;16(4):295–303.

18. Benson H, Kotch JB, Crassweller KD, Greenwood MM. Historical and clinical consideration of the relaxation response. Am Sci. 1977;65:441–445.

19. Azhar MZ, Varma SL, Dharap AS. Religious psychotherapy in anxiety disorder patients. Acta Psychiatr Scand. 1994;90:1–3.

20. Razali SM, Hasanah CI, Aminah K, Subramaniam M. Religious – sociocultural psychotherapy in patients with anxiety and depression. Aust N Z J Psychiatry. 1998;32:867–872.

21. Zhang Y, Young D, Lee S, et al. Chinese Taoist cognitive psychotherapy in the treatment of generalized anxiety disorder in contemporary China. Transcult Psychiatry. 2002;39(1):115–129.

22. Chaturvedi SK, Bhandari S. Somatisation and illness behaviour. J Psychosom Res. 1989;33: 147–153.

23. Koenig HG, Ford SM, George LK, Blazer DG, Meador KG. Religion and anxiety disorder: an examination and comparison of associations in young, middle-aged and elderly adults. J Anxiety Disord. 1993;74:321–342.

24. Androutsopoulou C, Livaditis M, Xenitidis KI, et al. Psychological problems in Christian and Moslem primary care patients in Greece. Int J Psychiatry Med. 2002;(32):285–294.

25. Flannelly KJ, Koenig HG, Ellison CG, Galek K, Krause N. Belief in life after death and mental health: findings from a national survey. J Nerv Ment Dis. 2006;194(7):524–529.

26. Goldstein J. Console and Classify: The French Psychiatric Profession in the Nineteenth Century. Cambridge: Cambridge University Press; 1987.

27. Charcot JM. Lemon d'ouverture. Progrès Médical. 1882;10:336.

28. Gilman SL, King H, Porter R, Rousseau GS. Hysteria Beyond Freud. Berkeley, CA: University of California Press; 1993:360–379.

29. Simonfay G. Stigmata: from religion to psychosomatics. Med Psicosom. 1988;33(4):289–302.

30. Carroll MP. Heaven-sent wounds: a Kleinian view of the stigmata in the Catholic mystical tradition. J Psychoanal Anthropol. 1987;10(1):17–38.

31. Pio of Pietrelcina. http://en.wikipedia.org/wiki/Pio_of_Pietrelcina.

32. Martinez-Taboas A. Psychogenic seizures in an Espiritismo context: the role of cultural sensitive psychotherapy. Psychother Theory Res Pract Train. 2005;42(1):6–13.

33. Koenig HG, Pargament KI, Nielsen J. Religious coping and health outcomes in medically ill hospitalized older adults. J Nerv Ment Disord. 1998;186:513–521.

34. Koenig HG. An 83-year-old woman with chronic illness and strong religious beliefs. JAMA. 2002;288(4):487–493 (quote from p 487).

35. Kabat-Zinn J, Lipworth L, Burney R. The clinical use of mindfulness meditation for the self-regulation of chronic pain. J Behav Med. 1985;8:163–190.

36. Koenig HG, McCullough ME, Larson DB. Handbook of Religion and Health. New York, NY: Oxford University Press; 2001.

37. Matthews DA, Marlowe SM, MacNutt FS. Effects of intercessory prayer on patients with rheumatoid arthritis. South Med J. 2000:93(12):1177–1186.

38. Hill TD, Burdette AM, Angel JL, Angel RJ. Religious attendance and cognitive functioning among older Mexican Americans. J Gerontol Ser B-Psychol Sci Soc Sci, 2006;61(1):P3–P9.

39. Kaufman Y, Anaki D, Binns M, Freedman M. Cognitive decline in Alzheimer's disease: impact

of spirituality, religiosity, and QOL. Neurology. 2007;68:1509–1514.

40. Lee BK, Glass TA, McAtee MJ, et al. Associations of salivary cortisol with cognitive function in the Baltimore memory study. Arch Gen Psychiatry. 2007;64:810–818.

41. Carrico AW, Ironson G, Antoni MH, et al. A path model of the effects of spirituality on depressive symptoms and 24-h urinary-free cortisol in HIV-positive persons. J Psychosom Res. 2006;61(1):51–58.

42. Dedert EA, Studts JL, Weissbecker I, Salmon PG, Banis PL, Sephton SE. Private religious practice: Protection of cortisol rhythms among women with fibromyalgia. Int J Psychiatry Med. 2004;34:61–77.

43. Ironson G, Solomon GF, Balbin EG, et al. Spirituality and religiousness are associated with long survival, health behaviors, less distress, and lower cortisol in people living with HIV/AIDS: the IWORSHIP scale, its validity and reliability. Ann Behav Med. 2002;24:34–48.

44. Hebert RS, Dang Q, Schulz R. Religious beliefs and practices are associated with better mental health in family caregivers of patients with dementia: findings from the REACH study. Am J Geriatr Psychiatry. 2007;15:292–300.

45. Rabins PV, Fitting MD, Eastham J, Fetting J. The emotional impact of caring for the chronically ill. Psychosomatics. 1990;31:331–336.

46. Rabins PV, Fitting MD, Eastham J, Zabora J. Emotional adaptation over time in care-givers for chronically ill elderly people. Age Ageing. 1990;19:185–190.

47. Lemere F. What happens to alcoholics? Am J Psychiatry. 1953;109:674–676 (quote from p 674).

48. Vailland GE. The Natural History of Alcholism: Causes, Patterns, and Paths to Recovery. Cambridge, MA: Harvard University Press; 1983 (quote from p 193).

49. Harris KM, Edlund MJ, Larson SL. Religious involvement and the use of mental health care. Health Ser Res. 2006;41(2):395–410.

50. Koenig HG, George LK, Meador KG, Blazer DG, Dyke P. Religious affiliation and psychiatric disorder in Protestant baby boomers. Hosp Community Psychiatry. 1994;45:586–596.

51. Koenig HG. Spirituality in Patient Care, 2nd ed. Philadelphia, PA: Templeton Foundation Press; 2007: 161–174 (Spirituality in Mental Health Care).

52. Pargament KI, Koenig HG, Tarakeshwar N, Hahn J. Religious struggle as a predictor of mortality among medically ill elderly patients: a two-year longitudinal study. Arch Int Med. 2001;161:1881–1885.

53. Propst LR, Ostrom R, Watkins P, Dean T, Mashburn, D. Comparative efficacy of religious and nonreligious cognitive-behavior therapy for the treatment of clinical depression in religious individuals. J Cons Clin Psychol. 1992;60:94–103.

15 Community Psychiatry and Religion

MARCUS M. MCKINNEY

SUMMARY

More people in the spiritual community around the world offer counseling and support to those suffering from mental illness than we can presently measure effectively. Yet these individuals collectively care for the soul in ways that our community relies on every day. When we think about where people go to access care when they are suffering from mental illness, we cannot overlook this group. Clinicians depend on sophisticated credentialing and training to provide their services. Although many in the spiritual community are also equipped to minister to their members, they often do not receive specialized training in counseling and even fewer have supervision available to them.

The inclusion of spiritual providers of care in training, collaboration, and referral with mental health providers provides challenges and opportunities for many communities. Both will be addressed in this chapter. Sustained recovery-oriented models of care can build on the unique resource of spiritual providers embedded in the community. In this section, we explore why people sometimes go to spiritual leaders for help, identify who the providers are, and discuss how to honor this point of access while adding quality to care. We will also offer ideas about developing locally relevant training and present ways to collaborate and establish a network of referral. Finally, we will offer resources to guide the process of ensuring quality for all providers sensitive to community psychiatry and religion.

Anyone who wants to know the human psyche will learn next to nothing from experimental psychology. He would be better advised to put away his scholar's gown, bid farewell to his study, and wander with the human heart through the world. There, in the horrors of prisons, lunatic asylums and hospitals, in drab suburban pubs, in brothels and gambling halls, in the salons of the elegant, the Stock Exchanges, Socialist meetings, churches, revivalist gatherings and ecstatic sects, through love and hate, through the experience of passion in every form in his own body, he would reap richer stores of knowledge than text-books a foot thick could give him, and he will know how to doctor the sick with real knowledge of the human soul.(1)

– Carl Gustav Jung

On any given day in any given town, odds are many people in distress will reach out to their local, trusted faith leader for help. In fact, about one-quarter of people with a psychiatric diagnosis will have first sought help from clergy.(2) Faith leaders ("Faith Leader" is a general term purposely used along with "spiritual leader" and clergy to signify the multiple important roles of religious/spiritual persons often sought by average people when in distress) do not often have advanced training to provide mental health services, yet they remain a primary access point of care for many. These faith leaders "care for the soul,"(3) an ancient notion that appreciates the root idea behind the "psyche." They are well acquainted with "real knowledge of the human soul" that Jung alludes to in the quote above.

We will consider how psychiatric care today challenges practitioners to learn how spiritual resources in communities provide collaborative opportunities and sustained support for individuals with mental illness. Although there is not adequate research on those local resources yet, with a little creativity and some training, those resources can be brought alongside clinical practice to aid and support patients.

This chapter requires us to be honest and take some risk. We need to be honest about where people go for help and to whom they go and why. We need to acknowledge the need to begin training spiritual caregivers who are seeking to attend to mental health needs in our communities. Let's help them do what they do better. This can be done while also inviting collaboration with other professional mental health providers. In so doing, we may develop a more clinically sound, spiritually relevant model of care for our communities.

This chapter also moves us one step closer to the streets, closer to our neighborhoods. Here we find that physical, emotional, and spiritual needs may not be differentiated. They come in the door at the same time. On these streets, you will find motivated spiritual leaders, often not trained, seeking to care for people as they are. We will look at existing and potential training opportunities of faith leaders in those neighborhoods as well as needed training for clinicians. This training will help us identify possible collaborators, but also help us become more understanding of the value in bridging the divide between the clinical and spiritual aspects of care.

When the idea of "provider of care" is broadened to include the natural, chosen network of patients and families in their community, several primary issues surface. Do the providers know how to maintain confidentiality? Are they knowledgeable about the patient's condition? Will they be accountable to the authorized medical team responsible for the patient's clinical care? Will they support the "treatment plan"? Will there be

sensitivity to the precept *primum non nocere*, do no harm?

With increasing economic and time pressures, the mental health practitioner might fairly ask, "In what way will collaboration truly help my clinical role?" We should honestly confront *barriers* to collaboration like having little time, as well as innovative *benefits* being considered now in recovery-oriented systems of care in behavioral health approaches. If a clinical practice depends on collaboration with colleagues in the *medical* community, how might the same kind of collaboration with *spiritual* "providers" of care assist the psychiatric plan? What concerns might arise?

Ideally, a clinical practice will include training, collaboration, and referrals responsive to the spiritual and mental health needs of the community. Regardless of the location of a practice, the community will have religious/spiritual ways of understanding and responding to psychiatric needs. This chapter recommends seven steps to build a local, spiritually relevant strategy of care. Along the way, we will hear from examples of spiritual leaders who reflect on the intersection of psychiatry and religion in their community.

I. STEP ONE: REALIZE PEOPLE ACCESS CARE THROUGH MANY PATHWAYS

Let's start by admitting that many people access care for psychological issues through local spiritual leaders. In many urban and rural settings, spiritual leaders are often the most accessible "providers" of care, even if they are not always trained. For a host of reasons, accessing mental health care may be challenging to average people. Economics, stigma (fear of discrimination), and the amount of time it takes to get an appointment with a "credentialed professional" all seem to push for creative options in mental health. If it takes weeks to get an appointment and I am limited to five visits, for thirty-minute sessions, I may find myself exploring who else I can talk to while waiting. Trends in community psychiatry are taking into account numerous modalities that broaden the notion of "providership." In addition, "wrap-around services" show interesting outcomes for people in recovery. Wrap-around services include services like supportive counseling, often provided by faith leaders (although they have less often been considered a "provider of care" in a collaborative sense). With a little work, a clinician can stimulate added supports for clients, understand the community better, and establish an ongoing training program that informs a clinical team and local spiritual leaders on ways to work together. In some regions, asset-based community development serves this purpose. This strategy involves incorporating natural, local resources and supports that are positive in nature, often identified by the client (and/or family) supplementing the expertise of mental health practitioners. In many instances family, faith leaders, elders, and physicians are the predominant first line of care for people suffering from mental health issues. Faith leaders and trusted spiritual elders who are commonly recognized as people who offer wisdom in the everyday problems of life can become part of the team whose center is patients themselves. Nazeh Natur, a psychologist in training, serving in Israel notes," People in our communities approach the 'old man' or 'old woman' in the village … they would try to treat the illness by reading from the Qura'n." (Nazeh Natur is a Ph.D. Candidate in Psychology. This quote is from our conversations at a federal conference on Arab/Islamic Behavioral Health issues. Used by permission.)

The local pathways a community chooses every day may not always be connected to other levels of mental health care.

In Connecticut, we have welcomed people from every imaginable religious tradition into pastoral counseling training. Aside from formal religious groups, many people see their role in a broader spiritual way. The increasing demand for these individuals to assess and care for people's emotional lives seems constant, and the importance of bridging these caregivers with professional mental health providers will not diminish. This chapter will introduce the field of pastoral counseling as a growing discipline addressing the need for community-based psychologically trained spiritual providers.

Every pathway of healing can potentially include specialized options in mental health care. Once we accept this, there is the potential to collaborate and refer for optimal care.

1.1. Reflection from India: Father Thomas Puthiyadom, Catholic Priest

"Average people in my country will try and hide mental illness until they find it impossible to manage by themselves. They might mention it to the local faith-leader and ask advice. Usually the priest sees them and refers them to the local psychiatric facility that can maintain confidentiality. The main barrier to getting treatment is the social stigma. Usually village people all know each other, so when people do seek treatment, they try to go where the care is hidden from the public. In my village, the family and the community provide a great deal of emotional support."

1.2. Reflection from Nigeria: Father Elias N. Menuba, Catholic Priest

"In my country it would be very uncommon for someone to go in search of a 'clinic' or hospital for mental problems. It is very hard to admit one has such problems. People are considered outcasts if they do. But people do go to their religious leader to seek help, for all kinds of problems. We (religious leaders) then often see them for a while and, as we need to, get them more help. I come from the Anambra State of Nigeria. In this region certain types of 'madness' are also treated by some native doctors (dibias) with native herbs. Many diseases, in fact, are treated at home. We do not have training opportunities in pastoral counseling, but I have tried to take such classes in the United States. In our tradition, both happiness and sorrow of individual members are shared by the entire family or community to which he/she belongs. Counseling needs to include more than an individual and it must avoid blaming.

"I believe if faith leaders could receive pastoral counseling the whole country would profit. Pastors are unable to help because they have not been taught. And while they do help many people, unless they get proper training they "burn out" and experience depression in their work.

"In general, faith leaders do not collaborate with physicians. The culture sees the two areas separate. Some faith leaders use their practices to try and bring healing instead of advising a person to seek medical attention. It would seem strange to imagine the two (doctors and clergy) working together. It would be great to have pastoral counseling offered to those suffering from mental illness in my country."

1.3. Reflection from Arab/Muslim Countries: Sameera Ahmed, The Family Youth Institute

"In most traditional Muslim countries the family (nuclear and extended) is the main support system that people go to when experiencing emotional difficulties. They often turn to their physician since many of the emotional illnesses are presented as somatic complaints. Depending on the religiosity of the family and their connection to the mosque, individuals may go to a Muslim scholar while others turn to people who claim to be able to do exorcism or homeopathy medicine, etc. In Western countries, Arab/Muslim individuals tend to rely on their local religious leader or Imam as well as their friends within the community. Depending on the level of acculturation of the individual or the desperation of trying to find a solution to one's difficulties, Muslims may seek the use of mental health services. Where Muslim mental health workers [are] present, sharing of religious and/or cultural similarity appears to help build trust with the individual. In addition, mental health workers that are engaged with the Muslim community aid in normalization and acceptance of mental health issues within the Muslim community."

2. STEP 2: GET TO KNOW SPIRITUAL CARE PROVIDERS

When the State of Connecticut embarked on a Faith-Based Initiative in Behavioral Health, something remarkable was revealed. Few behavioral health providers identified spiritual professionals they had existing relationships with for referral. Likewise, few religious leaders could identify behavioral health professionals whom they knew and collaborated with regularly. Breaking down the barriers to establish a meaningful referral network began with numerous conferences and training forums that included both audiences (faith leaders and mental health professionals). It began with a desire to meet others who serve the emotional needs of the community.

Consider for a few moments colleagues you have known who are mental health practitioners but, as you have come to know them, you discovered they were also active or knowledgeable in local religious practices. A person trained in mental health and participating in a religious group can have unique insight into clients. We call these practitioners "boundary spanners." In research and practice these individuals can often help bridge cultures (medical/psychiatric and religious) and the languages unique to both worlds. Identifying boundary spanners is an important first step to creative training in religious and psychological settings.

My experience has been very positive in this area. My career began with basic ministry training, then advanced training in hospital chaplaincy, and then specialized training in psychology. Each area brought its own "credentialing" process. I had an interest in teaching and found wonderful insight in bringing approaches from one field of study to another. On a deeper level, I found myself helping *translate ways of caring*. Psychiatry, for example, depends on "diagnosis." Ministry might make an assessment. Clinicians have "patients" or "clients," while faith leaders have members of a congregation or fellowship. If translation of culture is not attended to, one side may feel the other is labeling a person or judging them. Now, as a licensed therapist who is also a minister, I work to value both cultures (knowing neither is perfect). It is helpful to identify and acknowledge other people who serve as boundary spanners in the community: people who are credentialed mental health providers but might also be ministers or religious leaders.

Some health professionals have advanced training in mental health and spiritual practice. Chaplains, pastoral counselors, and faith leaders who also serve in professional behavioral health agencies are potential "boundary-spanners" who are trusted and recognized in the community, while able to "translate" languages (clinical and religious). The term *pastoral counselor* refers to an individual who blends insight from theology, spirituality, and behavioral health in ministry. In some areas, you will find pastoral counselors credentialed through professional organizations like the American Association of Pastoral Counselors (described at the end of our chapter). Other regions might have individuals who describe their ministry as pastoral counseling and might not even know of a professional category outside their own congregation or religion. In a similar way, chaplains are usually individuals who serve in (sometimes hired by) institutions to serve the spiritual needs of people within the institution, including families and staff members. Many chaplains have professional training and see their lifelong work in this specialized ministry. Yet many see their role in chaplaincy amending their other religious duties in the community. It is best to become acquainted with chaplains and pastoral counselors locally to better understand how they might work to serve patient/client spiritual and mental health needs. In many ways, the opportunity to provide holistic care lies in the art of translating those two powerful cultures.

Boundary spanners will likely know about the delicate issue of using their background and understanding in ways that assist care rather than drive a religious agenda. We encourage forums that invite leaders in the spiritual, psychiatric, and medical communities together to consider models of referral and collaboration. Maybe periodic talks can be arranged on aspects of each community's approach to healing that would be helpful

to everyone. An individual practice (not as a part of a group or institution) might consider offering to lecture on some evening to a local place of worship on a common issue in mental health. Even a brief talk followed by lively discussion can increase mutual understanding of what people believe helps and potentially reduce stigma.

Like the mental health and addiction fields, those in the spiritual field have increasingly "specialized" into a more stratified system over the years. For example, institutional spiritual professionals are held to different bodies of accountability than those in worship or congregational settings. Others are accountable to their own religious body only and may not have any counseling oversight. Yet their role remains critical because they are commonly chosen by congregants when seeking help. We are cautious not to call all of this "counseling." But let's be honest: Whatever we call it, people are attending to emotional needs. Consider the variety of "providers of care" in the spiritual community and the implications for the care of patients.

One way to increase awareness of a patient's support system is to offer a more in-depth spiritual assessment that would include a question like "who provides you with personal spiritual support?" This will likely elicit a more meaningful response than the typical spiritual assessment questions that are important but incomplete from the "every day" experience of a client. Sometimes people will offer a neighbor's name, a layperson in their religious congregation, or possibly a clergyperson. Their answer will reveal their chosen spiritual provider of care. The closer we get to the "personal" support the client is using, the more we will understand and support their healing.

We found in our pastoral counseling training programs that many people asking for training were coming at the permission of their religious authority (pastor, priest, imam, denomination) but who, long beforehand, had discovered they were the "kind of people everyone sought out for help." A more formal role for these individuals naturally followed. I am mindful that "titles" may not convey sufficiently the role spiritual leaders serve. But if we are collaborating, it is helpful to know how to identify spiritual leaders. Here are some of the titles you might look for in your community:

Abbot or Abbess: A title given to the head of a monastery in various religious traditions around the world.

Priest: A person having authority within a religion, usually in terms of liturgy and sacraments. In some traditions, a **priestess** is a similar designation. It is helpful to remember that most ministry roles invite personal support and counsel. When a person is sick in a parish, it is likely the priest will be sought and will attend to the person in need, even if there also are many others offering care in the parish.

Imam: An Islamic leader, usually a leader in a mosque or in the community.

Minister: A broad term used in many traditions for a person with responsibilities that might relate to worship or teaching as well as interpersonal support.

Healer: A broad term that would be defined by local religious groups. This term may also reference a growing category of practitioners whose self-identified caring role aims toward the healing of mind, body, soul/spirit.

Monk: A person usually devoted to celibate, contemplative living within a religious tradition. Living alone (from the word *monos*) or in a monastery is associated with this religious role. People in these roles are often felt to be helpful in the struggle people feel in religious and psychological life.

Bible teacher: A person with responsibilities to instruct scripture, often in class settings. These teachers often focus on age-specific students and are a primary support for everyday issues in a congregation.

Pastor: A leading role in congregations that includes the idea of shepherd. It usually is identified with clergy. The primary role is to lead the congregation. In some congregations, the pastor is involved in everyday emotional concerns of the congregants, while in others the role might be more administrative.

Deacon: A person (sometimes ordained) who assists a priest or pastor. The role might be to "serve" members of a congregation. Often this person is to be accessible to members for emotional concerns.

Elder: May refer formally or informally to a person with seniority in a religious setting. This title is also loosely applicable to those identified in a community who are valued as good counselors or guides.

Bishop: A senior member of a Christian Church, usually with oversight responsibilities of other pastors/priests/ministers.

Spiritual guide/advisor: Terms used in many traditions (for example, in India, Tibet, and Western Spiritualist traditions). Sometimes the term refers to a person trained in spiritual approaches of a variety of traditions.

Temple/tribal leader: Religious groups sometimes will have an informal designation of a person who might bear this title in their temple or tribe. Much like other less-formal positions, this role might only be known and defined locally, but can be an important liaison between the religious community and mental health provider.

Lay leader: The exact role of lay leaders can be almost any ministry. This title is often used to clarify that the person is not ordained as an official clergyperson, but has specific ministerial duties.

Evangelist: A person whose role is to evangelize, preach, and/or reach out to people. In some churches, this person may minister one-to-one to those in need.

Preacher: A title that signifies more of a pulpit or preaching role – one who gives sermons. But again, this title may be misleading, because many preachers also are associated with specific ministries within a congregation.

Chaplain: More often this is an institutional title for a person designated to meet the spiritual needs of patients (for example, in hospitals, prisons, homes, and assisted living settings) and link to local religious resources. Many institutions use professionally designated persons while others use volunteers from the community who may also have local religious responsibilities. Many congregations designate that chaplains or pastoral ministers go to local institutions to minister to their own members.

Pastoral counselor: As mentioned earlier, this category has unique implications for meeting the mental health and spiritual needs of people. From dealing with the everyday worries of life to complicated psychiatric situations requiring support in the community, this person can be a lifeline to recovery for someone suffering from psychiatric illness.

Heath-care institutions in a community may have designated spiritual care providers who have training in mental health. Typically they will be called chaplains and can be found in pastoral care departments. In times of economic challenge or in poor areas, there may be no one on the hospital staff with the role of pastoral caregiver. If there is a chaplain, he or she can be helpful in exploring community resources addressing spirituality and mental health. Generally speaking, however, a chaplain will not often have a community practice for referral. The work to access community resources will likely take a few more steps.

3. STEP 3: STRENGTHEN QUALITY AND EXPAND ACCESS

3.1. Reflection from the Republic of Trinidad: Reverend Elton Adams, Protestant Minister

"In Trinidad and Tobago the only place of resource for the mentally ill person is in the main hospital. A person with psychiatric illness might go first to a general hospital and, if needed, go to the long-term mental health facility. All costs for this care is born by the government.

"In our country it is often believed that a person with mental illness is 'filled with a demon or evil spirit.' This brings the experience of being shunned by family as well as the community. Medication is used a great deal. Seldom are patients seen by a pastoral counselor. We do not usually have chaplains in this role. Pastors, Pundits, and Imams visit their people.

"The main barriers to getting help seem to be stigma issues and shame, even felt by the whole family at times. Private counseling would be very costly. Often there is a sense of failure. A widely held belief is that illegal drugs are the main reason for much of the mental illness in my country."

People seeking psychiatric care usually value both clinical and empathic skills. Ideally they are all wrapped up in one provider. More realistically, we may find them in a mix of "providers" including professionals, faith leaders, and others. Not all caregivers, even if carefully chosen by a client, are necessarily "trained" to provide the empathic and clinical services needed. We must acknowledge the important value of sophisticated psychiatric training while appreciating that "real knowledge of the human soul" may be sometimes found in the caregiver who has less clinical training. And, of course, there are many who work to acquire skills both in psychology and spirituality.

It is also worthwhile to consider developing a community training program designed to build relationships and increase knowledge (spiritual and behavioral health) in ways that are not too time consuming or complex. It can be as simple as a single event for spiritual leaders, a forum to talk briefly on how to assess common mental health problems (depression, anxiety, dealing with stress), that invites spiritual insight into strategies for healing.

Usually faith leaders with responsibility for congregational leadership (like a youth pastor or priest) are trained in theological insight and ministry application. "Pastoral care" might best describe the intervention often required of their work with members. Typically the members themselves set the agenda. As leaders are trained for more "counseling" skills, the shift will move to hold the leader in more accountable roles. "Pastoral counseling" signifies a more psychologically rigorous training, sometimes performed by professionals whose single ministry is counseling in a religious, private, or institutional setting. Whether trained in listening skills for support or clinical assessment skills for treatment, faith leaders who have partnered with clinicians on care for their members refine their identity and effectiveness as an important "provider of care" in the community. It is no surprise that such collaborations allow clinicians to expand their referral base and expand their knowledge of spiritual resources. They may also increase their comfort in addressing spiritual issues in therapy to the extent such a partnership is established.

If we admit that stigma related to acknowledging one has an emotional struggle is a very common experience, then we might look in a more sophisticated way at what role people play in recovery and care. For example, part of our modern experience is to hold high the level of hard-earned training in any given field. So medicine and counseling (and governmental authorizing bodies) may have very strict guidelines giving license to levels of practice. Professional credentials, organizations, and extensive designations seek, appropriately, to raise the quality of care for people. However, we may have to consider ways to strengthen quality while broadening access at the same time.

Let's consider some of the barriers that might inhibit a person seeking help from seeing a fully credentialed psychiatric professional. First, economics. In addition to the stigma sometimes experienced by a person "admitting" they are ill or struggling with emotional issues, many people go to faith leaders in the community because they cannot afford the inevitable cost of seeing a "credentialed" mental health provider. The credentialing movement brings assumed quality *and cost.*

Second, people may ask for help, but resist treatment. With this in mind, a *movement to train and support people who are in the spiritual community seeking clinical skills to offer pastoral counseling* is worth considering. The Substance Abuse and Mental Health Services Administration in the United States has increasingly found good outcomes from "psychological first aid." (4) Some professional organizations have begun to incorporate a category of membership that embraces this level of intervention that comes closer to the network of trust and access that people seem to appreciate. For example, the American Association for

Pastoral Counseling (5) now offers an entry membership level designated 'Pastoral Care Specialist'. Some faith leaders find this movement validating their front line role as providers of care embedded in the community.

We also need to keep in mind that many people seek mental health services through their primary care provider, that is, people go to a physician often for emotional and psychiatric reasons, be it to seek medicine or ask for guidance. Most psychotropic medication in the United States is dispensed through a primary care physician. If we are serious about early detection, prevention, or even effective referral, the larger community of care must be reimagined. Informal links between physicians, mental health providers, and spiritual leaders represent a strong fabric of recovery for assessment, support, and care in our communities.

In the United States there is significant interest in how primary care physicians address mental health needs. For our purposes here, let me illustrate great potential in an integrative approach that can strengthen quality and expand access.

For decades, I have worked alongside physicians at a large acute care hospital in an urban setting (Hartford, Connecticut). First as a chaplain, then as a pastoral counselor taking referrals, I worked primarily in the hospital setting. I would hear from my physician friends how the counseling needs of patients had grown and the resources to get them help had decreased. The actual problem seemed to be that they could no longer refer a patient to their own preferred local mental health provider in their community. They had to keep a list of common insurance companies ... a "panel" of providers. Provider lists would change, sometimes every six months. The referral process would frustrate patients. Eventually many physicians simply gave up and suggested their patients call their own insurance company. Of course, that nonpersonal referral does not usually get followed up. And many patients came back to their physician with their symptoms worse.

We piloted a process to embed a pastoral counselor in some of the medical practices so the counseling referral process could be more personal and the site of care more familiar to patients. We included a sliding scale fee for most anyone, based on his or her ability to pay. The activity was significant. And the ability to refer to mental health providers was easier because the pastoral counselor understood the psychiatric process. Such an integrative approach does not have to be huge. But it probably needs to be personal.

A final word on quality: It is important to remind ourselves an individual who is credentialed (licensed, certified, or otherwise designated as authorized to provide mental health services) may not necessarily produce good outcomes for a person. In the same way, spiritual intention does not guarantee a desired outcome for people seeking mental health support. The best assurance of quality is accountability through having a caring supervisor. Supervision would be a place to safely address how to improve the counseling work. We believe this is a lifelong need for clinical and spiritual caregivers. And this enhances the likelihood that mutual referral will take place.

4. STEP 4: IDENTIFY REASONS TO REFER

What motivation(s) should we identify among clinicians and spiritual providers of care that might make referrals beneficial? "Referral" and "collaboration" take a common protocol in hospitals and among medical professionals. It is less common with religious leaders. That is not to say they would not jump at the opportunity. Both disciplines would have reservations, however. It probably only makes sense if you feel the patient could benefit and your work would be amended in ways that could sustain healing outcomes.

In a hospital setting, medical professionals refer frequently to other subspecialties. People know each other and their expertise pretty well. (Economic factors in Western Medicine may change this notion: The growing categories of Physician Assistant and Hospitalist may create more distance in the collaborative experience among even health practitioners.) Progress notes, often the residue of exhaustive assessment, are shared between peers. The language is common

and complex. There are lots of abbreviations. A *multi-disciplinary team* in a hospital shifts a little closer to "collaboration," although the team is likely also schooled in medical language.

From a patient's perspective, they may feel referral honors their desire to talk about spiritual issues safely. It can "normalize" their care to take into account their whole person.

When practitioners feel their care of clients and families will be enhanced by having spiritual issues addressed, many reasons to refer or collaborate with spiritual providers can be found that both facilitate care and honor the larger healing fabric that patients access frequently in everyday life. These reasons may have clinical and diagnostic implications and enhance client-centered approaches.

By using patient-approved collaboration, a practitioner will better "translate" spiritual themes. For example, if "guilt" is an issue frequently raised in therapy, a spiritual provider may shed light on how guilt is framed within the patient's belief system. Pathology can be differentiated more effectively. A faith leader may greatly appreciate simple, clinical clarification. Religion has a remarkable way of inviting pathological projections unless there is careful insight.

When clinicians are caring for more impaired clients who might benefit from socially meaningful activity, religious resources can build on any socialization tasks prescribed.

Spiritual themes permit the possibility of a shift away from the stigma associated with mental illness. Where the faith leader or religious environment is empathic, a "client" can find language that is dynamic for healing, helping them to feel that, as James Hillman notes, all humans have problems. To be human is a problem. We are all on that common ground.

But let's not be naïve. It must be acknowledged that some religious perspectives might *add* to stigma by (like some medical models) labeling the illness in such a narrow and negative way that the person is defined by the illness. This can put blame on the person. It is less likely, of course, that such a community would warm up to collaboration. But in any community, there will be challenges like this. Initiating a nonjudgmental relationship with spiritual leaders will serve to clarify common ground.

Referring to faith leaders can lighten the pressure clinicians and/or faith leaders may feel in caring for people. In our pastoral counseling training program (6) we have seen medical, psychiatric, and faith leaders benefit from the support they receive by a more collaborative style. They sleep better at night. They feel less responsible for "curing" the person and experience more of a caring role that has healing outcomes.

The life of a client seen from the perspective of a spiritual leader can fill in critical diagnostic and compliance information. A common reason for patients decompensating may be noncompliance with a treatment plan. Typically a person might stop taking a medication or going to therapy. Spiritual leaders may know well what is causing resistance with a patient. Sometimes a person may use their religion as a reason to justify noncompliance with a care plan.

Clinicians can learn key spiritual resources that make a difference to client outcomes. Spiritual leaders might know some common practices within their own traditions that help, for example, depression. Clinicians might be more limited to academic studies on spiritual resources. Groups that can assist people with talking about their illness, or about navigating employment, or finding housing can be initiated in the community. It is good practice to have readily available local contact information outlining such resources for patients. I suspect nothing is more valuable than local understanding of what helps a community with their mental health.

Aside from our propensity to think of "mental health" as individual in nature, it is advisable to assess the community mental health. By that I mean that culture and regional norms influence our individual mental health. Where do we learn about this? Collaboration with faith leaders who think in those terms can inform us better as we assess and treat mental illness. For example, a community might be very introverted. Not right or wrong, just is. The person with socialization needs might inappropriately seek to "cure" his or her introversion. A clinician might value weighing from different perspectives (spiritual, cultural, individual) insight that can shape assessment and care. In short, clinicians can learn from spiritual providers also.

Clients coming for psychiatric care might not know of an option to see a pastoral counselor. (Pastoral Counselor – This term refers to a minister who practices pastoral counseling at an advanced level which integrates religious resources with insights from the behavioral sciences. Pastoral Counseling – This term refers to a process in which a pastoral counselor utilizes insights and principles derived from the disciplines of theology and the behavioral sciences in working with individuals, couples, families, groups and social systems toward the achievement of wholeness and health.) Their contact with spiritual professionals may be limited to "official" clergy from their denomination or local place of worship. Many people desire a person who can preserve their spiritual life while not needing to defend any particular dogma, religion, or clergyperson.

A referral would also be recommended when a clinician feels very passionate about his or her own spiritual orientation (or, conversely, has been injured by a spiritual/religious experience) and a client presents in a way that tests the transference around their own issues.

Sometimes a client may simply ask about the clinician's religious faith. One way to hear this question is the desire of the client to feel safe or have common ground with his or her belief system. In many cases, the issue is addressed and no longer needs attention. However, this can be tricky, even if both clinician and the client are of the same religious tradition. If the client's care can be facilitated by having a faith-based counselor serve as his or her primary support person, this might be considered. If transference is an issue and it is not addressed, the alternative can sometimes be having this issue float around the room behind the scenes, popping out unexpectedly as topics are touched.

A final reason to refer is a bit controversial. Psychiatry and religion both can have a tendency to be practiced in "fundamentalist" ways. When one modality of care is the "only way to treat," or when "religious rules" become narrow and oppressive, we are appealing to the desire of average people for a simple solution. In fact, healing more often occurs (spiritually and medically) in a slow fashion. Of course there are exceptions. But the culture of "quick fix" feeds the way we view healing. Quick prayer would be nice. One unqualified pill (with no adjustments next month, please!) would be preferred. Mutually respectful collaboration over time between clinicians and faith leaders can assist in keeping perspective on this cultural tendency.

5. STEP 5: INTENTIONAL COLLABORATION, TRAINING, AND SUPERVISION

Collaboration doesn't just happen because we have chosen to work together. Collaboration is an art more than a strategy. If "parity" or mutual respect is not experienced by both providers of care, it may confuse rather than assist the client.

In my practice over the years, I have noticed some pastoral counselors and clergy abandon their empathic skills when ministering to people suffering with emotional illness in favor of a more distant approach they feel is appropriate and more acceptable in the medical world. Here it is worth emphasizing that *effective* treatment and care does not limit itself to clinical approaches or spiritual approaches. There are many paths to healing. Good spiritual responses will provide healing outcomes but will likely look a bit different than clinical strategies.

The best collaboration probably needs two individuals who appreciate supervision. I have noticed how students I teach (spiritual leaders and clinicians) do not often get the kind of supervision that might have been available a few years ago. I mean the kind of supervision that is supportive and feels safe enough for me to hear what *in me* is getting in the way of a good assessment. The idea of getting supervision in this way is foreign to some spiritual leaders, yet it can release the great burden they feel as "leaders expected to

have all the answers." And can we admit that, in some clinical settings, supervision looks more like administrative oversight than honest, supportive reflection on our own issues? Supervision, in this sense, is probably much less common than any of us would admit.

It is interesting that the history of some regions reveals why there is great distance between faith leaders and mental health practitioners. Stories may live in a particular region of "turf wars" between those who hold the "authority" to treat, or who can explain human behavior, or who are qualified to offer remedy. Sometimes historical events support religion as primary, while other regions might support medicine or science. Far too often the result is not a shared model of caring, but a polarized tension expressed by a critical eye that someone is not qualified. Lack of training or reckless lack of sensitivity can scar the possibilities of collaboration. However, creative models of training that incorporate spiritual and psychological insight matched with building relationships between the helping professions can go a long way toward forming a collaborative option for caregivers.

A couple of training models are worth mentioning here. Both nurture the kind of collaboration that helps to avoid polarization.

If mental health practices/agencies review their "continuing education" events (conferences, case presentations) as an outreach to local faith leaders who see their work as a pastoral counseling ministry, the chances increase for mutual understanding and insight. This is especially true, of course, if their insight is sought to understanding a case. This might be the first move toward collaboration. The required continuing education update in a clinical topic might need some attention to language (allowing for clinical and everyday language) for such an event. The avoidance of condescending attitudes will encourage honest discussion and ideas.

A program specifically designed to blend spiritual and psychological insight in training and case discussion is a second model that takes a bit more planning. The pastoral counseling program (6) in Connecticut falls into this category. A "middle ground" has been found in depth psychology. Carl Jung, the Swiss psychiatrist, wrote with a global respect for religion and medicine. A pastoral counseling program, from our experience, can welcome a wide variety of religious backgrounds, including very conservative religious groups that historically found the psychiatric world hostile to their views. And more and more health practitioners (integrative and complimentary practitioners) are seeking a middle ground as well and have found their way to the program. During the thirty-hour class, we include speakers from psychiatry, medicine, and religion. The class mix encourages networking that often ends in referral possibilities locally.

Given the paucity of mental health providers in many areas, an increasing "counseling" burden is now felt by average faith leaders (as well as professional pastoral counselors). Offering a training experience for these individuals to assist them in their roles, whatever they are, has proved to be energizing for clinicians and faith leaders alike. The goal in such training is modest but critically important: to provide a spiritually relevant and clinically sound forum for anyone who would benefit from pastoral counseling insight. Mental health practitioners, faith leaders, nurses, and lay leaders have all exhibited interest in these programs.

Mental health providers, complimentary practitioners, and spiritual leaders have participated in pastoral counseling training because they feel the nature of their work requires regeneration. All of these disciplines are in the helping professions. How do we care for ourselves? For many, the insights of ancient spiritual wisdom sustain the modern calling of caring for the soul. A spiritually informed training can add insight into ourselves and the culture we live in.

One of my clients who arrived late on his first appointment indicated he was "sent by his psychiatrist" because he had an obsessive-compulsive disorder (OCD). For an hour he spoke of his struggle with this malady. After a few sessions, he reflected on how our sessions forced him to slow down. He noted how he drove really fast on the highway to get to work. He felt guilty for slowing down, because it seemed he needed to keep pace with his world. The TV, the Internet, traffic, and even his cell phone seemed to be suffering, he said, from OCD.

Putting our culture in contact with the wisdom of the ages is not a bad idea. In a culture that suggests more information, especially the latest research, is best, where is the voice to slow down? Is more always better?

A male middle-aged patient in our cardiac rehabilitation class who built his career as an engineer gave our class some insight on this matter. He said he always minimized dreams. He felt they were simply caused by worry or bad digestion. When he discovered he had to go for cardiovascular surgery he got on the Internet to find out what it was like. After an hour or so he was full of information. Not all accurate of course. But the result was a feeling of panic. That night, just before surgery, he had a dream. Essentially it was calm and – in his mind – boring. But it stayed with him the next morning. Going into surgery, he felt one of the images of the "boring" dream calmed his nerves and gave him a sense all would be okay. In our class, he said it ran against all he believed that a dream could help him, especially as an engineer. But he could only say it made the difference. Spiritual leaders around the world might not be surprised at his story.

6. STEP 6: BUILDING A REFERRAL NETWORK

A faith leader who has participated in a training program that is integrated as noted above may return to his or her community setting talking in a different way. Before such an experience, he or she might have said to someone, "Go to Saint Francis Hospital, someone there can help you in the clinic," or "please check your insurance plan to find someone," or "have you looked into the yellow pages?" Now they are inclined to say, "Talk to Dr. Smith. Here is her number. I know her well and she can help."

Sometimes referral networks begin with a single contact within an institution. For clinicians attached to hospitals, a concerted effort to connect with a chaplain or pastoral counselor with advanced training can begin bridge building with other sources in the community. Knowing time is a precious commodity, a small initiative carefully planned can make a big difference. Public health agencies (local, state, and national) are frequently assigning a liaison to network with the spiritual community. Having a forum that honestly discusses the common resources and challenges of the helping professions in the mental health and faith communities can be in line with most public health missions and is worth recommending.

It's funny how large bureaucracies (like public/state agencies) sometimes become great barriers to networking. Middle managers can try and read the "political winds of the day" and feel anything religious is too sensitive to address. I have heard at times interesting explanations, for example, as to why a conference bringing spiritual and mental health leaders together is dangerous, even though patient-centered care often emphasizes the need of patients to have spirituality incorporated into care. A senior administrator can advocate for honoring the spiritual dimension of care, but mid-level anxiety dampens the actual implementation of any conference or assessment tool. Religion is too hot a topic for some. It can get you in trouble. Someone might be offended. All these worries might be addressed with carefully planned open forums in institutional settings. It is good to invite community providers to such forums.

7. STEP 7: IDENTIFY COMMON ISSUES IN SPIRITUALITY AND PSYCHIATRY

The chances are good that a person seeking a clinician's help has been to many others before. A common issue in counseling can be described as "bad experiences people have with providers of care." Those wounds are painful and seem to stay with us for a long time. In time, a person may seek help again out of necessity to deal with his or her pain. If the wound came from an experience with a religious leader, a person might address this to a clinician. Or if the wound was experienced while in therapy with a clinician, a person might seek help from a spiritual or religious leader

An example might be a client who shares a horrible experience he or she had while going to church, or seeing a spiritual leader, or counseling with their minister. That person cannot get over how damaging it was, and he or she wonders how people in places of responsibility like that can do such terrible things.

Or maybe a member of a church confides to his or her pastor how a psychiatrist completely misunderstood the expression "being in relationship with God." That person now feels unable to return to that psychiatrist.

Both people may get an empathic hearing. But a person (faith leader or clinician) who has a collaborative style might find a unique opportunity to offer some options for the client/member that doesn't lose the spiritual or psychiatric reason a person originally sought care.

Many of my clients have justified their intent to stop medication because of psychiatric unprofessionalism. Many clients have abandoned God because a faith leader was hurtful. Either result, of course, can have devastating consequences, even if we all understand why they responded a certain way. Developing a style that is informed by spiritual aspects of care, even if only by studying a text like this one, will support a more balanced assessment for patients.

Aside from inviting faith leaders into a setting, or participating in training programs, I suggest an old-fashioned approach: invite a faith leader to lunch. I recommend the same thing to faith leaders: invite a psychiatrist to lunch. Sound silly? One of the few ways to really ask the kind of questions needed to understand how you might collaborate is by exploring who the person is over lunch. Ask what they believe, what has been their experience? What does the faith leader feel about medication? What does the psychiatrist feel about prayer? And, reflecting on what patients might ask, take note of the approach the person takes.

Understanding that we are, as providers, only part of the healing equation will help us refer and collaborate more. If a clinician thinks they are THE answer (any discipline can take too narrow of an approach … a medicine, a theory, a spiritual practice … all can be viewed with such orthodoxy as to blind providers of care from the many streams of healing insight), or even the primary answer, they may miss the opportunity to participate in the mystery of healing. The symptom can be wrestled down. We can participate in the science but miss the art. Likewise a "formula" approach to religion can focus too narrowly on "right and wrong" or "how to behave" (admittedly important dimensions of life) but miss a healing assessment of what is going on deep inside.

One of my students in pastoral counseling was a 50-year-old Pentecostal minister. In his tradition, he was taught to be very skeptical of psychology. As he sat in our class, he would use his remarkable knowledge of scripture in addressing the counseling needs of his members. After awhile, he wanted to assess what was happening at a deeper level causing mental health suffering for his members. While in supervision, he recounted the story of a woman who came to him after many prayer requests for healing. She had spoken to him for months about her anxiety. He said, "Mrs. Jones (not her name), you would benefit from pastoral counseling. Let's meet this Tuesday at church at 7." Believing he would pray or read scripture she came and sat. When she began asking for Bible verses, he said, "Mrs. Jones, we both believe in God and will continue to pray, but for the next hour I want to know what is going on with you – tell me what is really going on." Only he could shift from one mode of religious care (prayer, scripture) to another (insight into her life). A mental health practitioner might not have been permitted to make that transition for some people.

A psychiatrist once reflected to me that the reasons he would not want to assess the spiritual life of patients is that he "felt so unqualified" and the subject was "so personal" and he admitted having some bias of what he called "skepticism" when people spoke of their "spiritual experiences." When a clinician feels this way, a referral should be considered. Again, an evolving list of known referral resources and a willingness to collaborate would help facilitate this process.

I recall being asked to lecture on psychology and spirituality to the staff of a large mental health agency. When I arrived, I was directed to a large empty room. As I set up my computer and projector, my anxiety increased. What controversial questions would they ask? Were they forced to attend?

To my surprise, a staff member began escorting into the room forty pleasant-looking folks who, I was told, were "consumers," people from the community who receive psychiatric services at the agency. "Okay," I thought, "let's go to plan 'B.'" I shut down my computer. I facilitated a remarkable discussion on how they get spiritual needs met. They were amazingly talkative and expressed how they felt therapists at the agency were not comfortable talking about spiritual things. They spoke of how important such a discussion was to them. And they talked about how they worked to find people in the community to have this addressed. The last person to speak suggested the staff be required to attend the next session.

We have a long way to go in understanding community resources, designing spiritually appropriate training, and responding to the spiritual needs of our patients. Agencies and individual clinicians can begin by listening to those they serve.

Research needs to be done regarding psychologically sound, spiritually relevant models of care and training around the world. Best practices, as they are developed, need to be broad enough to embrace a sophisticated notion of spirituality that is expressed in many forms: conservative religious orientations, liberal traditions, as well as forms of spiritual practice that are contemporary and local with no obvious connection with recognized faith groups.

The modern medical model, from which psychological theory and practice grows, needs to be examined for its strengths and weaknesses. We should revisit ancient spiritual lessons that assist our wounds and help in healing. The primary work of Thomas Moore, Ph.D., writer and therapist, is critically important for this reason. As a starting point, we invite readers to review the resources and curriculum of our pastoral counseling training web site.(6)

All helping professions that invite spiritual and psychological insight for healing are growing in our day. The people we seek to help are in search of a meaningful life. If we can walk "with the human heart through the world" taking lessons on "real knowledge of the human soul," we will surely help those who come to us for care. Take some time to engage the community that seeks to teach us these lessons.

I would like to suggest one final resource. We can build on the strong tradition of pastoral counseling. Next you will find important resources regarding standards and ethics that will be useful in providing care and cultivating relationships with spiritual leaders in your community. We invite clinicians to share these ideas, add to them, and join in conversation with others who are equally committed to care of the soul.

8. STANDARDS OF PASTORAL COUNSELING

Standards of pastoral counseling worldwide are always evolving. For the purposes of helping readers become acquainted with a primary organization in this field, I recommend becoming aware of the American Association of Pastoral Counselors (AAPC). The standards below (from the AAPC directory and Web site) delineate membership, ethical considerations, and issues of confidentiality.

The American Association of Pastoral Counselors

The American Association of Pastoral Counselors (AAPC) represents and sets professional standards for over 3,000 Pastoral Counselors and 100 pastoral counseling centers in North America and around the world.(7) AAPC was founded in 1963 as an organization that certifies Pastoral Counselors, accredits pastoral counseling centers, and approves training programs. It is non-sectarian and respects the spiritual commitments and religious traditions of those who seek assistance without imposing counselor beliefs onto the client.

AAPC Code of Ethics

As members of the American Association of Pastoral Counselors, we are committed to the various theologies, traditions, and values of our faith communities and to the dignity and worth of each individual. We are dedicated to advancing the welfare of those who seek our assistance and to the maintenance of high standards of professional conduct and competence. We are accountable for our ministry whatever its setting. This accountability is expressed in relationships to clients, colleagues, students, our faith communities, and through the acceptance and practice of the principles and procedures of this Code of Ethics.

In order to uphold our standards, as members of AAPC we covenant to accept the following foundational premises:

- To maintain responsible association with the faith group in which we have ecclesiastical standing.
- To avoid discriminating against or refusing employment, educational opportunity or professional assistance to anyone on the basis of race, gender, sexual orientation, religion, or national origin; provided that nothing herein shall limit a member or center from utilizing religious requirements or exercising a religious preference in employment decisions.
- To remain abreast of new developments in the field through both educational activities and clinical experience. We agree at all levels of membership to continue post-graduate education and professional growth including

supervision, consultation, and active participation in the meetings and affairs of the Association.

- To seek out and engage in collegial relationships, recognizing that isolation can lead to a loss of perspective and judgment.
- To manage our personal lives in a healthful fashion and to seek appropriate assistance for our own personal problems or conflicts.
- To diagnose or provide treatment only for those problems or issues that are within the reasonable boundaries of our competence.
- To establish and maintain appropriate professional relationship boundaries.

Confidentiality Statement of AAPC

As members of AAPC we respect the integrity and protect the welfare of all persons with whom we are working and have an obligation to safeguard information about them that has been obtained in the course of the counseling process.

All records kept on a client are stored or disposed of in a manner that assures security and confidentiality. We treat all communications from clients with professional confidentiality.

Except in those situations where the identity of the client is necessary to the understanding of the case, we use only the first names of our clients when engaged in supervision or consultation. It is our responsibility to convey the importance of confidentiality to the supervisor/consultant; this is particularly important when the supervision is shared by other professionals, as in a supervisory group.

We do not disclose client confidences to anyone, except: as mandated by law; to prevent a clear and immediate danger to someone; in the course of a civil, criminal or disciplinary action arising from the counseling where the pastoral counselor is a defendant; for purposes of supervision or consultation; or by previously obtained written permission. In cases involving more than one person (as client) written permission must be obtained from all legally accountable persons who have been present during the counseling before any disclosure can be made.

We obtain informed written consent of clients before audio and/or video tape recording or permitting third party observation of their sessions.

We do not use these standards of confidentiality to avoid intervention when it is necessary, e.g., when there is evidence of abuse of minors, the elderly, the disabled, the physically or mentally incompetent.

When current or former clients are referred to in a publication, while teaching or in a public presentation, their identity is thoroughly disguised.

We as members of AAPC agree that as an express condition of our membership in the Association, Association ethics communications, files, investigative reports, and related records are strictly confidential and waive their right to use same in a court of law to advance any claim against another member. Any member seeking such records for such purpose shall be subject to disciplinary action for attempting to violate the confidentiality requirements of the organization. This policy is intended to promote pastoral and confessional communications without legal consequences and to protect potential privacy and confidentiality interests of third parties.

REFERENCES

1. Jung CG. *Two Essays on Analytic Psychology.* CW 7 Appendix 1: "New Paths in Psychology." Princeton University Press; 1912:246–247.

2. Wang PS, Berglund PA, Kessler RC. Patterns and correlates of contacting clergy for mental disorders in the United States. *Health Serv Res.* 2003;38(2):647–673.

3. Moore, T. *Care of the Soul – A Guide for Cultivating Depth and Sacredness in Everyday Life.* New York: Harper Paperbacks; 1994.

4. Psychological First-Aid For First Responders. http://download.ncadi.samhsa.gov/ken/pdf/ katrina/Psychological.pdf. Accessed December 1, 2008.

5. The American Association of Pastoral Counselors. http://aapc.org. Accessed December 1, 2008.

6. The Pastoral Counseling Training Program at Saint Francis Hospital and Medical Center www.pastoralcounselingtraining.com. Accessed December 1, 2008.

7. The American Association of Pastoral Counselors. www.aapc.org. Accessed December 1, 2008.

16 Religious and Spiritual Assessment in Clinical Practice

SYLVIA MOHR AND PHILIPPE HUGUELET

SUMMARY

Spirituality/religion are rarely assessed in psychiatry. However, for many reasons, such an assessment is useful. The primary reasons are the many domains of interdependence between mental disorders and culture, including religion.

What should be evaluated in a spiritual/religious (S/R) assessment? Although several instruments have been developed for this purpose, the clinical interview, which allows clinicians to adapt their language to the beliefs of each individual, appears to be the most appropriate evaluation method.

Specific aspects elements of this assessment are detailed in this chapter, such as religious/spiritual background and preferences, the illness's effect on spirituality and/or religiousness over time, current spiritual/religious beliefs, religious practices in private and in the community, amount of support from the community, and the subjective importance of religion in the patient's life. Depending on how important religion is to the patient, further questions should be asked about the spiritual meaning of the illness, the way patients cope with symptoms, the degree to which their spiritual beliefs comfort them, and the relationship (that is, synergy versus antagonism) between spirituality/religiousness and psychiatric care.

Examples of individual situations warranting specific approaches are provided at the end of the chapter.

Evidence exists that spirituality and religion are rarely assessed by clinicians caring for psychiatric patients. A Swiss study aiming to assess clinicians' knowledge of the spirituality and religiosity of their patients suffering from chronic psychosis found that only one-third of them reported discussing spiritual and religious issues with their patients. Moreover, none of the clinicians initiated discussions of the topic themselves.(1) The replication of the study in Québec, Canada, elicited similar results.(2) In another Canadian study, only one-third of psychiatric patients reported that their psychiatrist had inquired about spirituality/religiousness.(3) Psychiatrists reported several reasons for not discussing religion/spirituality with their patients: insufficient time, concern about offending patients, insufficient knowledge/training, general discomfort, concern that colleagues would disapprove, and lack of interest from the patient.(3, 4)

Several factors may account for the neglect of spiritual and religious issues in psychiatric practice. First, religiously inclined professionals are underrepresented in psychiatry, as compared to the general population. This has been reported for United States,(5) Canadian,(3) British,(6) and Swiss psychiatrists.(1) Second, mental health professionals often lack the necessary education in religion/spirituality.(7, 8) Third, mental health professionals tend to pathologize the religious dimension of life (Lukoff, 1995).(8, 9) Fourth, the neglect of religious issues in psychiatry may also be linked to the rivalry between medical and religious professions that stems from the fact that both address the dilemma of human suffering.(10, 11) Clinical and existential concerns overlap across issues of identity, hope, meaning and purpose, morality, and autonomy versus authority.(12) However, in recent years, the historic division between psychiatry and religion has narrowed. In the United States, all psychiatric residencies must include didactic sessions on religion/spirituality,(13) and recent findings tend to indicate that psychiatrists may be more comfortable and have more experience in addressing religious/spiritual issues, as compared to other physicians.(4)

In the present chapter, we adopt a broad definition of religion, including spirituality (concerned with the transcendent, addressing the ultimate questions about life's meaning) and/or religiousness (specific behavioral, social, doctrinal, and denominational characteristics).(14)

1. WHY SHOULD SPIRITUALITY/ RELIGION BE SYSTEMATICALLY ASSESSED?

S/R assessment is recommended as part of psychiatric evaluation in several evidence-based guidelines for good clinical practices. According to the American practice guidelines for the psychiatric evaluation of adults, the developmental, psychosocial, and sociocultural history domain must be systematically evaluated. Religious and spiritual assessment is included in that domain with a question to consider: "What are the patient's cultural, religious, and spiritual beliefs, and how have these developed or changed over time?" Religion and spirituality are emphasized because they may give meaning and purpose to the patient's life and provide support. Moreover, cultural factors and explanatory models of the illness can affect attitudes toward, expectations of, and preferences for treatments. Therefore, the spirituality/religiousness assessment may play a crucial role in developing a therapeutic alliance, negotiating a treatment plan, and enhancing treatment adherence.(15) These issues are discussed in more detail below.

1.1. Religion/Spirituality as a Component of Cultural Sensitivity

Including spirituality/religion in the more general category of culture could suggest that it's of general interest but not worth spending valuable time on during the clinical encounter. Cultural psychiatry makes the opposite argument. Indeed, culture can "1) define and create specific sources of stress and distress; 2) shape the form and quality of the illness experience; 3) influence the symptomatology of generalized distress and of specific syndromes; 4) determine the interpretation of symptoms and hence their subsequent cognitive and social impact; 5) provide specific modes of coping with distress; 6) guide help-seeking and the response to treatment; and 7) govern social responses to distress and disability."(16) Religion and spirituality are considered cultural factors influencing the process of diagnosis and treatment. So, S/R assessment is a component of a clinical practice that is sensitive to culture.

1.2. Religion and Mental Health Are Interdependent Phenomena

Numerous studies have emphasized the relationships between religion and mental health.(17) These reviews have indicated that religion generally has a positive effect on mental health, well-being, drug and alcohol use, suicide, and familial issues. Religion may play a central role in the psychological recovery process in mental illness (18) and substance abuse.(19) So, the therapeutic approach should take into account the spiritual resources and needs of individuals in the recovery process.

However, not all spiritual/religious practices are healthy. Many patients cope with their illness through spirituality and religiosity, but this may take place in either positive or negative ways.(14) Therefore, the clinician needs to differentiate between religion as a resource and religion as a burden. Sometimes, patients do not benefit from needed psychiatric treatment due to religious beliefs (see Chapter 18), or spiritual crises may lead to emotional, behavioral, or social disturbances.

1.3. Motive for Psychiatric Consultation

In 1994, the American Psychiatric Association included the category "religious and spiritual problems" in the *Diagnostic and Statistical*

Manual of Mental Disorders, Fourth Edition (*DSM-IV*) to describe problems that may lead to psychiatric consultation and that are not to be avoided or considered as psychopathological. "Examples include distressing experiences that involve a loss or questioning of faith, problems associated with conversion to a new faith, or a questioning of spiritual values that may not necessarily be related to an organized church or religious institution"(20) (p. 685).

Spiritual life has been conceptualized as a process with stages of development. Problems may arise during transitions from one stage to another, which are often experiences involving a crisis of faith.(21) A loss or questioning of faith could be compared to the grief process with its associated clinical problems: anger, resentment, emptiness, despair, sadness, and isolation. For some individuals, a loss of faith involves questioning their whole way of life, purpose for living, and source of meaning. This problem can occur when an individual is ostracized by his or her religious community.(8) Struggling with religious beliefs during an illness diminishes the chances of recovery.(22) Changes in membership, practices, and beliefs often disrupt people's lives and may be misdiagnosed as mental disorder, especially when conversion to a new faith occurs. New religious movements may be dangerous and genuinely destructive. But these are not the rule. Membership in cults isn't necessarily oppressive and detrimental to mental health. Some cults are helpful to their adherents. Moreover, belonging to a new religious movement is typically a transient experience, because 90 percent of adherents leave within two years.(23)

Case Example

As an example of religious and spiritual transformation, a 45-year-old man with paranoid schizophrenia reported at baseline that he had greatly suffered when his religious community had rejected him. "What happened to me was very hard. The spirit group cannot put up with the fact that I go on to smoke cannabis. I tried to quit several times, but I failed. I have lost all my friends. I have lost the meaning of my life. I do not believe in spiritism any more." Three years later, he reported that he had spent a few months at the hospital after a suicide attempt. During his stay, he met the chaplain regularly and he joined a Christian community in his neighborhood. He said, "Now, when I feel very deep sorrow, I read the Bible and I find consolation in Jesus Christ. This is what helps me, what restores my hope."

Sometimes, spiritual experiences involve distress and may be misdiagnosed as psychopathological. The most common spiritual problems involving distress are related to mystical experiences, near-death experiences, spiritual awakening, meditation, and medical illness.(8) An S/R assessment is necessary to make a differential diagnosis, which is often not an easy task.

1.4. Satisfaction with Psychiatric Care

Psychiatric care is not only oriented toward psychopharmacology and psychosocial treatments, but also toward promoting psychological recovery for people with severe mental disorders. Despite persistent symptoms and disabilities, people may live fulfilling lives and develop a positive sense of self founded on hope and self-determination.(24) In a patient-centered approach, examining the individual's spiritual and religious history is a therapeutic tool in itself. Indeed, patients who value spirituality and religion will appreciate the doctor's sensitivity and feel understood and respected. As a result, the patient's satisfaction increases and the quality of therapeutic relationship is improved.(25) A qualitative study using a phenomenological approach showed that patients wish to have their spiritual needs addressed in mental health care.(26)

2. WHAT SHOULD BE ASSESSED?

Numerous scales and questionnaires have been developed to assess religion, which is a multidimensional construct.(27) Numerous studies have highlighted the relationships between religion and mental health.(17) These studies encourage the search for the specific dimensions of religion that may have an effect on mental health. The working group of the Fetzer Institute has identified some of the specific physiological, behavioral, psychological, and social mechanisms of spirituality and religiousness and provides a multidimensional questionnaire for use in clinical research (however, this should be distinguished from spiritual assessment tools used in clinical practice).

At the physiological level, religious practices prompt a relaxation response that reduces stress reactions. At the behavioral level, spirituality and religiousness may indirectly protect against disease by encouraging healthy lifestyles. In particular, a robust inverse relationship has been established between religiosity and substance misuse.(28) At the social level, religious and spiritual groups may provide supportive, integrative communities for their members. At the psychological level, spirituality and religiousness provide beliefs about life and death that can directly help patients to cope with illness.(29)

Any instrument devoted to S/R assessment must be adapted, because no questionnaire can fit every kind of religious belief and practice.(30) In clinical practice, the most appropriate evaluation method is the clinical interview, which allows clinicians to understand their patients' views on the world. Nevertheless, the research above has provided categories of spirituality and religiousness that are useful guidelines for clinical practice.

Psychiatric assessment is a time-consuming task. To minimize the time devoted to spiritual assessment, some authors suggest a short list of screening questions. For example, Koenig and Pritchett (31) refer to four systematic questions (FICA) developed by Dale Matthews and Christina Puchalski:

Faith: "Is religious faith an important part of your life?"
Influence: "How has faith influenced your life (past and present)?"

Community: "Are you currently a part of a religious or spiritual community?"
(A) Needs: "Are there any spiritual needs that you would like me to address?"

As a mnemonic reminder, Anandarajah proposed the HOPE questions, which systematically address four domains, that is, the sources of hope, strength, comfort, meaning, peace, love, and connection (H); the role of organized religion for the patient (O); private spirituality and practices (P); and the effects on medical care (E).(32) These instruments emphasize the dimensions of spirituality and religiousness that are relevant for patient care. In clinical practice, S/R assessment aims to understand this dimension in the patient's life. As spirituality and religiousness take on so many different individual meanings and evolve over the course of a lifetime, particularly with illness, a concrete framework helps the clinician to elicit relevant data.

3. HOW TO CONDUCT A SPIRITUAL ASSESSMENT IN CLINICAL PRACTICE

During the screening phase of the S/R assessment, we suggest establishing an outline of the patient's spiritual and religious history. Spirituality and religiousness are loose concepts, not only for clinicians, but also for patients. Creating a temporal organization of significant events and significant others in his/her spiritual/religious life helps the patient to clarify cultural influences, significant changes, current involvement and interaction with the illness. Domains and questions to consider can be found in Table 16.1.

3.1. Religious/Spiritual History

At the beginning of an S/R assessment, establish the patient's cultural background by asking a few open-ended questions about religious practices of the family of origin and significant others and about religious education. Spirituality is known to evolve over the course of a lifetime. What is of importance for the clinician is that these experiences may affect mental health

Table 16.1: Religious and Spiritual Assessment.

Religious/Spiritual history
Family background
  What were your father's religious or spiritual beliefs and practices?
  What were your mother's religious or spiritual beliefs and practices?
Childood
  In which religious tradition were you raised?
  When you were a child, what kind of religious practices were you involved in? How often?
Adolescence
  When you were a teenager, did you experience changes in your religious beliefs or religious practices?
  Which ones?
Adulthood
  In your adult life, have you experienced changes in your religious beliefs or practices? Which ones?

Effect of the illness upon spritiuality/religiousness
  Since you have been ill, have you experienced changes in your religious beliefs or practices? Which ones?

Current spiritual/religious beliefs and practices
Religious preference
  At the present time, what is your religious preference?
Beliefs
  What are your spiritual or religious beliefs today?
Private religious practices
  Do you have private religious or spiritual practices? Which ones? How often?
Religious practices in community
  Do you engage in religious or spiritual practices with other people? Which ones? How often?
Support from religious community
  To what extent, do people in your religious community help you cope with your illness?
  In which ways?

Subjective importance of religion in life
Salience
  In general, how important are your religious or spiritual beliefs in your day-to-day life?
  In which ways?
Meaning of life
  To what extent do your religious or spiritual beliefs give meaning to your life?
  In which ways?

Subjective importance of religion to cope with the illness
Meaning of the illness
  To what extent do your religious or spiritual beliefs give meaning to your illness?
  In which ways?
Coping with symptoms
  To what extent do your religious or spiritual beliefs help you to cope with your illness?
  In which ways?
Coping style
  To what extent do your religious or spiritual beliefs help you gain control over your illness?
  In which way?
Source of strength
  To what extent are your religious or spiritual beliefs a source of strength and comfort for you?
  In which ways?

Synergy of religion with psychiatric care
Medication
  To what extent are your religious or spiritual beliefs in conflict with your medication?
  In which ways?
Therapy
  To what extent are your religious or spiritual beliefs in conflict with seeing a psychiatrist?
  In which ways?
Comfort level
  How does it make you feel talking about your religious or spiritual beliefs with me?

status. Inquiries about life-changing spiritual experiences or religious practices are especially important to understand the impact of religion on mental health status. This initial investigation may uncover that drastic changes have occurred in the patient's spiritual and religious biography, such as significant growth or loss of faith, conversion, or apostasy.

3.2. How the Illness Affects Spirituality and/or Religiousness

The experience of the illness may also affect spirituality and religious practices. This is why the psychiatric interview inquires about relationships between the illness and changes in spirituality/religiousness. When confronted with mental illness, as with other stressful events, some people lean on their religious background to cope. Religious coping is not always effective; it can also lead to negative outcomes.(14) Some people may endow their delusions or hallucinations with spiritual meaning (see Chapter 7). Some people may seek spiritual healing in various religious communities (see Chapter 18). Some people may question or lose their faith when confronted with adversity.

3.3. Current Spiritual/Religious Beliefs and Practices

Exploring the spiritual and religious history leads to inquiries about current religious and spiritual status. Beliefs belong to the cognitive dimension of spirituality. By definition, beliefs differ from religion to religion. However, beliefs about the meaning of suffering and death are in some way central to all religions and therefore may be related to mental health status because they provide a framework of interpretation and expectation. Beliefs not only vary across religious traditions, but also among believers sharing the same tradition. For patients who believe in God or in a deity, it can be informative to ask about their image of God and their relationship with him. Asking the patient about his or her spiritual beliefs gives the clinician an understanding

of the appropriate spiritual language to use, making it possible to adapt subsequent questions accordingly.

3.4. Private Religious Practices

Private religious practices are individual religious behaviors occurring outside the context of organized religion, and not always at a set time or place. Praying, reading holy scriptures, listening to religious radio programs, watching religious television programs, or meditation are common private religious practices.

3.5. Religious Preference

Asking about religious preference elicits which religious community or tradition the patient identifies with. This preference doesn't imply current religious practices but rather a social or cultural identity. This cultural identity is of clinical interest because it may affect the patient's attitudes and behaviors toward substance use, sexuality, family, suicide, and other issues. It also indicates which religious community may support the patient if needed.

3.6. Community Religious Practices

Usually, community religious practices include organizational religiousness that encompasses behaviors such as membership in a congregation, frequency of attendance at religious services, involvement in other activities in the religious community (for example, choir practice, volunteer activities, participation in a special interest group). It is also important to find out if the patient meets individually with one or several religious leaders of the community and the frequency of nonorganizational social contacts with other members of the congregation. This leads to the question about the patient's relationships with members of the religious community. Because social isolation is so often associated with mental illness, this item focuses on religious practices that the patient shares with others.

3.7. Support from the Religious Community

Support from the religious community is founded on two dimensions: first, the social support that members of the religious congregation may offer, just like any other social network, and second, specifically religious support. The religious community may assist the patient at several levels (material, emotional, and informational). Moreover, many religions emphasize the importance of helping others, which may encourage the patient in a role of assisting others. This attitude is especially relevant to self-esteem and recovery. However, patients may also feel that their religious communities reject or judge them. They may be disappointed or angry with their religious communities. This potential negative aspect must also be elicited and elaborated, like other conflicts in relationships.

3.8. Subjective Importance of Religion

At this point in the interview, the clinician has already learned about the patient's spiritual beliefs. To gain a better understanding of the salience of spirituality and religiousness in the patient's life, the clinician must accommodate the patient's spiritual and religious language. For example, if the patient believes in God, the clinician will replace "your religious or spiritual beliefs" by "your belief in God" and ask, "In general, how important is your belief in God in your day-to-day life?" Given the variety and looseness of the concepts of spirituality and religiousness, appropriate language is essential. To help the patient express the salience of his or her spiritual beliefs, the clinician may suggest anchored points of importance, such as "not at all," "a little," "some," "very," or "essential." By providing support, spiritual or religious beliefs may bring hope, acceptance, joy, and meaning to life. But religious beliefs may also be a source of suffering and despair.

At this point in the interview, the clinician should be aware of the patient's religious preference, his or her spiritual beliefs and practices, major changes in his or her spiritual history, and

the salience of spirituality and religiousness in his or her life. But to what extent is this relevant to clinical outcome and care?

For the assessment of spirituality and religiosity, Huber (33) has pointed out the key concept of centrality. Centrality describes the hierarchical status of religion in personality. The more central the religion is, the more it can influence the person's experience and behavior. When religion is central, it has a powerful influence on every domain of life (health and illness, family, career, sexuality, politics, and other beliefs and behaviors). When religion is subordinate or peripheral, it influences fewer areas. At this point, the clinician can readily identify the patients for whom religion is marginal in their life, that is, for whom religion has never been important and who currently have no or few religious practices.

Case Example

As an example of low centrality, a 45-year-old man with paranoid schizophrenia reported, "I am a Catholic. I haven't gone to church since I was a teenager because I am not interested. I believe in God; this gives me hope for an afterlife. I don't think about it in my daily life or use it to help me."

For patients with low centrality, the spiritual assessment should end at this point for two reasons. First, assessment of these areas is not needed because there is no apparent relationship between religion and their psychiatric condition. Second, the clinician must respect every kind of spiritual stance, including a professed absence of belief. Addressing religious coping with patients with low religiosity could send the ill-fated message that they are missing something, and thus be harmful. Excessively concentrating on religion in this case may be the counterpart of the dismissive message about spirituality that is so frequently sent when the issue is not addressed with patients for whom it is central. The prevalence of low centrality varies according to area, cohort, and population studied. In Germany, one study found that religion was marginal for 26 percent of nontheological students and for none of the theological students.(33) For outpatients with schizophrenia or schizoaffective disorders, religion was marginal for 15 percent in Switzerland and 7% percent in Québec, Canada.(2)

3.9. Importance of Religion in Coping with Illness

For all patients with high centrality, the screening of spirituality and religiousness will be deepened by the assessment of spiritual or religious coping. This will give the clinician an indication of whether religion is an asset or a burden, and if some kind of intervention is needed.

3.9.1. The Spiritual Meaning of the Illness.

When confronted with illness, people look for meaning: "Why did this happen to me?" Biomedicine has no answer to this question. Some people turn to religion to find meaning. Some authors have even reduced religion to a meaning-making system.(34) Pargament (14) identifies four typical spiritual meanings of illness: a benevolent religious reappraisal (that is, redefining the illness through religion as benevolent and potentially beneficial); a punishing God reappraisal (redefining the illness as a punishment from God for the individual's sins); a demonic reappraisal (redefining the illness as the act of the devil); and a reappraisal of God's powers (redefining God's power to influence the illness). These different spiritual meanings have been associated with positive and negative outcomes in some studies. For example, a study among patients coping with psychosis found that benevolent religious reappraisals of the illness were predictive of stress-related growth and psychological well-being. Conversely, punishing God reappraisals and reappraisals of God's power were predictive of self-reported distress and personal loss.(35) The same trends were obtained with medically ill elderly patients.(22) However, it is not the religious content per se that automatically influences the outcome. For example, in the Pentecostal tradition, it is common to

attribute illness to demons, but if the patient is a born-again Christian, he or she has power over demons and, therefore, is in control. Hence, in this situation, the demonic reappraisal of the illness is linked with empowerment, a component known to be a key of psychological recovery.(24) This short digression aims to emphasize the need to understand the psychological meaning of spiritual beliefs for the patient. Moreover, the open-ended question about the spiritual meaning of the illness makes it possible for spiritual meanings lying outside the Judeo-Christian tradition to emerge. For example, a Buddhist woman with schizoaffective disorder answered this question with the concept of karma; she believed her illness was due to her wrongdoings in a previous life. This spiritual belief brought her hope for a better karma in her next life in reward for her current pro-social behaviors.

3.9.2. Coping with Symptoms

Spirituality and religiousness are not only effective in giving meaning to the illness, but also in alleviating psychiatric symptoms. When dealing with depression, people may find hope and comfort in spirituality/religion. When dealing with anxiety, people may find peace. A robust relationship has been established between reduced depression and anxiety and religion.(17) Emotional and behavioral disturbances associated with delusions and hallucinations may also be reduced by religion.(36) However, spiritual beliefs may also aggravate psychiatric symptoms. Worries about sin, hell, and demons may nourish anxiety, depression, and delusions. This item helps the clinician to determine whether spiritual or religious coping alleviates or aggravates symptoms.

3.9.3. Coping Style

Pargament (14) identifies three major spiritual or religious methods of coping to gain control over symptoms. The patient may rely on himself alone without God's help (self-directing religious coping style), he may rely passively on God or plead for direct intercession (deferral style), or he may do his best to collaborate with

God (collaborative style). These styles are not positive or negative per se, but depend on the scope of the individual's power to influence the course of the illness in the context of a specific situation.

3.9.4. Comfort

This item examines the emotional influence of spiritual beliefs. Inquiring about this aspect is especially necessary when the patient has recounted only the cognitive dimension of his or her spiritual beliefs. The strength and comfort provided by spiritual beliefs are associated with lower levels of depression.(29) Often, spiritual beliefs bring hope and comfort; however, they may be a source of suffering too. The illness may call attention to the fact that spiritual struggles are a necessary stage of any spiritual journey.

3.10. Synergy of Religion with Psychiatric Care

The literature examining the pathways to psychiatric care points out that spiritual and religious beliefs about mental illness may influence help-seeking behavior and adherence to psychiatric treatment.(37) Different kinds of relationships exist between spirituality/religiousness and psychiatric care. For some patients, the two areas have nothing in common; psychiatry and religion are two separate areas in their lives. However, when religion is central in people's lives, it encompasses almost all areas, including psychiatric care. This spiritual meaning may foster or hinder adherence to psychiatric treatment. Some patients believe that God gives knowledge to the clinician to care for them; thus, they trust in psychiatric care. Other patients first put their trust in religious professionals who advocated psychiatric care, thus allowing the patients to trust psychiatry. But other patients experience conflicts between their spiritual beliefs and psychiatric care. These conflicts may lead to noncompliance and distress, so this issue must be addressed.

4. S/R ASSESSMENT: OTHER ELEMENTS

The semistructured interview guide provided here (see Table 16.1) outlines a first spiritual/religious case formulation in a single assessment lasting about half an hour. Based on a global clinical impression, the first element to examine is the centrality of spirituality/religion. If it is low, the S/R assessment is of no importance for current clinical care. However, because spirituality and religiousness tend to change over time, especially in association with mental illness, drastic changes may occur over the course of a lifetime. We recommend regular checks of this dimension, like other areas assessed in long-term follow-up case management.

The second element to examine is the patient's relationships with his or her religious community. Does the patient currently belong to a religious community? Is he or she supported by this community or does he or she feel rejected or in conflict? Does the patient ask for support from the religious community for his or her mental illness or does he or she feel too ashamed or guilty? Do his or her symptoms hinder him or her from participating in religious activities? Do religious professionals from the religious community collaborate with the psychiatric care network or are they in conflict? Could they be integrated into psychiatric care? To summarize, is the religious community an asset or a burden?

Patients' relationships with their religious communities deserve special attention because they provide a natural social network that may be a powerful resource for social integration and psychological recovery. Like family, the clergy may need psycho-education and support from clinicians to deal with people suffering from severe mental illness.(37)

The third element to examine is the positive or negative role of spirituality and religiousness for the patient. Is spirituality/religiousness a source of hope, comfort, meaning in life, and joy or a source of suffering? Is the individual upheld in his or her identity by spirituality/religiousness or undermined?

If a patient's spirituality/religiousness is an uplifting force, it should be sustained throughout follow-up care. Spirituality and religiousness become key elements of psychological recovery when they are central in a patient's life and integrated into–not in conflict with–other fundamental dimensions of life. In this case, spirituality and religiousness give meaning to the person's life, foster acceptance of the illness and psychiatric care, and provide coping methods to cope with symptoms, social support, and guidelines for a healthy lifestyle.

Case Example

A 34-year-old man with paranoid schizophrenia reported, "As a child, I was sexually abused. God gave me the strength to forgive and restored my dignity to me. I hope God will heal me. God gives me the security I need. I pray to be relieved of sadness, the desire to die and anxiety. I still hear voices, but I don't mind any more. They are evil spirits who want to bring me down. I focus on God and I don't listen to them. Now, I see schizophrenia as a blessing. If I didn't have this illness that broke me down, I would live like everyone else: work, marriage and children. I would not long for God and to meet Jesus. God put psychiatrists and psychologists on my path to help me and to open my mind."

In such situations, the salience of spirituality and religiousness is associated with reduced psychopathology and enhanced social functioning.(36) However, spirituality and religiousness may be positive for the self without being integrated into the process of coping with the mental illness. In such cases, although religion plays a central role in the patient's life, it is not associated with coping with the mental illness.

Case Example

A 47-year-old woman with schizoaffective disorder reported, "When I was a teenager, I wanted to become a nun. I lived in a closed convent for two years.

But community life with other women was too hard for me so I left and worked in a Catholic organization for years. Finally, I also left this church because I can't stand feeling that I am part of a community, I was afraid of being imprisoned. Spirituality is the essence of my life, a personal experience; it belongs to me and nobody else. I pray every day; this is what holds me up. For several years, I had the vision a woman who tells me to end my life by killing myself. I don't know if she is right or not. I have tried to kill myself several times. Spirituality doesn't help me to cope with the voice, because I expect nothing from it. Medication reduces my anxiety so it hinders me from wholly experiencing my spiritual life."

Case Example

Similarly, a 30-year-old man with paranoid schizophrenia reported, "I have been unable to work for three years now; the only thing I do is go to the synagogue every day. Believing in God comforts me. The rabbi and the other students at the synagogue don't support me as I have never told them about my psychiatric condition."

Because spirituality and religiousness encompass several dimensions, they can have a positive impact at the level of the self and a negative impact at other levels. A spiritual belief in a life after death may facilitate suicidal behavior to end current, unbearable suffering.(38) Spirituality often plays a central role in recovery from substance addictions, but substance misuse may also be used to cope with spiritual suffering.(39) Patients may be tormented by conflicts between spirituality and psychiatric care.(40) An assessment of the various dimensions of spirituality and religiousness breaks the myth that all kinds of spirituality and religiousness are healthy. Some aspects may need to be targeted by clinical intervention. In other cases, spirituality and religiousness are negative for the self. When confronted with mental illness, individuals may feel abandoned by God or angry with God, or they may lose their faith. They report distressing spiritual struggles and conflicts similar to those that anyone may endure in times of hardship. In these cases, the S/R assessment helps the clinician to identify which religious professionals can best provide spiritual counseling to the patient. Spirituality and religiousness may be negative for the self when they intermingle with psychopathology. Indeed, current spirituality and religiousness may be by-products of the patient's disorder. This aspect is discussed in several chapters of this book. In manic states, patients sometimes present delusions of grandeur with religious content; for example, they believe they are Christ or Buddha. In persecutory delusions, the agents of persecution may be spiritual entities, especially demons (see Chapter 7). People with depression may lose all interest and motivation, including spiritual and religious involvement. In anxiety disorders, people may be excessively tormented by worry about sins and hell. In obsessive-compulsive disorder, religious rituals may become pathological, with an intense focus on avoiding sin or error (see Chapter 10). In personality disorders, spirituality and religiousness may be used in unhealthy ways to cheat others, serve personal needs, or dismiss the individual from personal responsibility (see Chapter 13). However, it is important to keep in mind that even if a patient's spiritual life may be distorted by the mental illness at times, this doesn't mean that the spiritual life of those patients is only – and always – psychopathological. Spiritual and religious assessment can provide some indication of how to orient treatment in those cases. In addition to the usual clinical care, the clinician can decide whether to address spirituality or not, in collaboration with clergy if needed.

5. SYNTHESIS

S/R assessment is an important part of the psychiatric evaluation. It should be performed at the beginning of treatment and at regular intervals in cases of mid- or long-term care. The principal elements of this assessment have been described in this chapter. Other elements specific to different diagnoses or clinical situations are described in other chapters of this book. What all these situations have in common is that (1) psychiatrists are confronted with patients' cultural/religious backgrounds even more than other clinicians, so this dimension must be taken into account; (2) particularly when involved in psychotherapy, the question of meaning should be addressed, including its religious/spiritual dimension; (3) the phenomenology of psychiatric symptoms may be characterized by religious elements; (4) when treating patients with persistent mental disorders, recovery-oriented care should involve a religious dimension when needed; and (5) all spiritual orientations must be respected when addressing spirituality/religion with patients, including a professed absence of belief.

REFERENCES

1. Huguelet P, Mohr S, Borras L, Gillieron C, Brandt PY. Spirituality and religious practices among outpatients with schizophrenia and their clinicians. *Psychiatr Serv.* 2006;57(3):366–372.
2. Borras LMS, Brandt P-Y, Gillieron C, Czellar J, Huguelet P. Religious coping among patients with schizophrenia in Quebec vs. Geneva, Switzerland. Submitted. 2009.
3. Baetz M, Griffin R, Bowen R, Marcoux G. Spirituality and psychiatry in Canada: psychiatric practice compared with patient expectations. *Can J Psychiatry.* 2004;49(4):265–271.
4. Curlin FA, Lawrence RE, Odell S, et al. Religion, spirituality, and medicine: psychiatrists' and other physicians' differing observations, interpretations, and clinical approaches. *Am J Psychiatry.* 2007;164(12):1825–1831.
5. Curlin FA, Lantos JD, Roach CJ, Sellergren SA, Chin MH. Religious characteristics of U.S. physicians: a national survey. *J Gen Intern Med.* 2005;20(7):629–634.
6. Neeleman J, King MB. Psychiatrists' religious attitudes in relation to their clinical practice: a survey of 231 psychiatrists. *Acta Psychiatr Scand.* 1993;88(6):420–424.
7. Shafranske EP. *Religion and the Clinical Practice of Psychology.* Washington, DC: American Psychological Association; 1996.
8. Lukoff D, Lu FG, Turner R. Cultural considerations in the assessment and treatment of religious and spiritual problems. *Psychiatr Clin North Am.* 1995;18(3):467–485.
9. Crossley D. Religious experience within mental illness. Opening the door on research. *Br J Psychiatry.* 1995;166(3):284–286.

10. Roberts D. Transcending barriers between religion and psychiatry. *Br J Psychiatry*. 1997;171:188.

11. Sims A. The cure of souls: psychiatric dilemmas. *Int Rev Psychiatry*. 1999;11:97–102.

12. Peteet J. Therapeutic implications of worldview. In: Josephson AM PJ, ed. *Handbook of Spirituality and Worldview in Clinical Practice*. Washington, DC: American Psychiatric Publishing, Inc.; 2004:47–59.

13. American Medical Association. Program requirements for residency education in psychiatry. Graduate Medical Education Directory 2002–2003. Chicago: AMA; 2002:218–225.

14. Pargament KI. *The Psychology of Religion and Coping: Theory, Research, Practice*. New York: The Guilford Press; 1997.

15. Vergare MJ, Binder RL, Cook IA, Galanter M, Lu FG. American Psychiatric Association practice guidelines. *Am J Psychiatry*. 2006;163(3):1–36.

16. Alarcon RD, Alegria M, Bell CC, et al. Beyond the funhouse mirrors: research agenda on culture and psychiatric diagnosis. In: Kupfer DJ, First MB, Regier DA, eds. A research agenda for DSM-V. Washington, DC: American Psychiatric Association; 2005:219–282.

17. Koenig HG. *Handbook of Religion and Mental Health*. San Diego: Academic Press; 1998.

18. Fallot RD. Spirituality and religion in recovery: some current issues. *Psychiatr Rehabil J*. 2007;30(4):261–270.

19. Galanter M, Dermatis H, Bunt G, Williams C, Trujillo M, Steinke P. Assessment of spirituality and its relevance to addiction treatment. *J Subst Abuse Treat*. 2007;33(3):257–264.

20. American Psychiatric Association. *DSM-IV: Diagnostic and Statistical Manual of Mental Disorders*. Washington: APA; 1994.

21. Fowler J. *Stages of Faith*. San Francisco: Harper and Row; 1971.

22. Pargament KI, Koenig HG, Tarakeshwar N, Hahn J. Religious struggle as a predictor of mortality among medically ill elderly patients: a 2-year longitudinal study. *Arch Intern Med*. 2001;161(15):1881–1885.

23. Mayer J-F. *Confessions d'un chasseur de secte*. Paris: Cerf; 1990.

24. Andresen ROL, Caputi P. The experience of recovery from schizophrenia: towards an empirically validated stage model. *Aust N Z J Psychiatry*. 2003;37(5):586–594.

25. D'Souza R. The importance of spirituality in medicine and its application to clinical practice. *Med J Aust*. 2007;186(10):57–59.

26. Koslander T, Arvidsson B. Patients' conceptions of how the spiritual dimension is addressed in mental health care: a qualitative study. *J Adv Nurs*. 2007;57(6):597–604.

27. Hill P, Hood, R. *Measures of Religiosity*. Birmingham AL: Religious Education Press; 1999.

28. Kendler KS, Gardner CO, Prescott CA. Religion, psychopathology, and substance use and abuse; a multimeasure, genetic-epidemiologic study. *Am J Psychiatry*. 1997;154(3):322–329.

29. Institute F. Multidimensional measurement of religiousness/spirituality for use in health research. US Department of Health and Human Services; 1999.

30. Wulff DM. *Psychology of Religion: Classic and Contemporary*. New York: John Wiley; 1997.

31. Koenig HG, Pritchett, J. Religion and psychotherapy. In: Koenig HG, ed. *Handbook of Religion and Mental Health*. San Diego: Academic Press; 1998: 323–336.

32. Anandarajah G, Hight E. Spirituality and medical practice: using the HOPE questions as a practical tool for spiritual assessment. *Am Fam Physician*. 2001;63(1):81–89.

33. Huber S. Are religious beliefs relevant in daily life? In: Streib H, ed. *Religion Inside and Outside Traditional Institutions*. Leiden, Netherlands: Brill Academic Publishers; 2007:211–230.

34. Park CL. Religiousness/spirituality and health: a meaning systems perspective. *J Behav Med*. 2007;30(4):319–328.

35. Phillips RE, III, Stein CH. God's will, God's punishment, or God's limitations? Religious coping strategies reported by young adults living with serious mental illness. *J Clin Psychol*. 2007;63(6):529–540.

36. Mohr S, Brandt PY, Borras L, Gillieron C, Huguelet P. Toward an integration of spirituality and religiousness into the psychosocial dimension of schizophrenia. *Am J Psychiatry*. 2006;163(11):1952–1959.

37. Leavey G, Loewenthal K, King M. Challenges to sanctuary: the clergy as a resource for mental health care in the community. *Soc Sci Med*. 2007;65(3):548–559.

38. Huguelet P, Mohr S, Jung V, Gillieron C, Brandt PY, Borras L. Effect of religion on suicide attempts in outpatients with schizophrenia or schizoaffective disorders compared with inpatients with non-psychotic disorders. *Eur Psychiatry*. 2007;22(3):188–194.

39. Huguelet P, Borras L, Gillieron C, Brandt P-Y, Mohr S. Influence of spirituality and religiousness on substance misuse in patients with schizophrenia or schizo-affective disorder. *Subst use Misuse*. in press.

40. Borras L, Mohr S, Brandt PY, Gillieron C, Eytan A, Huguelet P. Religious beliefs in schizophrenia: their relevance for adherence to treatment. *Schizophr Bull*. 2007;33(5):1238–1246.

17 Integrating Spiritual Issues into Therapy

RENÉ HEFTI

SUMMARY

The task of this chapter is to give recommendations on how to integrate religious and spiritual aspects into the treatment of persons suffering from mental illness, based on the evidence from past and recent research and from clinical experience.

Religious coping is highly prevalent among patients with psychiatric disorders. Surveys indicate that 70 to 80 percent use religious or spiritual beliefs and activities to cope with daily difficulties and frustrations. Religion helps patients to maintain hope, purpose, and meaning. Patients emphasize that serving a purpose beyond one's self can make it possible to live with what might otherwise be unbearable.

Religious coping is also prevalent among family caregivers and enhances emotional adjustment, lowers levels of depression, and fosters self-care. A substantial proportion of family members of persons with serious mental illness mobilize religious and spiritual resources to cope with their situation as caregivers.

Programs that successfully incorporate spirituality into clinical practice are described and discussed in detail. Studies indicate that the outcome of therapy in religious patients can be enhanced by integrating religious elements into the therapy protocol and that this can be successfully done by religious and nonreligious therapists alike.

I. SPIRITUAL PERSPECTIVES ON MENTAL ILLNESS

1.1. General Considerations

Previous chapters of this book have demonstrated the importance of religious and spiritual aspects in psychiatric disorders providing evidence of the therapeutic potential for integrating spirituality into mental health treatment. Nevertheless spiritual approaches in mental health care are still in their infancy, certainly in Europe but also in the United States. Due to concerns about harmful effects, a controversy is ongoing regarding whether or not to integrate spiritual elements into the treatment of persons suffering from mental illness. At the same time, a growing body of evidence shows beneficial outcomes of religious and spiritual approaches to psychiatric disorders with regard to the following aspects: seeing spirituality as a unique human dimension, (1) making life sacred and meaningful, (2) being an essential part of the physician-patient-relationship, (3) and the recovery process.(4, 5)

1.2. Spirituality and the Recovery Perspective

Persons suffering from mental illness have been exploring spiritually based approaches to mental health for decades. Most importantly, they emphasize that psychiatric diagnosis does not affect the deepest human drives, that is, to live with purpose and to flourish as a human being. Understanding one's problems in religious or spiritual terms can be a powerful alternative to a biological or psychological framework. Although reframing the issue in this manner may not change the reality of the situation, but having a higher purpose may make a big difference in an individual's willingness to bear pain, work hard, and make sacrifices. Given the fact that people with serious mental illnesses already struggle against widespread prejudice and discrimination, it would seem important to maintain or strengthen people's existing religious affiliations and support systems as part of their treatment or rehabilitation plan.(2)

Furthermore, mental health practitioners will increasingly be seeing clients who choose to view their mental health problems through a traditional, non-Western lens. Although a significant majority of Americans define themselves as Christians (76.5 percent), the percentage of the U.S. population that identifies itself with other religious and spiritual traditions is increasing.(6) Substantial increases are seen in the percentage of people identifying themselves as New Age (240 percent), Hindu (237 percent), Buddhist (170 percent), and Muslim (109 percent). The Christian population showed only a small increase (5 percent), and the Jewish population even declined slightly (-10 percent). As a consequence of this shift, many culturally based "alternative" treatments are widely accepted as beneficial, including prayer and faith healing.

1.3. The Voice of Persons Suffering from Mental Illness

Many individuals with psychiatric disabilities view spiritual activities as an integral part of their recovery process. They have consistently indicated that religion and spirituality can serve as a major resource in recovery.(5, 7–14) Lindgren and Coursey (15) interviewed participants in a psychosocial rehabilitation program: 80 percent said that religion and spirituality had been helpful to them. Trepper et al. (11) found that participants experiencing greater symptom severity and lower overall functioning are more likely to use religious activities as part of their coping. Symptom-related stress leads to greater use of religious coping, a phenomenon that has been shown in other studies too.(16, 17) Baetz et al. (18) demonstrated among psychiatric inpatients that both public religion (for example, worship attendance) and private spirituality were associated with less severe depressive symptoms. Religious patients also had shorter lengths of stay in the hospital and higher life satisfaction.

Koenig, George, and Peterson (19) followed medically ill older persons who were diagnosed with a depressive disorder and found that intrinsic religiosity (following religion as an "end in itself," rather than as a means to other end) was predictive of shorter time to remission of depressive disorder, after controlling for multiple other predictors of remission. Pargament (20, 21) has studied extensively the role of religious coping methods in dealing with stress. He found consistent connections between positive styles of religious coping and better mental health outcomes. Religious coping styles such as perceived collaboration with God, seeking spiritual support from God or religious communities, and benevolent religious appraisal of negative situations have been related to less depression,(19) less anxiety, (22) and more positive affect.(23)

1.4. Religious and Nonreligious Therapists

Can nonreligious therapists deliver religious therapy for religious patients, and if yes, how effective are they? Is religious therapy per se more effective for religious patients than nonreligious therapy? To answer these questions, Rebecca Probst from the Department of Counseling Psychology, Portland, Oregon, conducted a comparative study of the efficacy of religious and non-religious cognitive-behavioral therapy with religious and nonreligious therapists on religious patients with clinical depression.(24) She hypothesized that religious cognitive-behavioral therapy (RCT) might be more effective for religious patients than standard cognitive-behavioral therapy (CBT) because of higher consistency of values and frameworks.

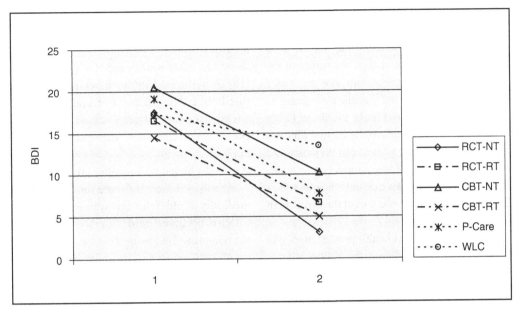

Figure 17.1. Reduction of BDI-scores during treatment period (1 = pre-treatment, 2 = post-treatment).

In that study, religious cognitive-behavioral therapy gave religious rationales for the procedures, used religious arguments to counter irrational thoughts, and used religious imagery procedures according to a manual published by Probst in 1988.(25) Furthermore, the study was designed to determine whether nonreligious therapists could successfully implement RCT.

Focusing on pre- and posttreatment results (see Figure 17.1) Probst et al. found that religious individuals receiving RCT reported more reduction in depression (BDI) and greater improvement in social adjustment (SAS) and general symptomatology (GSI, SCL-90-R) than patients in the standard CBT. Individuals in the pastoral counseling treatment group (PCT), which was included to control for the nonspecific effects of the treatment delivery system, also showed significant improvement at posttreatment and even outperformed standard CBT. This finding is analogous to the results obtained with a nonclinical population in a previous study.(26)

The most surprising finding in the recent study was a strong therapist-treatment interaction. The group showing the best performance on all measures was the RCT condition with the nonreligious therapists (RCT-NT), whereas the group with the worst pattern of performance was the standard CBT with the nonreligious therapists (CBT-NT). Less difference in performance was noted between the cognitive-behavioral therapy conditions for the religious therapists (RCT/CBT-RT). This pattern of therapist-treatment interaction suggests the following:

1 Effectiveness of CBT for religious patients delivered by nonreligious therapists can be enhanced significantly by using a religious framework.
2 Impact of similarity of value orientation of therapists/therapy and patients on outcome of therapy seems to suggest that neither extreme value similarity nor extreme value dissimilarity facilitates outcome.

Value similarity must be defined as a combination of the personal values of the therapist and the value orientation of the treatment. Done so, the RCT conditions with religious therapists and standard CBT with nonreligious therapists show the most value similarity. Neither of them, however, showed high performance.

The Probst study clearly indicates that the outcome of therapy in religious patients can be

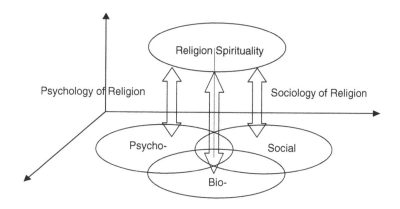

EXTENDED BIO PSYCHO SOCIAL MODEL

Figure 17.2. Extended bio-psycho-social model integrating religion/spirituality as a fourth dimension (published by Hefti R, 2003).

enhanced by integrating religious elements into the therapy protocol and that this can be successfully done by religious and nonreligious therapists alike.

2. A HOLISTIC AND INTERDISCIPLINARY MODEL FOR THERAPY

2.1. The Extended Bio-Psycho-Social Model

In psychiatry and psychosomatic medicine, the bio-psycho-social model, introduced by George L. Engel (27) is the predominant concept in clinical practice and research. It shows that biological, psychological, and social factors interact in a complex way in health and disease. Our book illustrates that there is a fourth dimension involved. Religion and spirituality constitute an additional, distinct, and independent dimension, interacting with biological, psychological, and social factors. I have called this model the extended bio-psycho-social model (Figure 17.2).(28)

The extended bio-psycho-social model is a useful framework to understand the religious and spiritual dimension in clinical practice as well as in religion, spirituality, and health research. It shows that religion and spirituality can be causing, mediating, or moderating factors on mental health and disease in the same way as biological, psychological, and social factors, constituting biology of religion, psychology of religion, and sociology of religion. The model illustrates that pharmacotherapeutic, psychotherapeutic, sociotherapeutic, and spiritual elements must be integrated in a holistic perspective, thus establishing a whole-person approach to mental health.

2.2. Religion and Spirituality as a Main Resource

In general, people who are more religiously or spiritually devout report better physical health, psychological adjustment, and lower rates of problematic social behavior.(29–32) Spirituality strengthens a sense of self and self-esteem, (5, 10, 33) of feeling more like a "whole person," and of being valued by the divine (as part of creation, as a "child of God"), countering stigma and shame by positive self-attributions and, through all of this, reinforcing "personhood."(34)

Spirituality is associated with decreased levels of depression,(35) especially among people with intrinsic spirituality or faith based on internalized beliefs.(36) Spirituality correlates with lower levels of general anxiety (31, 36, 37) and with positive outcomes in coping with anxiety.(38) Higher levels of spirituality among individuals recovering from substance abuse are related to resiliency to stress and optimism,(39) and spiritual coping methods are found to have positive effects for persons diagnosed with schizophrenia.(40) Participation in spiritual and religious activities helps to integrate individuals into their families.(41)

Religion and spirituality also deliver social and community resources (10, 33) being enhanced by the "transcendent nature" of the support. Belonging to and finding acceptance in a religious community may have special importance for people who are often rejected, isolated, or stigmatized.(42) Spiritual experiences facilitate the development of a fundamental sense of connectedness. Religion and spirituality foster a sense of hope and purpose, a reason for being, as well as opportunities for growth and positive change.(5, 33, 43) These are ways in which the patients have expressed the experience of enhanced personhood or empowerment.

2.3. Religion and Spirituality as a Burden

It is important to be aware of the "negative" (or at least challenging) effects that religion and spirituality can have on mental health outcomes and recovery.

Negative religious coping involves beliefs and activities such as expressing anger at God, questioning God's power, attributing negative events to God's punishment, and discontent with religious communities and their leadership. Negative religious coping in community samples has been linked to greater affective distress, including greater anxiety and depression and lower self-esteem (44) and more PTSD symptoms.(45)

Religious struggles involving interpersonal strain rather than social support, conflicts with God rather than perceived collaboration and support, struggles with belief rather than clear meaning and coherence, and difficulties related to imperfect striving after virtue have been linked to higher levels of depression and suicidality.(46) Negative experiences with religious groups can aggravate feelings of rejection and marginalization.(47)

Religious convictions can intensify excesses of self-blame and perceptions of unredeemable sinfulness. If they are woven into obsessive or depressive symptom patterns, they can be even more distressing. Furthermore, they can be reinforced by religious communities that see mental disorders as signs of moral or spiritual weakness or failure. Prayer or other religious rituals can become compulsive and interfere with overall daily functioning.(11) Finally, beliefs involving themes of divine abandonment or condemnation, unrelenting rejection, or powerful retribution may make recovery seem unattainable or unimportant.(48)

2.4. An Interdisciplinary Approach

Applying a holistic or whole person approach to mental illness demands an interdisciplinary concept. Different competencies have to be represented in the therapeutic team (*inpatient setting*, Figure 17.3).(28) The pastoral/spiritual counselor should be a full member of the interdisciplinary team with rights and responsibilities equal to the other therapists. This guarantees working on common therapeutic goals and prevents playing off pastoral counseling against the other disciplines, what we consider an important aspect in the psychiatric and psychotherapeutic context.

3. RELIGIOUS AND SPIRITUAL COPING IN MENTAL DISEASE

3.1. The Key Role of Religious Coping for Patients

Several surveys showed a high prevalence of religious coping among patients with severe and persistent mental illness. Tepper et al.(11) investigated 406 patients at one of thirteen Los Angeles County mental health facilities. More than 80 percent of the participants used religious

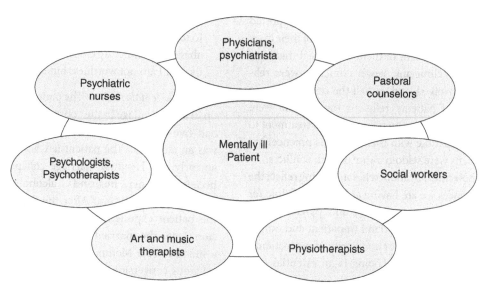

Figure 17.3. Model of an interdisciplinary team (inpatient setting).

beliefs or activities to cope with daily difficulties or frustrations. A majority of participants devoted as much as half of their total coping time to religious practices, with prayer being the most frequent activity. Specific religious coping strategies, such as prayer or reading the Bible, were associated with higher SCL-90 scores (indicating more severe symptoms), more reported frustration, and a lower GAF score (indicating greater impairment). The amount of time that participants devoted to religious coping was negatively related to reported levels of frustration and scores on the SCL-90 symptom subscales. The results of the study suggest that religious activities and beliefs may be particularly important for persons who are experiencing more severe symptoms, and increased religious activity may be associated with reduced symptoms over time.

This is not only true in the United States but also in Europe. The findings of Tepper et al. have been replicated by Mohr et al. in Geneva, Switzerland.(49) Semistructured interviews focused on religious coping were conducted with a sample of 115 outpatients with psychotic illness at one of Geneva's four psychiatric outpatient facilities. For a majority of patients, religion instilled hope, purpose, and meaning in their lives (71 percent), whereas for some, it induced spiritual despair (14 percent). Patients also reported that religion lessened (54 percent) or increased (10 percent) psychotic and general symptoms. Religion was also found to increase social integration (28 percent) or social isolation (3 percent). It reduced (33 percent) or increased (10 percent) the risk of suicide attempts, reduced (14 percent) or increased (3 percent) substance use, and fostered adherence to (16 percent) or was in opposition to (15 percent) psychiatric treatment. The results highlight the clinical significance of religion and religious coping in the care of patients with schizophrenia. Thus, spirituality should be integrated into the psychosocial dimension of care.

Huguelet et al. from the same public psychiatric outpatient department in Geneva investigated spirituality and religious practices of outpatients (N = 100) with schizophrenia and compared them with their clinician's knowledge of patients' religious involvement.(50) Audiotaped interviews were conducted about spirituality and religious coping. The patients' clinicians (N = 34) were asked about their own beliefs and religious activities as well as their patients' religious and clinical characteristics. A majority of the patients reported that religion was an important aspect of their lives, but only 36 percent of them had raised this issue with their clinicians. Fewer clinicians were religiously involved, and, in half the cases, their perceptions of patients' religious involvement were inaccurate. Some patients considered treatment to be incompatible with their religious practice, but clinicians were seldom aware of such conflicts.

These findings about religious coping reflect the experiences we are having at the SGM-Clinic for psychosomatics, psychiatry, and psychotherapy in Langenthal, Switzerland (inpatient and outpatient department). For a majority of our patients, religious or spiritual coping is an essential part of their coping behavior. Religion provides patients with a framework to cope with disease-related struggles. Existential needs such as being secure, being valued, and having meaning and purpose are addressed by clinicians and pastoral counselors, despite and beyond psychiatric conditions.(51) To illustrate this, I quote some passages from open, unstructured interviews that were performed with depressed patients as part of a qualitative study conducted in our clinic.(52)

32 year old male patient: The patient is married and has a 1-year-old son. He has been working in the same company for many years and is a member of a Protestant church. He was hospitalized because of a severe depressive episode. How did he use religious coping to overcome his depression?

- By reading scriptures/psalms: "Reading psalms helped me a lot to feel closer to God in difficult times. I realized that others (the writers of the psalms) had to cry also and felt desperate in their situation. They argued with God and pleaded to him."
- By getting spiritual support: "In the very dark moments, when I felt totally lost and abandoned by God, I couldn't cope with my situation any more. I couldn't fight negative thoughts about the future and

myself. I needed somebody from outside to tell me that these are lies, that I am not abandoned either by God or by my family, that I am not worthless but loved."

65 year old female patient: The patient grew up in a small village in the countryside. She had five brothers and sisters. Her father was an alcoholic. The patient left home at an early age. Her first marriage collapsed because of her husband's alcoholism. They had two children. After the divorce, the patient experienced her first depression. Later she married again and became a member of a Methodist church (after a religious conversion). Depressive episodes became less frequent and less severe. What did the patient do to help her cope with depression?

- Controlling depression by faith/prayer: "When I feel sad and my thoughts become gloomy, when I wake up early in the morning and can't sleep anymore then I go outside into nature and speak with God, thanking him for being in control and for not letting me go down."
- Not asking why: "In past times I always began to ask why, why did I marry this man, why did God let this happen? But this made things worse. I began to turn in circles. Today I stop this kind of thinking and focus on God."

Our task as a physician, psychotherapist, or mental health worker is to support the coping capacities of patients by understanding and empowering them.

3.2. The Key Role of Religious Coping for Family Caregivers

Research that has examined the outcomes of religious coping has generally found that religiosity among caregivers is linked to enhanced adjustment. For example, in a longitudinal study of sixty-two caregivers of persons with Alzheimer's disease or cancer, Rabins and colleagues (53) found that strength of religious belief at baseline was associated with better emotional adjustment among caregivers at two-year follow-up, even when personality variables, family functioning, and levels of anger and guilt were controlled for. In another study of 127 caregivers of elderly persons with disabilities, Chang and colleagues (54) found that caregivers who used religious or spiritual beliefs to cope with caregiving stress had a better relationship with care recipients, lower levels of depression, and better self-care; for example, they experienced less "submersion" in the caregiving role.

Only a few published studies have quantitatively assessed and examined the correlates of religiosity among family caregivers of persons with serious mental illness.(55) For example, sixty Hindu family members of patients with schizophrenia were recruited through a public hospital in India. These individuals completed measures of caregiving burden, coping activities, religious beliefs and practices, and adjustment. The results of the study highlight the prevalence of religious coping; 90 percent of participants reported praying to God, and 50 percent viewed religion as a source of solace, strength, and guidance in coping with caregiving demands. In multiple regression analyses, the authors found that strength of religious belief was linked to greater well-being among caregivers, with other types of coping and demographic characteristics controlled for. Although generalization of these results is limited by cultural context, these findings highlight the prevalence and potential benefits of religiosity among caregivers of persons with serious mental illness.

Johnson (56) interviewed a sample of 180 family members about their understanding of their relative's illness, sources of support, and ways of coping and found that family members often turn to religion to cope with the stress of caring for an ill family member. Bland and Darlington (57) echoed these results in their study of hope among family members of persons with serious mental illness. Five of the sixteen participants spontaneously identified religious beliefs and participation as a significant source

of hope. Thus, research points to the important role of religiosity among family caregivers of persons with serious mental illness. Moreover, these preliminary studies, along with work in other caregiving populations, suggest that religiosity may have salutary effects on caregiver adjustment.

A recent study aimed to characterize the nature of religiosity and sources of spiritual support in a sample of family caregivers of persons with serious mental illness in the National Alliance on Mental Illness (NAMI) Family to Family Education program.(58) Forty-four percent reported having a relative with schizophrenia, 50 percent had a relative with a major affective disorder, and the remaining 6 percent had a relative with another diagnosis. The mean rating of importance of religion and spirituality, on a scale of 1 to 4, was 3.43 ± .83±, which is halfway between "fairly important" and "very important." The mean rating of whether participants considered God to be a source of comfort and strength was 3.26 ± 1.03, falling between "quite a bit" and "a great deal." Overall, this was a moderately religious and spiritual sample, comparable to the general population.

Thirty-one participants (37 percent) reported that they had received religious or spiritual support in coping with their relative's illness in the past three months. The most frequent types of spiritual support were praying or meditating, reading the Bible or other religious literature, and watching or listening to religious programs on television or the radio. Notably, nineteen participants (23 percent) reported that they contacted clergy or a religious leader to talk about problems or concerns related to their relative's illness. Twenty-three participants (28 percent) reported relying on members of their congregation for support in coping with their relatives' illness during the previous three months. Personal religiosity was positively associated with level of mastery ($r = .26$, $p = .017$) and self-care ($r = .33$, $p = .003$) and negatively associated with level of depression ($r = -.25$; $p = .025$).

The major findings of this study are twofold. First, a substantial proportion of family members of persons with serious mental illness mobilize religious and spiritual resources to cope with their situation as caregivers. Second, higher religiosity was associated with greater self-esteem and self-care and less depression among family caregivers. This pattern suggests that religiosity may bolster the internal coping resources of family members who are caring for people with serious mental illness. The strongest relationship observed was the link between religiosity and self-care, suggesting a pathway whereby religiosity may contribute to enhanced well-being among caregivers by expanding the capacity or motivation for self-care.

3.3. The Key Role of Religious Communities (Faith-Based Organizations)

A recent survey of faith-based organizations in the Los Angeles area highlighted a high demand for mental health services in religious and spiritual communities but also identified significant barriers to the implementation of such services; for example, limited expertise and resources. In reporting these results, Dosset and colleagues (59) emphasized that partnerships between mental health providers and faith-based communities may be a particularly effective strategy for meeting the mental health service needs of populations that are underserved by the mental health system, such as persons with low incomes, ethnically diverse communities, and recent immigrants. In one attempt to include caregiver services within a religious congregation, Pickett-Schenk (60) conducted a church-based support program for African-American families coping with the mental illness of a family member. In a study of twenty-three caregivers, participants reported that they were highly satisfied with the group and perceived gains in knowledge and morale. In another vein, NAMI provides support to faith-based communities that are attempting to address the needs of persons with serious mental illness through projects such as the Faith Communities Education Project and Faith Net (www.nami.org/faithnet).

It is critical for mental health professionals to appreciate the role of religion and spirituality among persons with mental illness and their caregivers. Clinical interventions should include routine assessment of this area, and interventions should be appropriately tailored to build on relevant religious and spiritual resources, while respecting the diversity of background and beliefs. It is important for mental health professionals to effectively collaborate with clergy and other religious professionals in providing services to persons with serious mental illness and their caregivers. Collaborative partnerships between mental health professionals and religious and spiritual communities (61) represent a powerful and culturally sensitive resource for meeting the needs of family caregivers of persons with mental illness.

4. MENTAL HEALTH CARE PROGRAMS INTEGRATING RELIGION/SPIRITUALITY

4.1. An Overview of Past and Recent Programs

The first therapy group on spiritual issues was started by Nancy Kehoe in 1981 in the Department of Psychiatry at Cambridge Health Alliance and Harvard Medical School, Belmont, Massachusetts.(62) She felt the need to provide seriously mentally ill persons with an opportunity to explore religious and spiritual issues in relation to their mental illness. At first, the idea of having such a group generated anxiety, fear, and doubt among staff members. It brought out the ambivalence that many mental health professionals have about religious issues, an ambivalence reflected in Gallup poll findings.(63) In addition, Bergin and Jensen's work (64) has highlighted the marked difference between the religious beliefs and practices of the general population and those of the mental health professionals. Staff training and instruction alleviated some staff concerns about Kehoe's group. However, the long-term success of the group has been the strongest factor in staff acceptance. Group rules contributing to its success are tolerance of diversity, respect of others' beliefs, and a ban on proselytizing. Another factor is that membership is open to all, regardless of religious background or diagnosis.

At least three other programs integrating spiritual issues into mental health care originate from the United States. The main information on these four spirituality groups is presented in Table 17.1. The programs will be described in detail in the following paragraphs. In addition, the integrative concept of the SGM-Clinic as a European model will be discussed and illustrated.

4.2. "Spirituality Group" at the Hollywood Mental Health Center, Los Angeles

The study of Ana Wong-McDonald et al.(65) examines the results of a spirituality group that was offered at a psychosocial rehabilitation program at an inner-city community mental health center in Los Angeles. It was anticipated that, along with proper medication and psychiatric rehabilitation, the inclusion of spirituality as a therapeutic component would enhance the recovery of persons who wish to incorporate it as a part of their treatment services.

Of the forty-eight individuals included in the study, twenty attended the spirituality group (SG). All of the participants in the SG indicated that spiritual issues are important in their lives and that they wish to discuss them in the group. Eighteen participants professed adherence to some form of Judeo-Christian faith. The group members indicated that the following issues were pertinent in their recovery: finding hope again; dealing with depression, fear and anxiety, negative thoughts, self-doubt, and self-worth; emotional healing; and forgiveness.

The standard psychosocial rehabilitation program was conducted two days per week, five hours on each of the days, emphasizing skills training, psycho-education, community integration, and cognitive behavioral treatment.(66) In April 2003, however, a spirituality group was offered as a sixty-minute optional weekly session in the same time slot as the regular standard group. The spirituality group was open-ended. Each session focused on a topic of interest (for example, forgiveness). Spiritual interventions included discussing spiritual concepts (for example, raising awareness of God's promises of peace, love, and faith and helping participants to see their self-worth based in God's promises), encouraging forgiveness, referring to spiritual writings (for example, encouraging participants to read the story of the prodigal son to understand God's love and forgiveness), listening to spiritual music, and encouraging spiritual and emotional support among the SG members (for example, praying for one another and telephoning each other for support).

The general purposes of the interventions were to help participants understand their problems from an eternal, spiritual perspective, to gain a greater sense of hope, to emotionally forgive and heal past pain, to accept responsibility for their own actions, and to experience and affirm their sense of identity and self-worth. Participants were also encouraged to connect with their faith communities for social and spiritual support.

At time of entry into the psych rehab group and at six-month intervals thereafter, participants set treatment goals for symptom management, community integration, and improvement in their overall quality of life. Examples of goals included health-related wellness (such as lowering the frequency of panic attacks, losing weight, decreasing cigarette smoking, and lowering the number of hospitalizations), socialization goals (such as making at least one new friend, going out on a date, or saving money to go on vacations with friends), and vocational and educational goals (such as obtaining a driver's license, maintaining a car, earning a high school diploma, and obtaining a volunteer job).

All twenty participants (100 percent) in the spirituality group (SG) achieved their treatment goals, compared to sixteen out of twenty-eight people (57 percent) in the nonspirituality group (non-SG). The difference in goal attainment between the two groups was highly significant ($p = .0001$). Individual examples of how spirituality may enhance recovery give an idea of its

Table 17.1: Overview of Four Programs Integrating Religious and Spiritual Issues.

	Therapy Group on Spiritual Issues	Spirituality Group (SG)	Spirituality Matters Group (SMG)	Spiritual Issues Psychoeducational Group
Author(s)	Kehoe NC	Wong-McDonald A	Revheim N, Greenberg WM	Phillips RE, Laking R, Pargament KI
Center	Day treatment center	Hollywood Mental Health Center	Nathan Kline Institute, Clinical Research Evaluation Facility	Local community mental health center
Setting	Outpatient setting, chronically ill psychiatric patients, 22 to 60 years old	Community-based psychosocial rehab program, psychiatric outpatients, 2 days a week	24-bed state-hospital inpatient unit for persons with persistent psychiatric disabilities	Outpatient setting, people with serious mental illness (SMI), referred by mental health workers
Format of the SG	45 minutes weekly, ongoing, typically 10 to 12 clients, attending for 2 to 3 years	1 hour per week, 20 participants, open-ended, focusing on topics of interest	Continuous enrollment, typically 12 to 40 sessions, multi-disciplinary concept	Seven weeks, 1.5 hrs/week, psycho-educational program, 10 participants
Purpose	Foster tolerance, self-awareness, and nonpathogenic therapeutic exploration of value systems	Enhance recovery, support treatment goals, help participants gain a spiritual perspective	Promote spiritual and social support and improve coping resources, emotion-focused coping	Provide new information about spirituality and allow participants to share experiences
Spiritual key elements, interventions	Exploring ways in which beliefs and practices help or hinder coping with mental illness. Considering questions, problems, and feelings about religious belief. Strict group rules: tolerance and respect	Discussing spiritual concepts, encouraging forgiveness, referring to spiritual writings, listening to spiritual music, encouraging spiritual and emotional support among group members and with their faith communities	Structured group treatment approach addressing spirituality, promote using spiritual beliefs for coping, shifting perspective from victimization to resilience. Reading psalms and spiritual stories, reciting prayers	Presenting an inclusive set of spiritual topics: spiritual resources, spiritual strivings, spiritual struggles, forgiveness of others, and spiritual strategies to promote hope
Evaluation	Feedback of the group and co-workers	Degree of goal attainment	Evaluation period in the second year	Survey for feedback of the group
Result	Transcripts of group meetings: exemplification of group interactions	100% goal attainment in the SG vs. 57% in the non-SG	More qualitative, e.g., new insights: medication as a gift of God	Appreciation of the group, the unique opportunity to discuss spiritual issues
Personal statements of group members	"Group interactions reveal that individuals are more than their mental illness"	"By remembering that Jesus suffered more than I ever did kept me from self-pity"	As an outcome of a group discussion: "Oh Lord, your medication has brought me a sense of peace"	"I liked hearing from other spiritual beliefs and interests"
Conclusion	A group focusing on religious issues can provide an opportunity to explore topics usually ignored by mental health practice	Spirituality as a therapeutic component can enhance recovery of persons with severe mental illness	Reviewing activity plans and group notes identified themes consistent with an "emotion-focused coping" model	The intervention appeared to reach its original objectives and provided a safe environment to discuss spiritual concerns

role in psychiatric rehabilitation. One participant with a thirty-year history of agoraphobia and daily panic attacks shared that she was able to "push away" the symptoms by using a combination of prayer and relaxation techniques. Another group member with bipolar disorder and a history of risky sexual behaviors shared that by returning to God, he had stopped his behaviors for over a year. A third participant said that her hope in Christ empowered her to journey through her depression. Finally, a fourth group member said, "By remembering that Jesus suffered more than I ever did kept me from self-pity and on the course to getting better." Participants as a group stated that sensing God's presence helps lessen feelings of sadness, calms fears and anxieties, and helps in dealing with forgiveness and resolving daily problems.

The findings from the Wong study encourage inclusion of spirituality in psychiatric rehabilitation as a promising approach. Participants' self-report and goal-attainment outcomes point to the positive effects that spirituality has for people in recovery.

4.3. "Spirituality Matters Group" at the Nathan Kline Institute, New York

The Spirituality Matters Group (SMG) was developed in 2001 at the Clinical Research Evaluation Facility (CREF) of the Nathan Kline Institute for hospitalized persons with persistent psychiatric disabilities,(67) following the rationale that spiritual support fosters the recovery process. SMG is distinct from comparable groups (68) in its multidisciplinary leadership that focuses on integrating spiritual/religious, psychological, and rehabilitative perspectives over an extended treatment period. Staff concerns about potential deleterious effects (for example, increased psychopathology) were discussed in the context of staff resistance encountered by proponents of this treatment format.(62) SMG's purpose was described as strength-based, offering individuals personal choice, respect, and peer support, corresponding to accepted core principles for mental health recovery (www.samhsa.gov). The SMG is

made up of self-referred persons who join three group co-leaders (representing psychology, pastoral care, and rehabilitation) in exploring nondenominational religious and spiritual themes designed to facilitate comfort and hope, while addressing prominent therapeutic concerns. Patients are told this group "focuses on the use of spiritual beliefs for coping with one's illness and hospitalization."

The one-hour weekly SMG has had continuous enrollment over the last five years. Attendance ranges from six to eight members, with participants making a commitment to the group for the duration of their hospitalization at CREF, typically twelve to forty sessions. Group membership demographics during an evaluation period in SMG's second year included ($n = 20$): average age 35 years, education 11 years, first hospitalization age 21, and current inpatient stay 255 days. Seventy-nine percent were male; 33 percent black, 42 percent white, 12 percent Hispanic; 72 percent diagnosed with schizophrenia, 28 percent schizoaffective disorder; 80 percent had past substance abuse and 5 percent a history of pathological religious ideation. Participants identified themselves as Protestant, 25 percent; Catholic, 35 percent; Jewish, 2.5 percent; Muslim, 2.5 percent; other, 10 percent; multiple, 5 percent; and none, 20 percent. The highly-structured group format accommodates cognitive deficits and limited social skills, prevalent in persons with persistent psychiatric disabilities.

During each session's *initial phase*, members are introduced, the group's purpose reviewed, and seasoned group members orient newcomers on how the group can be used (for example, using spiritual beliefs to cope with daily stressors and for support with behavioral change). The multireligious and nondenominational nature of the group is affirmed. Spirituality is defined as "personal beliefs and values related to the meaning and purpose of life, which may include faith in a higher purpose or power."

In the *middle phase*, a topic with a related group activity or exercise is introduced, with warm-up questions for personal sharing and reflection, followed by distribution of handouts, readings, or other materials that are read aloud. Topics are selected by leaders on a rotating basis and carefully prepared so that both negative and positive emotions are addressed. For example, individual members' guilt, anxiety, and intolerance or cognitive distortions resulting from previous religious/spiritual experiences are explored. Group members are encouraged to share how the topic has relevance to the perception of their illness, previous behavior patterns, treatment failures (for example, medication nonadherence, rehospitalization), and future goals (for example, appropriate discharge planning, commitment to treatment recommendations). At least one group leader is familiar with the individual treatment plans and offers such input into the group process when appropriate to ensure integration with other clinical programming for goal attainment.

In the *ending phase*, group members summarize the session's emergent themes and new learning that influences goals and future choices, followed by a formal closing with a prayer composed by group members: "Give me light and insight so that I may trust. Let me learn the way of peace so that I may grow…. May those who find themselves off track, be guided. May those who are afraid, find comfort. And may we all find patience on our path." Topics for subsequent groups emerge from each week's discussion, which fosters continuity, repetition, and self-disclosure.

Group activities and exercises highlight using spirituality as a coping mechanism during recovery. The principal group activities are reading Psalms (consistent with most participants having Judeo-Christian identification), reading prayers, writing prayers, and telling stories from a variety of faith perspectives.

- *Readings from the Book of Psalms* (69) evoke the full range of human emotions from thanksgiving and praise to anger, fear, desperation, despair, abandonment, hope, and protection. Reading selected Psalms as a group, followed by personal sharing, emphasizes the universal nature of experiencing conflicts and struggles in daily life, while focusing on elements of

faith that maintain strength and perseverance during these difficulties.

- *Reciting prayers together* that are familiar and common ("St. Francis Prayer") or those specific for personal needs (for example "prayers to start the day") reinforce individuals' existing religious/spiritual practices. Using congregate prayers with individuals with limited social skills can enhance social support through focusing on a shared goal.

- *Writing original prayers* helps improve self-awareness of one's needs and allows articulation of one's experiences in a setting that brings comfort and a sense of closure. The use of templates or prayer formats (praise, thanksgiving, and intercession) assists individuals in this creative and empowering experience.

- *Reading spiritual stories, fables, allegories and personal narratives of others* allows group members to identify personal needs and values, and through identification, offers opportunities to express difficult emotions.

Reviewing activity plans and group notes identified themes consistent with an "emotion-focused coping" model.(70) Emotion-focused coping includes cognitive reframing, social comparisons, minimization ("looking on the bright side of things"), and behavioral efforts to feel better (exercise, relaxation, meditation, support, religion, humor, and talking). Emotion-focused coping is useful when a situation cannot be changed, and only the emotional response can be changed, which can be self-affirming and empowering. This coping style is congruent with both recovery and SMG goals and can coexist with problem-focused approaches.

4.4. "Spiritual Issues Psychoeducational Group" at a Community Center

This study describes an innovative program for people with serious mental illness (SMI) who are dealing with spiritual/religious issues.(68) The program was a seven-week semistructured, psycho-educational intervention in which participants discussed religious resources, spiritual struggles, forgiveness, and hope. The intervention was designed to provide new information about spirituality to participants and to allow them to share experiences and knowledge that they felt might be of value to others. An additional goal was to present a more inclusive set of spiritual topics to clients with SMI than has previously been described.

Group members were recruited through referrals from mental health workers at a local community mental health center. Potential members participated in individual interviews to determine whether their needs, expectations, and level of functioning were appropriate for the group. The interview examined their religious/spiritual background, the role that religion/spirituality has played in their experience with mental illness, and their expectations for the group.

There were ten participants, all Caucasian, and 70 percent were female. One-third of the group members reported a diagnosis of schizophrenia, one-third indicated a diagnosis of depression, and one-third reported personality disorders as their primary diagnosis. In terms of religious affiliation, 30 percent identified themselves as Roman Catholic while all others were affiliated with Protestant denominations. Two doctoral students in clinical psychology served as ongoing facilitators for each group session. Furthermore, each week (with the exception of the first and last weeks) an additional graduate student joined the group to introduce discussion on a specific topic. Therefore, on most weeks, three facilitators were present. The group took place once a week for 1.5 hours over the course of seven weeks.

Week One: Introduction. The facilitators gave group members an overview of the group format and what topics would be discussed. In addition, the group rules were reviewed and group members shared their "personal spiritual journey."(62) Questions revolved around the theme of their past and present spirituality, how their spirituality was affected by their mental illness, and vice versa.

Week Two: Spiritual Resources. This session was intended to elicit members' ideas of personal and community spiritual resources.(20) The session began by providing the group with definitions and examples of spiritual resources. Multiple resources were generated by participants, including prayer, reading religious literature, prayer groups, going to religious services, journaling, listening to spiritual music, burning candles, doing artwork, and just socializing with friends. In addition, potential barriers to using these resources were also explored, such as avoiding church when experiencing high levels of symptoms.

Week Three: Spiritual Strivings. The primary objective was to have group members explore ways to create and achieve meaningful, realistic goals related to their spiritual journey. Emmons (71) has discussed the importance and positive implications of spiritual strivings. The facilitator first discussed the importance of having strivings. To facilitate the discussion, group members generated personal lists of their strivings. These lists were based on what participants found meaningful.

Week Four: Spiritual Struggles. The overall goals were to emphasize the importance of expressing thoughts and feelings about spiritual struggles, validate and normalize anger with God or the church, and reframe struggles as a time of potential personal growth and change. Group members were given a list of common struggles with God (for example, feeling abandoned, spiritual emptiness, feeling sinful, and feeling frustrated) and church (for example, not feeling welcomed, feeling abandoned, stigma, and paranoia) and asked to circle ones that they have experienced. They then shared with other group members ways in which they have dealt with these struggles.

Week Five: Forgiveness of Others. The primary goal was to examine how forgiveness related to the members' lives. First, group members discussed the definition of forgiveness. They then explored what forgiveness is not; that is, forgiveness is not forgetting, reconciliation, acceptance or tolerance of injustice, letting go of anger, condoning, excusing, or legal pardon. Next, group members generated ideas about the costs and benefits of forgiveness. Then members reflected on incidents in their lives when they were hurt by another person or institution. Finally, the steps toward forgiveness were briefly outlined.(72)

Week Six: Hope. The primary goal was to explore spiritual strategies that could be used to hold on to hope. Facilitating questions were taken from readings on integrating hope and spirituality into treatment.(73) Group members first talked about the meaning of hope and reasons to retain hope. They then divided into pairs and discussed their personal hopes. The major pathways to keeping hope alive were through spiritual rituals (for example, hymns, reading the Bible), trusting that God has a greater purpose, and through supporting each other.

Week Seven: Wrap-up. In the final session, the two permanent facilitators reviewed the topics covered by the group, solicited feedback from group members, and shared their personal reactions. Emphasis was placed on maintaining confidentiality even after the group ended. A survey was also distributed to gather feedback. Participants were asked what they learned from the group, what they found most helpful and least helpful, and what suggestions they had for future groups. Most members spontaneously expressed that they wanted the group to continue. Although most members felt they did not necessarily learn new information, they enjoyed and appreciated the unique forum in which they could explore an area that is often neglected in the mental health services setting. Participants further reported that they liked hearing others' spiritual beliefs and interests.

In conclusion, this intervention appeared to reach many of its original objectives. It provided a safe environment for those with SMI to discuss spiritual concerns. This unique topic of intervention appeared to be highly valued by participants. Community mental health professionals may feel that it is not their place to employ a spiritual issues group in a publicly funded agency. Yet Richards and Bergin (74) (p. 159) note that there "are no professional ethical guidelines that prohibit therapists in civic settings from discussing religious issues or using spiritual interventions with clients." In fact, they assert, it is unethical to derogate or overlook this dimension.

Overall, this intervention holds promise as a useful addition to current community mental health practice. Such groups have been run by licensed nurse practitioners,(62) social workers, (75) and clinical/community psychologists.(15) With some training in the area of serious mental illness and spiritual concerns, professionals from diverse areas of training (for example, psychiatrists and hospital chaplains) could also lead groups or supervise the intervention.

4.5. The Integrative Concept of the SGM-Clinic Langenthal (Switzerland)

The scientific framework for our integrative concept is the extended bio-psycho-social model (28) as described earlier in the chapter. We believe that in mental as well as in physical illness there is always an existential and therefore a spiritual dimension that will influence therapy in an explicit or more implicit way. For this reason, we take a spiritual history from every patient. We want to know whether and how religiousness or spirituality determines the patient's understanding of his illness. Does the patient have spiritual resources in coping with his mental condition, or are his religious beliefs a burden and an obstacle in the therapeutic process?

If a patient doesn't consider himself religious or spiritual, he will get a state-of-the-art-treatment for his mental illness focusing on his or her personal treatment goals. If a patient is religious or spiritual, we try to understand how he wants to integrate these aspects into his treatment program. Spiritual treatment goals can be:

- Regaining hope and meaning
- Strengthen the relationship with God to better cope with mental illness
- Persevere in difficult circumstances
- Resolving anger, frustration, or disappointment toward God
- Understanding why God allows bad things to happen in patients' lives

Table 17.2: Overview of Spiritual Activities/Offerings for Patients in Addition to Their Standard Treatment Program. Bars Illustrate Patient's Appreciation of the Activity/Offering (from Left to Right: "It Helped Me a Lot," "It Helped Me Quite a Bit," "It Helped Me Some," "It Didn't Help Me.")

Activity/offering	Description/focus	Duration/ frequency	Evaluation
Psycho-educational group meetings	Integrating therapeutic and spiritual issues, focus on coping with life and mental illness	1 hour, 4x/week	
Spiritual singing and music group	Singing spiritual songs, listening to spiritual music, reciting prayers	1 hour, 1x/week	no evaluation
Spiritual issues discussion group	Discussing upcoming spiritual issues in an open group setting, led by a pastoral counselor, including religious rituals	1 hour, 1x/week	new activity/offering
Spiritual art therapy	Expressing spiritual topics in art therapy, e.g., creation, self-image and God image, psalms	1–2 hours weekly	
Spiritual counseling and psychotherapy	Integrating spiritual elements into counseling and psychotherapy, e.g., forgiving myself/others, individual prayers	individual	
Pastoral care	Individual pastoral counseling, delivering rituals and sacraments, anointing of the sick, Lord's supper	individual	
Patient Library	Containing a broad range of religious and spiritual books	1–2x/week	no evaluation

- Working toward forgiveness in difficult relationships
- Being more aware of God's presence and guidance in daily life

Spiritual needs and treatment goals are discussed in the therapeutic team, of which the pastoral counselor is a ordinary member. We then evaluate the best way to meet these needs and to help the patient attain his treatment goals. We also verify whether the spiritual goals are in line (don't conflict) with the other treatment goals. Spirituality can be a way of escaping from reality, which we would not support in the therapeutic context.

For many years we have been offering psycho-educational group meetings focusing on the integration of therapeutic and spiritual aspects and emphasizing the benefit and importance of religious and spiritual coping (see Table 17.2). (11, 20, 49, 70)

Typical topics of these interactive group meetings are:

- Developing life perspectives despite illness and limitations
- Coping with fear and depression; listening to the Book of Psalms
- Attaining personhood, spiritual identity ("I called you by your name")

■ Understanding healthy and unhealthy religiosity and spirituality

We also have a spiritual singing and music group. Patients can get actively involved by proposing songs, playing their own instruments, performing a dance, focusing on the presence of the divine, or just listening to the music. Singing helps patients to overcome negative feelings or thoughts.

Furthermore, we offer a spiritual issues discussion group led by our pastoral counselor (similar to groups discussed elsewhere).(62, 65) Participants can introduce spiritual topics, questions, or problems related to their illness or personal situation. They are discussed in the group, and the pastoral counselor shares insights from his spiritual background. Participants learn how to use their own spiritual resources, how to cope with spiritual questions and struggles related to their illness, and how to support others spiritually.

Another approach to spirituality is art therapy. Figure 17.4 shows a patient suffering from chronic pain and depression. Her chronic pain had two components, represented by the two human figures: a "red" one (middle) representing a burning type of pain difficult to sustain and a "black" one (right) expressing a dull type of pain making the patient depressive. Figure 17.5 demonstrates the patient's fight to maintain her relationship with God despite pain and depression. She mobilizes all her energy to grip God's outstretched hands while slowly sliding out of them – a picture of existential fight and despair. Figure 17.6 visualizes the further spiritual and therapeutic process. God lets her go and fall into a seemingly endless depth. But at the bottom of the hole, God is absorbing her smoothly, carrying her through the painful and dark valley. Deep relaxation and pain relief results.(76–78) Furthermore, the patient's relationship to God changes in character and depth.

The integration of spiritual issues in counseling and psychotherapy (24) represents another form of spiritual support. For example, a patient

in a submanic/psychotic state felt energized by God's overwhelming presence in his mind and body. The therapist discussed this "spiritual perception" in the psychotherapeutic sessions with the patient. Other topics are feelings of guilt, shame, being rejected or abandoned by the divine, and working toward forgiveness. If a patient has unhealthy beliefs, it is important to challenge them from a spiritual as well as a psychotherapeutic point of view.

We also provide pastoral care to meet the specific religious and spiritual needs of our patients. This includes rituals and sacraments, for example, anointing with oil or taking the Lord's Supper. The pastoral counselor is a member of the interdisciplinary team with equal rights and obligations. He reports back at the team meetings.

Finally, there is a patient library with a wide variety of religious and spiritual books patients can borrow, for example, "Canvas of Love – Reflections on a Rembrandt" by Henri J. M. Nouwen,(79) reflecting the story of the two sons and the father, known as the prodigal son parable (Luke 15, 11–32).

5. RECOMMENDATIONS AND GUIDELINES

5.1. Recommendations Based on Patients' Perspectives

Patients' hopes and concerns lead to specific recommendations about the place of spirituality and religion in mental health service contexts (80):

■ Mental health programs should adopt a holistic approach to both assessment and intervention, addressing patients' own understanding of religion and spirituality and the importance in their lives. They should ask whether or how patients would like to have spiritual concerns or goals included in their therapy and should develop structured ways to discuss spirituality in group or individual meetings.

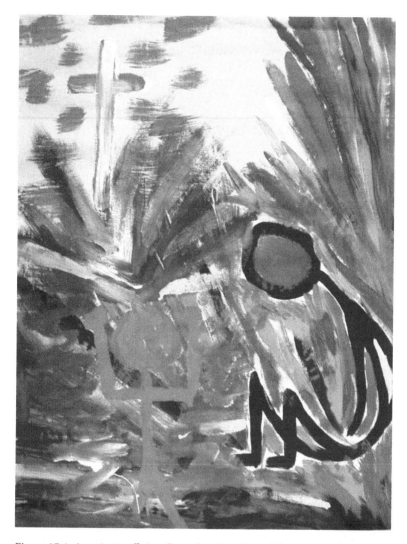

Figure 17.4. A patient suffering from chronic pain and depression. The drawing shows the patient's perception of her pain differentiating two main components: a burning and dull type of pain (burning = figure at the bottom in the middle; dull = figure on the right side).

- It is important for service providers and programs to have an open and inclusive understanding of religion and spirituality, sensitive to the many differences of experience and conviction among patients.

- Most patients want service providers to address spiritual and religious issues (81); but they do not want them to "push" either religion in general or a particular expression of spirituality or religion.

- For some patients, the experience of spirituality is profoundly personal, private, and meaningful. Many are cautious in discussing it with service providers.(15) Some fear that clinicians will "reduce" or trivialize their beliefs or that they will see them as a sign of pathology. This requires clinicians to take a respectful and individualized approach to spiritual and religious realities.

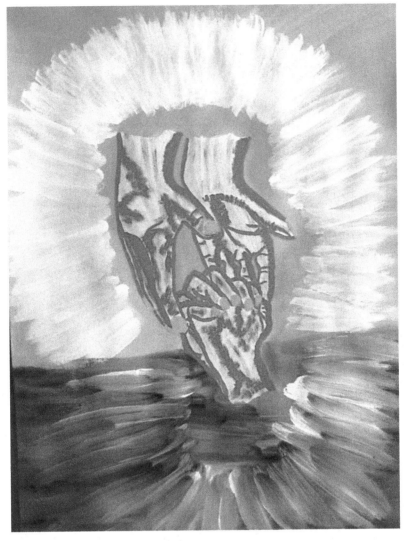

Figure 17.5. A patient suffering from chronic pain and depression. The drawing reflects the patient's fight to maintain her relationship with God.

5.2. Recommendations Based on Professional Perspectives

The most obvious recommendation is the need for more extensive training and education for human service providers (including psychiatrists, psychologists, social workers, and psychiatric nurses) on how to integrate religion and spirituality into patient care, training that is pertinent to the particular service setting in which staff and patients work together.(80)

Such training needs to address the following topics:

- Taking a spiritual history, understanding the ways in which religion and spirituality relate to patients' overall well-being, and evaluating whether patients' particular expression of spirituality is helpful or harmful for the recovery process
- Developing the ability to talk with patients about spirituality in a manner that is neither

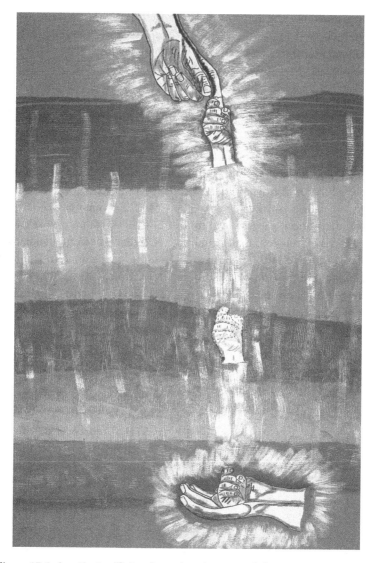

Figure 17.6. A patient suffering from chronic pain and depression. The drawing illustrates the further spiritual and therapeutic process. Finally, the patient finds herself in God's hand experiencing security, relaxation, and pain relief.

intrusive nor reductive but that communicates respectful openness to a patient's unique spiritual experiences, both positive and negative

▪ Supporting religious and spiritual coping, for example, prayer and meditation, reading psalms or other religious/spiritual literature, and attending religious services

▪ Reflecting countertransference reactions that can be influenced by the therapist's religious or spiritual experiences (p.165) (82)

▪ Encouraging family members/caregivers to use their spiritual resources (56–58)

▪ Delivering social and community resources and providing opportunities to expand the connections between religious or spiritual activities in the community and in the mental health program itself (59–61)

- Learning when and how to make referrals to religious professionals, to faith-based programs (www.nami.org/faithnet), or to centers of spiritual activity, based on an adequate understanding of the patient's needs and preferences

Programs integrating spiritual issues range from short-term psycho-educational groups designed to explore ways in which spirituality may enhance self-esteem and social support (15) to open-ended discussions of "religious issues" and the way they relate to mental health concerns. (62, 65) For additional information on how to incorporate religious and spiritual interventions in clinical practice, see the following list of books, addresses, and Web sites.

5.3. Recommended Books, Addresses, and Web Sites

Books

- Koenig HG. *Spirituality in Patient Care: Why, How, When and What*, 2nd ed. Philadelphia: Templeton Foundation Press; 2007.
- Miller WR, ed. *Integrating Spirituality into Treatment: Resources for Practitioners.* Washington, DC: American Psychological Association; 1999.
- Richards PS, Bergin AE, eds. Toward religious and spiritual competency for mental health professionals. In: *Handbook of Psychotherapy and Religious Diversity.* Washington, DC: American Psychological Association; 2000: 3–26.
- Shafranske EP. *Religion and the Clinical Practice of Psychology.* Washington, DC: American Psychological Association; 1996.
- Sperry L, Shafranske EP. *Spiritually Oriented Psychotherapy.* Washington, DC: American Psychological Association; 2005.
- Peteet J. Selected annotated bibliography on spirituality and mental health. *South Med J.* 2007;100(6):654–659.

- Hefti R, Fischer F, Teschner M, et al. *Glaube und seelische Gesundheit.* Langenthal: RSH-Publikationen; 2007.

Addresses and Web Sites

- NAMI (National Alliance for the Mentally Ill). Faithnet: Resources, Web pages, and Internet links for faith communities caring for the mentally ill. Address: Colonial Place Three, 2107 Wilson Blvd., Suite 300, Arlington, VA 22201, phone: 703–524–7600, fax: 703–524–9094, Web site: www.nami.org/faithnet
- Archdiocesan Commission on Mental Illness. Address: Deacon Tom Lambert, Our Lady of Mt Carmel Parish, 708 W Belmont, Chicago, IL 60657, phone: 773–525–0543, ext. 21, e-mail: olmcinfo2@aol.com, Web site: www.miministry.org
- Pathways to Promise, Faith community outreach. Address: 5400 Arsenal Street, St. Louis, MO 63139, phone: 314–644–8834, Web site: http://pathways2promise.org
- Center for Spirituality, Theology and Health (CSTH). Address: Duke University Medical Center, Box 3825, Busse Building, Suite 0507, Durham, NC 27710, phone: 919–660–7556, Web site: www.dukespiritualityandhealth.org
- Research Institute for Spirituality and Health (RISH), Switzerland/Europe. Address: Weissensteinstrasse 30, 4900 Langenthal, phone: 0041–62–9192211, fax: 0041–62–9192200, e-mail: info@rish.ch, Web site: www.rish.ch

REFERENCES

1. Frankl V. *Men's Search for Meaning.* New York: Washington Square Press; 1984.
2. Blanch A. Integrating religion and spirituality in mental health: the promise and the challenge. *Psychiatr Rehab J.* 2007;30:251–260.
3. Matthiews DA. *The Faith Factor: Proof of the Healing Power of Prayer.* New York: Penguin Books; 1998.
4. Russinova Z, Blanch A. Supported spirituality: a new frontier in the recovery-oriented mental health system. *Psychiatr Rehab J.* 2007;30:247–249.
5. Fallot RD. Spirituality and religion in recovery from mental illness. *New Dir Ment Health Ser.* 1998;80:25–33.

6. Barrett DA. *World Christian Encyclopedia*. New York: Oxford University Press; 2001.

7. Weisburd D. Spirituality: the search for meaning (Publisher's note). *J Calif Alliance Ment Ill.* 1997;8:1–2.

8. Sullivan WP. It helps me to be a whole person: the role of spirituality among the mentally challenged. *Psychosoc Rehab J.* 1993;16:125–134.

9. Bussema KE, Bussema EF. Is there a balm in Gilead? The implications of faith in coping with a psychiatric disability. *Psychiatr Rehab J.* 2000;24:117–124.

10. Longo DA, Peterson MS. The role of spirituality in psychosocial rehabilitation. *Psychiatr Rehab J.* 2002;25:333–340.

11. Tepper L, Rogers SA, Coleman EM, Malony HN. The prevalence of religious coping among persons with persistent mental illness. *Psychiatr Serv.* 2001;52:660–665.

12. Corrigan P, McCorkle B, Schell B, Kidder K. Religion and spirituality in the lives of people with serious mental illness. *Community Ment Health J.* 2003;39:487–499.

13. Fallot RD, Heckman J. Religious/spiritual coping among women trauma survivors with mental health and substance use disorders. *J Behav Health Ser Res.* 2005;32:215–226.

14. Fallot RD, Flournoy MB. Trauma among women with co-occurring disorders. Paper presented at the Conference on State Mental Health Agency Services Research, Program Evaluation, and Policy, Washington, DC; 2000.

15. Lindgren KN, Coursey RD. Spirituality and serious mental illness: a two-part study. *Psychosoc Rehab J.* 1995;18:93–111.

16. Koenig HG. Religious coping and depression in elderly hospitalized medically ill men. *Am J Psychiatry.* 1992;149:1693–1700.

17. Chang BH. Religion and mental health among women veterans with sexual assault experience. *Int J Psychiatry Med.* 2001;31(1):77–95.

18. Baetz M, Larson DB, Marcoux G, Bowen R, Griffin R. Canadian psychiatric inpatient religious commitment: an association with mental health. *Can J Psychiatry.* 2002;47:159–166.

19. Koenig HG, George LK, Peterson BL. Religiosity and remission of depression in medically ill older patients. *Am J Psychiatry.* 1998;155:536–542.

20. Pargament K. *The Psychology of Religion and Coping: Theory, Research, and Practice.* New York: Guilford Press; 1997.

21. Pargament K. The bitter and the sweet: an evaluation of the costs and benefits of religiousness. *Psychol Inq.* 2002;13:168–181.

22. Pargament K, Koenig HG, Perez LM. The many methods of religious coping: development and initial validation of the RCOPE. *J Clin Pyschol.* 2000;56:519–543.

23. Bush EG, Rye MS, Brant CR, Emery E, Pargament K, Riessinger CA. Religious coping with chronic pain. *Appl Psychophysiol Biofeedback.* 1999;24:249–260.

24. Propst LR, Ostrom R, Watkins P, Dean T, Mashburn D. Comparative efficacy of religious and nonreligious cognitive-behavior therapy for the treatment of clinical depression in religious individuals. *J Consult Clin Psychol.* 1992;60:94–103.

25. Probst LR. *Psychotherapy in a Religious Framework: Spirituality in the Emotional Healing Process.* New York: Human Sciences Press; 1988.

26. Propst LR. The comparative efficacy of religious and nonreligious imagery for the treatment of mild depression in religious individuals. *Cogn Ther Res.* 1980;4:167–178.

27. Engel GL. The need for a new medical model: a challenge for biomedicine. *Science.* 1977;196(4286):129–136.

28. Hefti R. *Unser Therapiekonzept.* Langenthal: Infomagazin; 2003.

29. Miller WR, Thoresen CE. Spirituality and health. In: Miller WR, ed. *Integrating Spirituality into Treatment: Resources for Practitioners.* Washington, DC: American Psychological Association; 1999.

30. Mulligan R, Mulligan T. The science of religion in health care. *Veterans Health Sys J.* 1994;55–57.

31. Richards PS, Bergin AE. Toward religious and spiritual competency for mental health professionals. In Richards R, Bergin A, eds. *Handbook of Psychotherapy and Religious Diversity.* Washington, DC: American Psychological Association; 2000:3–26.

32. Seybold K, Hill P. The role of religion and spirituality in mental and physical health. *Curr Dir Psychol Sci.* 2001;10(1):21–24.

33. Sullivan WP. Recoiling, regrouping, and recovering: first-person accounts of the role of spirituality in the course of serious mental illness. *New Dir Ment Health Serv* 1998;80:25–33.

34. Anthony WA. The principle of personhood: the field's transcendent principle. *Psychiatr Rehab J.* 2004;27:205.

35. Cosar B, Kocal N, Arikan Z, Isik E. Suicide attempts among Turkish psychiatric patients. *Can J Psychiatry.* 1997;42:1072–1075.

36. Mickley J, Carson V, Soeken L. Religion and adult mental health: state of the science in nursing. *Issues Ment Health Nurs.* 1995;16:345–360.

37. Bergin AE, Masters KS, Richards PS. Religiousness and mental health reconsidered: a study of an intrinsically religious sample. *J Counsel Psychol.* 1987;34(2):197–204.

38. Jahangir F. Third force therapy and its impact on treatment outcome. *In J Psychol Relig.* 1995;5:125–129.

39. Pardini D, Plante TG, Sherman A. Strength of religious faith and its association with mental health outcomes among recovering alcoholics and addicts. *J Subst Abuse Treat.* 2001;19:347–354.

40. Walsh J. The impact of schizophrenia on clients' religious beliefs: implications for families. *Fam Soc.* 1995;76:551–558.

41. MacGreen D. Spirituality as a coping resource. *Behav Therap.* 1997;20:28.

42. Fallot RD. Spirituality in trauma recovery. In: Harris M, ed. *Sexual Abuse in the Lives of Women Diagnosed with Serious Mental Illness.* Amsterdam: Harwood Academic Publishers; 1997:337–355.

43. Onken SJ, Dumont JM, Ridgway P, Dornan DH, Ralph RO. *Mental Health Recovery: What Helps and What Hinders?* Alexandria, VA: National Association of State Mental Health Program Directors; 2002.

44. Exline JJ, Yali AM, Lobel M. When God disappoints: difficulty forgiving God and its role in negative emotion. *J Health Psychol.* 1999;4(3):365–379.

45. Pargament K, Smith BW, Koenig HG, Perez L. Patterns of positive and negative religious coping with major life stressors. *J Sci Stud Relig.* 1998;37(4):710–724.

46. Exline JJ, Yali AM, Sanderson WC. Guilt, discord, and alienation: the role of religious strain in depression and suicidality. *J Clin Psychol.* 2000;56(12):1481–1496.

47. Bussema KE, Bussema EF. Is there a balm in Gilead? The implications of faith in coping with a psychiatric disability. *Psychiatr Rehab J.* 2000;24(2):117–124.

48. Exline JJ. Stumbling blocks on the religious road: fractured relationships, nagging vices, and the inner struggle to believe. *Psychol Inq.* 2002;13(3):182–189.

49. Mohr S, Brandt P-Y, Borras L, Gilliéron C, Huguelet P. Toward an integration of spirituality and religiousness into the psychosocial dimension of schizophrenia. *Am J Psychiatry.* 2006;163:1952–1959.

50. Huguelet P, Mohr S, Brandt P-Y, Borras L, Gillieron C. Spirituality and religious practices among outpatients with schizophrenia and their clinicians. *Psychiatr Serv.* 2006;57:366–372.

51. Längle A. The art of involving the person – fundamental existential motivations as the structure of the motivational process. *Eur Psychother.* 2003;4(1):25–36.

52. Schmidt T, Adami S. *Depression und Glaube – eine qualitative Studie an der Universität Freiburg.* Freiburg: Diplomarbeiten; 2008.

53. Rabins PV, Fitting MD, Eastham J. Emotional adaptation over time in caregivers of chronically ill elderly people. *Age Ageing.* 1990;19:185–190.

54. Chang BH, Noonan AE, Tennstedt SL. The role of religion/spirituality in coping with caregiving for disabled elders. *Gerontologist.* 1998;38:463–470.

55. Rammohan A, Rao K, Subbakrishna DK. Religious coping and psychological wellbeing in carers of relatives with schizophrenia. *Acta Psychiatr Scand.* 2002;105:356–362.

56. Johnson ED. Differences among families coping with serious mental illness: a qualitative analysis. *Am J Orthopsychiatry.* 2000;70:126–134.

57. Bland R, Darlington Y. The nature and sources of hope: perspectives of family caregivers of people with serious mental illness. *Perspect Psychiatr Care.* 2002;38:61–68.

58. Murray-Swank AB. Religiosity, psychosocial adjustment, and subjective burden of persons who care for those with mental illness. *Psychiatr Serv.* 2006;57:361–365.

59. Dossett E, Fuentes S, Klap R. Obstacles and opportunities in providing mental health services through a faith-based network in Los Angeles. *Psychiatr Serv.* 2005;56:206–208.

60. Pickett-Schenk SA. Church-based support groups for African-American families coping with mental illness: outreach and outcomes. *Psychosoc Rehab J.* 2002;26:173–180.

61. Cnaan RQA, Sinha JW, McGrew CC. Congregations as social service providers: services, capacity, culture and organizational behavior. *Admin Soc Work.* 2004;28:47–68.

62. Kehoe NC. A therapy group an spirituality issues for patients with chronic mental illness. *Psychiatr Serv* 1999;50:1081–1083.

63. Gallup G. *The Gallup Poll: Public Opinion.* Wilmington, DE: Scholarly Resources; 1994.

64. Bergin AE, Jensen JP. Religiosity of psychotherapists: a national survey. *Psychotherapy.* 1990;27:3–7.

65. Wong-McDonald A. Spirituality and psychosocial rehabilitation: empowering persons with serious psychiatric disabilities at an inner-city community program. *Psychiatr Rehab J.* 2007;30:295–300.

66. Reger G, Wong-McDonald A, Liberman R. Psychiatric rehabilitation in a community mental health center. *Psychiatr Serv.* 2003; 54(11):1457–1459.

67. Revheim N, Greenberg WM. Spirituality matters: creating a time and place for hope. *Psychiatr Rehab J.* 2007;30:307–310.

68. Phillips RS, Lakin R, Pargament K. Development and implementation of a spiritual issues psychoeducational group for those with serious mental illness. *Community Ment Health J.* 2002;38:487–496.

69. Weintraub SY. From the depths: Psalms as a spiritual reservoir in difficult times. In the outstretched arm. New York 1999: National Center for Jewish Healing of JBFCS (www.ncjh.org/downloads/Psalms).

70. Folkman S, Chesney M, McKusick L, Ironson G, Johnson DS, Coates TJ. Translation coping theory into an intervention. In: Eckenrode J, ed. *The Social Context of Coping.* New York: Plenum Press; 1991:70.

71. Emmons RA. *The Psychology of Ultimate Concerns.* New York: The Guilford Press; 1999.

72. Enright RD, Fitzgibbons RP. *Helping Clients Forgive. An Empirical Guide for Resolving Anger and Restoring Hope.* Washington, DC: APA; 2000.

73. Yahne CE, Miller WR. Evoking hope. In: Miller WR, ed. *Integrating Spirituality into Treatment.* Washington, DC: APA; 1999: 217–233.

74. Richards PS, Bergin AE. *A Spiritual Strategy for Counseling and Psychotherapy.* Washington, DC: APA; 1997.

75. O'Rourke C. Listening for the sacred: addressing spiritual issues in the group treatment of adults with mental illness. *Smith Coll Stud Soc Work.* 1997;67(2):177–196.

76. Benson H. *The Relaxation Response.* New York: Harper Torch Paperback; 2000.

77. Kutz I, Caudill M. The role of relaxation in behavioural therapies for chronic pain. *Int Anesthesiol Clin.* 1983;21(4):193–200.

78. Schaffer SD, Yucha CB. Relaxation and pain management: the relaxation response can play a role in managing chronic and acute pain. *Am J Nurs.* 2004;104(8):75–76, 78–79.

79. Nouwen HJ. *Canvas of Love – Reflections on a Rembrandt.* Freiburg: Verlag Herder; 1991.

80. Fallot RD. Spirituality and religion in recovery: some current issues. *Psychiatr Rehab J.* 2007;30(4):261–270.

81. D'Souza R. Do patients expect psychiatrists to be interested in spiritual issues? *Aust Psychiatry.* 2002;10(1):44–47.

82. Koenig HG. *Spirituality in Patient Care: Why, How, When and What.* Philadelphia: Templeton Foundation Press; 2002.

18 Explanatory Models of Mental Illness and Its Treatment

LAURENCE BORRAS AND PHILIPPE HUGUELET

SUMMARY

Despite overwhelming evidence that psycho-pharmacology is effective in the acute treatment and maintenance therapy of psychiatric disorders, 40 to 60 percent of patients do not take their medication and thus are at increased risk for relapse. Episodes due to nonadherence have negative consequences for both the patient (by lowering quality of life and treatment outcome) and society (by increasing costs). "How to find a cure?" is a question that these suffering people ask themselves, especially when medicine does not heal, or when one is facing a chronic disease. Many psychiatric therapies and mutual aid groups have their foundations in different religions and still use values, concepts, and therapeutic methods that have their origins in religious beliefs and practices. However, there are many people who resort to alternative therapies, over-the-counter products, and traditional approaches to healing. In this chapter, we will describe the treatment of mental disorders across history and according to various cultural settings. Then we will describe how religion may influence patients' perceptions of illness and its treatment. The positive and negative impacts of spirituality on the outcome of illness and adherence to treatment will be discussed. This will lead to considerations as to how clinicians should address these issues.

Many people with chronic mental disorder are in search of healing, living a deep identity crisis caused by their increasing marginalization. Understanding the individual's point of view by taking into account the biological, psychological, and social dimensions is essential, because it enables a better understanding of our patients and their pathologies. When referring to "social dimension," we mean culture in its broadest sense as well as the religion and spirituality that usually come along with it.

"Where to find a cure?" This is the question that most suffering people ask themselves, especially when medicine fails to heal or when some chronic disease takes hold of the individual. Many psychiatric therapies and support groups inspired by various religions promote values, concepts, and therapeutic methods that have their origins in religious beliefs and practices. In spite of this, many people continue to prefer alternative therapies. Do patients' spiritual and religious beliefs influence the understanding they have of their disorder? To what extent do religious beliefs about illness influence their understanding of the treatment and the relationship with the medical staff? Would it be possible to improve the patient-doctor relationship by taking into account the patient's religious beliefs? And if so, how?

In this chapter, we will attempt to describe the different understandings of mental disorders throughout history and according to various cultural settings. Then we will describe how these perspectives may influence patients' understanding of their disorders and treatments. This will lead to considerations of how clinicians should approach this issue.

1. MENTAL DISORDERS THROUGHOUT THE CENTURIES

A brief look into history will allow us to better understand the great number of theoretical perspectives on mental disorders that have preoccupied humanity since the beginning of time. Indeed, in every culture and at all times, the understanding of mental disorders, their treatment, and healing had their foundation in religion. In prehistory, illness, suffering, and death were probably already being interpreted in supernatural and magical terms. Therapy and healing were left to shamans and healers who, thanks to their privileged relationship with their gods, were thought to be able to cure madness and help people escape evil forces by using religious and magical rites (incantation, herbs, and physical therapy).(1)

During antiquity, while Pythagoras, Hippocrates, and Plato were laying the foundations for disease-based psychiatry, ordinary people would continue to associate medicine with magical practices and religion. Mental disorders were perceived as impurity, so healing and salvation were left to priests.(2)

During the Middle Ages, religious and the medical approaches to mental disorders coexisted. From a religious viewpoint, some patients suffering from mental disorders were considered to be possessed by demons. People suffering from psychosis often thought they were "possessed by the devil," to the point that they would proclaim it themselves. Therefore, rather than going to the doctor, would entrust their illness to the saints, who were thought to have the divine power to chase away the demons. Thus, people suffering from psychosis often found shelter in monasteries.(3)

In terms of health services provided to patients with mental disorders, the Renaissance was a mere prolongation of the Middle Ages, but it also marked the epoch of the first great humanist doctors. One of them, Jean Wier (1515–1588), of Belgian origin, defended the medical thesis of mental disorders and strongly rejected the satanic theory, protesting against "the practice of burning mad people at the stake."(4)

During the seventeenth and eighteenth centuries, the religious perspective on diseases continued to prevail. People believed that diseases were sent by God as a warning or a punishment and that they were meant to guide the spirit to its salvation. So a good Christian was expected to endure disease with patience and even with joy. Doctors and priests jointly took care of the patient; in addition, the doctor even had the duty to make sure that the patient confessed his sins. In 1712, according to a royal declaration, doctors could not visit severely ill patients more than three times, unless the patient provided his confession certificate. The priest himself had a therapeutic role. Beside its spiritual effects, the administration of the unction sacrament was thought to help restore the body's health.(5)

Along with the nineteenth century came the emergence of psychiatry and the classification of mental disorders. General psychopathology, psychoanalysis, phenomenology, biologic psychiatry, and sociocultural approaches also developed. However, the major schools of thought as well as the understandings of the disease and its treatment remained influenced by various religious and sociocultural factors.(4)

2. THE SOCIAL UNDERSTANDINGS OF DISEASE

Mental disorders are explained and studied via a medical discourse based on classification. However, mental disorders are definitely more than a mere medical inventory based on scientific research.

They actually point to a complex reality: For society and for social actors, disease is synonymous with sorrow or with an event threatening to disrupt one's personal life, social status, and meaning of life in general.(6) Suffering people tend to build their understanding of the disease according to social constructions collectively elaborated, which cannot be reduced to mere institutional or medical definitions. These understandings include religious, collective, existential, emotional, and sentimental dimensions. Hence, diseases can be described better by including the individual dimension in terms of severity, prognosis, and treatment options.(7)

Medical anthropology distinguishes among three realities under different words, defining health problems as biological abnormalities (disease), subjective experience of altered physical state (illness), and the process of socialization of pathological episodes (sickness).(8) Even though they belong to the same culture in its broad sense, doctors and patients have different visions of medicine and the way diseases affect individuals. Thus, when the doctor and the patient meet, there are actually two cultural and spiritual perspectives to reconcile through communication, confrontation, and sometimes even negotiation: the doctor's (disease) and the sick person's (illness). Unfortunately, medicine often has a selective approach to the patient's experience. The "key" symptoms enumerated by the *Diagnostic and Statistical Manual of Mental Disorders, Fourth Edition* (*DSM-IV*) (9) are considered to be more "real," more significant, and more interesting than the way in which patients perceive what they are going through. Doctors tend to create an objective reality of the disease based on causes, symptoms, and evolution, and they often try to impose it on patients via diagnosis. They very rarely ask patients questions about their own understanding of the disease.

On the other hand, patients develop a personal and therefore subjective experience (illness), mixing symptoms, emotional reactions, and impulsive interpretations of the disorders. Patients also try to find an explanation for their situation. They ask themselves questions such as, "Why do I deserve this?" In some cultures they ask, "Who wants to harm me?" The pattern serving as an interpretation grid for the disease is often included in a larger model, which attempts to explain feelings of unhappiness, misfortune, and adversity.(10) These three competing perspectives toward the disease are not always clearly distinguishable, and illness, sickness, and disease actually have more than one point in common. For instance, the subjective perception of the disorder (illness) is built mainly on social understandings (one of the sickness aspects), but also on biomedical understandings as conveyed by the media (bridge between illness and disease). These are not always clearly distinct from the popular understandings of the disorder (bridge between disease and illness).(8)

Herzlich (1969), a French sociologist, identified three types of understandings of illness, resulting from the integration of medical and profane knowledge. Illness is "destructive" when it entails the breaking of social bonds, as well as the loss of one's social role and ability to perform activities, which lead the patient to social exclusion. In this case, illness is interpreted in a fatalistic manner. Illness can be "cathartic" when it offers the individual the possibility to escape a social role perceived as suffocating, unbearable. Illness is therefore seen as an opportunity to give a new meaning to one's life. When really severe, illness can be experienced as a "profession": The professional activity of the individual is being replaced by a daily combat against the disease, which becomes the central focus of one's existence.(11) It is only natural to assume that the type of understanding patients have of their illness will deeply influence its evolution and the patients' views of the recommended treatment. Very often, doctor and patient have completely different interpretations of the disease. This can explain why sometimes patients leave the hospital for apparently no reason, and they turn to alternative medicine or healers or become noncompliant with treatment. In this respect, the ethno psychiatrist Jean Benoist (1996) said, "Once set in, the disease, starts growing its own double which is to be imagined as a subtle representation of itself, yet as persistent as the pain caused by the sick organ."(12)

A study led in Germany in 1992 by Gernd Mutz and Irène Künhlein indicated the different ways in which patients could combine the knowledge imparted by the doctor and their own knowledge to reshape their understanding of the disease. Patients tend to be quite selective in what they learn from their doctor. This information is used to fill in gaps in their previous knowledge and to normalize at a higher level the understanding they have of their disease. As for the rest, they would simply stick to their daily and traditional interpretations of the disease.(13)

Also, the patients' understanding is multifaceted and dynamic. Indeed, patients change their understandings quite rapidly, and sometimes they can use several explanatory models at the same time, under the influence of the events taking place in their lives and of the changing society they live in.(14) Williams compared several explanatory models of depression among three categories of population: the general community, people in the process of being diagnosed with depression, and people who already had an established diagnosis of depression. These three populations had different understandings of the disorder and of its treatment. These perspectives may evolve differently as illness is taking hold of the patient. Indeed, community surveys in Western societies tend to point to an explanatory model of mental health problems that is primarily social rather than biological.(15–17) On the other hand, most people today diagnosed with depression tend to consider it biological.(18) Perceptions of cause are also reflected in beliefs about the appropriateness of particular treatments. Out of a healthy community, less than 25 percent of the patients (16, 17) might benefit from an antidepressant treatment and more than half of them from talking therapies (16) whereas for more than two-thirds of the people diagnosed with depression, antidepressant treatment is necessary.(19) The data suggest therefore that a reformulation of beliefs and a transition in therapeutic perspectives may take place among people who develop mental disorders. Some researchers suggest that in the early stages of the mental disorder, there is a moment when change is most likely to take place. Indeed, Leventhal and Nerenz (1985) have suggested that when an individual faces a problematic psychological or physiological experience (or simply changes states), he will construct an understanding of

the problem based on five dimensions. These are identity (label), perceived cause, time line (how long it will last), consequences (physical, psychological, and social), and curability/controllability.(20) Such understandings may draw on explanatory models of diseases specific to the various cultures and societies. Those people facing a mental health problem for the first time in their life actively attempt to make sense of it. In doing so, individuals may explore and choose between a complex set of beliefs. However, such beliefs should not be regarded as taking the form of a coherent explanatory model but rather as a map of possibilities, providing a framework for the ongoing process of making sense and seeking meaning.

3. MENTAL DISORDERS IN DEVELOPING COUNTRIES

Clinicians meet patients with mental disorders who are embedded into various cultural/religious backgrounds. In many developing countries, there is a different approach to the understanding of the disease, as compared to that found in developed areas. In larger cities, we are increasingly dealing with patients belonging to migrant populations. In this context, it is important for the clinician to understand the perception patients have of their own disorder and to be aware of elements of their culture such as the understandings of disease, the body, and indigenous healing systems. Compared with Western societies, people in developing countries seem to attach more importance to the symbolic and spiritual side of the illness.(21) Empirical knowledge of the disease is influenced by a quasicompulsive search of the reason for the disease (the meaning of the disease). Generally speaking, the mental disease is not the result of a situation involving individuals in their personal organization. The environment, which historically helps determine the sick person's personality, is not concerned with the origin of the disease. Disease comes from somewhere else. Irrespective of ethnic groups or religious systems, mental disorders are considered to be the result of an aggression against the sick person or against the group to which this person belongs. Social changes brought by modernism or by imported religions (Islam and Christianity) have not always affected this primary model. Even if, according to their social origin, people may sometimes refer to a "vague" notion of "illness caused by a natural cause," the understandings of this attack are always very dynamic and are shared by the sick person, his or her entourage, and the healers. These modalities of understanding can be schematically reduced to two possibilities: the individual is being attacked by another individual or he is attacked by a spirit that is understood as a real creature and that is most often produced by the religious system.(22) In Africa, for instance, the attack by an individual is essentially set up according to two systems: anthropophagic-witchcraft and maraboutage. The attack by "spirits" is referred to in indigenous religions, as well as in imported religions. These explanations of mental disorders are found in most African societies.

Designations may differ, indeed, but what is important and constant in the understandings of diseases is the association of their causes with some attackers recognized by everybody. These models of understanding of mental diseases attempt to explain the phenomenon and to situate it in a familiar framework of categories, but it still opposes the biological explanation of the disease.(23) It follows that the sick person carries a message (the disease), which needs to be decoded and integrated into the symbolic language of the culture, a language shared by the individuals of the same social group.(24)

4. CONTAINING THE FLOOD OF UNDERSTANDINGS

The different representations of the disease as they are developed by patients may influence simultaneously or in turn the treatment choices. The logic of these choices can result from a combination of several signification areas, corresponding to the various ways of expressing pain. In developing countries, indigenous healers, religious therapists (priests and healing

prophets), doctors, or nurses are the "signification carriers."(25) Traditional therapists are the protagonists of traditional medicine. For them, "madness" may be seen as a sign that the family has deviated from cultural norms or as a form of harm instigated by some jealous third party, but it may also be understood as a form of social justice or a mere physical problem.(26, 27) They provide health care by using methods based on both religious and sociocultural foundations as well as on knowledge, behavior, and beliefs related to physical and mental well-being and to the etiology of disease and disabilities prevailing in the community.(28) In Africa, for instance, more than half of the population appeals to traditional therapists for health problems.(25) Their etiotherapeutic understanding of the disease is essentially of a magical-religious nature, and they share the same beliefs with their religious therapists as a basis for the healing process. Religious therapists are those who claim to be able to heal via the word of God and in his name. They attribute "madness" to the evil influence of Satan or of Jinnh.(26) There are two types of religious therapists: priests and healing prophets. For the first, healing is not immediate because it is considered in terms of hope; for the latter, healing is an end in itself. Being confronted with populations for whom healing is a process combining both supernatural elements of faith and medical elements, society entrusted priests with a therapeutic role. This repositioning of priests was accompanied by the birth of new practices with therapeutic purpose, with new names such as the "independent churches" and the "charismatic prayer groups." Interventions include prayers for deliverance and counseling.(29)

Doctors and nurses are trained in medical institutions and act according to a biomedical conception of the disease. They are official health professionals, unlike the indigenous and religious therapists, who are considered to be nonofficial practitioners.(30, 31) Anthropologists such as Helman or Good consider them to be the representatives of a distinct medical culture, which is the biomedical culture, taking into account not only the biological aspects, but also the scientific rationality.(32, 33) A study carried out by Wamba in Cameroon in 2005 (25) explored the impact of the coexistence of different interpretive models on the behavior of patients seeking health care as well as on the practitioners' conduct. On the one hand, some patients prefer religious therapists, who combine in their healing method both indigenous and religious means of healing. On the other hand, some patients would rather see indigenous healers, who work according to ancestral beliefs using medicinal plants. Other patients prefer to go to missionary hospitals because of the biomedical and religious therapy they provide (missionary priests practicing as nurses and doctors). In this list, secular allopathic hospitals are the last option, only when biological assessments and treatments are needed. Patients switch from one understanding of their illness to another, according to their personal history and to the evolution of the disease. Therapists are introduced to new systems of meaning made of elements selected from several levels of signification, which have a major impact on their daily practice. Indeed, some traditional therapists are now aware of the limits of their knowledge and feel they need additional medical training. Doctors want to continue practicing medicine by adapting their methods to the social mutations in terms of medical and sociocultural crossbreeding. They want to improve their knowledge of elementary medicine in their attempt to slow down the migration of patients from countryside to cities. Priests too are trying to enhance their medical knowledge and to adjust Christian healing practices to established religions. Bilu and Witztum (34) report their experience in Jerusalem with ultra-orthodox Jewish patients who were severely ill and spoke about the epistemological gap between the medical reality of mental health practitioners and the sacred reality of the patients. These patients turn to the mental health clinic as the very last resort, that is, after having attempted – and failed – to employ religious healing. Patients try to incorporate

religiously congruent elements composed of metaphoric images, narratives, and actions into the secular treatment modalities that they seek. The authors found that medications such as antipsychotics, initially ineffective, turned out to be quite potent when accompanied by a religiously informed intervention.

Khan and Pillay (35) reported that South Asian patients with schizophrenia living in the United Kingdom preferred home care because they wanted to continue practicing their faith and to have the possibility to add faith healing to their psychiatric treatment. The authors explain these motivations in terms of will to maintain their cultural identity (an important component of recovery), but also as a way to get a more holistic treatment. In Uganda, Africa, Teuton et al.(26) investigated qualitatively the conceptualization of "madness" across indigenous, religious, and "allopathic" healers and examined the relationships between service providers involved in the treatment of people with "psychosis." For indigenous healers, madness is a sign of a deviation, a form of harm instigated by some jealous party. Religious healers attribute it to the evil influence of Satan. Allopathic healers (that is, psychiatrists and specialized nurses) have fewer resources and provide services limited to psychotropic medication. The indigenous and religious healers had a rather tolerant attitude toward allopathic medicine, although religious healers often attributed its success to the Christian or Islamic influence. Unlike them, allopathic healers made little reference to religious healers and were ambivalent toward indigenous healers. Finally, the relationship between the religious and indigenous healers emerged as one characterized by conflict. Religious healers rejected the beliefs and methods of indigenous healers, whereas the latter regarded indigenous spirituality and evangelical Christianity as incompatible with their system. All the studies mentioned above underlined the necessity to improve dialogue between indigenous and religious healers and allopathic doctors to develop an integrative model of health care intended for individuals with mental disorders.

5. ALTERNATIVE THERAPY USE BY PATIENTS WITH MENTAL DISORDERS

In Western societies, patients feeling that their understanding of the disease and their personal perception of being ill are not properly understood have many different reactions, and we, as doctors, have to deal with them. Classical medicine defines diseases as a general or local failure within a complicated system of a physical and chemical nature. The spiritual factors related to health conditions are generally left out of this interpretation. Given this context, it is only natural for the patient to turn toward alternative and complementary medicine. A survey published in 2002 in the United States stated that 36 percent of the population resorts to "alternative and complementary medicine."(36) Chinese and ayurvedic medicine, acupuncture, meditation, hypnosis, tai chi, qi gong, chiropractics, praying, and spiritual healing are among the many practices that generate several billion dollars per year, which patients spend without hesitation and without any financial support. This is true for most Western countries because, according to surveys, the number of consumers seeking alternative health services varies between 20 percent and 50 percent, or even 65 percent in Japan.(37, 38) Chronic mental disorders represent a major reason why patients turn toward alternative therapies.(39) This is in response to their lack of satisfaction with conventional therapies, their desire to seek control over their health-care decisions, and their desire to include their philosophical values and religious beliefs in these therapies.(40, 41) Several studies revealed that health professionals tend to underestimate the extent to which patients turn to such therapies, which, in some cases, may worsen medical compliance and interaction.(42) On the other hand, as shown earlier, more and more general practitioners have been willing to entertain the idea of spiritual healing and include it in their daily practice or referral network. They have understood that recognizing patients' beliefs in the face of suffering is an important factor in health-care practice. The counseling methods incorporated in these medical approaches emphasize the person's concept of God, his or her sources of strength and hope, and the significance of religious practices and rituals for that person.(43) Twenty-five percent of the medical practitioners in the United Kingdom, 50 percent in Canada, and 80 percent in Victoria, Australia, regularly refer their patients to complementary medicine practitioners. In Victoria, 20 percent resorted to meditation, 5 percent to prayer, and 50 percent expressed their intention to attend training programs. A significant number of health professionals in the United States actually pray with their patients, because praying is recognized as an efficient coping strategy.(42) The treatment of alcoholism has historically included spiritual considerations.(44) Such treatments for alcohol abuse were often a composite of physical methods of relaxation, psychological methods of suggestion and autosuggestion, social methods of group support and service to the community, and spiritual techniques of prayer. Such procedures are still in use today and have been extended into the realm of chemical dependency and drug abuse.(45) Spiritual healing groups increase in number every day. In some regions of the world, they have organized themselves into confederations to practice in hospitals and take referrals from physicians. Their code of conduct covers legal obligations and emphasizes full cooperation with medical authorities.(46) Spiritual healing is practiced throughout Western Europe and the United States and occurs in two different ways. The first involves hands-on contact or near contact between the healer and the patient, similar to the church ritual of the laying on of hands. The second is distant healing, where a healer or group of healers pray or meditate for the absent patient.

There are various explanations for how spiritual healing works, including metaphysical, magnetic, psychological, and social. Most spiritual healers maintain there are divine energies that are transferred from the spiritual level by the healer and that produce a beneficial effect on the energy field of the patient. The notion of the energy field is a source of disagreement between orthodox researchers and spiritual healers.(46) Researchers argue that, if such a field exists, then it should be possible to measure it by physical means. However, the explanation of the energy field is as yet unsubstantiated by scientific research. Although spiritual healing is often dismissed as a placebo response, some studies claim there is a direct influence.(47, 48)

For the patient, it is vital to make sense of the experience when confronted with illness. There is a need to search for meaning in the face of chaos, loss, hopelessness, and suffering. New efforts for lay involvement in medicine and in the church and a call for spiritual (or holistic) understanding of illness are the expressions of individual calls for such meaning according to patient beliefs. Alternative therapies such as spiritual healing appear to be of particular benefit when requested by the patient. Recognizing a patient's beliefs and facilitating the practice of health that takes into account those beliefs appears to be an important initiative in the management of suffering and loss.(46)

6. EXPERIENCES OF PATIENTS IN RELATION TO THE SPIRITUAL ASPECTS OF BEING ILL

The experience that patients have of being ill strongly depends on one's personal understanding of the illness. Spiritual aspects are of vital importance to patients when they are dealing with their illness and their relationships, when they are making decisions and facing their loss due to illness, and when they are complying with their treatment. Spirituality may, in some cases, have a negative effect on the normal functioning of a person.(49, 50)

6.1. Religious Beliefs and Views on Life

Based on research by our group, we have found that themes according to religious beliefs and views on life can be both positive and negative and can influence or be influenced by the conceptualization of the illness and its prognosis. Positive influences are manifested in the sense that some of the patients during illness and treatment were trusting in God, believed

in miracles, and found strength in themselves, their faith, and nature.(50) A patient said, "What I read in the bible gave me lot of faith and rest. Yes, I could leave it in Gods hands easily. It has deepened my faith; my illness has enriched my life." Another patient said, "You have to pray and give it to God. He will take care of it." To the contrary, some patients talked about faith and their view of life in a negative way by saying that they were angry at God or could no longer draw any strength from their faith. A patient said, "I am not religious any more. I stepped out. I am angry with God because he sent me illness and pain."(50)

6.2. Goal in Life and Life Balance

Confrontation with their own vulnerability influences the patients' balance of life. Some of the patients experienced the illness as an experience of loss, because they could not go on living as they did before the illness. They were confronted with their own limitations. A patient said, "This disease makes me lose my abilities to resist and it is God who sent it to me perhaps in order to punish me for something I did."(50) Some patients experienced their situation as a fate, in which they could find rest or in which they could give their illness a place in their life. "Everybody gets his turn. Everyone has his own cross to bear. Everyone gets it in his own way on his own time. Let's make something of it."(49)

6.3 Humility

By confronting a severe disease, the patient becomes more aware of his personal history. A patient said, "Before, I was very full of myself. I felt I was the most beautiful and I would always outdo the others. This illness has turned me into a more humble person and has made me meditate upon what is really important in life and for me."(50) Patients said they were looking back on their life more and made up a kind of balance. Some of them took hope and strength out of earlier difficult life experiences that helped them to fight against this setback now.(49)

6.4. Courage, Hope, and Growth

"Acceptance" and "letting go" were important themes. It entails the belief that patients can give meaning to their disease, surrender themselves to the new situation, and seek new perspectives in life. The way in which patients handle this new situation differs for every person. Some patients could accept their situation easily, while others had more difficulty with it or could not accept it at all (at the moment). A patient said, "I have accepted my illness. I think God sent it to me in order to make me able to encourage the other persons suffering from the same disease."(50)

6.5. Guilt

When people are affected by a disease for a significant amount of time, they usually develop a subjective explanation for its causes. During our clinical practice, we have often been struck by the importance of guilt in some severely ill patients. In others, we noticed the will to understand. "Why is this happening to me? Have I done something wrong or bad? Am I a victim of someone or of something? Who is responsible for it?" The answers to these questions, taking into account the subjective explanation, are very important in the process of dealing with the disease. Patients' lack of understanding or guilt adds to the suffering just as much as their feeling that they are a victim of a more or less identified enemy. In response to this understanding, many dioceses in Europe have to set up exorcising teams to expel the enemy. This phenomenon clearly shows that, in Western cultures, the notion that disease is caused by an enemy is increasingly gaining ground. Mental health therapists are being asked for meaning and sometimes even for salvation. Spiritual leaders or praying groups are being asked for therapeutic services, while patients are dominated by guilt. In most cases, this is due to our religious education. It is also worth noting that certain pathologies, such as the obsessive-compulsive disorder or melancholia, have a higher incidence in religious countries, especially in Muslim and ultra-orthodox

Jewish cultures of the Middle East countries, where cultural identity and religious identity are inseparable.(51) Given these facts, the medical practitioner may find it useful to have some information about the understanding of illness that major religions of the world have.

6.6. Spiritual Understandings of Disease

As shown, the patient's understanding of illness can be influenced by religious beliefs.(52) Pargament describes four religious methods of coping to find meaning in negative events such as an illness. First, patients can define illness through religion as benevolent and potentially beneficial. The disease will then be considered as an ordeal sent by God or as a divine plan designed to turn the patient into a stronger person or to convey a message. It may also aim at activating the patient's spirituality or at making suffering acceptable. Second, patients can define the illness as a punishment from God for one's sins. Third, the illness can be defined as an act of the devil. Fourth, the patient redefines God's power to influence the stressful situation that can be a mental illness. A patient said, "I realized that God cannot answer all my prayers." At the beginning, patients may have a negative representation of their illness but in time, they may also start a dynamic process of coping with it positively by integrating it constructively. A 48-year-old patient suffering from schizophrenia said, "My illness was sent by the Devil; but I'm struggling to overcome it, to make Good win against Evil and I know that God is on my side in this struggle."(50) In some rare cases, the patient will reintegrate the illness in a negative manner by feeling guilty and being pessimistic about the prognosis. A patient said, "My illness is a punishment for my sins, I deserve it and I must endure it."(50) Yet it is quite rare that patients take a punishing God into account in their understanding of their illness. Most patients have a positive religious interpretation of their condition and feel guilty for what they go through without blaming God or others.(53) Patients' understanding of illness also has an impact on their acceptance of the recommended therapy and on the prognosis of the disease in addition to influencing their coping with its symptoms. Several studies have shown that there is a negative correlation between a negative representation of illness and the acceptance of the recommended therapy.(52, 54, 55)

6.7. Religious Delirium

In our research study, six to 10 percent of the patients with psychosis presented manifestations such as delusions or religious hallucinations, which obviously can influence the patients' understanding of their psychological processes and their understanding of illness and treatment. Some of these manifestations may be aggressive and lead to feelings of guilt, thus being a discouraging factor that can negatively influence the prognosis of the disease. A 30-year-old patient suffering from paranoid schizophrenia said, "I am transparent; everybody knows my thoughts, my feelings and my dreams. God wants to kill me; He wants to kill my soul. Everybody knows that God is planning to assassinate me. They're talking about it on the TV and on the radio too. I have tried to kill myself twice, but now I have given up, God will do it for me anyway."(52) Other manifestations of this kind may have a positive impact on the patients' coping with their illness. A 40-year-old patient suffering from paranoid schizophrenia said, "My illness opened my mind to spirituality. I do not talk about it to psychiatrists since they do not believe me. Before I received medication, I heard voices. Once I took refuge in a church, I prayed to the Virgin Mary and the voices felt silent. Since that day, she had protected me. Sometimes she appears to me; it is not a hallucination."(52)

6.8. Spiritual Understanding of Treatment

The understanding of medical treatment may also be influenced by religious beliefs. As shown earlier in this chapter, certain patients may consider medical treatment and psychotherapy as a divine gift intended to cure the disease. God is thus enlightening humans, whereas doctors are perceived as God's instrument. Thus, the recommended treatment will be more easily accepted. For others, treatment related to religious beliefs may be seen as destructive, being often perceived as a foreign body or as poison or even as a straitjacket. What they are trying to highlight is that the recommended treatment and their religious beliefs are not compatible. A patient said, "Only God can control people's thoughts. Doctors and drugs cannot do that." Another patient said, "People are the way they are because God wanted them to be this way, so we shouldn't try to change this through medication. Another said, "God thinks that this is not necessary." Some patients seek spiritual healing only, as often dictated by their religious leader. Other patients emphasize the incompatibility between what is being transmitted to them during psychotherapy sessions and their religious education. Taking care of oneself and learning to say no and to aspire toward self-accomplishment may enter into conflict with certain religious teachings. These teachings often encourage service to others and the community and the subordination of one's personal needs. Suffering and benevolence may be perceived as salutary.(54)

7. RELIGION AND MEDICAL TREATMENT: INTERFERENCE OR MUTUAL BENEFIT?

Over the last forty years, several articles highlighted the relationship between spirituality and understandings of illness. They also emphasized the need to take spirituality into account in the development of health-care services, especially aiming at improving the acceptance of the recommended therapy by the patient and the medical relationship with the patient. This issue was closely looked at in research studies concerning patients suffering from severe chronic somatic diseases (56–60) and patients with unipolar or bipolar mood disorders,(55) schizophrenia,(54) or substance addiction.(61) In most cases, a positive impact of religious beliefs on adherence to the treatment was reported, which facilitated the current integration of a spiritual approach into many health-care services. This positive impact also contributed to patients' improvement of their quality of life as well as to a more active social support and a more positive understanding of the disease in religious patients. Nevertheless, religious beliefs may interfere negatively with certain aspects of the treatment in several ways, for example, when the patient seeks spiritual healing only, when patients associate feelings of guilt with their religious understanding of the illness or of the treatment, or when there is incompatibility between religious education and psychotherapy. A study by Borras et al.(54) highlighted the fact that 57 percent of patients suffering from schizophrenia have an understanding of illness and treatment influenced by their religious convictions: positively in 31 percent ("test sent by God to put them on the right path," "a gift from God or God's plan") and negatively in 26 percent ("punishment of God, a demon, the devil, or possession"). The other 43 percent largely adhered to a medical understanding of disease and spoke about their condition in terms of genetic fragility or vulnerability. It is the patients rejecting the recommended treatment who generally develop a spiritual representation of their illness, whereas patients who accept treatment tend to favor a biological understanding of their suffering. Moreover, a third of nonadherent patients underlined an incompatibility between their religious convictions and medication and supportive therapy. Some patients reported to the evaluator that medical treatment or recommended behavior encouraged by the psychiatrist may enter into conflict with certain religious teachings of various religious groups. Certain religious groups promote spiritual healing exclusively. It is also worth noting that, in this study, the understanding of illness and the possible incompatibility between religious convictions and treatments were addressed in less than 20 percent of the cases, most of the medical practitioners having a tendency to overlook or underestimate the importance of their patients' spiritual dimension. The drug-addicted patients included in a methadone maintenance treatment program mention spirituality as a predictor for adherence to the treatment, spirituality being

thus a source of strength and self protection as well as a source of altruism and protection of the others. They highlighted the importance of taking into account this dimension in the recommended therapy, which represents an incentive to avoid risky sexual behavior while observing more closely the medical recommendations and growing hope for recovery.(61, 62) A study conducted on patients with bipolar disorders highlighted the importance of exploring the patients' understanding of their illness and of the treatment to observe, because they may be influenced by their religious convictions, with a direct impact on their observance of the treatment. Thirty percent of the patients with bipolar disorders actually connect illness to spirituality and 32 percent of them reported difficulties in reconciling their religious faith with the treatment recommended by the doctors. In such cases, interference of a spiritual leader against medical treatment may be suspected, along with an underlying desire to seek spiritual healing only. This may become an anxiety-producing dilemma for the patient.(55)

Concerning somatic and neuropsychiatry diseases, a review of literature analyzed twenty-seven studies addressing spiritual beliefs that could influence the treatment preferences of African Americans throughout the course of illness. The most frequently cited theme was the importance of spiritual beliefs and practices, particularly prayer, in coping with illness, a strategy of "turning it over to the Lord." Another frequently cited theme was the power of spiritual beliefs to promote healing: Many studies highlight the idea that prayer is the most helpful intervention, including medication. It was also mentioned as the most important help in their medication decisions. A third theme was the belief that God is ultimately responsible for physical and spiritual health: God's will appears to be the most important factor in recovery. The belief in miracles and faith healing as well as the preference to attend faith healing services rather than psychiatric therapy are obvious consequences of this. A final theme was the belief that the physician is God's "instrument" in promoting healing and that God acts through doctors to cure the disease. All these themes describing spiritual beliefs that may influence treatment throughout the course of illness seem to be more present in African American than Caucasian patients.(63) Pfeifer (64) pointed out that in Switzerland, 38 percent of the patients associate their psychological disorder with the fact of being possessed by an evil force, whereas 80 percent sought deliverance through prayers and exorcism. In most cases, these practices of spiritual healing are perceived as a positive experience that allowed these people to overcome their anguish and accept psychiatric treatment, as encouraged by their spiritual leaders. In some rare cases, these practices excluded other forms of treatment completely and induced feelings of distress, guilt, fear, isolation, and even psychotic decompensation, which needed hospitalization. Wilson (65) describes similar experiences of spiritual healing contributing to allaying anguish and violent behavior, but he also mentions a few cases of aggravation of the symptoms. In the same line, some authors (66) have described "possession" cases with dramatic outcome, due to the patient's rejection of neuroleptic medication. Thus, it is not the belief in a demonic origin of the disease that causes trouble, but rather the distress and the rejection of psychiatric treatment induced, in some patients, by their religious practices, as it is the case for certain sects.(67, 68)

A study of McCabe and Priebe (69) exploring explanatory models of disease in four different cultural frameworks highlighted the finding that white people are more likely to have a biological explanatory model, as compared to African-Caribbean, West Africans, and Bangladeshis, who are more likely to have a social or supernatural explanatory model. Having a biological explanatory model, especially compared with a social explanatory model, is linked with greater treatment satisfaction and better therapeutic relationships. People who cited supernatural causes for their disease were less open (that is, less likely to accept that they had a mental disorder) and therefore less compliant with treatment. A study by Saravanan et al. (70) assessing the explanatory models of psychosis in South India showed that patients' views of schizophrenia do not concur

with prevailing professional ideas, and this may be a source of conflict. Seventy percent of patients attributed schizophrenia to spiritual and mystical factors, whereas social and biological causes accounted for less than 20 percent of the overall attributed causes. The most individual folk causes reported are "black magic" and "evil spirits." Spiritual/mystical and social causal models were both associated with visits to indigenous healers. Thirty-five percent of patients held more than one treatment model for their psychosis, for example, "People may not improve with medications, so we go to the temple to pray for them." All these articles highlighted the importance of communication with patients regarding their representation of disease and treatment. On the one hand, this would help increase therapeutic trust as well as the patients' resources; on the other hand, it could help overcome the obstacles in the healing process.

8. CONCLUSION: THE ROLE OF THE MEDICAL PRACTITIONER

Given the vulnerability and the anguish that may be generated by mental disorders, therapists should feel concerned about the meaning of the disease to the patient, because it dramatically influences the therapeutic relationship as well as the healing process. The aim is to understand the religious (or nonreligious) and cultural understandings of the patient's disease. Unfortunately, in psychiatry, when patients talk about strange perspectives or understandings unknown by the doctor, the latter tends to overlook the meaning given by the patient to what he is experiencing. Even worse, the patient's account of the situation may be perceived as irrational or inconsistent because it refers to things that disturb the doctor. The doctor also may ignore the patient's account because it is dissimilar to his own belief pattern. A study by Hilton et al. (71) based on the observations of the physicians in an acute mental health unit for older people, showed that religious beliefs were only discussed with patients who had psychotic symptoms that had a religious content. Yet it is essential that the clinician is responsive to the patient's understandings of illness. Empirical evidence suggests that patients are more satisfied when their psychiatrist shares their model of understanding distress and treatment.(72) It has also been shown that patients are not less observant toward a clinician of a different culture.(73, 74) The success of strategies aimed at controlling the disease does not depend as much on the efficiency of the medical prescriptions (for example, medicines and traditional remedies) as much as it depends on the way the prescriptions are being prescribed and on the meaning attributed by the patient to the therapeutic process.(75) The clinician acts as a mirror, being simultaneously the recipient of the laments and the source of medical recommendations, of psychotherapeutic treatment and even of rituals. The clinician is also a mirror to himself because he has to ponder his own role as a specialist prescribing conduct and meaning, while realizing that his own sociocultural and religious heritage affects the therapy he recommends. The clinician must also take into account the therapeutic evolution of the patient, whose representations of the disease and its treatment may change, and along with them the patient's choices in terms of therapeutic solutions. Instead of calling these oscillations a therapeutic mistake, the clinician should remain open to the patients and join them in trying to understand the new interpretations determined by a set of complementary circumstances and explanations. When the clinician deals with a patient of a different origin or religion, it is interesting to have access to the elements specific to the patient's culture such as the representation of the disease, the body, and the healing system of his or her tradition to be able to adopt the most appropriate strategy and the best way to attend to the patient. It would be actually a good initiative to provide clinicians with an introduction to the general aspects of the culture of the immigrants. Nevertheless, as useful as this approach may seem in improving the understanding of differences, it cannot be generally applicable. In each country, there are cultural and religious variables between cities, regions, villages, regions, and ethnic groups. It is therefore

highly insufficient to take into account only the original culture of the migrant, while denying his or her own individuality and historical background. If therapists are informed of some essential aspects of their patients' culture and religion, they will be able to identify better the thin line between the healthy and the psychopathological expression of religious convictions to improve their approach to patients. However, the major recommendation for approaching patients in the best way is to have available someone who will listen. It is also true that, for our Western societies, listening is time-consuming and therefore economically problematic. Things are completely different in traditional allopathic medicine, which tends to promote a more deliberate and thorough approach to patients. In some cases, traditional allopathic medicine often takes into account, along with clinical symptoms, aspects such as personality, character, or the physical and the psychological environment, the living conditions, and the patients' relationships, as well as their moral issues and beliefs.

Kleinman and Becker (14) recommended that a patient's explanatory models of illness should be elicited using an ethnographic approach that explored their concerns: "Why me?" "Why now?" "What is wrong?" "How long will it last?" "How serious is it?" "Who can intervene or treat the condition?" Thus, the clinician would gather a better understanding of the subjective experience of illness and so promote collaboration and improve clinical outcomes and patient satisfaction.

REFERENCES

1. de Beaune SA. Chamanisme et préhistoire. Un feuilleton à épisodes, *L'Homme*. 1998; 38:203–219.
2. Sournia J-C. *Histoire de la médecine et des médecins*. Paris: Ed. Larousse; 1991.
3. Nicoud M. *Éthique et pratiques médicales aux derniers siècles du Moyen Âge*. Médiévales, n° 46, Paris, PUV; 2004:5–10.
4. Pichot P. *Un siècle de Psychiatrie*. Paris: Editions les Empêcheurs de penser en rond; 1983.
5. Marion M. *Dictionnaire des institutions de la France au XVIIème et XVIIIème siècle*. Paris: Ayer Publishing; 1968.

6. Carbonnelle S. La santé, la maladie comme représentation. Dans des Savoirs qui s'ignorent. *Santé conjuguée*. 2001;16:23–26.

7. Kleinman A. *Patients and healers in the context of culture*. Berkeley: University of California Press; 1980.

8. Cathébras P. Qu'est ce qu'une maladie? *Revue Médecine Interne*. 1997;18:809–813.

9. American Psychiatric Association. *Diagnostic and Statistical Manual of Mental Disorders*, 4th rev. Washington, DC: Author; 1994.

10. Zempleni A. La « maladie » et ses « causes ». Introduction. *L'Ethnographie* 1985;81:13–44.

11. Herzlich C. *Santé et maladie: analyse d'une représentation sociale*. Paris (France): Mouton; 1969.

12. Benoist J. Une médecine ou des médecines? A propos de la dimension culturelle de la maladie. *Nouvelle Revue d'Ethnopsychiatrie*. 1996;30:148.

13. Gerd M, Kühnlein I. Utilisation des savoirs quotidiens et scientifiques dans la construction scientifique de l'évolution d'une maladie, in Flick Uwe, La perception quotidienne de la santé et de la maladie, (ouvrage collectif), collection l'Harmattan, Paris; 1992.

14. Kleinman A, Becker AE. The contributions of anthropology to psychosomatic medicine. *Psychosom Med*. 1998;60:389–393.

15. Williams B, Healy D. Perceptions of illness causation among new referrals to a community mental health team: "explanatory model" or "explanatory map"? *Soc Sci Med*. 2001;53:465–476.

16. McKeon P, Carrick S. Public attitudes to depression. *J Ment Health*. 1991;4:369–382.

17. Priest RG, Vize C, Roberts A, Roberts M, Tylee A. Lay people's attitudes to treatment of depression: results of opinion poll for Defeat Depression Campaign just before its launch. *Br Med J*. 1996;313:858–859.

18. Kuyken W, Brewin CR, Power MJ, Furnham A. Causal beliefs about depression in depressed patients, clinical psychologists and lay persons. *Br J Med Psychol*. 1992;65:257–268.

19. Rogers A, Pigrim D. Service users' views of psychiatric treatment. *Soc Health Ill*. 1993;15:612–631.

20. Leventhal H, Nerenz D. The assessment of illness cognition. In: Karoly P, ed. *Measurement Strategies in Health Psychology*. New York: Pergamon; 1985:517–554.

21. Brelet C. *Médecines du monde: histoire et pratiques des médecines traditionnelles*. Paris: Ed Robert Laffont; 2002.

22. Loubières C. Comportements et pratiques thérapeutiques chez les migrants d'Afrique Noire dans le 18ème arrondissement de Paris. Monteillet N (dir), Maîtrise d'ethnologie, Université Paris 8, 2002–2003.

23. Pays JF. Relation avec les malades originaires d'Afrique Noire. In: Durand H, Biclet P, Hervé C, eds. *Ethique et pratique médicale*. Paris: Doin; 1995:18–21.

24. Dozon JP, Sindzingre N. « Pluralisme thérapeutique et médecine traditionnelle en Afrique contemporaine ». In: La santé dans le Tiers Monde, ed. *Coopérative d'édition de la vie mutualiste*, coll. Prévenir; 1986:43–52.

25. Wamba A. Education, thérapeutes et différentes cultures médicales. Du sens de l'interaction praticiens/praticiens dans la construction des savoirs médicaux en approches interculturelles des soins au Cameroun. *ARIC Bull*. 2005;41:44–54.

26. Teuton J, Dowrick C, Bentall RP. How healers manage the pluralistic healing context: the perspective of indigenous, religious and allopathic healers in relation to psychosis in Uganda. *Soc Sci Med*. 2007;65:1260–1273.

27. Jacobsson L, Merdasa F. Traditional perceptions and treatment of mental disorders in western Ethiopia before the 1974 revolution. *Acta Psychiatr Scand*. 1991;84:475–481.

28. World Health Organization. *Médecine traditionnelle africaine (série de rapports techniques)*. Brazzaville; 1976: Afro n°1.

29. Ensink K, Robertson B. Patients and family experiences of psychiatric services and African indigenous healers. *Transcult Psychiatry*. 1999;36:23–43.

30. Hacking I. *The Social Construction of What?* Cambridge, MA: Harvard University Press; 1999.

31. Horwitz AV. *Creating Mental Illness*. Chicago: University of Chicago; 2002.

32. Helman C. *Culture, Health and Illness*. London: Butterworth and Heinmann; 1994.

33. Good B. *Comment faire de l'anthropologie médicale? Médecine, rationalité et vécu*. Institut Synthélabo: Le Plessis-Robinson; 1998.

34. Bilu Y, Witztum E. Working with Jewish ultra-orthodox patients: guidelines for a culturally sensitive therapy. *Cult Med Psychiatry*. 1993;17:197–233.

35. Khan I, Pillay K. Users' attitudes towards home and hospital treatment: a comparative study between South Asian and white residents of the British Isles. *J Psychiatr Ment Health Nurs*. 2003;10:137–146.

36. Guiraud GG. Le recours aux médecines parallèles. *Presse Méd*. 2003;32:1638–1641.

37. Eisenberg DM, Davis RB, Ettner SL, et al. Trends in alternative medicine use in the United States, 1990–1997: results of a follow-up national survey. *JAMA*. 1998;11:1569–1575.

38. Lasell L. New data suggest importance of alternative medicine. *Manag Emp Health Benefits*. 1998;6:32–40.

39. Knaudt PR, Connor KM, Weisler RH, Churchill LE, Davidson JR. Alternative therapy use by psychiatric outpatients. *J Nerv Ment Dis*. 1999;187:692–695.

40. Astin JA, Marie A, Pelletier KR, Hansen E, Haskell WL. A review of the incorporation of complementary and alternative medicine by mainstream physicians. *Arch Intern Med*. 1998;23:2303–2310.

41. Millar WJ. Patterns of use – alternative health care practitioners. *Health Rep.* 2001;13:9–21.

42. Pirotta MV, Cohen MM, Kotsirilos V, Farish SJ. Complementary therapies: have they become accepted in general practice? *Med J Aust.* 2000;7:105–109.

43. Hopper I, Cohen M. Complementary medicine and the medical profession: a survey of medical students' attitudes. *Altern Ther Health Med.* 1998;3:68–73.

44. McCarthy K. Early alcoholism treatment: the Emmanuel movement and Richard Peabody. *J Stud Alcohol.* 1984;45:59–74.

45. Buxton M, Smith D, Seymour R. Spirituality and other points of resistance to the 12-step recovery process. *J Psychoactive Drugs.* 1987;19:275–286.

46. Aldridge D. Spirituality, healing and medicine. *Br J Gen Pract.* 1991;41:425–427.

47. Byrd R. Positive therapeutic effects of intercessory prayer in a coronary care unit population. *South Med J.* 1988;81:826–829.

48. Harris WS, Gowda M, Kolb JW, Stychacz CP, Vacek JL, Jones PG. A randomized controled trial of the effects on remote, intercessory prayer on outcomes in patients admitted to the coronary unit. *Arch Intern Med.* 1999;159:2273–2278.

49. van Leeuwen R, Tiesinga LJ, Jochemsen H, Post D. Aspects of spirituality concerning illness. *Scand J Caring Sci.* 2008;22:4.

50. Borras L, Mohr S, Brandt PY, Gilliéron C, Huguelet P. Religious coping among outpatients suffering from chronic schizophrenia: a cross-national comparison (submitted), 2008.

51. de Bilbao F, Giannakopoulos P. Effect of religious culture on obsessive compulsive disorder symptomatology. A transcultural study in monotheistic religions. *Rev Med Suisse.* 2005;1:2818–2821.

52. Mohr S, Brandt PY, Borras L, Gilliéron C, Huguelet P. Toward an integration of spirituality and religiousness into the psychosocial dimension of schizophrenia. *Am J Psychiatry.* 2006;163:1952–1959.

53. Pargament KI. *The Psychology of Religion and Coping: Theory, Research, Practice.* New York: Guilford Publications; 1997.

54. Borras L, Mohr S, Brandt PY, Gilliéron C, Eytan A, Huguelet P. Religious beliefs in schizophrenia: their relevance for adherence to treatment. *Schizophr Bull.* 2007;33:1238–1246.

55. Logan M, Romans S. Spiritual beliefs in bipolar affective disorder: their relevance for illness management. *J Affect Disord.* 2002;75:247–257.

56. Muthny FA, Bechtel M, Spaete M. Lay etiologic theories and coping with illness in severe physical diseases. An empirical comparative study of female myocardial infarct, cancer, dialysis and multiple sclerosis patients. *Psychother Psychosom Med Psychol.* 1992;42:41–53.

57. Patterson S, Balducci L, Meyer R. The Book of Job: a 2,500-year-old current guide to the practice of oncology: the nexus of medicine and spirituality. *J Cancer Educ.* 2002;17:237–240.

58. Kaasa S, Loge JH. Quality of life in palliative care: principles and practice. *Palliat Med.* 2003;17:11–20.

59. Salaffi F, Stancati A. Disability and quality of life of patients with rheumatoid arthritis: assessment and perspectives. *Reumatismo.* 2004;56:87–106.

60. Powell-Cope GM, White J, Henkelman EJ, Turner BJ. Qualitative and quantitative assessments of HAART adherence of substance-abusing women. *AIDS Care.* 2003;15:239–249.

61. Marcotte D, Avants SK, Margolin A. Spiritual self-schema therapy, drug abuse, and HIV. *J Psychoactive Drugs.* 2003;35:389–391.

62. Arnold R, Avants SK, Margolin A, Marcotte D. Patient attitudes concerning the inclusion of spirituality into addiction treatment. *J Subst Abuse Treat.* 2002;23:319–326.

63. Johnson KS, Elbert-Avila KI, Tulsky JA. The influence of spiritual beliefs and practices on the treatment preferences of African Americans: a review of the literature. *J Am Geriatr Soc.* 2005;53:711–719.

64. Pfeifer S. Belief in demons and exorcism in psychiatric patients in Switzerland. *Br J Med Psychol.* 1994;67:247–258.

65. Wilson WP. Religion and psychosis. In: Koenig HG, ed. *Handbook of Religion and Mental Health.* San Diego: Academic Press; 1998:161–173.

66. Hale AS, Pinninti NR. Exorcism-resistant ghost possession treated with clopenthixol. *Br J Psychiatry.* 1994;165:386–388.

67. Eckholm E. China's crackdown on sect stirs alarm over psychiatric abuse. *NY Times.* 2001;18:NE1.

68. Hoyersten JG. Possessed! Some historical, psychiatric and current moments of demonic possession. *Tidsskr Nor Laegeforen.* 1996;10:3602–3606.

69. McCabe R, Priebe S. Explanatory models of illness in schizophrenia: comparison of four ethnic groups. *Br J Psychiatry.* 2004;185:25–30.

70. Saravanan B, Jacob KS, Johnson S, Prince M, Bhugra D, David AS. Belief models in first episode schizophrenia in South India. *Soc Psychiatry Psychiatr Epidemiol.* 2007;42:446–451.

71. Hilton C, Ghaznavi F, Zuberi T. Religious beliefs and practices in acute mental health patients. *Nurs Stand.* 2002;16:33–36.

72. Callan A, Littlewood R. Patient satisfaction: ethnic origin or explanatory model? *Int J Soc Psychiatry.* 1998;44:1–11.

73. Desclaux A. L'observance en Afrique: question de culture ou "vieux problème de santé publique ? In: Souteyran Y, Morin M, Dir. *L'observance aux Traitements du VIH/sida : Mesure, Déterminants, Évolution.* Paris: ANRS; 2001:57–66.

74. Farmer P, Léandre F, Mukherjee J, et al. Community-based approaches to HIV treatment in resource-poor settings. *Lancet.* 2001;358:404–409.

75. Benoist J. *Petite bibliothèque d'anthropologie médicale. Une anthologie.* Paris: Amades; 2002.

19 Psychiatric Treatments Involving Religion: Psychotherapy from a Christian Perspective

WILLIAM P. WILSON

SUMMARY

In this essay, we observe that most religious therapies have as their goal the cognitive restructuring of the minds of those who seek therapy. Thus, cognitive-behavioral therapy is done by most practitioners. It is also true that the holy writings of each faith are used to teach their version of the "truth" to the person being treated. Islam believes that the patient should reconnect with their Muslim faith before therapy is undertaken. Christianity believes that a personal relationship with the living God is necessary for Christian therapy to be used. The goal of therapy in all faiths is to transform the mind of the believer so that they may have meaning and purpose in their relationship with a higher power. In some faiths, another goal is for them to encounter their higher power.

Christian psychotherapy differs in one major aspect. It seeks to enable patients to have a relationship with the living God who comes and dwells with them and in them. This is possible because the mind of man is supernatural and because the supernatural God can install himself in the mind. This means that God then can, with the believer's permission, guide and direct their thinking and activity in a positive way. Christian practices and interventions can then bring about the transformation of the mind we so earnestly seek.

Reviewing the literature concerning psychotherapy in the major religions of the world, one finds that there is very little information that describes in detail the psychotherapeutic process. Nevertheless, what information does exist helps us to understand that most cognitive restructuring is done in the context of the religion. An Islamic author (1) believes that therapy must be done after the patient has become devoutly Muslim. The restructuring is then done using the teachings found in the Koran. In Hinduism and Buddhism, it is assumed that the believer seeking therapy accepts the teachings of that particular faith. Hindu and Buddhist psychotherapy uses meditation focusing on a higher power and on right thoughts. Cognitive restructuring in all is done using the principles espoused in their holy writings. There also is an effort to contact a higher power through meditation, by good works, or through ascetic practices. Christian psychotherapy is a discipline that uses the teachings found in the Bible with an integration of current secular concepts. Therapy is facilitated by the power of the Holy Spirit to transform lives. The goal is transformation of the person so that he or she has a life with less conflict and symptoms as well as more happiness. In the light of the fact that there are similarities of practices in the psychotherapeutic approach of all faiths, we will take a detailed look at a psychotherapeutic approach into which Christian concepts have been included to achieve this transformation.

1. ANALYZING PSYCHOTHERAPIES

In an overview of current secular methods of psychotherapy, Karasu (2) noted that at least 140 claim to be distinctive. Certain factors, however, are said to be common to all methods. Among these are (1) an emotionally charged, confiding relationship; (2) a therapeutic rationale that is accepted by the patient and the therapist; (3) provision of new information, which may be transmitted by precept, example, and/or self discovery; (4) strengthening of the patient's expectation of help; (5) provision of success experiences; and (6) facilitation of emotional arousal.(3)

After discussing the differences claimed for each method, Karasu reduced the 140 varieties of psychotherapy into three groups: the dynamic, the behavioral, and the experiential. He then summarized the following themes of these three groups as follows: (1) prime concern, (2) concept of pathology, (3) concept of health, (4) mode of change, (5) time approach and focus, (6) type of treatment, (7) the therapist's task, (8) primary tools and techniques, (9) treatment model, (10) nature of therapeutic relationship, and (11) the therapist's role and stance. In none of these areas did he consider spiritual aspects, although he later recognized that they should have been considered.(4)

Because the proponents of each technique of psychotherapy tend to focus on certain aspects of their therapeutic approach, it is difficult to determine whether their claims have merit and whether significant differences really do exist. Karasu's scholarly analysis produced some order out of the chaos that appears to exist in the field of psychotherapy and provides us with a framework within which we can evaluate each therapeutic technique with standardized dimensions. It is within this framework that I shall attempt to evaluate Christian psychotherapy.

The title of this chapter presupposes that there is such a thing as Christian psychotherapy and that it differs significantly from secular forms of therapy. A casual reader of the literature on pastoral counseling, or Christian psychology, would probably not be convinced that there is a distinctively Christian form of psychotherapy, for he would find that many Christian therapists use Freudian dynamic therapy, Rogerian client-centered therapy, Adlerian individual psychological therapy, Jungian analysis, and other secular methods. Only a few writers such as Tweedie,(5) Collins,(6) Adams,(7) Minirth,(8)

and Crabbe(9) begin with a distinctive base, the Bible, and describe a counseling technique based on biblical teachings. From their books, articles, and the Bible, as well as my own observations, I have attempted to determine the fundamental theses of Christian psychotherapy.

2. FUNDAMENTAL THESES

First, we have to have a cosmology. The Christian's cosmology includes a transcendent God. It also includes a worldview. A worldview is a comprehensive conception or apprehension of the world especially from a specific standpoint. The Christian's standpoint is contrasted with that of the agnostic or atheist. It is, therefore, important for us to understand our worldview because it affects our view of the planet, our society, the nature of man, and our place in the world. The most important of these is the nature of man. There is no question that our view of man's nature affects our approach to psychotherapy. What then should our worldview be?

Leo Apostel,(10) a Belgian philosopher, hypothesized that there are five fundamental components to a worldview. The first is a model of the world that allows us to understand how the world functions. This includes (1) the universe, (2) the earth, (3) life, (4) the mind, (5) society, and (6) culture. Second, there should be an explanation for it all. We should know why it is the way it is, where it all comes from, and where we come from. Third, we need a futurology. This is an extrapolation of the past into the future to help us answer the question as to where we are going. Fourth, we need values. Values are things, especially beliefs, that make a favorable difference in our lives.(11) We need to know what is good and what is evil. When we know this, we can have a code of ethics or morals. Fifth, we need knowledge. Our actions can be based only on what we know and the information available to us. We can then formulate plans based on theories and models describing the phenomena that we encounter. Knowledge acquisition allows us to distinguish between better and worse theories. Values will help us distinguish between what is true and what is false.

Karasu commented that the starting point or foundation of all psychotherapies is a concept of the nature of man. Christians believe that man's human nature has three functional units: body, soul, and spirit (1 Thess. 5:23). The *body* is more than the various organ systems and flesh. They use the term *flesh* here to describe the muscles, bones, and skin. It is also made up of the biological drives such as psychomotor activity, sex, sleep, and appetite that are hardwired into the brain. These give rise to certain behaviors that will satiate the appetites. The *soul* is made up of (1) the emotional reflexes; (2) the intellect, which includes knowledge, memories of events, and the emotions elicited by them; (3) the values we have learned; and (4) our ability to process, compare, evaluate, and respond to incoming stimuli. The *spirit* is, in the biblical sense, an animating force that resides in man and operates through the flesh and soul. In the past it has been called the life force or *elan vitale*. On careful inspection, it may be concluded that the spirit does have undifferentiated feeling tones, those of pleasantness and unpleasantness.(12) Unfortunately, secular therapists have a more limited view of man's nature and of the factors determining behavior. The best secular effort made to formulate a concept of man's nature to date has been that of Freud, who divided it into three parts: the id, the ego, and the super-ego. His concept ignores the spiritual aspect of man's nature and includes only incomplete ideas of the flesh and the soul.

The *behaviorists* focus on the soul. Both Skinner (13) and Glasser (14) pay only minimal attention to the spirit or the body in their writings. The *experientialists*, on the other hand, focus on the transcendental or spiritual aspect of man and minimize the importance of the body and the soul.

Tournier,(15) who is considered the dean of Christian psychotherapists, has based his counseling approach on a holistic view of man. He has chosen to view man biblically and has postulated that his nature has three parts: body, psyche, and mind. The *body* includes the instincts, appetite, and physiological functions. It grows old, gets sick, and dies. The *psyche* is the part of man

that experiences emotion and is able to imagine things. The *mind* is the part that thinks, reasons, wills, and deals with abstract ideas. Tournier's ideas differ in many details from those of other Christian writers, but the major defect in his view of man is his failure to include the concept of man's spirit as a specific entity, even though he is aware of the transcendental and emphasizes its role. Nevertheless, Tournier's theories and techniques have had a profound influence on the field of Christian psychotherapy largely because he reconciles secular and biblical concepts in a way that reveals the essential truths of both. He believes that man does have a mind that contains the spirit and it is in his mind that God communicates with him.

Among secular psychotherapists, only the experientialists take into account the possible existence of a prime mover,(16) which they conceive of as a vague universal consciousness. In contrast, Christian psychotherapy is based on the certain knowledge that a prime mover does exist and that he (God) is more than simply consciousness. He is the great I AM (Rom. 1:19, 20), a person, who manifested himself in the form of a man, Jesus Christ (Col. 1:15). This Jesus died, was resurrected, and after returning to the Father sent his Spirit (the Holy Spirit) to live in believers to reveal the truth, to give power (Acts 1:8), and to fill them with love for their fellow man. Man experiences God transcendentally through his Spirit (1 Cor. 2:12) and his Word (2 Tim. 3:16). In the biblical record of his dealings with the Israelites and in Jesus, God has revealed his own personality attributes, provided guidelines for right living and emotional control, and has given a set of rules for right living that will make a favorable difference in human life (2 Tim. 3:15–17). One of the most important ideas in the Christian belief system, however, is that God gives his followers the power to live these values (Rom. 8:5–8).

Having outlined the major differences in the metaphysical anthropology of psychotherapists, let us now compare the thematic dimensions of Christian psychotherapy with those of the three other streams of therapy. In Table 19.1, I have summarized these thematic dimensions.

Table 19.1: Summary of Thematic Dimensions of Four Kinds of Psychotherapy.

Theme	Dynamic (D)	Behavioral (B)	Experiential (E)	Christian (C)
Prime concern	Sexual repression	Anxiety	Alienation	Alienation from God – incompleteness (sin)
Concept of pathology	Instinctual conflicts; early libidinal drives and wishes that remain out of awareness, i.e., unconscious	Learned habits; excess or deficit behaviors that have been environmentally reinforced	Existential despair; human loss of possibilities, fragmentation of self, lack of congruence with one's experiences	A combination of D, B, and E, along with sin and its consequences (death); inability to control behavior; painful emotional state
Concept of health	Resolution of underlying conflicts; victory of ego over id, i.e., ego strength	Symptom removal; Absence of specific symptom and/or reduction of anxiety	Actualization of potential; self-growth, authenticity, and spontaneity	A combination of D, B, and E; wholeness-(holiness) with peace and love and fruits of love; ability to control behavior
Mode of change	Depth insight; understanding of the early past, i.e., intellectual-emotional knowledge	Direct learning; behaving in the current present, i.e., action or performance	Immediate experiencing; sensing or feeling in the immediate moment, i.e., spontaneous expression of experience	A combination of D, B, and E; reconciliation with God; receipt of Holy Spirit; creation of pleasant emotional state; increased selflessness and control of behavior; adoption of new value system
Time approach and focus	Historical; subjective past	Nonhistorical; objective present	Ahistorical; phenomenological moment	A combination of D, B, and E; historical, nonhistorical, ahistorical, subjective past, objective present, phenomenological moment
Type of treatment	Long-term and intense	Short-term and not intense	Short-term and intense	Any time and any intensity
Therapist's task	To comprehend unconscious mental content and its historical and hidden meaning	To program, reward, inhibit, or shape specific behavioral responses to anxiety-producing stimuli	To interact in a mutually accepting atmosphere for arousal of self-expression (from somatic to spiritual)	Determination of relationship with God; spiritual growth, to relate to person in love, to uncover conflicts, to assist in resolution; to program, reward, shape responses
Primary tools and techniques	Interpretation; free association, analysis of transference, resistance, slips, and dreams	Conditioning; systematic desensitization, positive and negative reinforcements, shaping	Encounter; shared dialogue, experiments or games, dramatization or playing out of feelings	Conversion; prayer, determination of historical origins of conflicts, analysis of dreams, free association, interpretation, conditioning, education

(continued)

Table 19.1 *(continued)*

Theme	Dynamic (D)	Behavioral (B)	Experiential (E)	Christian (C)
Treatment model	Medical; doctor-patient or parent-infant (authoritarian), i.e., therapeutic alliance	Educational; teacher-student or parent-child (authoritarian), i.e., learning alliance	Existential; human peer-human peer or adult-adult (egalitarian), i.e., human alliance	Teacher; friend, fellow struggler, essentially egalitarian but at times authoritarian but as an agent of God
Nature of relationship to cure	Transferential and primary for cure; unreal relationship	Real but secondary for cure; no relationship	Real and primary for cure; real relationship	Transferential but real and primary for cure; real relationship
Therapist's role and stance	Interpreter-reflector; indirect, dispassionate, or frustrating	Shaper-adviser; direct, problem-solving, or practical	Interactor-acceptor; mutually permissive or gratifying	Interpreter, shaper, adviser, interactor, acceptor, reality orientor, teacher, limit setter

Modified after Karasu.(2) Reprinted with permission from the *American Journal of Psychiatry* (copyright 1977). American Psychiatric Association.

3. THEMATIC DIMENSIONS

3.1. Prime Concern and Concept of Pathology

Karasu observed that the prime concern of the dynamic psychotherapist is with sexual repression. The behavioral psychotherapist is primarily concerned with anxiety. The experiential therapist is concerned with alienation. I would propose that the Christian therapist is primarily concerned with man's alienation from God, which leads to alienation from man and society as well. His alienation from God is an outgrowth of sin. This sin is either original sin or acts of rebellion against God's authority, or both.

Becoming a Christian is purported by some to produce wholeness without other interventions. They argue that Christians should not need psychotherapy if they are truly "saved." But in spite of their admonitions, many authentic (17) Christians do consult psychiatrists or other professionals for psychotherapy. Why then do Christians need psychotherapy? Our response to the question is to say that if an ideal Christian community existed and was populated only by perfect Christians, psychotherapy might not be needed. But there are no perfect Christian communities and there are no perfect Christians, so the need exists. The reason it exists is that, in the past, most Christians believed in a kind of inherited sin. Many still do today. This inherited sin outweighs the good (Rom. 3:23). These same people also believe that there is a personal supernatural force for sin in the world (Satan) that seeks to destroy (1 Pet. 5:8). Such a belief is in contrast to the ideas held by the dynamicists and behaviorists, who see man at birth as a blank personality (tabula rasa). He learns to be bad either by the actions and teachings of parents, society, culture, or circumstance. The experientialists do not consider sin in their discussion of man's predicament.(18) They do mention man's revolt as a way of responding to his alienation. This revolt manifests itself in a rejection of God and society's values.

Most Christian psychotherapists admit the existence of a tendency to revolt. They call it original sin. Jay Adams (a theologian), Lawrence Crabbe, Jr., and Frank Minirth, mentioned earlier, all consider sin as a primary cause of man's neuroses and spiritual problems. But what is sin? Most persons would define sin as a set of specific behaviors such as drinking, smoking, cursing, sexual indiscretions, and other such misbehaviors. These are, to be sure, manifestations of sin, but sin is more than specific behaviors. It is *conscious rebellion against the authority of God*. Because of this rebellion, man indulges his biological drives and relates to others in ways that are contrary to the rules God has given him. These rules command that he relate to God and other men in love. Being alienated from God by his rebellion, man is not whole. His life is empty and meaningless.

Sin has consequences that result in pathology. The Bible used the term *death* to describe this pathology. The biblical concept of death has several interpretations. The most important aspect is alienation from God. A second is failure to receive the abundant and eternal life that the Bible promises. A third is the emotional pain, which results from man's inability to control his behavior and his failure to respond to the love of God. McKay (19) has called this lack of control moral paralysis. C. S. Lewis (20) has pointed out, "Until the evil man finds evil unmistakably present in his existence in the form of pain, he is enclosed in an illusion. Once pain has roused him, he knows he is in some way or another up against the real universe: he either rebels … or else makes some attempt at adjustment which, if pursued, will lead him to religion." The painful emotions of sorrow, fear, anger, emptiness, confusion, shame, jealousy, or disgust are manifestations of pathology. More recently, Moshe Spero (21) has pointed out that the pain arising from sin manifests itself as neurosis. In contrast, because neurosis results in a preoccupation with self, it is sin.

Finally, the Bible makes it plain that the final consequence of sin that is not dealt with is eternal separation from God and punishment (Matt. 25:46).

3.2. Concept of Health

The concept of health usually considered characteristic of Christian psychotherapy is holiness. Tournier is the leading proponent of holiness in today's psychotherapeutic world, a world in which the word holiness often suggests emotional instability and religious fanaticism. But this is not what holiness originally meant. John Wesley,(22) who was an outspoken proponent of holiness, believed that holiness, or sanctification, begins with a transcendental experience (salvation), but is at the outset incomplete. Wesley believed that confession, reproof, instruction,

and the performance of good works in love are all part of the process through which behavior is modified and men are made whole. In a world where medical care was almost nonexistent, Wesley went to the trouble to write a book on home medical care. He did not omit the body from his concern for the spirit and soul. Tournier's therapy of the whole man is in the same tradition.

The three secular systems list resolution of underlying conflicts, symptom removal, and actualization of potential as the primary goals of therapy. All these are goals of the Christian therapist. He knows that to attain wholeness they must be achieved. But there is more. The patient must also be reconciled to God and continue to be transformed as he matures in his faith.

3.3. Mode of Change

The mode of change in Christian psychotherapy involves a synthesis of the various mechanisms used by the proponents of the three kinds of psychotherapy. Not only is depth of insight necessary, but also direct learning and behaving as well as immediate experiencing are also necessary. In addition, the Christian therapist's goal is reconciliation with God, if this has not already taken place. A transcendental experience with God is one of the primary effectors of change (2 Cor. 5:17, John 3:3). The joining of God's Spirit to man's mind is essential if therapy is to become truly Christian. It is unfortunate that other writers have not emphasized this point. Reconciliation to God provides power to change (Rom. 8:7, 8).

3.4. Time Approach and Focus

Even in Christian therapy, however, we have to realize that the "present is viewed through the past in anticipation of the future." Therefore, an understanding of the past is necessary to determine what changes must take place before new patterns of thinking and behaving, determined by the patient's Christian value system, can be established.(23) Christian psychotherapy should use a variety of methods to bring about the necessary changes. It is conceptual narrowness of the worst kind to assume that all patients can be treated with the same approach.

At this point, we must emphasize the understanding that we derive from the Bible about time. In the dimension of the supernatural, there are no dimensions of time and space as we know them. Therefore, God is the Lord of time. This means that he can take us back in time, in a way that is impossible without his involvement. God's intervention allows us to heal events in the past as we relive them. This ability to supernaturally warp time back on itself is the basis for what is called inner healing. Because change is to be effected in different ways, we should also know that the time approach and focus would be variable. Christians cannot ignore the past, for in it are buried the experiences that determine responses in the present and their anticipation of the future. Christian therapists must, therefore, examine the objective reality of the patient's present situation to determine the significance of the subjectively remembered past. The intellectual and emotional knowledge thus gained can be used to help the patient understand his current dysfunctional thinking and behavior. After the therapist and patient together have examined their findings in the light of the biblical ideal, it is then possible to undertake the necessary modifications in thinking and behavior.

3.5. Type of Treatment

Little has been written about the type and duration of treatment that Christian psychotherapists should employ. Secular therapists use long-term intense, long-term not intense, short-term intense, or short-term not intense. As we have examined the activities of Christian therapists, it appears that they use different types determined by the patient's need. In many instances, a single encounter may be sufficient. In others, it may be necessary to see the patient up to sixty times to bring about healing. Patients with addictions, eating disorders, deviant sexuality, and borderline personalities are most likely to require long-term therapy.

3.6. The Therapist's Task

The task of the Christian psychotherapist is more formidable than that of the dynamic, behavioral, or experiential therapist. He must not only be able to determine the meaning of unconscious mental conflict, but he also must program, reward, inhibit, or shape behavioral responses to anxiety-producing stimuli. In addition, he must interact in a mutually accepting atmosphere to help arouse of self-expression. He begins by establishing an atmosphere of mutual acceptance to encourage the patient's self-expression. To be effective in this task, the therapist must be a mature Christian who is able to interact with the patient in a nonjudgmental, caring way. He has to accept the patient as he is and care for him in spite of his problems.

Such caring demands nothing and has as its concern the best interests and welfare of the other person. It is nonsexual, not exploitive, and eternal (Ps. 136:1). The bond established will be greater if both the therapist and patient are Christians. At the beginning, the therapist must determine the nature of the patient's relationship with God and/or his level of maturity in the Christian faith. This demands a thorough knowledge of spiritual development. Because of the relationship, the therapist is able to shape behavioral responses when necessary.

3.7. Primary Tools and Methods

Once the appropriate atmosphere has been established and the therapist has determined the level at which he and the patient can relate, he must explore the areas of conflict and determine their genesis. In many cases, it will be necessary to strip away defenses by which the patient maintains repression of the experiences that have given rise to his or her symptoms. Christians are particularly prone to deny conflict, simply because it is not compatible with their idea of Christian perfection. Having been taught that Christians should not get angry or hate, think lustful thoughts, should always love, and should not fornicate or commit adultery, the patient who considers himself a Christian may deny or repress thoughts, feelings, or behaviors that are not Christian because of shame and guilt. The therapist must be familiar with these defense mechanisms and know how to get around them. He can then comprehend (like secular therapists) the patient's conscious and subconscious mental conflict and its historical and hidden meanings. Next, the therapist has the task of helping the patient understand how this subconscious conflict is influencing his or her current behavior. By responding to the patient in ways that do not reward the behaviors that produce pain and anxiety, the therapist helps to bring about extinction or inhibition of such behaviors. He then must teach (or program) new behavioral patterns that will provide the patient with positive reinforcements. Because the Christian therapist will use biblical guidelines in his selections of new behaviors, familiarity with the Bible is essential. The use of journaling, psychodrama, visualization techniques, role playing, and gestalt techniques helps the patient "get in touch" with his long repressed feelings, so that he can take some definitive action to deal with them. Of particular importance is the management of shame and anger. In many cases, the patient's symptoms or behavioral aberrations are derived from profound shame and guilt, hate, or resentment. These emotions are derived from what the Bible calls a record of wrongs against oneself or others (1 Cor. 13:5 Good News Bible (TEV)). The only way to deal with these records of wrongs is to use God's forgiveness. Dynamic therapists believe that understanding results in forgiveness. Behaviorists believe that people are somewhat helpless in dealing with their past conditioning. Even so, they are responsible. Experientialists regard man as inherently good and, therefore, do not consider the need for forgiveness. For the Christian, it is impossible to deny moral responsibility. When a person has broken God's laws, he is guilty of transgression and must deal with the guilt. Tournier, Hyder, Crabbe, Adams, and Minirth all emphasize the role of forgiveness in Christian psychotherapy. Biblically, God is the source of all forgiveness (Luke 5:21), for forgiveness can come only out of the infinite love he has for mankind.(24) It is the task of the therapist to use this forgiveness for dealing with the anger he has toward others and the shame he feels about his own transgressions (John 20:23). Once the patient has accepted God's forgiveness for himself, he can develop a realistic self-concept. When he has forgiven those persons who he feels have wronged him, he can relate to them in love.

The primary tools and techniques of Christian psychotherapists are those used by dynamic, behavioral, and experiential psychotherapists, with several additions. The most vital addition is conversion. Biblically based Christian therapy takes seriously the statement of Jesus that "you must be born again" to enter the kingdom of God (John 3:3). Regeneration, or conversion, is the sine qua non of truly Christian therapy. If the therapist and the patient have not been born again, Christian therapy cannot take place. Wholeness in the patient cannot be attained without it. Even nonbelievers attest to the importance and the usefulness of conversion in some healings.

Another unique tool available to the Christian therapist is a reward system that produces a highly motivated patient. The promises of love, joy, and peace (Gal. 5:22, 23), to say nothing of abundant and eternal life (John 10:10, Mark 10:30), are powerful incentives for working toward healing. In a like manner, Jesus' promise to heal creates an expectation in the patient that he will be healed. The patient and his therapist believe that healing is more than a promise (something called disparagingly "pie in the sky by and by"), it can happen now.

Finally, the Christian therapist can use prayer, Bible study, worship, and the Eucharist (the means of grace) to help him in his teaching and conditioning tasks. One of the advantages of prayer is illustrated in Norman Grubb's statement that prayer is not intended to convince God, but to convince the person offering the prayer.(25)

3.8. Treatment Model

The treatment model used by dynamic and behavioral therapists tends to be authoritarian. The model used by experiential therapists is egalitarian. The Christian may use an authoritarian model, but he prefers an authoritative egalitarian model. Because the Christian therapist is a fellow struggler in the quest for holiness, he does not see himself as always having answers, neither does he have power to effect change. He is fully aware of the wisdom and power of God to work through him to bring about healing in the person under his care. He assumes many roles in his relationship with the patient, but he is always a teacher and a friend. He is working to bring about a complete change of the patient's mind (Rom. 12:2). This is done by restructuring the patient's thoughts, but also by decathecting (detaching) damaging emotions accumulated in the past. This will liberate the patient from the influence of these emotions over his thinking and behavior. If the damaging emotions are decathected, the patient's anticipation of the future will be changed. In short, patients will be released from their bondage to thoughts and behavior determined by their past experiences and will have hope for the future.

3.9. Nature of Relationship

For the Christian therapist, the nature of relationship for cure is the same as for any secular form of therapy. It must be real and primarily directed toward cure. The relationship is, however, one of love, otherwise it is not Christian.

If Christian psychotherapy is to be effective, there must be something unique about the therapist-patient relationship. Paul's statement that Christians are not to consider themselves better than others clearly commands us to have an egalitarian relationship (Phil. 2:3). This is in keeping with Jesus' commandment to love one another as he has loved us (John 13:34). In an egalitarian relationship, we will love our patients and authoritatively use the knowledge we possess to help bring about their healing. It is interesting that Meltzoff and Kornreich,(26) in their summary of research in psychotherapy, observed that "caring" was the single most important factor in achieving good treatment results. The relationship of therapist to patient should be, therefore, one of loving acceptance. The therapist should not see himself as superior or as having special powers, but should be humble. Humility is being able to see yourself as God sees you with all your vices and virtues, your perfections and imperfections as well as your assets and liabilities. In humility, he will accept the fact that he is just as human as the patient, but will understand that he has been given gifts of knowledge and healing to use to heal fellow strugglers in a broken and harsh world.

3.10. The Therapist's Role and Stance

Because most physicians and mental health professionals have a tendency to adopt an authoritarian role, they have a proclivity to adopt a priestly or prophetic role, but avoid a pastoral one. Psychiatrists, psychologists, ministers, and other therapists who adopt the priestly role may forget that they themselves are human. The humanity of some, however, is all too obvious to those who carefully inspect their lives. They have more suicides and some of them have just as many divorces and problems with alcoholism, drug addiction, and sex as society at large. It is a fact that they too frequently have "messed up" children. If they adopt a priestly role, it is likely that their human desire to appear strong will keep them from relating in an honest, real, and open way with their patients. This will hinder their therapeutic efforts.

Assuming that the pastoral or egalitarian role is the most desirable, what other roles should the therapist assume while treating his patients? Carl Rogers (27) promoted the idea that the therapist is to be nondirective and patient centered. He is to be genuine and open in dealing with the patient. He should have an unconditional positive regard for the patient as well as an accurate, empathic understanding of the patient's feelings, sentiments, and attitudes. This allows the patient to express his thoughts and feelings and increasingly be able to listen to his own communications. As he progressively accepts the therapist's feelings toward him, he can be more open and grow toward self-actualization. Although this approach to treatment has been accepted and practiced widely, it is only partly biblical. Jesus did relate this way with all the hurting people he came in contact with, but he assumed many other roles while he unconditionally accepted them.

Carlson (28) has described the many roles Jesus took while relating. He was critic, preacher, teacher, interpreter, mediator, confronter, admonisher, advocate, sustainer, supporter, lecturer, adviser, burden-bearer, listener, reprover, warner, helper, consoler, and pardoner. If we compare this list with the roles listed by Karasu, we find that the roles adopted by therapists using secular systems are quite limited. The roles adopted by Jesus included those used by secular therapists, but went far beyond. Because we are to treat persons using biblical insights, we should model our therapeutic role after the greatest healer of all.

The stance of the Christian therapist should be as variable as his role. There are times when he will have to be loving, comforting, accepting, permissive, confronting, gratifying, direct, problem-solving, and practical. At other times he will need to be indirect, dispassionate, or frustrating.

4. SPIRITUAL DISEASE

To a physician, the concept of spiritual disease is not difficult to accept if he or she believes that man has a spirit. However, theologians may have a problem with such a concept. Even so, it was recognized in Jeremiah 8:22 when it was said that the people of Israel needed healing for their idolatry and rebellion. The concept is also found in Christian hymnody in the use of the term "sin sick souls" to describe people who need Christ.

If we analyze the scriptures, we are able to identify four spiritual diseases. The first of these is a congenital one that all are born with, and that is to be unregenerate (i.e., not regenerated and therefore requiring to be born again into the

spiritual life). This came about because Adam and Eve sinned in the Garden of Eden when they wanted to "be like God." We are rebellious from the beginning. All one has to do to confirm this is to watch a child in the first two years of life. One of the first words he learns is "no." His rebellion will continue throughout his life. Before the fall, man lived in union with God; afterwards, he was alienated. This alienation is only relieved by a conversion experience.

A second spiritual disease is sin. Jay Adams made sin the center of his pastoral counseling approach. He was, however, a spiritual reductionist and did not consider man's other spiritual diseases. We have already defined sin as conscious rebellion against God. It occurs in both unregenerate and regenerate persons. W. M. McKay saw sin as a disease as did Moshe Spero. McKay said the thing that most characterized sin as a symptom was that it gave rise to moral paralysis. It also gave rise to deceit because the sinner did not want others to know of his moral dereliction. It also gives rise to negative emotions. Most commonly these are shame, fear (anxiety), and sorrow. The latter is due to the existential despair of morality that develops secondary to the moral paralysis.

Sin pollutes the environment. McKay recognized this and said that moral pollution makes the environment infectious. I need only refer to the drug-ridden environments of our schools today, which are as infectious as they can be for children who spend their time there. This is why we have an epidemic of drug use by teenagers.

A third spiritual disease is demonization. Satan's existence has been controversial for many years.(29) The Bible makes the existence of Satan explicit as it describes his person and works. Jesus was said to have come to destroy the works of the devil (1 John 3:8).

Satan's intimate interaction with mankind is called demonization. Satan uses his minions (demonic spirits) to accomplish this. Demonization has three forms. There is possession, oppression, and obsession. In possession there are diagnostic features. These have been summarized by Nevius.(30) The primary manifestation of this state is the regular appearance of another personality, who has a name, behaves in a manner compatible with his name, and has supernatural knowledge and power.

Oppression causes the afflicted to be in a state that is similar to depression. There is a grayness (gloom) that surrounds the person. One patient admitted because she was suicidal that she had been a witch, but kept her witch's paraphernalia after she had renounced witchcraft and became a Christian. The oppression occurred while in her apartment. Every time she entered, a grayness would descend on her. It lifted when she exited. When she disposed of the satanic bible, her cauldron, her cookbook for brews, and the ingredients for brews, she no longer experienced the gloom surrounding her. Another patient who had been oppressed for years had the gloom disappear when he was delivered from the oppression.

Mature Christians have spiritual immunity from all forms of demonization, but especially possession. They must, however, maintain an adequate level of piety. In doing so, they maintain spiritual immunity. Spiritual immunity is maintained by practicing regular prayer, Bible reading, and worship.

Obsession is to be abnormally preoccupied with some thing. It is almost universally one of ideology. There were many communist leaders who were obsessed. We see it among Christians, Muslims, and Hindus and, in our day, among the extreme animal rights people and environmentalists.

Finally, there is fanaticism. It can be an extreme form of demonic obsession, although it is usually a psychological state. We see it among Christians, Muslims, and Hindus and, during World War II, among the Japanese. Fanaticism also occurs in mental illness. This is especially true of some forms of schizophrenia and occasionally in mania where it occurs as one of the symptoms.

In completing this section, I must say that all spiritual disease is psychospiritual. It has to do with beliefs that we call cognitions, but have emotions connected to them. The behaviors that arise out of these beliefs are then good or evil, correct or erroneous, constructive or deleterious, and pleasant or painful. They will then determine the degree of happiness a person will experience in his life.

Spiritual disease can be both primary and secondary. There is no question that to be unregenerate is a primary disease. It gives rise to a secondary disease of sin. But sin may occur as a primary disease in the regenerate. Demonization is usually a primary disease occurring mostly in the unregenerate, but under certain circumstances it also occurs in the regenerate. Fanaticism can occur in the regenerate or the unregenerate.

Psychospiritual problems almost always occur in psychiatric diseases described in the *Diagnostic and Statistical Manual of Mental Disorders, Fourth Edition (DSM-IV)*. The writers of the Bible saw man as a unity, and one must use a systems approach to recognize that if one part of the system is not functioning correctly then it will affect all other parts of the system. Von Bertanlanffy,(31) who was the great proponent of General Systems Theory, said that psychiatry and psychology needed to consider it in its diagnosis and treatment of mental problems. In the light of his ideas, we can say that all illness has a psychospiritual component. We must recognize that to treat one aspect of illness and neglect the other two is an omission.

5. CHRISTIAN INTERVENTIONS

5.1. Evangelism

Just as the Muslim therapist feels the patient must be correct in his Islamic faith before therapy can be carried out, the Christian therapist must ascertain the spiritual state of the patient and determine whether the patient would benefit from Christian psychotherapy. Schizophrenics and some bipolar disorders (manic phase) should be treated without reference to Christianity.

If a patient is unregenerate and is not opposed to Christian therapy, they should be offered the choice of what form of therapy they desire. The therapist must always remember that the human will does not tolerate the imposition of another will above its own, so one must make an appeal to their will. It is not possible to forcibly evangelize someone! There is the criticism that Christian therapists who do evangelism are taking advantage of vulnerable people. In most instances have not found this to be true. Most patients realize that their therapist has their best interests at heart and readily agree to be evangelized. Even if a person submits unwillingly, they will not benefit from the experience, and one still cannot use Christian interventions and have them be effective.

The most effective form of evangelism is personal witness. One-third of all persons who become Christians come as a result of the personal witness of another believer. Personal witness of healing is especially desirable in the treatment of alcoholics and drug addicts. If one is dealing with a person who has a borderline disorder it is sine qua non. If the patient is willing to accept Christ as his Savior, then the therapist must know the plan of salvation that should be revealed to the patient. The plan is that the person is a sinner, that Christ died to take his punishment, and that he can receive pardon if he asks him into his life. The patient and therapist pray a prayer of surrender together. To illustrate this point, I cite the response of twenty-one Malagasy alcoholics. The lecturer was asked to preach to them. He chose as the basis for his lecture the scripture 2 Corinthians 5:17. It says that if anyone is in Christ he is a new person. These men were in a Christian healing community, so it was appropriate for him to deliver his message using scripture. After he had explained the scripture, he asked how many of the men had become new persons. No hands went up. He then asked how many of them would like to become new persons. All hands went up. He next asked if they knew the plan of salvation. None of them did, even though two of the men were Roman Catholic priests. He then explained the plan of salvation to them and asked them to pray the prayer of salvation with him if they desired to become a new person. They all did pray as he recited it. After the service was over, the two priests came and asked the lecturer if they could use this plan with their catechists.

He told them that they would be remiss if they didn't.

Sometimes if the patients have been regenerated but have grieved the Spirit with their sin, they may need to rededicate their lives to the Lord to regain their ability to be healed.

On occasions God will act sovereignly in a person's life and will reveal himself to the person, who then has the opportunity to accept or refuse the offer. Lord Kenneth Clark,(32) the producer of the BBC series *Civilization,* had such an experience. He was standing in the church at San Lorenzo in Italy when " for a few minutes my whole being was irradiated with a kind of heavenly joy, far more intense than anything I had known before. This state of mind lasted several minutes, and wonderful though it was, it posed an awkward problem in terms of action. My life was far from blameless: I would have to reform. My family would think I was going mad, and perhaps after all it was a delusion for I was in every way unworthy of receiving such a flood of grace. Gradually the effect wore off and I made no effort to retain it. I think I was right; I was too deeply embedded in the world to change course." Most accept such an offer.

5.2. Discipleship

Like any newborn baby, the newborn Christian needs to be taught how to live a Christian life. Just as a child needs to learn how to communicate with his parents, the newborn Christian needs to learn how to communicate with God and to understand who God is and how he relates and communicates with him. The process of teaching the skills necessary to do this is called discipleship.

It has been shown that only 5 percent of members of mainline denominational churches have any training at all. It is clear that if the therapist is to be effective in transforming lives with Christian psychotherapy, he must disciple his patients or make sure they are discipled. What do they need to learn? This is described in detail in my book entitled *The Nuts and Bolts of Discipleship.*(33)

5.3. Prayer

Most effective persons in the Christian world are people of prayer. In an unpublished study of people who were effective Christian leaders, I found that all prayed at least two hours a day. Jesus prayed more than that. Christian therapists also need to be men and women of prayer.

To cooperate in therapy, a believer has to know how to pray. Prayer is described as a conversation between two people who love one anther–God and man. It is the single most effective intervention in the Christian therapist's armamentarium. It has to be carried out to initiate the spiritual life of a patient, but it also has to be used in the transformation of the person's mind.

Other faiths also practice prayer as a means of communicating with the divine but in most of them they use prayers composed by their leaders or pray their particular holy writings. They also have certain behavioral rituals that they perform as part of their prayers. Islam is notable for its ritualistic prayer. Orthodox Jews also write out their prayers and lay them before God by putting them into crevices at the Wailing Wall while bowing. Buddhists inscribe them on wheels that they twirl. Hindus repeat a mantra. However, it is not clear what the content of the mantra is except it is usually taken from their holy writings and is quite varied. The frequent repetition of their prayers has a transforming effect on their minds. All prayer has as a goal putting the person praying in contact with his higher power.

Christian prayer is designed especially to put the person praying in contact with the triune God (Father, Son, and Holy Spirit). It has two aspects. The most commonly practiced is spoken prayer. The mature Christian does, however, more than talk, he also listens. There is one prayer that Jesus taught us to pray that is formal. It is called the Lord's Prayer. Most of his recorded prayers, however, were conversational. Christian prayer should be conversational.

God speaks to us in two ways. He puts illuminated thoughts into our minds, and he illuminates his message in the Bible. This illumination results in eureka or ah-ha experiences. He may also speak to us through his current prophets. The main reason why most prayer is a one-way conversation is that people do not intently listen. An example of God's communication was observed in a young Christian woman who was miserable in her bondage to her mother. She had never separated and individuated and was trying to free herself, but could not find a way. Her therapist told her to listen to God and find out what he would say. She was reminded in the ensuing silence of a scripture story that had a stubborn person in it who became obedient and was healed. She realized that she had to be obedient too. When she took steps to free herself, she was freed and healed.

Prayer does many things that facilitate transformation of a person's mind. It may reveal truths not perceived before. This is especially true if scripture is prayed. Prayer also reveals the errors in misbeliefs (or lies) that the person has learned in his early life so they can be corrected with the truth. This is not to say that the therapist as an authority can do the same, but prayers of thanksgiving for the truth will facilitate the change in thinking.

Prayer also facilitates the release of damaging emotions. This occurs when prayer visualization or prayers for the healing of memories are carried out.

5.4. Healing of Memories

This form of prayer is uniquely Christian.(34) It is a prayer in which the therapist uses the patient's ability to remember and visualize to bring into consciousness the traumatic event and have the Holy Spirit release the damaging emotion(s) by divine intervention and heal the memory.

Memories of traumas suffered in the past or, as the case above illustrates, of sins we have committed can be healed using an intervention called inner healing or healing of memories. It can also be used to bring about a release of bondage to the living or dead. In the post-abortion syndrome, one has the patient try to discern the sex and name of the fetus. To illustrate the use of this kind of prayer, I will relate the following case.

A wife of a physician in her late forties came because of depression of three years duration. It had not responded to several different antidepressants prescribed by a psychiatrist in her city. Her illness began when she was involved in a wreck while taking her son to reading therapy for his dyslexia. She had all the classical symptoms and signs of major depression. She was tried on a new antidepressant, but she did not respond to it either. Continuing cognitive behavioral therapy was of no avail, so it was decided to review her history to see if something of dynamic significance has been missed.

She said in this session that she was driving a small Volkswagen with her son when she lost control of her car and rolled it several times. With further questioning, she remembered that as the car rolled she thought, "I will have killed both my sons." The therapist said, "But you only have one son." "Oh!" She said, "I did not tell you. I had an abortion." She then guiltily explained her reasons for having one.

When she was asked how she knew it was a boy, she said that she "just knew." "I was going to name him Christopher." After she had finished her story she was told that she needed to commit Christopher to the Lord. She agreed and in a ceremony called "requiem healing" she committed Christopher to God.(35) A modified standard Eucharistic service in the Book of Common Prayer was used. The liturgy contains a request for forgiveness. She then committed Christopher to the Lord for his eternal destiny. As she did, she visualized standing at the threshold of the kingdom of God with the light of God's presence in the background. An angel then came out of the light and took Christopher off into the light of God's presence. At this point she wept for a few minutes. They then celebrated the rest of the Eucharistic service for closure. She was instantly healed of the depression and taken off medication. She has remained well for the last twenty-five years.

5.5. Use of the Bible

The Bible is for the Christian the authoritative word of God and the source of all truth. Because it is considered sufficient to lead a person to salvation and as a guide to right living, it is useful in helping the therapist transform the mind of the patient he is counseling. Almost all persons have a distorted image of God and themselves. One job of the Christian therapist is to help them see who God really is and who they really are. Most persons view God as they view their father. Most of them appraise themselves as they have been appraised. Some have low self-esteem and feel unworthy, whereas some are prideful with distorted views of their actual worth. All persons need to see God rightly. It is easy to correct their distorted view because God revealed himself when he sent Jesus to live among us (John 14:9).

Throughout the Bible, there are statements of who a person is in Christ and how God sees him. Neil Anderson, in his book *Living Free in Christ*,(36) has listed these so that they can see themselves as God sees them. If they have a distorted image of who they are, then praying these scriptures will facilitate a change in their view of who they are and their security in God's love.

There are many other things the Bible does when we read it. They include:

1 It provides a correct image of God. He is revealed to the believer.
2 It makes him wise for salvation. Each step of the plan of salvation has a scriptural reference.
3 It speaks to the person's security.
4 It provides knowledge about meaning and purpose for life.
5 It speaks on how to deal with sin by
  a Urging confession.
  b Calling to repentance.
  c Providing the offer of forgiveness.
  d Instructing how to meet and master temptation.
6 It condemns selfishness and teaches selflessness.
7 It teaches how to maintain right relationships.
8 It provides rules for a successful marriage.
9 It speaks negatively about divorce.
10 It provides directions for family life.

11 It teaches how to nurture children.

12 It enunciates rules of sexual behavior.

13 It enhances our self-esteem.

14 It teaches how to avoid diseases.

15 It teaches how to control greed.

16 It teaches good dietary habits.

17 It provides the basis for emotional healing.

18 It provides real values.

19 It defines real humility.

In these and many other ways, the Bible teaches a healthy way of living.

5.6. Worship

The purpose of worship is to bring us into an encounter with the living God. Having queried many who have left a church, I find that most leave because they do not encounter God there. An alive church will foster such encounters. People will encounter God in the music, in prayer and scripture reading, occasionally in the proclamation of God's Word, and especially in the witness of other believers. All should encounter him in the Eucharist.

Encountering God will result in access to a new experience of the Holy Spirit. All need this from time to time. God's Spirit guides and reveals Christ to the person. With these encounters, the person is spiritually renewed. The need for refilling by God is best stated by Dwight Moody. He was asked if he was filled with the Holy Spirit. His response was, "Of course I am, but I leak." I doubt that anyone understands why this occurs, but it may be the same thing that is true of all relationships. The need to be constantly renewed with regular encounters is true of almost all intimate relationships, and this is probably the reason for the need for repeat encounters with God.

People encounter God in music. Music elicits emotions. In worship, music will elicit the emotions of love and awe. The music that most commonly brings about an encounter is music in the idiom of that culture. Karen Boring, an ethnomusicologist with Wycliffe Bible Translators, said in one of their newsletters, "Music, although a universal phenomenon is not a universal language. It carries cultural meaning." I have seen African natives respond to music expressed in their heart language with behavioral evidence that they are encountering God. I agree with Charles Wesley that the devil should not have all the good music.

Prayer, whether solitary or corporate, can bring about an encounter with God. It is important that the prayer be of praise and not petition. When petitionary prayer is self-centered, it may not have the intimacy that brings about an encounter. Because music is a form of prayer, it is easy to understand why nonmusical prayers of praise will also be stimulating.

J. B. Phillips has commented that the purpose of the Eucharist is to provide a refilling with the Holy Spirit. Even so, it rarely elicits an encounter. The problem is not with the sacrament, but has to do with the celebrants. They do not understand its real meaning and the necessity of preparing for the sacrament. Therefore, they come to the table unworthily (1 Cor. 11:27, 28).

5.7. Confession, Repentance, and Forgiveness

These three spiritual interventions usually go together, so they will be described in the order I have listed them. Most patients come to a therapist with the expectation of confessing their wrongdoing. They may not consider it as such, but they will still confess it. In the course of the history taking, they will reveal their most inner thoughts and describe past behavior and its consequences in detail. In a like manner, they may feel that they deserve punishment to atone for their wrongdoing. This gives rise to the despair of morality. To alleviate their suffering, they must repent, that is, they must realize that they have sinned against God (Ps. 51:4) and intend to amend their ways. They do, however, need to be forgiven. Forgiveness can only come from God (Luke 5:21). Fortunately, Jesus deputized his followers to pass on God's forgiveness to repentant sinners (John 20:23). Thus, the therapist can effectively forgive in the name of Jesus. Human forgiveness does not have the effect of spiritual forgiveness. The following is a case that illustrates the healing power of forgiveness.

This patient was a Vietnam veteran who had been regenerated early in life, but in time because of cultural influences became an alcoholic and addicted to marijuana. He also, while stationed in Korea for a short time, got a woman pregnant but then deserted her when sent to Vietnam. He had a wife and two children back in the United States. He was sent to Vietnam in a noncombat role. In time he was issued a new rifle that he took with a friend to the rifle range to learn how to shoot it. He was drinking a pint of whiskey a day and smoking two to four joints of marijuana at the time. On their way back, they stopped by the roadside to shoot at random targets. They saw an old man and woman approaching them. His friend said, "Hey look, there's a couple of targets." With that, he fired two shots and killed them both. The next day, he was a psychiatric casualty. Eventually, he was evacuated to Okinawa, Honolulu, San Francisco, and finally discharged to a Veterans Administration (VA)hospital where he spent six months. Finally he was discharged from the VA, essentially unchanged, and returned home, but soon he chose to move and work in our community. For eleven years he lived with his guilt and shame. A month of treatment ten years later did not help, and one year later during a vacation he finally came back to our local VA hospital to find out if anything else could be done for him. The resident felt he did not know what to do. His supervisor then suggested he present him to me because I had done research on posttraumatic stress disorder (PTSD).

When I interviewed the patient he admitted to his sins. I asked if he felt he could be forgiven. He said no. He said he had prayed that someone would kill him to punish him for his sins. When reminded that he could commit suicide he said, "No I deserve to be punished for what I did." I chose not to debate the issue with him, but instead dismissed him. I then discussed the existential despair of morality and death that he suffered from with the residents and medical students who were in attendance.

After my teaching session, I told the resident that I had unfinished business with the patient, and wanted to see him again. In the company of the resident and a medical student, I took him in an office and asked why he said he could not be forgiven. He said that he had committed an unpardonable sin. I told him that it was only unpardonable if he attributed his murder of the two people to God. He responded, "No, I did it." I then told him that if Jesus could forgive his murderers as they were crucifying him, surely he could be forgiven. Then I said, "In Jesus' name and by his power you are forgiven." Big tears teetered on his lower lids for a moment and then trickled down his cheeks. With this he began to sob and weep profusely. He spontaneously embraced me and laid his head on my chest saying, "Are you sure?" "Yes," I replied. "The Bible says that if we confess our sins he is faithful and just to forgive us of our sins and cleanse us of all unrighteousness"(1 John 1:9). After he wept for at least ten minutes and thoroughly soaked my shirt with his tears, he asked me if there was anything else he needed to do. I told him he needed to rededicate his life to the Lord. He did and was totally healed.

5.8. Exhortation

Exhortation was commonly practiced in the early church and is still considered a gift of the Spirit. Exhortation as a gift is the ability to help others to reach their full potential by means of encouraging, challenging, comforting, and guiding. Christian therapists should remember that they are not to be neutral when transforming minds. To achieve the change they have to positively exhort a patient because it is difficult to refute many misbeliefs.

Exhortation (strong encouragement) was useful in a woman with three children who consulted me because her husband was divorcing her. He left her to marry a much younger woman. This man was obsessed with building an estate, so he wanted to divorce her and not have to pay any alimony or child support. The woman was very depressed and hopeless so she wanted to agree to the settlement that he proposed. This would have cheated her out of everything she had helped to accumulate. At the time, our state did not have a law requiring an equitable division of assets in divorces. There was a bill pending in the legislature, but it had not been passed. Feeling that what he proposed was unjust, I exhorted her to refuse to agree until he relented. She did so, but it took constant exhortation because he did not relent. In time, the equitable division bill passed in the legislature. Her lawyer then forced an equitable division and justice was done.

5.9. Deliverance

Authentic Christians have no difficulty in believing that personified supernatural evil exists. Satan uses his demons to harass man. I have already described his means, but it is well to point out that unregenerate and even regenerate persons can be demonized. Authentic Christians do, however, have to strongly believe that Satan can exploit to demonize them. The only way his forces can be dealt with is deliverance. It is true that Jesus deputized all of his disciples to cast out demons. We have the same power today if we are mature Christians.

A mature Christian can deliver a possessed individual with a simple command to the demon(s) to depart and be taken to Jesus for disposition. If the person (the one commanding the demon to leave) is not a mature Christian, he or she may be attacked as the sons of Sceva were in the Bible (Acts 19:14) when they tried to cast out demons.

In our culture, demon possession is rarely seen, but in the third world demonization is much more common.

5.10. The Holy Spirit and Christian Psychotherapy

To a nonbeliever, the above discussion of the Holy Spirit and demons will probably seem quite bizarre. But we have to realize that when the mind-brain problem is discussed, there are two opposing views. There are those that believe that

the mind exists above the brain, or that the mind and brain are one. The former is called dualist interactionism, the latter monism. In his discussion of the supernatural, C. S. Lewis (37) said that the mind is supernatural. Wilder Penfield,(38) the neurosurgeon, Sir John Eccles,(39) the neurophysiologist, and Karl Popper,(40) the philosopher, subscribe to dualist interactionism. Thus, the work of the Holy Spirit and Satan is relevant to Christian psychotherapy because Christians believe that there is a supernatural dimension to existence and that it is inhabited by supernatural beings.

It is unfortunate that the church has not given more importance to the transforming power of the Holy Spirit in the lives of believers. Instead, most churches have done everything they could to quench the Holy Spirit and eradicate any attention to its presence. This began in the third century when Montanus and Tertullian emphasized the work of the Holy Spirit. Admittedly some of their beliefs were heretical, but the belief in the presence of the Holy Spirit had truth and persisted in their followers for centuries. The charismatic movement was present from time to time in other isolated parts of the church, but recurred with the Huguenots who were put to the sword by the French king because their beliefs were thought to be heretical. At approximately the same time, people were filled with the Holy Spirit in the Wesleyan revivals, but they were not persecuted.

Jesus was emphatic about the role of the Holy Spirit in the life of the believer. On two occasions he said that we would first be clothed (Luke 24:49) and then filled (Acts 1:8) with power when the Holy Spirit came upon us. This happens with salvation. We may not get a full measure of the Holy Spirit, but we get enough to bring about the changes described by William James. There is more of course, and we can ask for a new measure of the Holy Spirit anytime we wish. God often responds.

The fullness of the Holy Spirit is given when a person absolutely surrenders. Jesus demanded that we be absolutely surrendered to him if we were to be his followers (Luke 14:33). This did not mean that we were to give up just a few things. He said all! Then he told Peter that having given up everything he would get it all back (Mark 10:29, 30). It is with absolute surrender that one gets filled with the Holy Spirit. This act adds to the power and increases fruits of the Spirit (Gal. 5:22,23). The fullness of the supernatural presence of the Holy Spirit installed in our lives is the source of power and gifts that makes the Christian therapist so effective.

REFERENCES

1. Islamic Psychology. http://islamic-world.net/psychology/psy.php?ArtID+174. Accessed November 23, 2008.
2. Karasu TB. Psychotherapies: an overview. *Am J Psychiatry*. 1977;134:851–863.
3. Frank J. *Persuasion and Healing: A Comparative Study of Psychotherapies*. Baltimore: Johns Hopkins University Press; 1971.
4. Karasu TB. Spiritual psychotherapy. *Am J Psychotherapy*. 1999;53:143–162.
5. Tweedie DF. *The Christian and the Couch: An Introduction to Christian Logotherapy*. Grand Rapids, MI: Baker; 1963.
6. Collins GR. *Psychology and Theology: Prospects for Integration*. Nashville, TN: Abingdon; 1981.
7. Adams J. *Competent to Counsel*. Nutley, NJ: Presbyterian and Reformed; 1971.
8. Minirth FB. *Christian Psychiatry*. Old Tappan, NJ: F. H. Revell Co.; 1977.
9. Crabbe L. *Basic Principles of Biblical Counseling*. Grand Rapids, MI: Zondervan; 1975.
10. Aerts DL, Apostel B, DeMoor, et al. *Worldviews from Fragmentation to Integration*. Brussels: VUB Press; 1994.
11. Baier K. The concept of value. In: Lazlo E, Wilbur J, eds. *Value Theory in Art and Science*. New York: Gordon and Breach; 1973.
12. Wilson WP. Man's human nature. Unpublished lecture, 1973.
13. Skinner BF. *About Behaviorism*. New York: Vintage Books; 1976.
14. Harris TA. *I'm OK You're OK: A Practical Guide to Transactional Analysis*. New York: Harper and Row; 1969.
15. Collins GR. *The Christian Psychology of Paul Tournier*. Grand Rapids, MI: Baker Books; 1973.
16. Frankl V. What is meant by meaning? *J Existentialism*. 1966;7:21–28.
17. Ryle JC. *Practical Religion*. Auburn, MA: Evangelical Press; 2001.
18. Kobasa SC, Maldi SR. Existential personality theory. In: Corsoini R, ed. *Current Personality Theories*. Ithaca, IL: Peracock; 1987:243–276.
19. McKay WM. *The Disease and Remedy of Sin*. London: Hodder and Stoughton; 1918.
20. Lewis CS. *The Problem of Pain*. New York: The Macmillan Co.; 1948.
21. Spero M. Sin as neurosis and neurosis as sin, further implications of a halachic metapsychology. *J Relig Health*. 1978;17:274–287.
22. Wesley J. *Primitive Physic*. London: R. Hawes; 1774.
23. Marias J. *Metaphysical Anthropology*. Lopes-Murillo M, trans. University Park, PA: Pennsylvania State University Press; 1971.
24. Wilson WP. The Psychological Significance of Forgiveness, Unpublished Manuscript.
25. Grubb N. *Once Caught, No Escape. My life Story*. London: Lutterworth Publishing; 1969.
26. Meltzof J, Kornriech M. *Research in Psychotherapy*. New York: Atherton Press; 1970.
27. Rogers C. Perceptual reorganization in client centered therapy. In: Blake R, Ramsey G, eds. *Perception: An Approach to Personality*. New York: Ronald Press; 1951.
28. Carlson DE. Jesus style of relating: the search for a biblical style of counseling. *J Psychol Theol*. 1976;4:181–191.
29. Barnhouse D. *The Invisible War*. Grand Rapids, MI: Zondervan; 1965:156.
30. Nevius JL. *Demon Possession*. Grand Rapids, MI: Kregel Publications; 1968.
31. Beranlanffy V. *General Systems Theory: Foundations, Development, Applications*. New York: Braziller; 1968.
32. Clark KM. *The Other Half: A Self Portrait*. London: J. Murray; 1977.
33. Wilson WP. *The Nuts and Bolts of Discipleship*. Lima, OH: Fairway Press; 2007.
34. Seamands D. *Healing of Memories*. Wheaton, IL: Victor Books; 1985.
35. Mitton M, Parker R. *Requiem Healing*. London: Daybreak; 1991.
36. Anderson N. *Living Free in Christ*. Ventura, CA: Regal Books; 1991.
37. Lewis CS. *Miracles*. New York: The MacMillan Co.; 1947: 10–16.
38. Penfield W. *The Mystery of the Mind*. Princeton, NJ: Princeton University Press; 1975.
39. Eccles JC. *The Human Psyche*. New York: Springer International; 1980.
40. Popper K. *Knowledge and the Mind Body Problem*. New York: Routledge; 1994.

20 Psychiatric Treatments Involving Religion: Psychotherapy from an Islamic Perspective

SASAN VASEGH

SUMMARY

Religious thoughts and behaviors can play an important role in the relief or exacerbation of psychopathologic symptoms in Muslim patients; therefore, every successful psychotherapist needs to be familiar with Muslim culture in his or her country. Furthermore, some clinical trials show that adding religious psychotherapy to the usual secular therapy can accelerate clinical improvement in religious Muslim patients. In this chapter, I will (a) provide a short description of the basic tenets of Islam, (b) describe important points in initial assessment of Muslim clients, addressing transference and countertransference issues, and (c) discuss several Islamic concepts useful in treatment of depression, anxiety, and interpersonal problems in Muslim clients. Clinical examples are also provided to show how these concepts can be used in psychotherapeutic settings.

Defining psychotherapy is difficult (pp. 6–7).(1) Although there are many kinds of psychotherapy(2) and many differences between them, it seems that all of them have at least one common goal: decreasing clients' overall suffering. Each client coming to a psychotherapeutic session has some problems, that is, some issues that cause (usually serious) negative feelings such as depression, anxiety, or anger. The more a psychotherapist succeeds in helping the patient overcome these negative feelings and prevent their recurrence, the more successful is his or her psychotherapy.

There are about 1.2 billion Muslims in the world and Islam is the second largest religion in Europe and anticipated soon to be the second largest religion in the United States.(3) Whether psychotherapists are Muslim or not, if they are to help their clients, they need to be familiar with Muslim clients. If not, they may try to apply unmodified Western theories of psychology and psychotherapy and apply their own stereotypes of Muslims to Muslim clients, which can cause therapeutic failure and frustration (p. ix).(4) Moreover, unfamiliarity with Muslim culture can cause serious diagnostic errors. For example, some Muslim patients may fear invisible creatures called Jinns, and this fear could be falsely diagnosed as psychosis by inexperienced clinicians.(5) Also, the collectivist nature of Muslim culture may be interpreted as "dependent personality disorder" (p. 73)(4) and Muslim women's hair coverings as a sign of their oppression.(6) Attempts to free Muslim clients from this perceived dependency or oppression may cause them to feel misunderstood and may cause them to drop out of therapy.

Muslims come to psychotherapy for various problems, including anxiety and depressive disorders or family and cultural problems. In addition, after the September 11 terrorist attacks, many Muslims in Western countries suffered increased social pressures such as physical or verbal attacks and discrimination (7) and experienced adjustment problems.

There is no single, best type of psychotherapy for all Muslim patients, and many of them need an eclectic approach. Although theoretically all kinds of psychotherapy can be used with Muslims, cognitive and behavioral interventions seem to be more suitable for most Muslim patients (p. 100).(4) Psychoanalysis or insight-oriented psychotherapies have sometimes been regarded as counterproductive in Muslim clients, leading to premature dropouts or worsening of the patient's condition.(6) Indeed, cognitive-behavioral therapy is also the psychotherapy with the most empirical evidence.(8)

Is Islamic psychotherapy really effective? Unfortunately, there are only a few studies in this regard. These show that Islamic-oriented cognitive-behavioral psychotherapy, when added to the usual secular therapy, leads to significantly faster recovery in anxious or depressed Muslim patients.(9–11) But to use Islamic concepts in the treatment of Muslim patients, the therapist needs some expertise in Islam, and most clinicians are not experts in Islam. The way to partially overcome this problem is to be aware of this lack of knowledge and seek more information regarding the patient's religious and ethnic background from trusted sources. There are case reports that show this approach can be very helpful. For example, Ali et al. (12) report an interesting case in which a non-Muslim male counselor could effectively help a young Muslim female client only after using this approach (see below).

The goal of this chapter is to suggest important clinical points and psychotherapeutic techniques helpful in therapy with Muslim clients. Both Islamic teachings and psychotherapy are so extensive that it is impossible to fully describe them in this chapter; therefore, I will begin with a short introduction to Islam basics and then I will briefly describe several Islamic techniques useful in problems common to Muslim patients.

I. ISLAM BASICS

Islam literally means *submission*, that is, submission to the word of God. Muslims believe that all previous prophets, such as Jesus, Moses, Noah, Abraham, and others, were Muslims, for they really obeyed God (who Muslims refer to as Allah). According to the Koran (Islam's holy book), the Prophet Muhammad is the last prophet, and the only religion acceptable to God is Islam.

The *pillars of Islam* are five fundamental beliefs or behaviors that are shared by almost all Muslim groups. These are *Shahadat* (the profession that there is no God but Allah, and Muhammad is his Prophet), *Siyam* or *Sawm* (fasting in the holy month of Ramadan), *Salat* (Islamic five-time daily prayers), *Zakat* (a tax providing financial help to the poor), and Haj (a pilgrimage to Mecca) (p. 16).(4) The first pillar is the most important and is enough for one to be regarded as a Muslim, that is, one need only acknowledge that he or she believes there is no god but Allah, and that Muhammad is Allah's messenger. Because Islam's official language is Arabic, these two acknowledgments usually are said in Arabic and are referred to as *"shahadatain,"* that means, "the two acknowledgments."

Just as some Christians apply their knowledge of Jesus's life and try to model their behavior after his,(13) religious Muslims try to follow the Prophet Muhammad. So the Prophet Muhammad's *Sunnah* (meaning his sayings and deeds) is one of the main sources of Islamic laws. The other source is the Koran, the holy book of the Muslims. The Koran is believed to be God's words revealed to the Prophet Muhammad by the angel Gabriel. Only ten years after the foundation of Islam in 610 AD, it became accepted by most people in the Arabian Peninsula in spite of strong opposition. The Koran was one of the most important factors in the fast spread of Islam because it sounded so beautiful that many Arabs accepted Islam after hearing only a few verses from it. Indeed, Koranic verses were so effective that when some of the early Muslims immigrated to Abyssinia (present-day Ethiopia) and recited verses from the Koran about the Blessed Virgin Mary in front of the Abyssinian king and his Christian clerics, the latter were highly impressed and began to weep (p. 181).(14) In addition, Islam announced equality and brotherhood for all people and prohibited violent acts such as burying their daughters alive and torturing slaves, thus making it more attractive.

Islamic rules are very extensive and cover all aspects of a Muslim's life: marriage, education, private and group worship, politics, eating, drinking, clothing, and so on. Some rules are mandatory, and others are recommended. For example, it is mandatory for a Muslim to pray the five Islamic daily prayers and to avoid consuming alcohol, but it is recommended that a Muslim marry, pray night prayers, and not sleep or eat too much. People usually depend on Islamic clerics to learn about their religious duties.

Islamic laws are remarkably flexible. For example, although consuming alcohol is strictly forbidden, if a trusted physician prescribes it as necessary to treat an important disease, it can be temporarily consumed. Or if a Muslim cannot do Islamic daily prayers in the usual standing position, she or he can do them while sitting or even lying down in bed. This flexibility is inferred from the two sources of Islamic laws: the Koran and the Sunnah. During his life, Prophet Muhammad had many situations in which his deeds and sayings indicated his flexibility. Some sayings of the Prophet Muhammad and verses of the Koran may seem inconsistent on a particular subject, for example, women's rights and the rights of parents and children. These Koranic verses and deeds of the Prophet may be interpreted differently by Islamic clerics. Usually, Islamic clerics within each Islamic division infer similar rules and orders regarding basic Islamic elements; so Islamic divisions have many similarities (in basic elements). They also, however, have differences (usually in details). For example, all religious Muslims believe in the five Islamic prayers, but some parts of the prayers differ between Islamic divisions. Usually the more they deviate from the basic rules, the more controversial they will be, even in a particular division. For example, there may be different attitudes toward details of parenting, women working , acceptable relationships with God, and forgiveness in a given Islamic division. This flexibility plays an important role in psychotherapy with Muslim patients, because most seemingly rigid issues causing psychological distress are really in fact flexible.

There are two main Islamic branches: Shia (about 15 percent) and Sunni (about 85 percent).(3) Shias predominate in Iran and Iraq. Although describing the similarities and differences between Shias and Sunnis is beyond the scope of this chapter, some points deserve brief description. The most important difference between Shias and Sunnis is that most Shias believe in twelve Imams (religious leaders) after the Prophet Muhammad and believe that their deeds and sayings (Sunnah) are the continuity of the Prophet's Sunnah and must be used as a root for Islamic inference. This belief is similar to what Christians believe about Jesus's Apostles. These Imams begin with Imam Ali (cousin of the Prophet Muhammad) and end with Imam Mahdi (born 869 AD), who is believed to be still alive and will come someday in the future to save the world from oppression. Interestingly, they believe that Jesus Christ will return and will be one of his special aides. So in addition to the Prophet Muhammad's Sunnah, Shias have many years of Shia Imams' Sunnah and volumes of books of their sayings and prayers that can be used in psychotherapy.

Many nonfunctional thoughts and behaviors of Muslim patients are rooted in their culture and not in their religion. However, they may think that these thoughts and actions are religiously justified (15) and may use them to resist change. Furthermore, despite many adaptive thoughts and behaviors in Islamic sources, a Muslim client may not be aware of or pay enough attention to them. If a psychotherapist can use his or her knowledge of Islam to show this to the Muslim client, adaptive changes may be more easily brought about.

But what can non-Muslim therapists who are not experienced with Islam do? As some cases show,(12) if non-Muslim therapists become aware of their lack of knowledge, respect the patient's culture and religion, and seek information from trusted sources, they may effectively help these clients. Indeed, some Muslim clients with religious conflicts may prefer non-Muslim therapists.(12)

In the following sections, I will describe some Islamic concepts useful in psychotherapy for common problems in Muslim patients. It should be noted that effectively using the Islamic concepts in psychotherapy also depends very much on the psychotherapist's own characteristics and experience with psychotherapy. Like other cognitive and behavioral approaches, specific religious concepts are better used indirectly through Socratic questioning and guided discovery (pp. 43–86)(16) to help the clients change more effectively toward more functional cognitions and behaviors.

2. COMMON FACTORS AND INITIAL ASSESSMENT

Surprisingly, despite wide theoretical differences between various psychotherapeutic approaches, some meta-analyses have shown all of them are more or less effective.(8) This research emphasizes the importance of the so-called "common factors," that is, factors such as warm and positive involvement with the patient, instillation of hope, and offering new perspectives to the patient's problems. Some of these factors and other first session issues relevant to Muslim patients are described here under broad concepts of "countertransference" and "transference."

2.1. Countertransference and Therapist's Misunderstandings

Because Muslims are minorities in most Western countries, they are usually stereotyped.(7, 12) After the terrorist attacks of September 11 and negative media attention, misunderstandings have become more common and may unconsciously affect the therapist's feelings toward Muslim patients.

There are many differences between Islamic culture and individualistic Western culture. Muslims often live in extended families and believe they must respect and obey their parents unless their orders oppose God's orders (Holy Koran 31:15). Muslim people usually are involved with and are ready to provide help to other family members. Islam has different laws regarding some rights and duties of men and women. For example, according to Islam, a Muslim man must provide for almost all of his wife's needs, but a Muslim woman does not have to work at home or outside to compensate. Although Muslim women must cover their bodies or hair in front of strange men, recommendations for Muslim men's clothes are much more lax. These rules have been interpreted by Islamic clerics as measures to strengthen family love and ties and to prevent sexual immorality of both men and women.(17) The non-Muslim therapist facing these differences may automatically assume that the Western culture is always more adaptive to the patient, an assumption that is not supported by empirical evidence (pp. 26–28).(4) Many Muslim women are successful at work and in their family and do not want to change their culture. Assuming that Muslim women should be saved from their "oppressor" culture, religion, or husband ignores their interest in their family and religious/cultural background and may cause them to feel misunderstood and to leave the therapy. On the contrary, some Middle Eastern women believe that Euro-American women working both inside and outside the home are greatly oppressed and that Euro-American men are not accountable enough for their families.(18)

Even if a Muslim client accepts the therapist's point of view, this may result in severe interpersonal conflicts and may end in a more disturbed and distressed patient. Therefore, although for some patients it may be better to modify some of their cultural or religious attitudes, if they show resistance to such modification, therapists can cautiously offer the pros and cons of these changes and then let patients decide for themselves.(12)

2.1.1. Female Muslim Client
When a Muslim woman consults a non-Muslim male therapist, some areas may cause misunderstanding because Islam affects all aspects of a Muslim woman's daily life.(19) For instance, Islam discourages men and women from

looking at the bodies of persons of the opposite sex (except one's spouse), supposedly to prevent sexual immorality and marital damage. Looking at the face is a lesser matter, although even this may be discouraged in many Islamic religious societies. Islam encourages sexual relationships between wife and husband, but prohibits any sexual relationships outside this boundary. In addition, in many religious Muslim families, women and men have more or less separate social groups. For example, when they attend a family party, most conversations occur within each sex group, and many parties may be exclusively for men or for women. Also, many Muslim women do not work outside the home and have little contact with strange men. All of these factors may cause the Muslim female patient to have less than usual eye contact with her male therapist, which can cause negative attitudes in the therapist or may be interpreted by him as a sign of depression, avoidant personality, or lying.

Islam also prohibits any bodily contact between non-relative opposite sexes. For example, a Muslim man is allowed to shake hands with his wife or sister but not with his female cousin or teacher. In a case described by Ali et al.,(12) the male counselor visiting Mona (a Muslim Arab girl) for the first time wanted to greet her by shaking hands with her, but this approach caused distrust in Mona and turned out to be his first mistake. Nevertheless, he was eventually able to help Mona after he showed more interest in her Muslim culture and after Mona felt that he was not going to rescue her from "her religion that is oppressive to women."

When a Muslim family immigrates to a Western country, the man often comes first and, after a period of stressful anticipation and preparation, other family members follow. Even if they immigrate together, men usually work outside and women at home. Therefore many immigrant Muslim women are not fluent in English and may bring a relative or child as a translator. This may also be interpreted as excessive dependency and create negative feelings in the therapist.

2.2. Transference

Physicians are highly valued in Islamic culture. In addition, consultation with a physician or therapist is generally favored and recommended to Muslims and even to the Prophet Muhammad in the Koran (Holy Koran 3:159 and 42:38). These recommendations can be used to facilitate the development of a working alliance with Muslim patients. However, Muslim clients may have negative stereotypes about Western culture and Western therapists resulting from their feeling of oppression by Western politicians and may use terms such as you (Westerns or Americans) and we (Muslims or Arabs) (p. 23).(4) Therapists should not take these statements personally but rather should help the clients think less categorically. For example, the therapist may say to the patient, "I understand you! I know some Western policies may have hurt you. But … may you have negative feelings toward me because I am also a Westerner? Because this negative feeling may adversely affect the success of our sessions, can I do anything to make you feel easier with me?"

Muslim clients in Western countries are under pressure of the dominant Western culture, so they may also feel shame and inferiority and fear punishment from the Western therapist. By adopting a sensitive and warm attitude, the therapist may help decrease these negative feelings.

2.2.1. Warm Greetings

When meeting a Muslim for the first time, warm greetings usually help to establish a more positive transference. In many Muslim cultures, standing up from a sitting position when someone arrives implies respect for him or her and is encouraged. Shaking hands with the same-gender client is also helpful.

2.2.2. Admiring Strong Points

At the end of the first session, we should have determined and negotiated the therapeutic goals with the client, and the client should have gained enough hope and developed a good enough transference to continue therapy. This good impression also usually needs to be impressed upon the client's family because the client may be dependent on them to come to psychotherapy. One important tool to instill hope and a good transference in the client or her family is to admire and encourage them and reinforce their positive characteristics and strong points. For example, the therapist can say to the client's husband, "Supporting your wife to come to psychotherapy shows that you feel responsible and love your family, because it may not be easy nowadays to come to a psychiatrist or psychotherapist." Dwairy (pp. 116–117)(4) has described that this approach helped his clients remain in therapy and receive effective help. If the client feels positive toward his or her religion or culture, admiring and showing respect for the religion/culture is another important way to create a positive transference.

2.2.3. Admitting to One's Lack of Knowledge

Admitting to one's lack of knowledge about the patient's culture or religion is another way to establish a positive therapeutic alliance. This can decrease the client's inferiority feelings and encourage more open communication. The following statements indicate a non-Muslim psychotherapist's sincerity and respect toward a Muslim client: "Because I am not a Muslim, my knowledge about Muslims' practices and beliefs is limited and there may be some misunderstandings. I would be glad if you would let me know should I make a mistake regarding your culture or religion."

2.2.4. Paying Attention to Negative or Positive Cues

Even when we try our best to help our clients, there may be some misunderstandings (pp. 31–41)(15); therefore, it is important to be sensitive to the clients' verbal and nonverbal cues. If a negative cue appears, help the patient to clarify it. Say, "You seem somewhat troubled. Was there anything in what I said or behaved that caused a negative feeling in you? Could you please explain your thoughts?" In addition, at the end of each session, it may be appropriate to ask about the client's feelings and thoughts about the session.

2.2.5. Predicting and Anticipating Reactions

Some Arabs or Eastern Muslims may have difficulty speaking about intimate or sexual subjects to therapists of the opposite sex. They may also expect the therapist to offer them direct advice and may expect the number of therapeutic sessions to be quite limited. If given homework or tests, they may think that this is childish. Anticipating such thoughts, feelings, or behaviors in the course of the therapy is another effective way of increasing clients' compliance and preventing them from dropping out. For example, the therapist may say, "Some clients may feel that doing homework is childish. The exercises may sometimes seem useless. How do you think we should handle these thoughts should they occur?" Or the therapist could say, "You said you had marital problems for about five years. How would you feel if I told you that it may take up to six months to control these problems? Does this seem too long to you?" Such questions can help clients anticipate their own reactions and manage them better.

2.2.6. Similarities *and* Differences

All Muslims are not the same. Although there are many similarities, these shouldn't blind us to the differences. One difference is related to Muslims' countries of origin. Usually the longer a Muslim has lived in a specific country or region, the more similar are his or her attitudes to the culture of that country. For example, Christian Arabs are culturally very similar to Muslim Arabs (p. 5),(4) but when they immigrate to Western countries, both gradually move toward the Western culture. Yet Arabs account for only 20 percent of all Muslims (3) and other Muslims may differ culturally from Arabs.

Another important dimension is their religiosity. Muslims differ in their acceptance of various Islamic beliefs and practices and in the degree of this acceptance. So before using religion-related techniques in therapy, we should first take a religious history.(20) If the patient agrees, the therapist should also obtain information from other significant family members because this may yield a very different picture of the patient's problem.

2.3. Two Important Questions Before Using Religious Techniques

Two important questions must first be answered before using religious techniques in therapy. First, "Are religious conflicts important as part of the client's problems?" For example, if religious guilt plays an important part in the client's depression or anxiety, the therapist should take time to help the client resolve her or his religious guilt; but if the problem is a specific phobia, religious techniques may be less helpful to the patient.

The second and more important question is, "How much is a religious technique really meaningful to the client?" For example, if a Muslim client has negative attitudes toward religious scriptures or Islamic daily prayers, trying to use them in therapy may cause negative feelings and resistance, while the same client may have private prayers and nonritualistic relationships with God that may be more effectively used in therapy. Therefore, in addition to taking a religious history at the first session, it may be necessary to collect more information about the client's attitudes toward specific religious techniques before using them.

Depression, anxiety, and various interpersonal conflicts are among the most common problems seen in Muslim clients, so I will briefly explain Islamic concepts useful in each of these problems. Reyshahri (1992)(21) has summarized and classified thousands of sayings of the Prophet Muhammad and Shia Imams using many Sunni and Shia books as references in his ten-volume Arabic book میزان الحکمة (balance of wisdom). My Hadiths quotations will be from this book. Related verses from the Holy Koran will also be provided, along with clinical examples of techniques.

3. ISLAMIC CONCEPTS USEFUL IN PSYCHOTHERAPY OF DEPRESSION

3.1. Believing in an Afterlife

According to cognitive theory, thoughts concerning an important loss cause sadness.(22)

Examples of these thoughts are: "I wish my wife was still alive!" or "It is terrible that I have diabetes!" Every time clients attribute much importance to an unattainable object, they feel sad. Many Muslim patients cope with these unattainable wishes or inevitable losses by believing in an afterlife where life will be much better. Believing in an afterlife, along with believing in one omnipotent God and the prophetic mission of Prophet Muhammad, is one of the fundamental beliefs of Islam. Afterlife issues are recurrently repeated in the Holy Koran, and almost all Muslims believe in some kind of reward and punishment after death, although the interpretations may vary. Some accept the Koranic verses about afterlife reward or punishment literally, while others may believe that these verses have more symbolic meanings.

According to the Koran and Sunnah, afterlife rewards are not only considered for Muslims' good deeds, but also for their good intentions or wishes and even for sufferings from problems such as poverty or death of loved ones, provided that these sufferings are not caused voluntarily or unduly by Muslims themselves. So there are many circumstances in which these religious beliefs can be used to lessen clients' sufferings.

3.1.1. Poverty

One example of a situation where believing in an afterlife and stating the Prophet's sunnah can be used to decrease the patient's suffering is poverty or monetary need. Although poverty is not regarded as good by itself in Islam (7:495),(19) showing patience when in this state and trying to overcome poverty by honest work are seriously encouraged. In addition, great afterlife rewards have been promised to poor believers who cannot afford things that they wish. One example from Prophet Muhammad Sunnah is: "Some poor Muslims said to Prophet Muhammad that sometimes they saw fruits in the bazaar and liked to buy them but hadn't any money, and asked him if this would result in afterlife reward for them. The Prophet said: 'Isn't the reward exactly for these things?'" (7:521).(19) The Holy Koran recommends the Prophet Muhammad to support the religious poor Muslims and to not reject them and turn toward the wealthy (Holy Koran 18:28). The Prophet himself loved the poor, and many famous Muslims were poor at some time during their lives. These statements show that God and his Prophet love poor Muslims who patiently endure, so the psychotherapist may use them to increase patients' self esteem.

3.1.2. Death of a Beloved

Another important example of loss is the death of one's beloved. For instance, great rewards are promised to parents suffering loss of children, and it is stated that the lost children will protect their parents against hellfire.(7) Interestingly, positive concepts are also found in Christianity regarding the death of a child.(13)

3.1.3. Diseases and Disabilities

Showing patience when suffering diseases and disabilities is also rewarded in the afterlife according to Islamic teachings. Because having patience is not an all-or-nothing phenomenon, all patients have some patience and therefore deserve afterlife rewards, and this reappraisal can lessen their suffering. In addition, suffering from disease is believed to atone for sins (9:122–126).(19)

3.1.4. Reward for Daily Usual Activities

Even many daily and usual activities are in Islam regarded as good and deserving of great afterlife rewards. Examples are greeting each other, helping parents, helping one's spouse, having good intentions (even when not able to practice them), having sexual relationships with one's legal partner, and so on. According to the Holy Koran, reward of each good deed is ten times the punishment of a bad deed. "Whoever does a righteous work receives the reward for ten, and the one who commits a sin is punished for only one and no one suffers injustice" (Holy Koran 6:160). When patients' attention is drawn to these rules, many of them feel better and can better tolerate their losses.

3.2. Prayer and Asking God

Asking from God is usually a central part of prayers, although prayers have other purposes too.(23) Many religious people turn toward God when disturbed, and ask him to relieve their distress. Theoretically, asking God and saying prayers can have different consequences. If the prayer is perceived as granted, it can increase the person's faith and optimism. If the prayer is perceived as rejected (for example, when the problem continues or worsens), it can lead to negative thoughts that in turn lead to feelings of guilt and hopelessness.

Asking from God is seriously encouraged in Islam. The Holy Koran says, "And your Lord says, Pray unto ME; I will answer your prayer" (Holy Koran 40:60) and "Say: My Lord would not care for you were it not for your prayer" (Holy Koran 25: 77).

There are many points and recommendations in Islamic scriptures regarding various aspects of the prayers, (3:243–281),(19) but two interesting points especially are useful in psychotherapy:

1) All prayers have effect.

Among other similar Hadiths, it is quoted from the Prophet Muhammad that, "No Muslim does pray to the eminent Allah, provided that he does not pray against his family or for a sin, unless the eminent Allah will give him one of these three things: expedites what he prays for, or reserves it in the afterlife for him, or will remove an equivalent trouble from him" (3:279).(19)

2) We may pray against ourselves!

It is stated in the Holy Koran, "But you may dislike something which is good for you, and you may like something which is bad for you. God knows while you do not know" (Holy Koran 2:216).

Although sins are considered as obstacles for prayers to be complied with, the forementioned points provide useful alternative interpretations that, if used appropriately in therapy, can prevent excessive guilt feeling and hopelessness in the troubled client.

3.3. Guilt Feeling

Guilt, like other negative feelings, is natural and sometimes helpful. For example, people with antisocial personality disorder have minimal guilt, insufficient to prevent their violence against their victims. Excessive guilt feeling, on the other hand, is one of the most important cognitive components of depression. According to Beck's theory, depressed people have prominent negative interpretations regarding themselves, their environment, and their future.(20) Guilt is part of negative self-esteem in depressed patients and may lead to hopelessness, self-destructive behavior, anxiety, and fear of punishment in this world and the afterlife. Depressed religious clients may selectively focus on God's punishments and thereby enhance their guilt feelings. Thus, drawing attention toward the following hopeful scriptures showing God's mercy can help them.

3.3.1. There Is No One Who Does Not Sin

"There is no one who does not sin" is a common positive concept between Christianity (Kings 8:46) and Islam against the negative thought in religious depressed patients, which may be expressed in words something like, "I have sinned so much, so I am bad." Shia and Sunni Muslims both believe that all people are needful of God's forgiveness and mercy (Holy Koran 35:15), and all people (except the twelve Imams, the Prophet Muhammad, and his daughter Fatimah in Shia belief) may sin. So sinning does not mean that one is totally bad.

3.3.2. Mercy and Beneficence of God

Drawing clients' attention to many verses from the Koran that help them realize the great mercy and beneficence of God is another way to decrease guilt feeling. For example, of the 114 sections *(Suras)* of the Koran, 113 start with "In the name of Allah, the beneficent, the merciful." Other examples of God's mercy from the Koran are, "O my servants who have acted extravagantly against their own souls! Do not despair of the mercy of Allah; surely Allah forgives the sins altogether; surely He is the Forgiving the Merciful" (Holy Koran 39: 53); and, "Surely Allah does not forgive that anything be worshiped with Him, but forgives what is besides that to whomsoever He pleases" (Holy Koran 4:48, 116).

3.3.3. Number of Good and Bad Deeds

Another way to decrease guilt is to count number of good and bad deeds that one has done during his or her life. As mentioned above, many ordinary activities are regarded as good in Islam, so the client's good doings usually greatly outnumber the sins, leading to decreased guilt.

3.3.4. Thoughts Are Not Punished

Sometimes guilt is related to blasphemous or shameful thoughts. Usually, the more patients try to control these thoughts, the more they become intrusive and obsessive. According to Prophet Muhammad sayings, people are not punished because of their thoughts, provided that they not put them into action. Sometimes religious obsessional thoughts are regarded as a sign of strong faith (10:448–450).(19)

3.3.5. Feelings Are Not Sins

Some religious clients have guilt related to their inability to control their negative thoughts and associated feelings. For example, they may feel guilt because they cannot accept their fate or their loss of dear ones, and therefore feel sad.(7) Mehraby has used the Prophet Muhammad Sunnah successfully with these patients.(7) She said to these patients that the Prophet Muhammad cried publicly on several occasions for the loss of his dear ones, without feeling guilt. He cried over the death of his mother, his son, and his wife Khadijah. Khadijah was very helpful to the Prophet and the Prophet loved her so much that even several years after her death, he cried every time he remembered her. Also it is quoted from him while burying his little son Ibrahim, "The eye weeps and the heart is sad, but I do not say anything that angers God" (p. 360).(13)

3.3.6. Physicians' Credit in Islam

Sometimes guilt is the result of a sin that the clients cannot quit. Such excessive guilt can cause hopelessness and decreased self-esteem, resulting in even more repeating of that sin. One way to decrease this guilt is to use the physicians' credit in Islam. One Islamic rule is that if a trusted physician recommends a basically prohibited action to treat an important disease, doing that action is not regarded a sin anymore and even may become mandatory. For instance, breaking one's fasting at Ramadan holy month is not regarded a sin if it is prescribed by a trusted physician as necessary for a patient's health. Similarly, some Muslim patients feel excessive guilt and are severely anxious or depressed because of doing masturbation. If a trusted physician considers this to be an important element in a patient's severe anxiety or depression and recommends that he or she occasionally perform masturbation to decrease his or her tension, this act is not regarded a sin anymore and can sometimes be done.

3.4. Hopelessness and Suicide

Suicide is regarded as an unforgivable great sin by almost all Muslims.(24) It is unforgivable because one has no time to repent from and compensate for it, for repentance is only allowed until death. In an aggregate study involving seventy nations (1989), it was found that after controlling for a large number of socioeconomic variables, the percentage of Muslims in the population was negatively correlated with suicide rates.(22) Considering suicide a great sin may be the only factor preventing some Muslim patients from committing suicide, so it should be encouraged in these patients.

Losing one's hope in God's mercy too is regarded as one of the worst sins in Islam (Holy Koran 12:87). Some patients think of suicide because they feel hopeless, and considering hopelessness a great sin may aggravate their guilt and hopelessness. The following example shows how to use Socratic questioning to decrease this guilt feeling.

Patient (crying): I am completely hopeless. No one can help me. I know hopelessness is a great sin so I have lost both my life and afterlife.

Therapist (sympathetically): Certainly this feeling hurts you so much. It is a very unpleasant feeling. How many sessions have you come to therapy by now?

Patient: About eight sessions.

Therapist: Are you going to continue your sessions?

Patient: I think yes.

Therapist: You have patiently come to eight sessions, and you want to continue. Do you think this could be a sign that you hope that these sessions may be helpful?

Patient (stops crying): Yes. Actually if I thought these sessions were useless, I never would have attended them.

Therapist: That is definitely true. So, can we say that you have not lost your hope, but you have been bravely fighting hopelessness by continuing your sessions?

Patient (after a pause): I don't know. I never thought of it that way before.

Therapist: If someone like you fights against a great sin, doesn't she deserve God's reward and great mercy in spite of punishment, as promised in Koran?

Patient: Maybe that is true. Yes, I have not lost all of my hope.

3.5. Saints as Examples

Prophet Muhammad himself, all Shia Imams, and other significant Muslims suffered a great deal in their lives. They tolerated many kinds of economic and social pressures and physical tortures.(25) Some of them were martyred and others remained, both fates being regarded as victories in Islamic culture. This can be used in psychotherapy, because when religious Muslims compare their difficulties with those of the Prophet Muhammad and significant Muslims, they usually feel somewhat relieved. One Iranian woman who had lost her children in the Bam earthquake (2003) said on Iranian television, "My sufferings never reach Zaynab's sufferings, so I'll try to be patient." Zaynab was Imam Hussein's (the third Shia Imam) sister. Her brothers, her sons, and many of her family members were martyred in front of her eyes during their unequal battle against thousands of the enemy, and she was taken captive, but she bravely tolerated it and even fearlessly lectured against the enemy sovereign.

3.6. God's Wisdom and Love

When a problem occurs, several kinds of thoughts may come into a religious person's mind, for example, "This is a punishment from God because of my sins" or "It is a trial for me to be revealed whether I will be patient or not" or "It can be a prevention from more serious problems in the future" or "God loves me and wants me to have a better afterlife and to forgive my sins." None of the above sentences can be proven logically, but those who see preferentially God's wisdom and love through a problem (the last two thoughts) may better tolerate it. The second sentence can increase self-esteem should the client see herself as tolerant, but if she feels that she could not pass the trial, it can lessen self-esteem and worsen her guilt feeling.

Many verses of the Koran imply God's love for several kinds of people, for example, "the beneficent people" (Holy Koran 2:195), "those who repent and want to purify themselves" (Holy Koran 2:222), "the pious" (Holy Koran 3:76), "the equitable" (Holy Koran 5:42), and others. Because these characteristics are not all or none, almost all clients can be helped by showing that they are significantly "good" and deserve God's love.

3.7. Loneliness

Feeling alone often worsens sadness. According to Koran, God is always with us. For example, God says to Moses and Aaron, "Fear not, surely I am with you both, hearing and seeing" (Holy Koran 20:46). Another verse promises, "He is with you everywhere you may be, and Allah is seer of what

you do" (Holy Koran 57:4). Therefore, repeating these phrases and strengthening this belief through praying and talking with God can help religious people.

3.8. "Thanks to God!"

According to the Holy Koran, "If you would count the graces of Allah, never could you be able to count them. Truly! Allah is Oft-Forgiving, Most Merciful" (Holy Koran 16:18). Some religious people use this belief to emotionally cope with the problems (losses). For example, if they have a car accident, they may think, "Thanks to God, we are still healthy and can recover from it." Even when they are injured, they say, "Thank God, it could be worse, someone could be killed"; and if someone has been killed, "It could be worse. Thank God that most of us are still alive!"

Even when there is a disaster, *cautiously* pointing to many important things that one still has through Socratic questioning can instill hope in and love for one's God and decrease religious conflicts. Sometimes, however, increasing the clients' awareness of God's blessings invokes guilt feelings because the patients feel they have not been thankful enough. This guilt feeling can be dealt with through paying attention to the fact that God's blessings and gifts are so numerous that no one can completely thank God, because thanking God in itself is another gift from God!

4. ISLAMIC CONCEPTS USEFUL IN PSYCHOTHERAPY OF ANXIETY

Anxiety and depression are usually found together. Many thoughts causing depression can also cause anxiety and vice versa. It depends on one's point of view. A loss considered as certain is usually associated with sadness; the same loss considered as probable is more associated with anxiety. For example, the thought "surely I will be in the hell. God will never forgive me" may cause more sadness, but the thought "maybe God doesn't forgive my sins. What should I do now?" causes more anxiety. So most Islamic concepts described in psychotherapy of depression are also useful in treating anxiety. Here some other Islamic concepts useful in psychotherapy of anxiety in religious clients are described.

4.1. Afterlife: Causing or Preventing Anxiety

4.1.1. Probable Losses

Because anxiety is provoked by perceiving a *significant probability* of an *important* loss, thoughts or concepts decreasing the subjective importance or probability of the losses can decrease anxiety.

According to Islam, all losses in this world can lead to afterlife rewards for a faithful Muslim, provided not caused intentionally and if the Muslim shows patience. The Holy Koran says, "And we shall certainly try you with something of fear and hunger and loss of property and lives and fruits. And give good news to the patient!" (Holy Koran 2:155). Because patience is really a relative concept, almost all clients can be shown to have some significant patience. This reappraisal can lessen the significance of probable losses and religiously decrease anxiety.

4.1.2. Probable Punishment

Alternatively, afterlife thoughts can themselves cause anxiety or fear if the client's mind turns toward the negative side of the coin, that is, punishment for the sins. Although this anxiety can have positive consequences, such as trying more to avoid sins, it can decrease the client's functionality if excessive and should be controlled. So all previously mentioned Islamic concepts for decreasing guilt feeling are of use here. For example, paying attention to the Islamic rule "Whoever brings a good deed, he shall have ten like it, and whoever brings an evil deed, he shall be recompensed only with the like of it, and they shall not be dealt with unjustly" (Holy Koran 6:160) and to the great mercifulness of God can lower the subjective probability of afterlife punishment and decrease anxiety.

4.1.3. The Grave Anxiety

Some religious Muslim patients have anxiety regarding the grave. Some may have excessive thoughts that they will be alive again soon after death, and must answer harsh questions from the angels regarding their faith in Allah and the Prophet Muhammad, and will be punished if not able to answer correctly. Although there are sayings of the Prophet Muhammad and Shia Imams pointing to in-grave interrogation (not pointing to becoming alive, but pointing to souls being asked questions), there are other sayings that say not all Muslims undergo such a trial, and that the grave will turn into a wide and beautiful place for the good and faithful Muslim's soul (8:11).(19) Again, having faith and being good are relative subjects, and evidence for goodness and faithfulness of the client can usually be found.

4.2. Reliance on God

Anxiety-provoking thoughts usually consider only one side of the event: the worst one. Some Muslims try to think more positive probabilities by repeating religious phrases such as "God is great" or "I rely on God" (Arabic: الله على توكلت). These conceptually mean, "I'll try my best to prevent the harm but I also try to accept whatever happens because it is God's will and God is great enough to protect me or to strengthen me enough to tolerate it." Such clients' adaptive religious behaviors should be encouraged and appreciated in the psychotherapeutic session.

4.3. Fear of Jinns

According to Koran, there are invisible creations named *jinns* that resemble human beings in that they have faithful or infidel groups or may sometimes have unusual powers.(26) Some Muslim religious people (mostly uneducated) fear that they may see jinns or jinns may hurt them. No routine religious ritual is widely practiced in Islam regarding protection against jinns or relationships with them. This fact can be used in these patients, saying to them, "If relationship with jinns or protection against them was really important in Islam, shouldn't there be some widely accepted rituals in this regard?" or "Could you state some Islamic evidence that emphasize the importance of doing some actions to protect against jinns? Is there any evidence that jinns can usually be seen? If not, can we say this is not really an important thing in real life?"

5. ISLAMIC CONCEPTS USEFUL FOR INTERPERSONAL PROBLEMS

Islam is, in fact, a social religion because there are many Islamic laws and recommendations regarding interpersonal relationships, most of them emphasizing unity and love. The following examples from the Koran and Hadiths demonstrate this issue:

> And of His signs is that He created for you helpmeets from yourselves that you might find rest in them, and He ordained love and mercy between you. Surely there are signs in this for a people who reflect. (Holy Koran 30:21)

> (O Muhammad!) It was mercy from GOD that you became compassionate towards them. Had you been harsh and mean-hearted, they would have broken away from about you. (Holy Koran 3:159)

> Those who have daughters and don't annoy and intimidate them and don't prefer sons to them, God will enter them heaven for this (from the Prophet Muhammad) (10:705)(19)

> As a thank for (God's) favor to you, do favor to the one who did evil to you (from Imam Ali, the first Shia Imam) (2:445)(19)

> God never permits carelessness in three circumstances: returning the deposit to its owner whether righteous or wicked, faithfulness to one's promise whether to

the righteous or to the wicked, and doing favor to one's parents whether righteous or wicked (from Imam Baagher, the fifth Shia Imam) (10:710)(19)

Although religion is an important part of Muslims' culture, many interpersonal behaviors are determined by local Muslim culture and do not really have their roots in religion. So when Muslims are informed from a trusted source about Islamic concepts opposing their nonfunctional cultural view, they usually are surprised and can better accept more adaptive thoughts or behaviors. Some psychotherapists report successful interventions using this approach in marital conflicts.(6, 17)

Here some common interpersonal problems in Muslim clients that can be addressed using this approach are briefly discussed.

5.1. Sensitivity to the Opinions of Others

Some patients are unusually sensitive to other's suggestions. This sensitivity can cause anxiety in disorders such as social phobia or avoidant personality disorder, or frustration and rejection sensitivity in other personality disorders. In Islam, it is important to be righteous, regardless of what others may think, as the Holy Koran says. "Allah will bring a people whom He loves and who love Him … striving hard in Allah's way and not fearing the blame of any blamer" (Holy Koran 5:54). Also, it is believed in Islam that if anyone says something against another Muslim, for instance, publicizing a wrongdoing of another Muslim, then the accuser's afterlife rewards will be transmitted to the accused, and the accused Muslim's sins are transmitted to the accuser's afterlife dossier (7:337).(19) These concepts may help the client to reappraise others' negative views of them and thus better tolerate the situation and maintain his or her self-esteem.

5.2. Oppression and Forgiveness

Some clients feel oppressed and are angry toward the perceived oppressor(s). Although this anger may strengthen the client in efforts to receive his or her rights, often it can be destructive in close relationships and lead to more provocative behaviors and even greater oppression. For example, a woman's anger toward her mentally and physically abusive husband may cause her to behave in such a way that irritates her husband more and results in her being even more abused. In Islam, oppression and being passively oppressed are both condemned, but the oppressed are encouraged not to abandon righteousness in the requital. It is also recommended that the oppressed try to forgive the offender, despite having the right to retaliate. The Holy Koran says, "And [believers are] those who, when suffering a great injustice, seek to defend themselves.⊙ The just requital for an injustice is an equivalent retribution, but those who pardon and maintain righteousness are rewarded by God. He does not love the unjust.⊙ There is no way [to put blame] on those who defend themselves after they have been wronged.⊙ The way (of blame) is only against those who oppress mankind, and wrongfully rebel in the earth. For such there is a painful doom.⊙ And whoever is patient and forgiving, these most surely are actions due to courage⊙" (Holy Koran 42:39–43).

To avoid unwanted consequences, therapists should not impose their own view of oppression or life on the clients. For example, a Muslim woman may not view seeking her independence and obtaining a divorce as a suitable solution to her marital conflict. Similarly, she may or may not see her husband's insistence on her Islamic head cover as oppression. A therapist's one-sided insistence on these issues may result in the client dropping out of therapy and so should be avoided.

5.3. Doing Good in Response to Evil

Sometimes, quarrels and bitter arguments result in pathogenic cycles in the family, so that memories of the arguments will cause more arguments and so forth. Breaking these cycles needs one or both of the partners to stop responding negatively to the other's negative stimuli. This may not be easy, especially when negative arguments have continued for a long time. One way for religious Muslim clients to accept this logic and try to alter their negative relationships is to draw their attention toward the Islamic concept of "doing favor in response to the evil." One example from the Holey Koran is, "And not alike are the good and the evil. Repel (evil) with what is best, so he between whom and you was enmity would be as if he were a warm friend. ⊙And none is granted it but those who are patient, and none is granted it but the owner of a mighty good fortune⊙" (Holy Koran 41:34, 35).

5.4. Duties in a Muslim Marriage

Islam offers a hierarchical system in which every Muslim has duties and rights according to his or her position. For example, according to Islamic law, men have a duty to cover all monetary needs of their wives including their food, clothes, and health expenses, even if the women are themselves wealthy (p. 261).(16) Alternatively, a Muslim woman should go nowhere without her husband's consent unless absolutely necessary or otherwise agreed on in the marital contract. In Islam, it is not mandatory for women to do housework, and they have the right to request salary even for breastfeeding their own infants (Holy Koran 65:6). In practice, usually both husband and wife need to renounce some of their rights. For example, most husbands need their wives to work inside (and sometimes outside) the home, and therefore need to give up most of their controlling rights.

These Islamic laws are usually modified by culture, so that Muslim men or women may act culturally but think of their behavior as religious. For example, some Muslim men expect their wives to work both outside and inside the home as their duty. Although similar to Christianity (Col. 3:18–19), women are exhorted in Islam to obey their husbands; husbands, too, are encouraged to respect their wives and not oppress them (Holy Koran 4:19). Likewise, men cannot force their wives to do housework. It has been shown that cautiously drawing the attention of husbands to these Islamic rules and Sunnah of the Prophet Muhammad related to the treatment of women can help them modify their expectations and result in decreased marital conflict.(17)

5.5. Muslim Women and Extended Family

Most Muslim psychotherapy clients are women (p. 120),(4) and among the most common problems they face are those related to interpersonal relationships with their husbands and the families of their husbands. Parents have a high position in Islam so that Muslims are encouraged not to say even the slightest harsh words to parents, especially their mothers and especially when they have become old (Holy Koran 17:23 and 31:14). Furthermore, Muslim women in many families have to take care of their own parents as well as their husband's parents. Fighting this situation and trying to help the client toward more independence may result in negative feelings both in the client and her husband and lead to the termination of therapy. The therapist instead can first try to learn about the family dynamics and then use those dynamics to help the client without unnecessarily confronting them. For example, Daneshpour (2008) reports a case in which she helped the client use her mother-in-law as an ally to alter her husband's behavior.(17)

5.6. Polygamy

Having more than one wife is allowed in Islam, but because the polygamous men usually have difficulty complying with their duties to their wives, it is restricted in many Islamic countries and is therefore rare. For example, in Iran and several other Muslim countries it is allowed only by means of court order that either requires the first wife's consent or her right to divorce.(27)

Although this law may be interpreted as oppression against women, Islamic clerics argue that not allowing legal polygamy may be more oppressive against women. They say that young women usually outnumber men, because more men work outside the home (especially in Islamic countries) and more men die due to accidents or wars. Thus, allowing polygamy gives widows and single women more chance to marry legally and be eligible for support. Second, abandoning legal polygamy does not prevent men from having multiple sexual partners because there are easier but more unsafe ways for this (pp. 363–454).(16)

Again, therapists should be aware of their own possible negative feelings and not allow these feelings to interfere with their effort to professionally help their clients.

6. CONCLUSION

Given the complexity of psychotherapy itself, psychotherapy of a client from another religion or culture will be more difficult and more complex. Naturally, psychotherapeutic skill and experience play an important role in success. However, of the many other variables, obtaining sufficient knowledge about the client's culture and religion seems vital. Although this chapter can help therapists to better understand and help religious Muslim clients, it is to be regarded only as a short introduction that by no means is complete. Thus, searching for more information from other valuable sources is always recommended.

REFERENCES

1. Sommers-Flanagan J, Sommers-Flanagan R, eds. *Counseling and Psychotherapy Theories in Context and Practice*. New Jersey: John Wiley & Sons; 2004.
2. Hersen M, Sledge W, eds. *Encyclopedia of Psychotherapy*. New York: Academic Press; 2002.
3. Riggs T, ed. *Worldmark Encyclopedia of Religious Practices*, Vol 1. New York: Thomson Gale; 2006:349, 350.
4. Dwairy M. *Counseling and Psychotherapy with Arabs and Muslims: A Culturally Sensitive Approach*. New York: Teachers College Press; 2006.
5. Husain SR. Religion and mental health from the muslim perspective. In: Koenig HG, ed. *Handbook of Religion and Mental Health*. San Diego: Academic Press; 1998:289.
6. Badri M. Can the psychotherapy of Muslim patients be of real help to them without being Islamimized? In: Fadel HE, ed. *FIMA yearbook 2004*. Jordan: Jordan Society for Islamic Medical Studies; 2005:61–87. Also available at http://www.islamic-world.net/psychology/psy.php?ArtID=204.
7. Mehraby N. Psychotherapy with Islamic clients facing loss and grief. *Psychother Australia*. 2003;9(2):30–34.

8. Aveline M, Strauss B, Stiles WB. Psychotherapy research. In: Gabbard GO, Beck JS, Holmes J, eds. *Oxford Textbook of Psychotherapy*. New York: Oxford University Press; 2005:449–462.

9. Azhar MZ, Varma SL. Religious psychotherapy in depressive patients. *Psychother Psychosom*. 1995;63:165–173.

10. Azhar MZ, Varma SL, Dharap AS. Religious psychotherapy in anxiety disorder patients. *Acta Psychiatr Scand*. 1994;90:1–3.

11. Razali SM, Hasanah CI, Aminah K, Subramaniam M. Religious – sociocultural psychotherapy in patients with anxiety and depression. *Aust N Z J Psychiatry*. 1998;32:867–872.

12. Ali SR, Liu WM, Humedian M. Islam 101: understanding the religion and therapy implications. *Prof Psychol Res Pr*. 2004;35(6):635–642.

13. Carone DA, Barone DF. A social cognitive perspective on religious beliefs: their functions and impact on coping and psychotherapy. *Clin Psychol Rev*. 2001;21(7):989–1003.

14. Rasuli Mahallati SH, ed. (In Persian) محمد (ص) زندانی حضرت (Biography of Prophet Muhammad [PBUH]), 11th ed. Tehran: دفتر نشر فرهنگ اسلامی (Office of Islamic culture publications); 1998.

15. Daneshpour M. Lives together, worlds apart? The lives of multicultural muslim couples. *J Couple Relat Ther*. 2003;2(2/3):57–71.

16. Sudak DM, ed. *Cognitive Behavioral Therapy for Clinicians: Psychotherapy in Clinical Practice*. Philadelphia: Lippincott Williams and Wilkins; 2006.

17. Motahari M., ed. (In Persian) حقوق زن در اسلام نظام (*Organization of Women Rights in Islam*), 14th ed. Tehran: Sadra Publication; 1991. Available at http://www.motahari.org/asaar/books.htm.

18. Daneshpour M. Couple therapy with Muslims: challenges and opportunities. In: Rastogi M, Volker T, eds. *Couple Therapy with Ethnic Minorities*. Sage Press. (in press).

19. Carter DJ. and Rashidi A. (2004). East meets west: integrating psychotherapy approaches for Muslim women. *Holistic nursing practice*, Volume, 152–159.

20. Koenig HG, Prichette J. Religion and psychotherapy. In: Koenig HG, ed. *Handbook of Religion and Mental Health*. San Diego: Academic Press; 1998;324–335.

21. Reyshahri M, ed. (In Arabic) میزان الحکمه (balance of wisdom), 4th ed. Qom: الاعلام الاسلامی مکتب;1992.

22. Beck AT, Rush AJ. Cognitive therapy. In: Sadock BJ, Sadock VA, eds. *Kaplan and Sadock's Comprehensive Textbook of Psychiatry*. Philadelphia: Lippincott Williams and Wilkins; 2000:1267–1277.

23. Koenig HG, Mccullough ME, Larson DB, eds. *Handbook of Religion and Health*. New York: Oxford University Press, 2001:21.

24. Anees MA. Salvation and suicide: what does Islamic theology say? *Dialog J Theol*. 2006;45(3):275–279.

25. Basit A. An Islamic perspective on coping with catastrophe. *South Med J*. 2007;100(9):950–951.

26. Babaii A. (In Persian) برگزیده تفسیر نمونه (Chosen parts of The Example Interpretation [of Koran]), Vol 5. Tehran: دارالکتب الاسلامیة; 1998: 308–310.

27. Mir-Hosseini Z. Polygamy. In: Martin RC, *ed. Encyclopedia of Islam and Muslim World*. New York: Macmillan Reference; 2004:552–553.

21 Psychiatric Treatments Involving Religion: Psychiatric Care Using Buddhist Principles

CHARLES KNAPP

SUMMARY

The Windhorse Therapy approach was developed in 1981 by Chogyam Trungpa and Dr. Edward Podvol. It is based on the Buddhist understanding of fundamental health and sanity and the inseparability of one's entire life from one's environment, while integrating applicable Western psychology. The primary activity involves creating individually tailored, therapeutic living environments for people with a variety of mental health issues. Within these comprehensively coordinated arrangements, clients are able to significantly reduce the chaos and confusion of mental disturbances and improve life functioning. Briefly outlining this approach, we will discuss foundational training, roles, and some therapeutic elements of a recovery environment. A case example is provided that illustrates the theoretical underpinnings and what a representative recovery process can look like. A version of this paper was published in 2008 in the book *Brilliant Sanity*.

I. WINDHORSE THERAPY

The Windhorse Therapy process is a unique multi-layered and comprehensive treatment approach for people with a wide variety of mental health recovery needs. In this approach, for every client, we create an individually tailored therapy environment, addressing his or her needs in a whole person manner. This whole person approach also includes, whenever possible, the voice and needs of the client's family.

Windhorse Therapy is based on ancient understandings of the fundamental nature of human health and the energy it takes to recover from mental and life disturbances. With this as its foundation, Windhorse incorporates a combination of ordinary common sense, twenty-seven years of clinical experience with the treatment process, and the application of fitting psychological therapy or therapies. A key element of potency in this approach, both in its view and our experience, is that no matter how severely confused a mind has become, recovery is possible.

The term *windhorse* refers to an energy that is naturally positive, confident, uplifted, and, according to the Buddhist tradition, fundamental to human beings as a "life force" energy. Our individual connection to this energy can wax and wane depending on what's happening in our environment and inside ourselves. And *windhorse energy* can be deliberately roused and cultivated. When our connection to this energy is strong, we feel confident that our life is workable. *Windhorse* was chosen as the name of this type of therapy because it is the energy that is essential for people to discover and rouse to recover from mental illness and difficult life problems.(1)

A simple snapshot of a Windhorse Therapy looks like the following: A client lives in a house or apartment with a housemate who is part of a treatment team. Their relationship resembles a normal roommate relationship. There are a number of clinicians on the team who spend time with the client on a regularly scheduled basis, sometimes one "shift" per day or more, doing a wide variety of activities, from keeping the house in order to helping him or her to get out and connect with interests in the world. These activities are elements of an individually tailored environment to help the person live in an ordinary and healthy way, with good relationships and meaningful pursuits. The client may work, see friends and family, and be part of the normal community in which she or he lives. The schedule usually includes meeting with a psychotherapist and with a psychiatrist if medications are used. There is a system of meetings that all members of the team, including the client and his or her family, participate in to keep the activity of the therapy, household, and treatment team coordinated and up-to-date. Most treatments last six months to two years.

2. HISTORICAL ROOTS

The Windhorse Project, as it was originally called, arose out of the powerful environment of the early 1980s at Naropa University and the atmosphere and teachings of its Buddhist founder, Chogyam Trungpa. At that time, many outstanding and accomplished people had been drawn to him, and his influence invariably had the effect of helping experts to see their respective disciplines in a new light and larger context. Scholars, poets, dancers, musicians, and many involved with psychology found these experiences not just enlivening, but revolutionary in the way they now saw their activities. The late Dr. Edward Podvoll, who had had a distinguished career as director of psychiatry at the inpatient psychiatric hospital Chestnut Lodge, was one of these people. Through years of inpatient psychiatric work, Podvoll knew about the benefits and deficits of the inpatient environment. That knowledge, coupled with his developing contemplative perspective, showed him that there were other ways one could work with people in extreme mental states. In 1981, with the help of Trungpa and a group of committed students, Podvoll founded the Windhorse Project.(2)

Windhorse Therapy was originally designed only for individuals with acute mental disturbances, and many treatments are still conducted for people with extreme and chronic major mental health issues: schizophrenia, schizoaffective disorder, bipolar disorder, and major depression. Over time, we have also found Windhorse Therapy effective in treating milder forms of mood disorders, substance abuse and addictions, eating disorders, autism, head injuries, and issues of old age.

Given the range of the types of treatments we conduct, there is a wide variation in size, and related to the size is cost. At the extremely structured end of our care continuum, expenses can approach those of inpatient services. At the lightly structured end, expenses resemble outpatient psychotherapy. It is common that costs may be high at the beginning of treatment, due to the need for more contact and support at that transition. And, as recovery progresses, our teams adjust the level of contact so that costs can fluidly reduce.

3. THERAPEUTIC FOUNDATIONS

Windhorse Therapy is based on three healing principles. The first is that all human beings are fundamentally sane and healthy. As Trungpa states, "Mental confusion exists and functions in a secondary position to one's basic health."(3) This first principle is not about just adopting an optimistic attitude toward human beings. Confidence in basic sanity is a direct experience that results from the clinicians' exposure to contemplative discipline, which we will discuss later.

The second principle of the Windhorse Therapy process is, because human beings are inseparable from their environments,(4) if a healthy environment is created for the treatment, then clients will have a greater probability of recovery. As stated by Trungpa, "The basic point is to evoke some gentleness, some kindness, some basic goodness, some contact. When we set-up an environment for people to be treated, it should be a wholesome environmental situation. A very disturbed or withdrawn patient might not respond right away – it might take a long time. But if a general sense of loving kindness is communicated, then eventually there can be a cracking of the cast-iron quality of neurosis: it can be worked with."(5) As we will see, creating tailored healing environments is the core therapeutic methodology of the Windhorse Therapy process.

The third principle of Windhorse Therapy is that recovery is discovering and synchronizing with one's own fundamental health and sanity.(3) As our clinical results show, the client gains health, skills for his or her particular life needs, confidence, and independence as this discovery and synchronization take place and stabilize. For Windhorse Therapy clinicians, recovery is characterized by a significant, stable, and heartening increase in the client's "windhorse" energy.

A thoroughly trained Windhorse Therapy clinician has a confident and practical understanding of all three of these core principles, plus therapeutic expertise for treating specific psychological disorders.

4. CONTEMPLATIVE ROOTS

Windhorse Therapy is a treatment process whose innovations are founded in the practice of a contemplative tradition. Whatever its form, contemplative discipline invites a progressively more intimate relationship with one's own mind and life in a fresh, moment-to-moment way.(3) For our purposes, it's important to note that a typical individual's contemplative path follows the basic pattern of a typical process of mental health recovery.(4) This parallel has great implications for the design of our tailored recovery environments and for how a client's recovery process is understood, nurtured, and achieved.

One's contemplative path often begins with the distinct sense that something is not right with the way one's life is going. For some individuals, a safe, simple, and attractive method to interrupt this repetitive confusion is to adopt a contemplative practice such as meditation, tai chi, or yoga. Most Windhorse Therapy clinicians have experience with the contemplative practice of Buddhist/Shambhala meditation. This is a simple discipline of attending to or watching one's state of mind without judgment. This can be done formally in periods of "sitting meditation" and also informally in the midst of ordinary activity as clinicians go about their day.(6)

To begin, one simply learns to tolerate how it feels to be aware in the present moment, and how it feels to be with whatever is going on in one's life without self-conscious judgment. Over time, one develops the ability not to be overly carried away by strong positive or negative thoughts and feelings. As one's mind becomes more settled, clarity and awareness develop. With this comes vivid insight, or *islands of clarity,* as this experience is referred to in Windhorse Therapy.(7) The ability to tolerate and appreciate insight is a basic life skill and is essential to any process of recovery. As a typical contemplative path continues, healthy self-love begins. This is called "maitri" in the Buddhist tradition.(8) *Maitri* is the experience that one has basic intelligence, warmth, compassion, good intentions, and the brilliant capacity to love and forgive oneself for not living up to unrealistic judgments. This healthy self-love is also a basic life energy, and the discovery and experience of maitri is frequently a turning point in the path of recovery.

In the contemplative process, one also discovers a naturally confident energy, *windhorse,* that can be used in the service of countering hopelessness, depression, and the mindless repetition of habitual patterns. In contemplation, as in recovery, the more we see our lives and ourselves clearly, the more we have a sense of which actions and thoughts lead to harmonious living and which lead to suffering and unnecessary confusion. Making skillful choices, and rousing the confidence to implement them, becomes an emerging discipline.(9) In Windhorse Therapy we refer to this emerging discipline as having an *allegiance to sanity.*(2) With the recognition and discipline of one's allegiance to sanity, it's natural to feel that recovery from a confused state is not only possible, but likely.

A thoroughly trained Windhorse Therapy clinician has direct experience of the process described above. One result of this contemplative foundation is the clinician's personal conviction that synchronization with one's basic sanity and health is possible for all human beings. It is also clear that the more one knows one's own mind, the more one has insight into and compassion for how others' minds are working. This is not academic knowledge for the clinician, but lived experience.

As one's contemplative path progresses, it becomes apparent how much we affect and are affected by our friends, family, household, and the world around us. We see clearly that as individuals we are inseparable from the powerful effect of our environment. This insight influences the methodology of Windhorse Therapy treatment environments, because our clinical work with a person's specific mental health recovery issues, such as schizophrenia or bipolar disorder, is inseparable from how we "treat" the person's environment to make it a healthier place to be.

From contemplative practice, we also know directly that there is no end point after which we have an absence of problems or suffering. Instead, we have tools to work with whatever comes up in our life. Attempting to synchronize with our fundamental sanity and health becomes a way of life in relationship to ourselves, our friends and family, and our environment as a whole. Fundamentally, we haven't become something different. We have become a more synchronized version of who we basically are. This is how recovery is defined in the Windhorse Therapy process: A person achieves a way of life, unique to himself or herself, that is synchronized with his or her fundamental health and sanity.

5. RECOVERY ENVIRONMENT

Windhorse Therapy is often conducted by a small number of clinicians, using the same fundamental principles as large teams. However, for the purposes of this paper, the following discussion will relate to fully developed teams.

To clarify the therapeutic methodology of "treating" the client's environment, Windhorse Therapy defines environment as having three aspects: *body, speech, and mind.*(10) Very simply, *body* has to do with a person's body, how they dress, and any aspect of their immediate physical world. This includes their home, how they eat, how they exercise, their use of drugs and alcohol, and their use of money. *Speech* is about literal communication with the world, emotions, creativity, and relationships. *Mind* has to do with how

one thinks, attitudes toward oneself and others, spirituality, and schedule.

When we are called to meet with someone who has been struggling with mental health and life issues, it is very common to see the following kind of situation. On the body level, the person's home may have become a very disorganized place. It's difficult to maintain a good place to live when you don't feel well, or are somehow absorbed into states of mind where you don't notice what's around you. There may not be regular cleaning going on so the home feels dirty and uninviting. Clothing is not being washed enough. Shopping and preparing food aren't regularly done, and what is eaten may not be nutritionally sound. Any form of exercise, even going for walks and getting enough fresh air, can be neglected. It's very common for money to be a problem as well. Even if one has enough, without a sense of budget or adequate tracking of what one has and what is spent, the chaos of running out of money, bouncing checks, and not feeling clear about what one has is a very unsettling stressor. Drugs and alcohol are often a contributing factor to one's life circumstances being in disarray.

On the speech level, communication is often very strained between this person and his or her parents. It's not that they don't love each other, but there are so many problems that need working with, it's become almost impossible to have a normal conversation due to everyone's anxiety and fear. On the part of the son or daughter, he or she may be angry and frustrated because of wanting to be independent from the parents, but still needing help in many ways. And the parents may be the only really reliable people in his or her life. It's very common for this person to be socially isolated, and what friends she or he has may have a variety of problems themselves, which can create negative consequences when they get together.

On the mind level, this person may have had a creative and meaningful intellectual life. Now she or he is cut off from these disciplines and all the feelings of success and confidence that come from engaging in these aspects of intelligence. There may not be enough meaningful activity to engage in, like a job or school, and his or her schedule is highly irregular. All this combines to make one feel very disconnected with the world and terrible toward oneself. If she or he is a sensitive person, and so many who are struggling like this are profoundly sensitive, the intricacy of how interconnected and self-sustaining the problems of environment are creates a hopeless state of mind. At this point, the person's windhorse energy is deflated and there is little loving kindness toward oneself. When one feels this bad, you really believe that you are bad. This person and family feel at a loss as to where to begin the recovery process. We know that if we want to help a person and his or her family to break out of the variety of cycles and compounding feedback loops built into this life predicament, it will be far more effective to work with all aspects of personal needs and the environment concurrently. By creating individually tailored recovery environments, the unique strengths and difficulties of each client and family can be simultaneously engaged.(11)

When we create a recovery environment, we are actually forming a very specific arrangement of elements and relationships, with a beginning, middle, and end. We attempt to create an environment that holds all aspects of the client's life, within optimal boundaries that are permeable yet containing, between him or her and the outer world. This environment is a comprehensively coordinated organization of body, speech, and mind, comprised of the household, the people and relationships, therapeutic methodologies, schedules, intentions, and awareness. Influenced by the Buddhist concept of "mandala," defined as a total environment, association, "orderly chaos," or "gestalt,"(12) a recovery environment functions as a compensatory, external, organizing entity.

In many ways, families naturally work this way. If a family member has a life situation – for instance, a woman has a baby – it is very hard for the first few weeks for the mother to be able to shop, cook, clean house, and take care of all the baby's needs. There is a good chance the mother's sleep is disrupted, and there is simply not enough energy to do the tasks of life in the way that has

been normal. It is very common under these circumstances for partners to take time off from work to make sure that everything in the life of the mother and child can be accomplished as necessary. Other family members may also help out. In this case, the mother and the baby are the focus, but anyone who is helping out will do their best to help in a balanced way, so they themselves don't lose their health in the process. Like a Windhorse Therapy recovery environment, this family system is compensating for a change that has occurred, and there is a sense that this is a transitional phase.

6. THERAPEUTIC ELEMENTS AND ROLES

To create a recovery environment, a team is created made up of the clinicians, the client, and whenever possible, the family. These people work in a complementary system of roles, each carrying out a range of functions and therapeutic activities that develop, maintain, evolve, and "are" a large part of the environment. The cohesion and communication of this "whole person system" is carried out within the household, the meetings, and the relationships of the team. To understand the context for much of the relationship activity of the team, we will now look at basic attendance.

6.1. Basic Attendance

A highly flexible and innovative clinical practice, "basic attendance" is the most active, apparent, and principal therapeutic activity in a Windhorse Therapy recovery environment. Influenced by the Buddhist practice of being attentive or simply watching the mind without judgment in the midst of everyday activity, basic attendance is being actively and with helpful intention in relationship with someone in the broad spectrum of his or her life activities, to promote the synchronization of body, speech, and mind, and connection to his or her fundamental health.(2) Its possibilities range from being with a client in the ordinary domestic activity of a household, doing artwork, signing up for classes, looking for employment, or simply having time to relax and play. The work of "basic attendance" may look very simple to the untrained eye, but a seemingly simple task for the client, such as cooking a meal, can stimulate a powerful profusion of conflicting thoughts, emotions, and growth frontiers. It can take a great deal of skill and sensitivity on the part of the clinician in a "basic attender" role to create a safe and successful experience.

6.2. Clinician Roles

Most of the direct clinical contact in Windhorse Therapy is performed by a *basic attender*, as described above. He or she will usually have two shifts per week, generally two to three hours in length.

The *team leader,* also doing basic attendance, is the primary coordinator and a major participant in the direct clinical contact. He or she oversees the day-to-day flow of activity for the team as well as being a sturdy, dependable, and knowledgeable reference point in the life of the client.

The *housemate's* job has two primary functions. The first is simply to live, with good boundaries, in the therapeutic household and support the functioning of a normal and uplifted domestic setting. The second is to be in relationship with the client in that ordinary and earthy way that tends to occur when people share a home. As with all roles, but particularly for the housemates, we are very careful to establish appropriate therapeutic boundaries, prohibiting sexual contact between the staff and clients.

The *psychiatrist* is often a part of a recovery environment, because frequently our clients are using medications. Some psychiatrists may only be doing medication management, so their involvement with the team could be minimal. Others, particularly those whom we have worked with over many years, can be a critical part of the treatment management. As it is often the case when a client is in one of our teams, she or he is able to be on less medication, and his or her needs change over time. We find that the psychiatrist will have a more subtle knowledge of who the client is and what his or her needs are if

the psychiatrist is an integrated part of the team structure.

Usually meeting once or twice per week with the client, the *psychotherapist* is looking for the intelligence and patterns that reside below and within the often-confused behaviors of the client. He or she learns this through the work done in sessions with the client as well as through experience in meetings where the housemate, basic attenders, team leader, and psychiatrist describe their client contact. Likewise, the insights about the client that the psychotherapist provides in the meetings help inform the entire clinical team.

The *team supervisor* watches the dynamics and patterns of the team as the treatment progresses, often working with the family members as they make their own recovery journey. The team supervisor also has a key role in creating a "visualization" for the team and the entire Windhorse Therapy plan, while holding the overall activity of the recovery environment in his or her awareness.

6.3. The Therapist-Friend Relationship

In most psychotherapeutic disciplines, therapy occurs in an office. For some roles in a Windhorse Therapy recovery environment, the formality and boundaries that are a normal part of how most psychotherapy operates would seem altogether unnatural and stiff. In fact, the basic attenders intentionally acknowledge and cultivate client relationships that are part friendship and part therapist. With this in mind, basic attenders are carefully chosen to match a client's interests, deficits, and diagnosis, with an eye toward whether they might actually like one another.(2)

The therapist–friend relationship brings a number of benefits to the recovery environment. First, it can make basic attendance more relaxing and fun, much more like normal life than therapy. Second, many of our clients have had a very difficult time forming treatment alliances. For these people, having clinicians who share at least a slight mutual attraction as friends may make it possible to join and stay in treatment. And as with ordinary friendships, as the therapist-friend relationship develops, it is common for shared interests to "jump-start" dormant passions and interests in each other's life. Third, it opens up the possibility of being able to bring a client into a team member's household. Whenever appropriate and in well-considered measure, a Windhorse Therapy clinician will often invite a client into the world of their family and home. This can provide a powerful experience of acceptance and role modeling for the client as he or she enters the home and relationships of the "therapist-friend."

6.4. Mutual Recovery

A therapeutic element related to the therapist-friend relationship is called "mutual recovery."(2) This originates with the contemplative training of a Windhorse Therapy clinician, and his or her own process of recovery and eventual lifestyle of synchronization. As Trungpa stated in *Creating Environments of Sanity*, "You don't just regard psychology as a J.O.B."(12) This means that the Windhorse Therapy clinician aspires to conduct his or her professional work in fundamentally the same way that he or she lives life. This training promotes a sense of inclusion of everything in one's personal discipline, a "sacred world" orientation, to borrow a Buddhist concept, where "sacred" doesn't mean precious or rare, but what reminds one of basic sanity and goodness.(13) Because everything is included in one's view of how to live and work with life, the relationship with the client and his or her recovery environment is naturally part of this. Instead of "I'm well, you are sick, and I'm going to fix you," there is a sense that we are in this together, and we all are working on our humanity.

6.5. Meetings

In a recovery environment, meetings play a completely critical role. There are a variety of meetings, and all are designed with complementary functions to enhance the communication, cohesion, synchronization, and awareness of the team, the client, and the family. The dynamics of mind in meetings are remarkably energetic, complex, often subtle, at times not, and can generate a wide range of feeling experiences. For those who are paying attention, a wealth of information about how the client is doing and what is going on altogether in the recovery environment is available.(14) Of the types of meetings generally conducted in the course of Windhorse Therapy, these four – the house meeting, the supervision meeting, the team meeting, and the family meeting – have the most central roles.(15)

Attended by the team leader, client, and housemate, and held in the home once a week, the *house meeting* supports the operation of the therapeutic household. Helping the client and the housemate work with relationship and communication issues is a large part of the work of this meeting.

The *supervision meeting* is held at an office, usually every other week in alternation with the team meeting. The entire team, except the client and family, attends. These meetings typically have a relaxed but precise focus, often with good humor. Aside from issues of recovery environment coordination, this meeting is a place where the team can freely discuss the experience of his or her work and develop further understanding of the treatment issues. While checking in, we encourage clinicians to take risks by saying whatever he or she is thinking and feeling, because it is so often the odd and even embarrassing experiences that are most informative about how the client is doing. This meeting also covers the next steps the therapy may need to take and how to best care for the health of the entire team.

The clinicians and the client attend the *team meeting*. When possible, it is held in the client's home. Because of this, the team is very careful to tailor the meeting to the client's needs and sensitivity. Some clients can comfortably participate, with all of us being relatively direct and forthcoming in our communication. Others need more emotional insulation and a less stressful meeting environment. And some can't, or won't, participate for some time. A team meeting is a holding environment that allows the client and clinicians to be comfortable, but also sustains enough tension to produce therapeutic work.

The *family meeting* includes whatever combination of client and family is most relevant to the recovery process, plus the clinician or clinicians who specifically work with them. Because family circumstances and their readiness for therapy have so much variation, these meetings are carefully tailored in their form and frequency.(16)

6.6. The Phenomenon of Group Windhorse

The team often shows up for meetings having done a lot of individual work since the last gathering. Some may be feeling isolated and road weary. The basic attenders, team leader, psychotherapist, housemates, team supervisor, and psychiatrist have all had their experience of client and family, and of each other. Clients and family members likewise have had to deal with the team, themselves, and each other. Feelings have developed, questions have come up, perhaps a troubling observation needs to be discussed with the group. Intense emotional energy may have arisen for some. In these varieties of meetings, the team has a chance to hear and feel what is going on with each other and to explore personal experience in the work. A significant task for the group is to help everyone say what's going on for him or her. Once again, no matter how negative, painful, or hopeless it might sound, the team members need to feel heard and to be connected to the whole. From there, the team tries to make sense of feelings and experiences as they relate to the common developing understanding of the recovery environment, the client, and this unique shared path of recovery. Once team members feel heard and connected to the whole, feelings aren't experienced as being quite so solid, and people tend to relax.(17) With relaxation and clarity often comes the experience of heightened compassion and windhorse energy being aroused in the group. This phenomenon of "group windhorse" is an experience of certain qualities of mind being heightened – upliftedness, confidence, compassion, not being fixed on a thought. Windhorse Therapy clinicians recognize this experience, and

it is directed back to the client and family in our individual contacts after the staff-only meetings. In the meetings involving the client and family, everyone is participating in this heightened positive atmosphere of mind, which promotes an arousal of windhorse energy. Through meeting practice, confident life energy is strengthened in the team, and the entire recovery environment is affected positively. Meetings maintain the pulse and breath of a recovery environment.

7. CASE STUDY

Given the complexity of Windhorse Therapy, it is hoped that this case study will provide a useful sense of how treatment actually looks and works.

Julie was a 27-year-old woman whom Windhorse Therapy worked with for about two years. Five years prior to our first meeting, she had experienced her first manic episode. By the time we met, she had been hospitalized seven times, while maintaining that she did not need psychological treatment. What was different about her current hospitalization was that for the first time she said she was tired of being "thrown in the hospital" and wanted some help. The hospital thought Windhorse Community Services could be a good resource, and her mother, Beth, called us.

Beth was in a guardedly hopeful state of mind, but also heartbroken, bewildered, and exhausted. Because she had never heard Julie say she needed treatment, this was stunning. While being careful not to create false hope, I described the Windhorse Therapy approach, which made great sense to Beth. We agreed that I should go to the hospital to meet Julie.

Even in hospital pajamas, Julie looked like an athlete. She was 5'8" tall, weighed around 145 pounds, and looked physically strong. She had a pleasant face, and the ruddy, fair complexion of someone who had spent a lot of time outdoors. Our initial meeting in the hospital didn't last long because she immediately told me that her mother had described what Windhorse Therapy does and that sounded fine to her, "just to get everyone off my back." She said she really didn't need treatment but agreed to work with us for six months. It felt like she was commanding me to listen, not interrupt, and not to make eye contact or say anything that would put her on the spot. I complied with her "commands," asked her if it would be OK if I started introducing her to potential team members while she was in the hospital, and she said a bit dismissively, "of course." She reported no preference for men or women on the team and "anything else you need to know my mom can tell you. Are we done?" Though she was outwardly a bit hostile, I found her quite likable. I could see it was unspeakably difficult being in her situation and thought she did a good job of getting to the point and taking care of herself. I left with the impression that Julie was terrified, feeling completely vulnerable, and making a tremendously courageous effort to try something different in her life.

From all we could gather in our ensuing assessment, including, importantly, her history of sanity and success,(2) Julie had grown up quite normally as an energetic, intelligent, athletic, and creative person. She had begun to experience mood instability late in high school, at times needing to withdraw a bit from her usual lively flow of activity, seeming depressed with lower energy. Once in college, Julie continued to do well in all areas, but her mood irregularity became more pronounced. Sleeping was often difficult, and it was harder for her to keep an energetic schedule. Her art at times became more brilliant and subtly expressive, but she also did less of it. She tried medications for a brief period, but rapid weight gain and unimpressive results convinced her that they weren't worth the trouble and she stopped. In the meantime, Beth and Julie's father were in the midst of a fairly amicable divorce, which resulted in her father moving out of state and essentially out of her life.

After a heroic struggle to stay in school, and with her life badly deteriorated from how she had been at the beginning, she finally graduated from college. Shortly after that, Beth visited her and immediately knew that something was terribly wrong. Julie was talking in a rapid and

pressured way, was very irritable, and was speaking in an urgent manner about what sounded like Christian mysticism. Her apartment looked like someone had ransacked it, and it appeared that Julie might not have been sleeping for awhile because her bed was now under many layers of oddly arranged artistic creations that appeared to constitute a shrine. When Beth urged her to see her old psychiatrist again, Julie stormed out of the apartment and recklessly drove off. She was picked up later that day by the police and was taken to the psychiatric hospital on a mental health hold. Thus began the cycle that would become her life for the next five years: brief periods of stability interrupted by involuntary hospitalizations, medications, weight gain, and "stupidity," sometimes a job that was hard to cope with, no friends, no meaning, "mom worried about me all the time," "wanting my life and freedom back," and almost dying on two occasions after intentionally stepping into traffic.

The consensus of the assessment was that Julie needed a fully developed team and two shifts per day to begin with. This is a lot of contact, which could be overwhelming, but we also sensed that we needed a very solid structure for her to actually stabilize and be safe. The shifts would be relatively brief, an hour and a half in the morning, to help her get breakfast and organize the day, and another shift at around 6 to 8 p.m., to get dinner and to make the transition from the day to evening. With the day book-ended in this manner, it was also designed to get Julie's sleep cycle stabilized with her being awake during the daytime. We had worked on this plan as best we could with her, but she was not interested in the details of what we would all do. She just said, "I'll do whatever for six months."

As with so many of our clients, Julie was highly ambivalent toward psychiatric medications. Windhorse Therapy does not have a policy that dictates or prohibits the use of medications. Rather, we attempt to approach each client's needs and desires, without pre-judgment, from a place of "taking a fresh look." From what we heard in Julie's case, it was reasonably clear that medications had helped to settle her moods for brief periods in the past, and she was currently on mood stabilizers that seemed to be having a positive effect. She had not tried these before, and significantly, she seemed to be getting benefit without feeling "like my head is full of concrete." We were very careful not to push the idea of medications toward her, but rather to help explore whether or not now was the time to try an experiment with them, within a more structured environment. Consistent with her resolve to break out of the familiar, destructive cycle, Julie opted to try medications, "for six months."

The immediate work at hand was creating the recovery environment. For the psychotherapist, a man named John was chosen and for the team leader a woman named Sandy. Both were very experienced Windhorse Therapy clinicians with strong expertise in bipolar disorders. Because Julie was quite intelligent and had a severe and deadly mood disorder with psychosis, we knew the team likewise needed skilled basic attenders with experience in bipolar disorder. We wanted them to be in their late twenties or early thirties, and the team needed a gender balance. Fortunately, just such candidates were available, and after the first interviews, Julie accepted them all. The team had three women basic attenders and two men. There was also a woman housemate available immediately whom Julie really liked. Rounding out the team was a psychiatrist with extensive Windhorse Therapy experience, and myself in the role of team supervisor. With the team selected, it was now time to gather for the first supervision meeting to assemble the schedule and create a vision for the beginning phase of the journey we were about to take.

As the treatment began, Julie 's terse guardedness with me was in stark contrast to how she spoke in one-on-one situations with John, the therapist, and with Sandy, the team leader. She related to them as if they were her students, and she was a spiritual teacher. She was a little formal, tolerant, and "patient" with how distracted they were by mundane life activity. At any given opportunity, she would teach about the spiritual aspects of life, relationship, the universe, and anything at hand that had inspired her. She

would let John and Sandy do their work, and she would cooperate and teach them when she could. She related to the basic attenders in a similar manner.

Our shift contact began when Julie was still in the hospital, and shortly after she was discharged, the schedule began in full. A good deal of the early shift activity, especially for the team leader and Donna, the housemate, was spent finding an apartment and shopping for furnishings. Of anyone on the team, Donna seemed to have the most relaxed relationship with Julie. It was the least professionally oriented relationship, and they often were just in the house together in a quiet way. They both enjoyed working together to make a comfortable home, and she did very little teaching with Donna.

Julie settled into the basic attendance schedule in what appeared to be a surprisingly unconflicted manner. She was on time for shifts, didn't seem to get particularly close to people, still did a lot of teaching, and tended to be pretty organized about how the time was spent. She would typically use shift time to do errands, get coffee, take a walk, or organize her art studio. Her psychotherapy sessions, which were once per week, were rapidly evolving in a less comfortable way. She and John would meet in his office, and she began to be either completely silent or would show the same kind of guardedness she had with me in the beginning. When she did talk it was mostly to teach.

Julie declined to be part of the family meeting to begin with, although she spoke with her mother several times per week.

Although things were going well for a beginning phase, in the supervision meetings some basic attenders expressed feeling useless and irritated. The shifts felt like a waste of time. My experience was almost always one of vigilance. Despite how easy almost everything about the treatment was, I felt like we were constantly on the verge of something dangerous happening, some disaster. We were also easily able to see what a lovely person Julie was, and her good-heartedness showed in many ways. Even her teaching felt like a generous offering to us. It had a touch of a psychotic flavor, but you could see that she really cared about what she was saying. We all liked her and sensed she had been, and continued to be, in a terrible life predicament.

The team meetings were held at her house. These were generally not very comfortable, a difficult variation on a basic attendance shift, with Julie needing to keep the relationships at a safe distance. The house meetings, also held at the home, were more comfortable and productive as they focused on details of running the home with Donna.

Julie continued showing up for every shift, but as time passed, she was beginning to let it be known that we were all nice enough people but quite useless as therapists. Especially John. There were many sessions where they would just sit with a lot of silence. A little teaching would happen, and then Julie would tell John what a waste of time therapy was. She didn't need therapy, and John was a lousy therapist anyway.

One morning Julie didn't want to get out of bed. Her polite demeanor had been slowly changing over the last month, and she stopped teaching. This morning she looked withdrawn and terrified, like she was really suffering, as if it were difficult for her to breathe. She spent the morning in bed but seemed to appreciate the quiet company of the basic attender, who brought her tea and food and read a book while Julie lay in bed, not wanting to talk. Later in the day she had a therapy session with John, and strangely, she seemed interested in seeing him. At the beginning of the therapy session she was quiet, but it had a completely different feeling about it. Instead of angry and guarded, she appeared completely vulnerable and fearful, very uneasy. Finally in a quiet tone she said, "I can't believe this is who I am." Then in a steady and measured flow of words, she described how horrible it had been over the last five years to see life as she thought it would be, completely washed down the drain. She couldn't count on herself, and nobody else could count on her, except to do something crazy, destructive, and stupid. She had wanted to ignore it, but the mania kept coming back. She wanted to leave everything, but the

police kept bringing her back. Now she was here and having more awareness than she wanted and John, after having survived so much of her anger, felt like the safest person to be with. At least for right now. Caught between the depression, which made her feel like a hopeless and utterly bad, worthless person, and the insight of what she had lost, and without having any sense of a way out of this horror, she saw no realistic option but to kill herself. She had no immediate plan, but she promised that if she tried again, it would be successful. It was clear that she meant it.

John quietly listened to her. When she appeared to be done, he said that he was glad she came in that day. The simplicity of him just being there listening to all this horror and then genuinely communicating that he was glad to be with her, spoke straight to the level of her experience where she felt utterly lonely and unlovable, cut off from everyone, unspeakably afraid and out of control in a world without allies. She cried for most of the rest of the session until John took her home. Once there, Sandy, the team leader, joined Julie and John to talk about what was going on. After believably agreeing not to hurt herself, they all felt it would be best to increase her shift support for at least the next week. Because we had expected her to get depressed at some point and thought this was likely to be a positive development, no medication changes were indicated.

Waking up to who you are and how your life has been is a critical part of the recovery process. This dramatic shift in Julie's awareness was very sudden, which is a dangerous place for a lot of people to be. It can be extremely difficult to tolerate how it feels to be suddenly that aware. Often, a person needs to diminish awareness through cultivating psychosis again, finding other ways of being defended, or killing oneself. But Julie was able to tolerate this experience and use it as a reference point throughout the rest of her time with the team. It was very striking to her that the team did not shy away from the painful intensity of her emotional state, but actually seemed to appreciate her all the more in her vulnerability and for being genuine. Julie's awakening was a dramatic example of an *island of clarity*, an insight or experience that interrupts confusion and helps one to become oriented to the reality, potential sanity, and promise of the here and now. Stated succinctly by Trungpa in *Creating an Environment of Sanity*, "Earth is good."(18)

Julie's first shifts with each clinician after this breakthrough were a little awkward. She was embarrassed that people had seen her act the way she had and was very touched that everyone stood by her. It seemed to her that we had more confidence in her than she had in herself. It appeared that she genuinely no longer wanted to die, but instead was connecting with energy and passion to be physically active and to resume her artwork.

This middle phase felt like an unleashing of her pent-up desire to have a normal life again. If that were simply a matter of her taking medications and having some therapy to help recover from five years of life trauma, we could have ended the team. But having had a radically unstable mood for such a long time, it took Julie about a year and a half to get her moods, and the persecutory voices that came along with them, to settle. As hard as it was for her to be patient with this continued mood cycling, it was encouraging when she noticed that, as she became more stable and closer to her normal mood baseline, the quieter and at times nonexistent the voices became.

As her mind became less chaotic, Julie continued to become clearer about what she valued in her life and to pursue reengaging activities that reflected these. Volleyball and tennis, first with the team members, later with the city's Parks and Recreation leagues, became great opportunities to get her weight back down to where she felt more comfortable, had more energy from being in shape, and felt more like her competent self. These activities also helped her to meet new people outside the team.

At this point, a major part of the work of the team was helping her learn that how she engaged with her physical world, including medications, how she related to people, how she worked with meaningful activities, and how she worked with her thinking had a profound effect on whether her moods were more or less stable. She

learned that sleep was connected to appetite, that her relationship world affected how she ate and slept, and that her thinking was related to everything. As this understanding grew, she was beginning to have more of a sense of maitri toward herself. She was developing unconditional confidence that she was not a bad and hopeless failure of a person. She was feeling better, more alive, and more positive and she liked herself again. She was gaining windhorse energy.

Julie was also becoming a peer on the team to all of us, and she did not hesitate to confront us on our blind spots. For instance, she felt that for all our nice attitudes about the *therapist-friend* relationship, she often found us to be arrogant, as psychotherapists can be, about the fact that she was the "client" and we were the "mature professionals" who have their lives together and, therefore, could help her with how to live hers. As uncomfortable as this was at times, we also appreciated the piercing accuracy of her observations and her confidence to speak directly to us. Our team meetings were now almost always lively, sometimes intense, as we were all not holding back as much. That shift in honesty with all of us was the outer reflection of a shift in her interest and capacity to be more honest with herself. She was gaining strength in unflinchingly identifying which of her actions and thoughts led to more confusion and suffering, and which to more health and harmony in her life. It was clear that her *allegiance to sanity* was becoming a reliable reference point.

Julie never felt compelled to be an ongoing part of the family meeting as the tension between her and her mother, Beth, seemed to resolve through their informal contacts. Between the infrequent face-to-face meetings we had with Julie and Beth, and Beth's more frequent phone conversations and visits, they did manage to establish a much more natural relationship tone and distance for a mother and her adult daughter. This was largely possible because Julie was being "held" by the recovery environment. She was healthier, and Beth was not induced into so much vigilance and protection. Beth could behave more like a mother and not as a caretaker. Also, in a parallel process with Julie, Beth's confidence in Julie's recovery was strengthening. She was very appreciative of how the team was being helpful to Julie and could see the lessening of her dependence on the compensatory nature of the team as her health became more resilient.

By the end of eighteen months, Julie had developed a reasonably energetic schedule of ordinary community activities outside the team structure. This allowed the schedule to be reduced to four basic attendance shifts per week and one psychotherapy session per week. With fewer shifts, we were able to reduce the number of basic attenders needed.

There was one more significant life development that occurred in this phase that shouldn't have been a surprise. Once Julie was more confident in her ability to be in complex social environments outside the team, she found a progressive Christian church to attend that practiced meditation and centering prayer. Besides participating in many social activities and making some nice friendships, she began a daily meditation practice.

The end phase of Julie's Windhorse Therapy treatment was brief, and it began with an argument. Her sister Lisa was coming to town for a visit, and this seemed like an opportunity to have her join a family meeting. Julie really liked that idea. Her life was in a much better place. She was physically healthier, was more mood stable, and the voices had almost entirely disappeared. She was now doing most of the organizing of her life that the team had done. She continued to work on relationships both in and out of the team in a wonderfully direct and honest way, and she had learned for the first time how to live with someone her age in relative harmony and be close with them at the same time. Once we settled into the family meeting, Lisa said in a heartfelt way how amazed she was to see her having such a good life. Julie exploded. "You think this is my life! I'm in treatment and have paid friends! Don't try to make me feel good because I've learned to tie my shoes and you've got your life so together." Lisa was stunned. She was glad that Julie was doing this well and tried to express it. Julie accepted

her apology and over the next hour and a half they were able to resolve the immediate tension between them. Something that was particularly meaningful to Julie was an insight that both Beth and Lisa had when Julie had become angry and essentially declared that having half a life was not going to be settled for: "This feels like we've got our Julie back."

Very significantly, we all noticed that Julie did not experience any mood instability from this very intense emotional event, as she previously might have. She too was surprised by this and later said, "This showed me that I was ready to leave treatment."

In the next week's team meeting, Julie announced that she was leaving the team in one month. She had been researching colleges where she could get a master's degree in physical education and had found one that she liked in a small city out of state, about an hour from where her father lived. School would be starting in nine months and she wanted to move there, get her life established, and apply to school. Once there she would also look for a psychiatrist and a psychotherapist to continue the work she had done with us. She expressed appreciation for all we had done together, "I think you actually saved my life," but said she was tired of having training wheels and paid friends, and needed to get on with her life. "I think I've learned the care and feeding and thinking of Julie, and have a good toolbox for when things come up that I need to deal with." Once she finished talking, she seemed to glow with a quiet resolve, confidence, and a bit of defiance.

To say we were stunned was an understatement. Also, we knew this was absolutely the right thing for her to do. But *we* were not ready for her to leave. We had a more graduated plan for the eventual team reduction and how we could continue to see her for years to come. We really liked her. We wanted to feel appreciated and valued. As is usually the case in the life of a family, artificial or not, emancipation isn't how the parents planned it. And as is usually the case with a successful treatment, recovery is almost always more intelligent than the clinician imagines and certainly not in the clinician's control. John was the first to speak, and much like once before, he said something simple, that "this sounded really right." Others expressed support. Someone else said, "What took you so long to figure this out?" from which we all got a good laugh.

The last month went quickly while we said our good-byes and packed up the house. Julie was busy making her plans and saying good-bye to friends. Without a lot of sentimentality, she ended with us as individuals, as part of the group, and as the host of a lovely going away party. Then she was gone.

In summary, this case shows the compensatory recovery environment in action. Julie entered treatment in a highly disturbed state, in which she was not able to care for herself and had no sense of how to get back to a meaningful and recognizable life. In a very real way, Julie's recovery began as she became part of a recovery environment that allowed her to have a life that functioned, because the recovery environment functioned in a comprehensive and synchronized manner with her and her mother fully integrated into it. Simultaneously, the recovery environment provided specific and integrated psychological treatment that identified and disorganized confusion-producing life patterns and behaviors, helped establish new ones based on health, and over time stabilized those new behaviors.

In the beginning we saw Julie explore whether she could trust the team, knowing that she needed to do something different or die, either literally or die to herself as she knew herself. She then learned to tolerate difficult, life-changing insight, becoming fearless and attentive to the islands of clarity that she had previously avoided. She was also continuing to live as an integral part of a sane environment. This was a world with good body and domestic practices, strong and healthy relationships, good rhythms that tended to support the harmony of the total environment, and adaptable intelligence and awareness. The mind experience of the environment was strong with a sense of allegiance to sanity, maitri, and windhorse. By herself and in the varieties of dyadic and group relationships, the practice of waking up to her sanity and developing confidence in her

path of recovery became a compelling and lived experience, not unlike the contemplative and life experience of the Windhorse Therapy clinicians.

As Julie grew healthier and more independent, we collaboratively reduced the structure of the environment. This reduced the compensatory effect, and she progressively lived a less protected and more normally engaged life, at a more comfortable relationship distance with her mother. With solid skills around working with her mood stability and with confidence in her health and that she was on a resilient recovery path, Julie left treatment. By then, she had internalized a treasure of healthy experience gained from being part of the recovery environment.

In Julie's case, recovery included an abatement of her primary destabilizing symptoms and a return to normal life at a higher level of functioning. To herself and her family, after treatment Julie looked like a mature and wiser version of that bright and good-hearted child they knew growing up.

8. CONCLUSION

After twenty-seven years and hundreds of treatments, much has been learned about Windhorse Therapy. We know it is a highly adaptable form of psychological treatment that can work with a wide variety of complex mental health and life problems. We create compensatory recovery environments that range in size from being quite small to being like small towns. Not everyone needs or wants this type of treatment, but for many who do, it can really work. It works for the client, it works for the family, and it works for the team itself. Those of us who have been fortunate to participate in this process find each team, in its own way, to be a health-promoting and clarifying experience for our own growth as human beings and as clinicians. A significant reason for this is the ability to cultivate individual and collective windhorse energy, which promotes staying committed, continually learning, and being unconditionally confident in each person's possibility of recovery and growth, including our own.

We also know, based on our personal contemplative experience as well as from conducting treatments, that Windhorse Therapy is based on a powerful integration of elements central to the well-being of human beings. Succinctly put, Windhorse Therapy connects the fundamental health of a human being, which is naturally inclined toward recovery, with finely tuned treatments for the psychological disorders that are present, within a highly adaptable recovery environment. This makes Windhorse Therapy particularly effective for complex and difficult-to-treat conditions.

Looking forward, we believe Windhorse Therapy has tremendous potential to evolve over time and be ever more relevant to individual and social well-being. We believe this can occur as the complementary therapies included within the recovery environments continue to advance, as new applications for whole person recovery environments become apparent, and as we continue to deepen our understanding of this promising therapeutic process.

REFERENCES

1. Trungpa C. *Great Eastern Sun*. Boston: Shambhala Publications; 1999.
2. Podvoll E. *Recovering Sanity*. Boston: Shambhala Publications; 2003.
3. Trungpa C. *The Sanity We're Born With*. Boston: Shambhala Publications; 2005.
4. Epstein M. *Going to Pieces without Falling Apart*. New York: Broadway Books; 1999.
5. Trungpa C. *The Collected Works of Chögyam Trungpa: 2:254*. Boston: Shambhala Publications; 2003.
6. Mipham J. *Turning the Mind into an Ally*. New York: River Head Books; 2003.
7. DiGiacamo AM, Herrick M. *Beyond Psychiatry: The Windhorse Project*. Berlin: Peer Lehman Publishing; 2007.
8. Chödrön P. *When Things Fall Apart*. Boston: Shambhala Publications; 1997.
9. Kneen C. *Awake Mind, Open Heart*. New York: Avalon Publishing Group; 2002.
10. Rabin B, Walker R. A contemporary approach to clinical supervision. *J Contemplat Psychother*. 1987;9:135–146.
11. Almaas AH. *Facets of Unity*. Boston: Shambhala Publications; 1998.
12. Trungpa C. *The Collected Works of Chögyam Trungpa, vols. 2 and 6*. Boston: Shambhala Publications; 2003.
13. Kneen C. *Shambhala Warrior Training*. Boulder: Sounds; True 1996.
14. Knapp C. Windhorse therapy: creating environments that arouse the energy of health and sanity. In: Kaklauskas FJ, Nimanheminda S, Hoffman L, Jack M, eds. *Brilliant Sanity: Buddhist Approaches to Psychotherapy*. Colorado Springs: University of the Rockies Press; 2008:275–297.
15. Fortuna J. The windhorse project: recovering from psychosis at home. *J Contempl Psychother*. 1994;9:73–96.
16. Miklowitz DJ, Goldstein MJ. *Bipolar Disorder: A Family Focused Treatment Approach*. New York: Guilford Press; 1997.
17. Weisman A. *Gaviotas: A Village to Reinvent the World*. New York: Chelsea Green Publishing; 1998.
18. Trungpa C. *The Collected Works of Chögyam Trungpa: 2:255*. Boston: Shambhala Publications; 2003.

22 Teaching Religious and Spiritual Issues

ELIZABETH S. BOWMAN

SUMMARY

United Kingdom, American, and World Psychiatric Association guidelines for education of psychiatry residents recommend teaching religion-spirituality. Elsewhere, educational guidelines implicitly subsume religion-spirituality under cultural competence recommendations. American ethical guidelines require knowledge of religion-spirituality for psychiatrists and psychologists. In the United States and Canada, approximately 25 percent of psychiatry residencies teach religion-spirituality. Training of North American psychologists lags but has risen to about 15 percent of programs. Virtually no information is available about religion-spirituality education of African, Australian, or Middle Eastern psychiatrists or psychologists. I review psychiatry and psychology education availability in eight African and eleven Middle Eastern countries. Interest in religion-spirituality in Australia is rising but lags behind that of North America. Religion-spirituality is taught to medical students in 101 American and Canadian medical schools, but information is unavailable on medical student education in religion-spirituality elsewhere. I discuss education grants, an English religion-spirituality curriculum for psychiatry and psychology residents, other teaching resources, teaching methods, faculty qualifications, and recommended content prioritized into essential, important, and helpful categories. This chapter also addresses resistance to curricular integration of religion-spirituality. Religion-spirituality education of psychiatrists and psychologists is low, but rising, and would be more common if educational and ethical guidelines were followed.

This is a book for clinicians. This chapter is about teaching religious-spiritual[a] issues to psychiatric and psychological trainees. Did it take the wrong exit on the editorial freeway and end up in this book instead of an educational one? Clinician colleague, before you decide to skip this chapter, consider this: Why did you decide to read this book? Was it because your clinical training didn't teach you enough about religion-spirituality? If teaching about religion-spirituality in clinical mental health care was inadequate in your training, do you want the future generations of your colleagues and their patients to suffer the same fate?

I. RATIONALE FOR TEACHING RELIGION-SPIRITUALITY

1.1. Scope of Issue and Rationale for Teaching

Religion and spirituality are nearly ubiquitous in human life, and mental illness afflicts approximately 500 million people worldwide.(1) No country lacks religion or mental illness. Thus, the education of mental health professionals must address treatment of illnesses in people of all religions. But why teach it to psychiatric, psychological, and other trainees? I propose three reasons: for our field, for our patients, and for our colleagues in training.

---

[a] For ease of expression, this chapter refers to religion and spirituality with one hyphenated term. This implies inclusion of both, but not equivalence. This chapter conceptualizes religion as institutional or organized and spirituality as a connection to the transcendent or sacred.

1.1.1. For the Mental Health Field

I will state this bluntly: Someday we are all going to die. If we do not teach our knowledge to a new generation, it will die with us. The next generation will lack the skills and knowledge we have acquired. If we mental health professionals cannot provide care for religious-spiritual issues, our patients will go (and already are going) elsewhere.(2–4) Either we provide treatment relevant to our patients' needs, or we die as a field. Training in this field, like training in other topics, will improve the competence of mental health clinicians and will strengthen the healing power of our professions. In fifteen years of teaching religion-spirituality to psychiatry residents and psychology interns,(5) I have observed that trainees exposed to religion-spirituality teaching are usually more well-rounded clinicians than unexposed ones.

1.1.2. For our Patients

People who seek mental health care are as religiously oriented as the general populations in which they live.(6) Mental illness causes intense suffering. People cope with suffering by seeking meaning in their suffering, very often through religion, which provides a system of meaning.(7–9) Morally and professionally, we owe our patients and clients the best possible care. That includes care for religious-spiritual issues, which patients view as essential to their overall health.(8) If *you*, the reader, are a person for whom faith is essential, wouldn't you want a therapist for yourself or your family who was skillful in dealing with religion-spirituality?

1.1.3. For our Colleagues in Training

The World Psychiatric Association's recommended curriculum for psychiatry residents worldwide (discussed below) explicitly recommends teaching religion and spirituality (p. 10).(9) The training requirements of psychiatrists in the United States and Canada require teaching of cultural issues such as religion.(10, 11) Standards for training of United Kingdom psychiatrists and American psychologists refer to teaching cultural competence, which includes religion.(12, 13) The

ethical guidelines for American psychologists and psychiatrists(14–17) require competent treatment of religious and spiritual issues in treatment. The American Psychological Association's ethical code 18 (section 2.01b) explicitly states that "psychologists have or obtain the training, experience, consultation, or supervision necessary to ensure the competence of their services" and expects them to be competent in "factors associated with ... religion ... essential for effective implementation of their services." Ethical requirements dictate that we educate our younger colleagues to meet competency requirements in religion-spirituality.

We can ensure good care for the next generation of patients by providing skilled clinicians to help them with their religious-spiritual issues. Those clinicians are not going to absorb this knowledge by osmosis. They have to be taught religion-spirituality, just as each of us had to be taught assessment and psychotherapy techniques. If we don't educate them about a topic as universal as religion-spirituality, we have failed in our duty to give them the best possible education. We wouldn't dream of neglecting to teach trainees about common and important conditions such as depression, anxiety, or psychosis. The same is true of religion-spirituality: It is a core human issue and is more prevalent in the population than all mental illnesses combined. We can't be silent about it and pretend to be educating fully competent colleagues.

1.2. Why Focus on Students and Trainees?

Given the reality that few practicing psychiatrists and psychologists were given adequate training in religion-spirituality, why focus on education of students and clinical trainees? Surely we have enough education to do with clinicians already in practice. That's true, but it's short-sighted. First, it is far easier to initially teach someone a skill correctly than to struggle to reshape inadequate skills practiced for decades. Old dogs *can* learn new tricks, but it's much easier to teach the puppy. If we teach residents, interns, and students about religion-spirituality, we can form their lifelong attitudes and practice skills toward competent treatment of religion-spirituality.

Second, if we teach this topic to trainees, some of them can become the next generation of researchers on religion-spirituality in mental heath. All vibrant fields need to mentor their next generation of researchers while they are young. My interest in this topic blossomed in my first year of residency after I attended a conference on psychiatry and religion-spirituality where I was exposed to academicians working in this field. My interest grew into an academic career, years of educating residents, and mentoring at least one to an academic career in religion-psychiatry.

Third, this chapter focuses on teaching psychiatric and psychological trainees because that is already occurring in increasing numbers of programs with success. Grant funding,(18) a curriculum,(19) and ample research data (20, 21) are available to support evidence-based education in religion-spirituality. Religion-spirituality is now a viable academic option for psychiatric and psychological faculty.

2. EDUCATIONAL STANDARDS FOR TEACHING RELIGION-SPIRITUALITY

2.1. International Standards for Psychiatric Education of Medical Students

The World Psychiatric Association's (WPA) (22) psychiatry curriculum for medical students (1) grew out of the 1988 Edinburgh World Conference on Medical Education.(23) This curriculum describes the minimum requirements in psychiatry for medical students who will enter further training in either primary care or any medical specialty. It emphasizes that medical education that concentrates on curative medicine is no longer enough; disease prevention and health promotion must also be taught.(1, 24–25) This curriculum is directed primarily at medical school teaching of psychiatry.

The WPA-World Federation for Medical Education (WMFE) medical student curriculum does not explicitly mention teaching about religion-spirituality, but renders it necessary via numerous expectations regarding education on the social setting of mental illness. Like most curricula, it emphasizes teaching attitudes, skills, and knowledge. This curriculum includes religion-spirituality relevant objectives of integrating "humanistic, scientific and technological aspects of knowledge of psychiatry," teaching "the context of an integrated biological, psychological and social approach," and teaching the "skill to evaluate the role of personal and social factors in the patient's behaviour."(1)

The medical student curriculum also expects medical students to communicate with "nonmedical agencies involved in the care of patients," learn "teamwork skills necessary for the doctor to … work in conjunction with non-medical staff," and learn the "principles of psychiatric care in non-psychiatric settings and in the community."(1) In many countries, these agencies would include religious groups or clergy. These requirements implicitly include teaching of the religious-spiritual aspects of psychological sciences to medical students.

2.2. Standards for Education of Psychiatrists

The WPA also has produced a Core Curriculum for Postgraduate Training in Psychiatry.(26) Unlike the medical student curriculum, the residency training curriculum explicitly includes a recommendation to teach "religion and spirituality" as one of seventeen areas of "special aspects" of curricular knowledge (p. 10).(26) Another recommended special aspect is "cross-cultural psychiatry." This curriculum is general enough to be applied to training in the WPA's 104 member countries, so further details are not offered. What is important is this: The world's foremost psychiatric authority has recommended all psychiatry residents be taught religion and spirituality.

2.2.1. Guidelines for American Psychiatrists

American guidelines mandate or encourage teaching of religion and spirituality in the training of psychiatrists. The most influential American guideline encouraging teaching of religion and spirituality in psychiatry residencies is the 1994 training requirements for accreditation of U.S. psychiatry residency training programs, published by the American Medical Association's Accreditation Council for Graduate Medical Education (ACGME).(10) This document requires education of residents about religious and spiritual factors in psychiatric care and prescribes inclusion in the didactic curriculum of "religious/spiritual" factors influencing development. The ACGME guidelines also include religion/spirituality among issues to be taught as part of competence in cultural understanding. Thus, teaching religion-spirituality has been mandated for accreditation of American psychiatric residencies for fourteen years.

In 1990, the American Psychiatric Association (APA-psychiatry) approved ethical guidelines for possible conflict between psychiatrists' religious commitments and psychiatric practice.(15) These guidelines specify that psychiatrists respectfully address their patients' religious and spiritual beliefs. In 1994, the fourth edition of the *Diagnostic and Statistical Manual of Mental Disorders* (*DSM-IV*) (27) included a category "Religious or Spiritual Problem" among nonpsychopathological Conditions that May be a Focus of Clinical Attention. Neither the ethical guidelines nor the inclusion of "Religious or Spiritual Problem" in the *DSM-IV* mandate training in religion and spirituality, but each provides a rationale for training.

2.2.2. Guidelines for Canadian Psychiatrists

Psychiatric training in Canada occurs under the auspices of the Special Committee in Psychiatry of the Royal College of Physicians and Surgeons of Canada (RCPSC). The RCPSC's psychiatry training requirements (11) do not specifically mention spirituality or religion. The RCPSC's standards for accreditation of psychiatry residency programs (28) do not mention religion or spirituality but make room for it: They require facilitation of "the acquisition of knowledge, skills, and attitudes relating to aspects of … culture and ethnicity" (28) (part B.4, p. 2) and mandate "opportunities for consultations to … community agencies" (28) (part B.4.3c, p. 4). Religion is an aspect of culture and ethnicity. Consultations with pastoral

caregivers and religious congregations would fall under community agencies. These references are quite spiritually and religiously nonspecific, but these requirements are Canadian applications of a more religiously and spiritually specific set of curricular requirements from the Royal College of Physicians (RCP) of the United Kingdom.(12)

2.2.3. Guidelines for United Kingdom (UK) Psychiatrists

The Royal College of Psychiatrists (RCP) is the psychiatric organization of the Royal College of Physicians in the UK, which is the parent organization of Royal Colleges of Physicians of British Commonwealth nations. The Competency-Based Curriculum for Specialist Training in Psychiatry of the RCP (12) is the standard for psychiatry residency training in England and Northern Ireland and is used in Canada and other current or former Commonwealth nations. In two places in the competency standards of these guidelines, residents are expected to "take into account …spiritual … factors in service development and delivery" (12) (section G.a.11) and to "take account of the complex … religious … issues that play a role in the development and delivery of services" (12) (section G.d.11). In addition to these two specific references to religion and spirituality, this curriculum frequently mentions delivery of service in "culturally diverse" or "multicultural" settings, terms that include religion and spirituality. The psychiatry residency curriculum of the United Kingdom is clear that residents should learn competency in spiritual factors and religious issues in clinical care, but it is not explicit that residency programs teach it.

2.3. Standards for the Education of Psychologists

2.3.1. American Psychologists

The American Psychological Association (APA-psychology) standards for accreditation of graduate school programs in psychology include religion by requiring focus on "cultural and individual diversity … with regard to personal and demographic characteristics. These include but are not limited to age, color … *religion*, sexual orientation"(13) (p. 5, italics added). APA training standards require programs to inform the student of relevant knowledge and experiences in the area of diversity. This means religion-spirituality should be taught to all American psychologists in training.

3. WHAT TRAINEES ARE ACTUALLY BEING TAUGHT

3.1. Limitations of Available Data

Our field is still in the stage of convincing the larger scientific community of its clinical importance. Accordingly, the scientific literature on education of mental health clinicians about religion-spirituality is still quite limited. Most research on religion-spirituality in health care is clinical, not educational, in focus. Research on religious-spiritual training in psychiatry and psychology consists mostly of surveys of the prevalence and extent of such education. Few teaching outcome data are available. Most research on mental health religion-spirituality education has come out of psychiatry and psychology in North America and former British Commonwealth nations. Accordingly, this chapter focuses primarily on those professions, but includes some information on religion-spirituality training for medical students. Unfortunately, addressing the fields of social work, marriage and family therapy, and pastoral counseling is beyond the scope of this chapter.

3.2. Religion-Spirituality Training: Psychiatry and Psychology

Information on actual training in religion-spirituality in psychiatry and psychology across the world is limited. This chapter reviews available information on training efforts arranged by continents.

3.2.1. North American Psychiatry Training: Canada

The RCPSC is the Canadian society of the Royal College of Psychiatrists of the UK. Canadian psychiatric training uses the 2006 standards of the Royal College of Psychiatrists,(12) discussed above. The RCP psychiatry standards encourage teaching of religion and spirituality. Is this actually happening?

A majority (78 percent) of Canadians endorse belief in God.(29) Among Canadian psychiatric inpatients, 59 percent believe in a personal God and 27 percent attend worship services frequently.(30) Canada has sixteen accredited general psychiatry residency training programs.(31) In a 2003 survey, fourteen of these programs reported on spirituality and religion training available to residents.(32) Four programs (25 percent of all Canadian programs, 28 percent of responding programs) offered no formal or informal training in this area. Four programs (25 percent of all, 28 percent of respondents) reported mandatory didactic teaching, but the maximum hours offered was four in one program and one hour in two programs. Nine programs (56 percent of all, 64 percent of respondents) offered case-based supervision to interested residents (three of them in programs with didactic teaching). Two programs (12.5 percent of all, 14 percent of respondents) offered clinical electives related to religion and spirituality. Residents in three programs (19 percent of all, 21 percent of respondents) were involved in related research endeavors under the supervision of faculty experts. Thus, a maximum of one-fourth of psychiatry residents in Canada receive mandatory training in religion and spirituality, and the time allotted to training is quite brief. In response to reports from Canadian psychiatry residents that they support introduction of formal lectures on religion and spirituality, Grabovac and Ganesan (32) offered a ten-session proposed psychiatry residency curriculum on religion and spirituality specific to Canadian cultures.

Religion and spirituality are taught to about half of Canadian psychiatric residents, but the dose of religious-spiritual education that Canadian psychiatric residents receive appears small, perhaps because few Canadian residencies have applied for the Templeton Foundation psychiatry curricular awards discussed later in this chapter. Two Canadian psychiatry residencies have received these awards, which encourage religion-spirituality education in all years of residency. Ample opportunities exist for the expansion of training in religion and spirituality for Canadian psychiatry residents.

3.2.2. North American Psychiatry: United States

A 1988 survey of American psychiatry residency training directors found that very few residency programs had either frequently or always offered didactic course work (12 percent) or provided clinical supervision (33 percent) that usually addressed religious issues.(33) Two-thirds of directors reported rarely or never offering courses on religion-spirituality. Few residents received training in the dynamics of religious beliefs, or were supervised regarding the dynamics of their own or their patients' religious beliefs, regardless of the program's association with religiously affiliated institutions.

In 1992 and 1993, Waldfogel et al.(34) surveyed the religious lives and didactic and supervision experiences in religion-spirituality of 121 American psychiatry residents in five programs not affiliated with religious institutions. They found 86 percent of residents had a religious affiliation, higher than the 76 percent found in 1990 by Bergin and Jensen.(35) This level of religious affiliation may have been elevated by African American psychiatry residents who reported considerably more religious participation and personal religious belief than white residents. Waldfogel and colleagues found that 49 percent of residents prayed at least weekly, although only 22 percent attended religious services weekly, compared with 32 percent of a national sample of persons of similar age.(36) Twenty-seven percent of residents and 29 percent of third-year through fifth-year residents reported that religion was discussed or presented in their didactic program. A significant relationship was found between having either didactic (p < 0.005) or supervision exposure (p < 0.001) and residents stating that religion is important in the clinical setting. A high percentage of residents reported feeling "somewhat (72 percent) to very (12 percent)

competent" in their ability to recognize and attend to a patient's religious and spiritual issues. Feelings of clinical competence in recognizing and dealing with patients' religious-spiritual issues were significantly correlated with didactic or supervisory education in religion-spirituality (p < 0.05). Waldfogel's sample,(34) although moderate in size, shows that religious-spiritual education of psychiatry residents can affect clinical attitudes. It is not known if residents' clinical skills increased along with their confidence.

These studies indicate that American psychiatrists, like Canadian ones, remain less religious than their patients, but are more religiously affiliated than reported in the past. Even in intensely religious America, in the early 1990s, at most 30 percent of residencies were teaching about religion-spirituality. However, that began to change as funding of religious-spiritual education became available.

This author believes two major factors – guidelines (discussed above) and education grants – and two less influential factors have generated increased interest in teaching religion and spirituality in American psychiatry residency programs. Before the 1994 accreditation requirements, the majority (67–75 percent) of psychiatry residents in the United States were exposed to little or no training about this topic. Is this still the case? Not since grants for religion-spirituality education have been available.

More U.S. psychiatry residencies began to teach religion-spirituality after 1997 when the John Templeton Foundation (37) inaugurated an award program for religion and spirituality curricula in psychiatric residency training for accredited American and Canadian adult and child psychiatry residencies. This program was administered by the National Institute for Healthcare Research (NIHR) until it ceased operations around 2002. Since then, this program has been administered by the George Washington Institute for Spirituality and Health (GWISH) (18) of Georgetown University in Washington, DC, which funds three to five psychiatry residency program awards yearly. Since 1997, at least forty-nine American and two Canadian psychiatry residencies have received awards. Far more residencies have created curricula to apply for these grants, but the number of unsuccessful applicants who teach their curricula without monetary support is unknown. Standards for receiving awards are high: Awardees must teach religion and spirituality to nearly all years of residents, use a diverse array of teaching methods, and have visibility in the community. The infusion of monetary support into education on religion-spirituality in psychiatry has greatly accelerated interest in teaching it to residents. But what proportion of American psychiatry residencies does this represent?

The Accreditation Council on Graduate Medical Education (ACGME) lists 181 accredited psychiatry residencies in the United States and Puerto Rico.(38) The fifty-one programs (forty-nine American; at least two Canadian) that have received Templeton awards account for 27 percent of accredited American residencies. If even half of the approximately fifty unsuccessful applicants for Templeton awards are teaching the curricula they developed, seventy-six (42 percent) of accredited American psychiatry residencies are involved in teaching religion-spirituality to their residents. This is not a majority of American psychiatry residencies, and we have no actual data that more than 27 percent of residencies teach religion-spirituality. The proportion of psychiatry programs teaching religion-spirituality is quite similar in Canada and the United States, probably because of cultural similarities.

A third factor that may have encouraged teaching of religion-spirituality in U.S. psychiatry residencies is the availability of a 1997 curriculum specifically for psychiatry residents. Funded by the Templeton Foundation, the 105-page *Model Curriculum for Psychiatric Residency Training Programs: Religion and Spirituality in Clinical Care. A Course Outline* (19) (hereafter referred to as the *Model Curriculum*) was developed as a guide for residencies applying for the Templeton psychiatry curricular awards. This ready-to-use curriculum is applicable to psychology or social work training programs in any English-speaking country, and for use in continuing medical education

(CME) presentations. It contains three core modules (overview, assessment, and human development), eight accessory modules, discussion of learning formats, and a sample evaluation form. It is unknown how many residencies are using this curriculum.

A fourth factor, the intense religiousness of American culture, may also contribute to the willingness of American psychiatry residencies to offer courses in religion-spirituality. Surveys of Americans consistently show high endorsement of religious belief and practice: 95 percent of Americans endorse belief in God (39), 90 percent pray, and 50 percent pray daily.(40) Almost three-quarters of Americans say their religious faith is the most important influence in their life. (35, 36) The religiousness of American society is not necessarily shared by American psychiatrists, who are much more likely (21 percent) than the general U.S. population (6 percent) to consider themselves atheist or agnostic (36) and less likely (40–70 percent) than their patients to believe in God.(14) However, Bergin and Jensen (35) found psychiatrists (40 percent) no less likely than the general American public (42 percent) to regularly attend religious services.(36, 41)

3.2.3. Psychology Training: United States and Canada

Psychology is a mental health discipline that prides itself on its objective scientific base. Thus, we might expect psychology training to be devoid of education on religion-spirituality and few psychologists to be personally religious. Do data support these predictions?

The picture of religion-spirituality education in North American psychology has not been pretty. A quarter century ago, Bergin (42) noted that "training in the clinical professions is almost bereft of content that would engender an appreciation of religious variables in psychological functioning." In 1990, Shafranske and Maloney (43) reported that as few as 5 percent of American clinical psychologists reported having had religious or spiritual issues addressed in their professional training. The next year, Lannert (44) reported that no psychology internships offered education on religious or spiritual issues. Brawer et al. (45) noted psychology's "general negative stance" on religion and spirituality. Despite this, they noted that psychology is following the U.S. trend toward addressing religion-spirituality in medical training, but not to the degree seen in medical schools and psychiatry residencies. Brawer and colleagues note more journals and more research devoted to psychology and religion-spirituality and the creation of Division 36 of the APA (psychology) devoted to religion-spirituality in psychology. The latter development indicates a considerable number of psychologists with a primary interest in religion-spirituality. But does this translate into attention to this topic in training?

Brawer and colleagues (45) investigated this question with a survey of education in religion-spirituality in the APA-accredited clinical psychology programs in the United States and Canada. They considered course work, research, and clinical supervision in a survey of directors of training of the 197 programs accredited as of 1998. Among ninety-eight respondents, they found that 13 percent of programs offered a specific course on religion-spirituality in psychology. Twenty-four more programs were considering adding such a course. In the 77 percent of programs that addressed religion-spirituality in clinical supervision, coverage was often inconsistently incorporated into the usual supervisory process. In 61 percent of programs, religion-spirituality was covered as part of another course not devoted specifically to religion or spirituality: in cultural diversity courses (57 percent), ethics courses (41 percent), psychotherapy courses (32 percent), psychopathology courses (19 percent), and courses on psychology history, family, and assessment. Brawer and colleagues concluded that psychology training programs tended to incorporate religion-spirituality into multiple course offerings. More than 30 percent of the training programs had a faculty member who had published scholarly work on religion-spirituality, and 22 percent had a faculty member who identified this field as a major area of interest. Forty-three percent of programs had a student whose major area of interest was religion-spirituality. This study did not specify if programs were masters or doctorate level. Data collection methods for Brawer et al.'s study and for research on psychiatry residencies are too different for meaningful comparison of religious-spiritual education of psychiatrists and psychologists in North America.

The data of Brawer and colleagues' study need replication, but indicate that religion-spirituality training, while infrequent, is becoming more available to Canadian and American psychologists. Systematic training in this field still occurs only in a minority of psychological programs (systematic in 17 percent),(45) but interest appears to be rising, and a corps of faculty members is forming to mentor research in religion-spirituality for future generations of psychologists. Still, the majority of programs do not offer much education in this area. Further evidence that North American psychology is more interested in religion-spirituality comes from the APA's (psychology) recent publication of several books dealing with religion in therapy: Shafranske's *Religion and the Clinical Practice of Psychology* (46) and Richards and Bergin's *Handbook of Psychotherapy and Religious Diversity*.(47) Like our polar ice caps, the frostiness of psychology to religion-spirituality appears to be melting somewhat.

3.2.4. European Psychiatry Training: United Kingdom

Little information is available on whether religion-spirituality courses are actually taught in U.K. psychiatry residencies. As in the United States, U.K. psychiatrists are considerably less personally religious than the general population: 27 percent of 231 London teaching hospital psychiatrists and psychiatric residents reported a religious affiliation (versus two-thirds of the residents' parents) and 23 percent (versus 70 percent of the U.K. population) endorsed a belief in God.(48, 49) Among respondent psychiatrists, 87 percent attended religious services once a year or not at all. Psychiatrists who trained outside Europe tended to report a belief in God more than those who trained in Europe (35 percent versus 20 percent, p = NS). In practice, about half

(48 percent) of these London psychiatrists and residents usually or always inquired about their patients' religious beliefs, but only 42 percent had ever initiated a referral to clergy. Psychiatrists who regularly attended religious services were significantly more likely (p $<$ 0.005) to have made a referral to clergy. The attitudes of these London psychiatrists toward religion and mental illness were diverse, with a minority holding positive views of the effect of religious belief on mental health. Neeleman and King's (48) data are not a direct survey of training on religion-spirituality in the United Kingdom, but suggest it is unlikely this group of academic psychiatrists and residents had received effective training in religion-spirituality.

3.2.5. Australian Psychiatry Training

As a group, Australians are less religious than Americans: 61 percent of Australians believe in God, 67 percent pray at least sometimes, and 25 percent attend religious services at least monthly.(50) Interest in spirituality and general health may be rising in Australia, as evidenced by conferences on this topic in July 2005 and August 2007 and publication of the proceedings of the 2005 conference as a supplement to the *Medical Journal of Australia* in 2007.(51) This author was not able to find information on teaching religion-spirituality to Australian psychiatry residents.

3.2.6. Australian Psychology Training

Australian psychologist Passmore (52) holds that Australian psychologists have been less active than their American colleagues in stimulating debate, conducting research, and making clinical application in religious issues in psychotherapy. She called for training Australian psychologists to sensitively deal with religious issues in therapy.

3.2.7. African Psychiatry and Psychology Training: Uganda

Uganda has few psychiatrists. Kenyan psychiatrist Njenga (53) describes the ranks of Ugandan psychiatry being decimated "in the dark

days of consecutive dictatorial regimes" via migration elsewhere. The Department of Psychiatry of Uganda's Makerere University Faculty of Medicine in Kampala offers Uganda's only postgraduate program in psychiatry. Makerere University trains psychiatrists for clinical work and trains them to train other mental health professionals and primary health-care providers. Makerere University's psychiatry training program is centered in Butabika Hospital, a national referral government hospital in Kampala that provides inpatient and outpatient psychiatric and general medical care.(54) This author found no information available about religion-spirituality education in Butabika's or Makerere University's psychiatry programs or any information on psychology training in Uganda.

3.2.8. African Psychiatry and Psychology Training: Tanzania

Njenga (53) reports mental illness was traditionally linked to demon possession and spiritual factors in indigenous Tanzanian society. Modern psychiatry also is present in Tanzania. The Muhimbili National Hospital in Dar Es Salaam is the main teaching and referral hospital and the only psychiatry training facility in Tanzania.(53) The Department of Psychiatry of the School of Medicine of Muhimbili University of Health and Allied Sciences (MUHAS) (55) offers a master of medicine in psychiatry degree (equivalent to a Western psychiatry residency). MUHAS distinguishes itself by having an Institute of Traditional Medicine for the study of indigenous healing practices, which are often linked to religion or spirituality, but this institute does not appear to provide education on mental health. The Tanzanian Ministry of Health has a section of traditional medicine, but its focus is not on education. Njenga (53) reported that in 2001, Tanzania had ten psychiatrists total working in the public sector. Mental health is taught in all five years of medical school training at MUHAS, but details of the curriculum are not available.

The people of Tanzania have a single training program in psychiatry, but no information is available about whether trainees are educated about religion-spirituality. However, the existence of the Institute of Traditional Medicine indicates Tanzanian academic medicine is likely aware of traditional healing practices that may be linked to spiritual beliefs. This author was not able to find information about psychology training in Tanzania.

3.2.9. African Psychiatry and Psychology Training: Kenya

The medical director of Mathari Hospital in Nairobi, Dr. Frank Njenga, reported in 2002 (53) that all psychiatrists in Kenya were Europeans at the time of the country's independence in the 1960s. In 1971, the Department of Psychiatry of Nairobi University School of Medicine (NUSOM) was founded in Nairobi.(56) In 1982, this department began to train adult and child psychiatrists at Kenyatta and Mathari National Hospitals for certification in the United Kingdom and established a three-year master of medicine in psychiatry degree. At Mathari Hospital, most of the patients are Christian; treatment is Western and biological.(53, 57, 58)

The first indigenous Kenyan qualified in psychiatry in 1970 from the United Kingdom. In 1975, NUSOM arranged with the University of London to place four Kenyans each year for psychiatric studies in the United Kingdom, training under U.K. psychiatry standards.(53) In 2008, the NUSOM Department of Psychiatry was also training medical students and nursing students and was offering degrees in other mental health specialties, including a master of science in clinical psychology, a master of medicine in psychiatry (psychiatry residency), and postgraduate diplomas in psychiatry, substance abuse, and social work. This author was not able to find information on whether religion-spirituality are addressed in these degree programs, but found a required course in social and transcultural psychiatry in the master of medicine in psychiatry curriculum.

Kenyan psychiatrists use Western approaches in large hospitals where the most severely ill patients are treated. However, in much of Kenya,

traditional healers are used more than psychiatrists. In regional health centers across Kenya, psychiatrists work collaboratively rather than competitively with traditional healers such as herbalists and spiritualists, and even offer them training.(58) Publications by Kenyan psychiatrists often refer to indigenous beliefs and practices that are effective in treating many mental illnesses. It is unknown if Kenyan psychiatry residents are taught about religion-spirituality issues, but their faculty appear well aware of these issues. A second Kenyan medical school, Moi University, established in 1990 does not offer psychiatric training.(59)

3.2.10. Psychiatry Training: South Africa

Emsley (60) reports "qualification for registration as a psychiatrist" [in South Africa] can be accomplished either by completing a university-based master's degree in psychiatry – MMed(Psych), or completing the fellowship of the College of Psychiatrists of the Colleges of Medicine of South Africa– FCPsych. Both the Mmed(Psych) and FCPsych degrees require a 4-year full-time training period in an approved registrar post. Admission requirements include an MBChB degree, a year of internship, and an additional year as a medical practitioner. Psychiatry is a popular specialty among South African physicians.(60) Training programs have waiting lists. Psychiatric treatment takes a biological approach, but South Africa also has a Jungian Psychoanalytic Institute.

In 2001, South Africa had eight medical schools, with approximately 130 registrar (resident) posts. Since the national regulatory body, the Health Professions Council of South Africa, recognized psychiatry as the fifth major clinical specialty, a clinical rotation in psychiatry is required in the sixth year of MBChB training. Most medical schools, in spite of staff shortages, provide undergraduate teaching courses in psychiatry. South African academic psychiatrists spend an average of 7.5 hours weekly teaching while managing large clinical loads.(61)

3.2.11. African Psychiatric Training: Malawi

British psychiatrist Herzig (62) visited Malawi as a missionary in the 1990s to find himself the only psychiatrist in the country and the only psychiatric hospital staffed primarily by nurses and orderlies. He opined that specialist psychiatric education was a luxury beyond the means of the poorest countries where clinical services are too inadequate to provide experience for trainees. Malawi's situation rendered Western psychiatric curricula unusable. Most mental and behavioral problems are treated by traditional healers, with the most disturbed patients being brought to the hospital or left untreated. Herzig recommended Malawi's College of Medicine approach of focusing on teaching medical students to treat common mental illnesses in outpatient primary health-care clinics and on supervising and training psychiatric nurses to provide mental health care in hospitals and in rural clinics. Herzig's (62) only reference to religion-spirituality in training was to recommend medical students be taught to consider "local cultural explanations for abnormal behavior such as bewitchment and spirit possession." No information on psychological training in impoverished Malawi is available.

3.2.12. African Mental Health Training: Morocco

Mohit (63) reports Morocco's World Health Organization (WHO) Collaborating Centre in Casablanca conducts psychiatric research and was active in collaborating with WPA-WFME in the development of the medical student core curriculum for psychiatry.(1) Morocco contains more than 2000 psychiatric beds and offers psychiatric training in Casablanca and Rabat. Psychiatric nursing courses are also available. No information is available about religion-spirituality education in training in Morocco.

3.2.13. Psychiatric and Psychological Training in the Middle East

The vast Middle East, stretching from northern India to northern Africa, contains a rich array of religions. Its ancient cultures spawned Zoroastrianism, Judaism, Christianity, and Islam. After the rise of Islam in the sixth century CE, medicine and mental health treatment flourished. Currently, psychiatric education in many middle east countries occurs in conjunction with the WHO and WFME. Numerous Muslim-associated mental health groups exist in the Middle East. The Muslim Mental Health Association (64) publishes the *Journal of Muslim Mental Health*. The MMHA web site (http://www.muslim mentalhealth.com/index.php?option=com_ weblinks&Itemid=14) features links to nineteen related Muslim mental health groups worldwide, including the International Association of Muslim Psychologists and the World Islamic Association for Mental Health.(65) The Arab Board of Psychiatry offers certification of psychiatrists in a number of Middle Eastern countries. Very little, if any, information is available on education in religion-spirituality in most of these predominantly Muslim countries, so this chapter discusses mental health training.

3.2.14. Egypt

Egypt has approximately 9000 psychiatric beds and 500 to 1000 psychiatrists.(66) Psychiatric training is offered in major medical schools and certification is given through national examination and the Arab Board of Psychiatry. The Institute of Psychiatry at Ain Shams University, a WHO Collaborating Centre, offers training in child psychiatry. Egyptian training is available in psychiatric nursing and clinical psychology. No information is available on teaching religion-spirituality to Egyptian psychiatrists or psychologists.

3.2.15. Iran

The Islamic Republic of Iran has 9200 psychiatric beds, about 1000 psychiatrists, 350 masters and doctoral level psychologists, and more than 50 psychiatric nurses.(63) Currently, ten universities offer specialty training in psychiatry, and several centers offer subspecialization in child psychiatry. Psychiatric certification is granted through the Iranian Board of Psychiatry. Iran also offers doctoral and masters degrees in psychology, a doctoral degree in child psychology, and masters degrees in social work, psychiatric nursing, and occupational therapy. Details of training requirements were not available to this author. Doubtless, the overwhelmingly Islamic milieu of Iran affects training.

3.2.16. Iraq

Iraq has psychiatric facilities in at least three locations, one of which, the main Shamaeeah hospital, is from the mid-twentieth century. Mohit (63) reports the conditions of psychiatric treatment deteriorated after the 1991 international embargo. With Iraq now in the sixth year of war, it is likely that mental health training, about which little information is available, may be severely disrupted. No information was available to this author about mental health training in Iraq.

3.2.17. Lebanon

Psychiatric training for physicians has been available in Lebanon since the mid-nineteenth century from American University in Beirut and the Lebanon Hospital for Mental and Nervous Disorders. The Lebanon Hospital has provided British-oriented training to numerous international psychiatrists. In the twentieth century, Deir El-Saleeb (Hôpital de Croix), affiliated with the French Faculty of Medicine, has trained psychiatric nurses and other auxiliary psychiatric workers.(63) A one-year, postgraduate mental-health nursing course is available. Lebanon also has a twentieth century Muslim psychiatric hospital. This author could find no information about religion-spirituality in mental health training in Lebanon. The mixed Christian and Muslim population likely leads to salient religious issues in treatment.

3.2.18. Jordan

The country of Jordan has about 330 public and private psychiatric beds and 50 psychiatrists.(63) Mental health services are often provided in general outpatient health clinics. Mental health training is available to general physicians. This author found no information on psychiatric or psychological training in Jordan,

whose population includes primarily Muslims (over 90 percent) and Christians.

3.2.19. Pakistan

At present, eighteen medical colleges have departments of psychiatry, psychiatric hospitals, and specialty training programs.(63) Psychiatric research is conducted in Rawalpindi by the Institute of Psychiatry. Master degree training in mental health nursing is available in Pakistan. The Pakistan Board of Psychiatry offers certification of mental health specialists. Pakistan has master's degree training for mental health nursing. Pakistan's mental health system offers integrated care. Naeem and Ayub (67) include "loss of religious values" and "prejudices based on … sect" among factors contributing to high rates of mental health problems in Pakistan, a country that is 97 percent Muslim.

In 2004, Pakistan had about 870 teaching hospital psychiatric beds, four mental hospitals and about forty psychiatric units attached to medical colleges, most of whom have psychiatry departments.(67) Psychiatry is recognized by the Pakistan Medical and Dental Council (PMDC) as part of the medical school curriculum. The PMDC lacks a prescribed curriculum for teaching behavioral sciences, so medical school psychiatric curricula vary widely. No information is available regarding inclusion of religion-spirituality in the medical school curricula.

Postgraduate medical training in Pakistan is regulated by the College of Physicians and Surgeons of Pakistan (CPSP), which accredits training institutes and sets curricula for specialties. Few general practitioners receive postgraduate training in psychiatry.(67) The CPSP offers fellowship (FCPS) exams in psychiatry that allow physicians to practice psychiatry. Candidates may sit for the first part of the FCPS exam after obtaining a MBBS or equivalent degree and completing a one year "house job" (internship) in any clinical area. Candidates must complete four years of psychiatry training in a recognized institute before they qualify to take part two of the FCPS psychiatry examination. Psychiatry training consists of registering with a tutor approved by a college with an accredited department of psychiatry. Information is not available on the content of the curricula of psychiatric postgraduate training in Pakistan.

3.2.20. Saudi Arabia

Saudi Arabia has inpatient psychiatric treatment available at Shahar Hospital in Taif, and in Jeddah, Riadh, and other large cities.(63) As in much of the Middle East and Africa, Saudi mental health treatment is integrated into primary health care. Specialty training in psychiatry is available, as are national certification and certification through the Arab Board of Psychiatry. Information on psychological training or inclusion of religion-spirituality in psychiatric training was not available to this author.

3.2.21. Syria

The Syrian Arab Republic has two twentieth-century psychiatric hospitals in Damascus and Aleppo. Psychiatric training is conducted by medical schools.(63) No curricular information is available.

3.2.22. United Arab Emirates (UAE)

The UAE boasts a newly built psychiatric hospital in Abu Dhabi. Psychiatric training is offered by the United Arab Emirates University College of Medicine and Health Sciences Department of Psychiatry and Behavioral Sciences, which oversees an eight-week junior medical student psychiatry clerkship, a child psychiatry rotation, psychiatric CME, psychiatric training of primary health care trainees, and a four-year postgraduate psychiatry training in hospitals accredited by the Arab Board of Psychiatry.(68) Psychiatry trainees complete two years of adult and child psychiatry in Al-Ain before rotating for training in subspecialty psychiatry in the Psychiatric Hospital in Abu-Dhabi. Neither the four-year didactic curriculum in psychiatry nor references to religion-spirituality were available to this author.

3.2.23. Palestinian Territories

In 2001, Mohit (63) reported the Palestinian Authority was operating a Ministry of Health,

with a community mental health center and small inpatient unit in Gaza and a 320-bed inpatient unit in the West Bank. At that time, Palestine had psychiatrists, psychologists, social workers, and trained psychiatric nurses. The dire current conditions imposed on Palestine by Israel in their political conflict render it impossible to state whether these facilities are still operating or if psychiatric or medical education is available in the Palestinian territory.

3.2.24. Israel

Founded mostly by European Jewish refugees, Israel is aligned with Western medicine. It is one-sixth Muslim and contains a population of orthodox Jewish patients, for whom religious factors may require treatment modifications.(69) Mental health training in Israel might be expected to include religion-spirituality.

Israel has a system of mental hospitals, outpatient clinics, and community mental health centers operated by the government and private organizations.(70) With one psychiatric bed for every 1,000 people in the population, its services appear advanced compared to its Middle Eastern neighbors. Enosh (71) (Israel's Mental Health Association) provides a wide array of community-based support and advocacy services.

Psychiatry residency training is available from a number of universities. Child psychiatry is the only psychiatry subspecialty recognized by the Israel Medical Association, but other subspecialty training is available. Tel Aviv University operates a two-year postgraduate program in forensic psychiatry,(72) programs in infant psychiatry, child/adolescent psychiatry, and basic and advanced level three-year programs in psychotherapy for psychiatry residents, psychiatrists, psychologists, and social workers.(73) The Department of Psychiatry of Hadassah Hebrew University in Jerusalem offers psychiatric training from its two massive Hadassah University Medical Center hospitals.(74)

Little information is available about religion-spirituality teaching in Israeli mental health training. Blass (75) described a framework for teaching psychiatry residents to assess and treat religious patients, but did not describe efforts that had actually been carried out in that direction. Lev-Ran and Fennig (76) mentioned "the increasing popularity of different spiritual movements" in a list of issues not adequately addressed in contemporary psychiatric residency programs in Israel. Israel appears well-situated in providing mental health care and training, but efforts at including religion-spirituality may be spotty, despite this nation's Jewish-Muslim-Christian mix.

3.3. Training of Medical Students

The WPA curriculum for psychiatry for medical students does not specifically mention religion-spirituality, but strongly emphasizes the worldwide trend toward integration of psychosocial and community issues in medical care. Are medical students being taught the religious and spiritual aspects of psychosocially integrated care?

3.3.1. United States and Canada

Templeton grant support for teaching religion-spirituality in medical schools has spurred curricular development in the United States and Canada.(18) More than 100 U.S. and Canadian medical schools (up from only five schools in the early 1990s) (77) have developed courses (70 percent required) to teach students to do spiritual assessments with patients, to integrate spiritual concerns into therapeutic plans, and to provide guidance on when to refer patients to chaplains.(78)

3.3.2. Australia

In 2003, Peach (50) called for more research to improve the "current superficial knowledge of Australian spirituality" and concluded, "The proportion of physicians who currently enquire into their patients' spirituality is unknown, but is probably small. Spirituality has a place in Australia's medical courses, but perhaps not in practice until more data are available." It appears doubtful that many Australian medical students are trained in religion-spirituality. This author found no data on this topic in Australia.

3.4. Training of Primary Care Physicians in Religion-Spirituality

Primary care physicians (family physicians, general practitioners, pediatricians, and internal medicine specialists) deliver considerable mental health care across the world and 54 percent of mental health care in the United States.(4) Their training at both the medical school and residency levels should include religion-spirituality education. Since 2000, the Templeton-GWISH program has given at least twenty awards to North American primary care residencies for curricula in religion-spirituality.(18) This is a drop in the bucket compared to the number of primary care residencies, but these efforts are a solid start toward educating primary care practitioners. Less is known about religion-spirituality education training of primary care physicians worldwide, but the WPA-WFME advocates such training.(1)

4. WHO SHOULD BE TAUGHT RELIGION-SPIRITUALITY IN MENTAL HEALTH CARE?

My answer to this question is simple: Any clinician who performs clinical mental health evaluations or delivers mental health care needs education in religion-spirituality. Most guidelines are explicit about the need for training of psychiatrists and psychologists in religious-spiritual aspects of clinical care. This author advocates religion-spirituality training for clinical social workers, marriage and family therapists, inpatient psychiatric nurses, inpatient and outpatient mental health counselors, advanced practice psychiatric nurses, emergency mental health workers, and substance abuse treatment workers. Because education on this topic has been scarce, postgraduate clinicians in these disciplines also need education via CME courses.

5. WHAT SHOULD BE TAUGHT?

5.1. Educational Goals

The content of a curriculum depends on its educational goals, which are determined by the target learner population. I offer recommendations from my experience teaching a religion-spirituality course to psychiatry residents and from the *Model Curriculum*.(19) Three broad goals are key for all student clinicians who will provide psychological assessments and psychotherapy: (1) to recognize and distinguish pathological from normal religious and spiritual life; (2) to acquire skills, knowledge, and attitudes enabling them to deal therapeutically with religion-spirituality in mental health care; and (3) to acquire clinical competence in addressing religion/spirituality in actual treatment settings. Although the broad educational goals are identical for all disciplines, tailoring of content is indicated. Education of psychiatry residents should include religious attitudes toward medication and somatic treatments of mental illness, as well as toward psychological therapies. Marriage and family therapy students especially need education about religious group practices and beliefs about marriage, families, and sexuality. In the education of all mental health clinicians, knowledge, but also skills and attitudes, need to be taught.

Undergraduate course work in psychology, social work, and counseling also should require education about religion-spirituality. The goals for undergraduates should be: (1) raising awareness of the central role of religion and spirituality in human life and society (sociology of religion-spirituality); (2) communicating respect and basic knowledge about diverse religious traditions and spiritual practices (world religions); and (3) teaching evidence-based interrelationships between psychology and religion-spirituality (psychology of religion).

5.2. Curricular Content

"If there is one law of curricular development, it is that the material always exceeds the allotted curricular time" (5) (p. 369). The amount of training time given to religion-spirituality in a residency curriculum is likely to be small, so prioritizing content is critically important. Content priorities should be guided by the overall goal of assisting trainees in recognizing normal and pathological religious and spiritual life and assisting them in developing ethical and sensitive assessments and responses. I recommend setting priorities and teaching in order of decreasing importance.

Several approaches to teaching this topic have been published. Israeli psychiatrist Blass (75), advocates a pragmatic teaching framework. He holds it is more effective to focus on teaching knowledge of phenomenology and information-gathering skills rather than broad knowledge of many religions. For instance, he suggests teaching trainees the components that define a delusion and the skills to seek collateral information from local informants (family, clergy, and other believers) on normative religious beliefs. Blass's approach to education would not include didactics on the content of major faith groups.

Canadians Grabovac and Ganeson (30) advocate teaching basics of major world religions and indigenous religion in their proposed eleven-session academic curriculum for Canadian psychiatry residents. Their recommendations for teaching on indigenous religion could be adapted to African, South American, or Middle Eastern settings, but their curriculum, like the *Model Curriculum* (19) is best suited to Europe and North America.

Puchalski and Romer (79) suggest a simple formula of content that fits into a single session of education and applies to medical students and primary care health professionals: FICA. This is a four-question assessment of *Faith*, its *Importance*, whether the person has a religious-spiritual *Community*, and how the person wants the provider to *Address* these issues as part of health care. Sample questions of the FICA model are available at http://www.gwish.org. This approach can be adapted for single or in-service CME presentations or brief education for nurses and primary care residents. Psychiatrists and psychologists can use FICA, but need more religion-spirituality training.

This author recommends dividing content for clinical care students into three categories of decreasing priority: essential, important, and helpful.(5) The content of these categories differs from the core modules of the *Model Curriculum*. First, teach essential information, then important information if time permits, and finally provide helpful information in longer undergraduate pre-clinical courses. New instructors don't have to re-invent the wheel to teach this topic: The 105-page *Model Curriculum* is available for teaching psychiatry residents, psychologists, or social workers and would require only an updated literature search for new mental health-religion research data. The *Model Curriculum* is too long to be taught in most residency curricula, but contains three core modules that would fit into most postgraduate clinical didactic programs and has optional modules (for example, trauma, gender issues, and substance abuse) for other settings.

5.2.1. Essential Content

The goals of essential material are to help trainees gain enough skills and comfort to take religious-spiritual histories from their patients and to mold attitudes with scientific data on religion-spirituality. This author recommends dividing this essential content into two sections: (1) general information on data on religion-spirituality in health, and (2) gathering and interpreting a religious/spiritual history. Address knowledge by teaching general information that includes definitions of religion, spirituality, religious demographics in the surrounding general population, and the gap in interest between mental health practitioners and the population (outlined in reference 20). Address attitudes and counter preconceived beliefs by including basic research data on the relationship of religion-spirituality to physical and mental health. Teach essential skills by presenting a live or recorded religious-spiritual history with a patient. Essential self-knowledge can be gained by asking students to interview

each other or present their personal religious history to a small student group. Appendix A of the *Model Curriculum* contains sample history questions; Appendix B contains criteria for evaluating a religious biography.(19)

5.2.2. Important Content

This author recommends three topics as high priority after essential material has been covered. The most important is examination of psychodynamics by which religion and spirituality operate to enable students to interpret clinical data. Trainees should learn the characteristics of psychotic, neurotic, and healthy expression of individual religion-spirituality and the dynamics of religious group processes. Important material includes ethical standards in addressing religion-spirituality in treatment and case examples of therapeutic responses to religious-spiritual issues. Adult learners respond best to practical educational approaches, so this author advises using case examples of healthy and pathological uses of religion.(80, 81)

5.2.3. Helpful Content

Here we arrive at the luxury section for curricula blessed with ample teaching time. This author recommends three topics. Most important is further differential diagnosis of religious-spiritual material and psychodynamics, best taught via case discussion augmented with didactic instruction. Inpatient, psychiatric emergency workers, and primary care students will encounter religious material in psychosis, mania, severe depression, substance abuse, and organic brain illness. Psychiatrists, psychologists, and therapists conducting outpatient psychotherapy will encounter those topics and neurotic and personality disorder manifestations of religion-spirituality. Clinical trainees are notoriously content-bound, so this author highly recommends teaching simultaneous attention to religious-spiritual content and process in small groups and individual supervision.

Second, this author recommends teaching religious-spiritual development across the life cycle, perhaps as part of a development course (19) (Module 3). This author has taught this material by asking students to place themselves in Fowler's (82) stages of religious development after presenting their own religious-spiritual histories. Development of conscience can be taught in child psychiatry or psychology fellowships.(83, 84)

Third, for longer courses or curricula taught across years of clinical training, the eight accessory modules of the *Model Curriculum* provide assistance.(19) Content (abuse issues, women's issues, sects/cults, consultation-liaison, substance abuse, and dynamics of God/Deity images) should be tailored to specific needs of training programs and trainee levels. Many of these topics will be optional and can be addressed in individual supervision or in single sessions in other training courses.

The amount of material available to teach trainees need not be overwhelming if priorities are set and education is offered at multiple training levels and in different learning formats. We now turn to these topics.

6. WHEN SHOULD RELIGION-SPIRITUALITY BE TAUGHT?

Teaching is like an effective interpretation in psychotherapy: it is helpful only when the content and timing are both correct (p. 374).(5) Thus, religion-spirituality should be taught when trainees are ready and able to use such learning. Content of education is linked to educational timing. Trainees need antecedent clinical knowledge or experience to render a topic practical and relevant.

For psychiatry residents and psychology interns, no single "correct" approach exists; residencies have successfully taught this material in "single dose" (one course) and "multiple dose" (graded exposure) formats. Because residents and interns are doing clinical care, content should be tailored to their current clinical level and type of patient. The ideal is to teach psychiatry residents across all years of training. In a single year of psychology internship, a single short course will likely be more realistic.

For four-year psychiatry residencies, this author recommends the following: in the first year, teach definitions of religion-spirituality, basic data on religion and mental health, and molding positive attitudes. For the second year, educate students in history-taking skills, personal religious-spiritual histories, and differential diagnosis of healthy and unhealthy religion-spirituality. In the third year, residents are ready for a higher level of psychodynamic understanding of religious-spiritual life and groups, along with some special topics such as trauma or substance abuse. In the fourth year, teach finer techniques of addressing this topic in psychotherapy and additional special topics as listed above. In undergraduate curricula, religion-spirituality will likely be covered in upper-level university classes or in medical student clerkship didactics. The author suggests trying different teaching strategies to determine the best approach to specific programs and students.

In summary, adapt content to the available time and students' needs. If one session is available, consider demonstrating the FICA approach to assessment (79) and discussing assigned reading on data about religion and spirituality in mental health. If four to ten teaching contacts are available, consider using the core modules of the *Model Curriculum* (19) or selected topics from Grabovac & Ganesan's (30) curriculum. For longer courses, consider use of the *Model Curriculum* supplemented by chapters from recent books, including this volume.

7. HOW RELIGION-SPIRITUALITY CAN BE TAUGHT: TEACHING FORMATS

Educational formats, like timing, depend on the training program and student population. Baccalaureate, master, and doctoral level preclinical training programs for psychotherapists will need a different format than medical/psychiatric residencies and psychology internships. Formats are discussed in detail elsewhere.(5) The most common format is didactic courses or seminars, but such time is often severely limited in postgraduate clinical training. Other brief teaching formats can include offering intermittent in-service training to nurses and inpatient personnel (usually best if case-based), ongoing case conferences, departmental Grand Rounds, film clubs or journal club discussions, or CME formats. In training programs, brief formats have the disadvantage of nonsystematic education but the advantage of high clinical relevance. Adult students need practical applications for learning, so case material is essential in lecture formats. Clinical supervision of psychotherapy is ideal for teaching skills and attitudes toward religion-spirituality, but faculty members with such interest and expertise may not be available. Teaching skills can be addressed in faculty development or provision of consultation to supervisors. Trainees learn best by doing, second best by observing, and least from listening to lectures.

In teaching a religion-spirituality course to psychiatry residents, it is valuable to include chaplains or chaplain students as co-learners. This author's experience has been that exposure to clergy desensitizes residents to anxiety about interacting with clergy, increases their respect for chaplains, and has led to more patient consultation requests from residents to chaplains. Chaplains offer clinical viewpoints that enrich courses, and they themselves benefit from increased psychiatric knowledge. This author's residents gave high ratings to inclusion of chaplains in their religion-spirituality course. Chaplains and community clergy can serve as guest presenters or discussants in trainee education, especially in sessions on the clergy's religion.

Formats for post-training education can include CME lectures, CME courses that include literature and case discussions, or ongoing case discussion/peer supervision groups to develop collegial support. These groups can develop the skills of colleagues who could eventually become a team of faculty for trainee courses.

7.1. Post-Learning Evaluation of Educational Effectiveness

Evaluation of educational offerings is helpful to answer the question of whether teaching religion-spirituality to trainees is effective in improving patient care. Evaluation also provides essential feedback to help faculty improve teaching skills and understand how to modify curricula. A sample evaluation form is available in the *Model Curriculum* for adaptation.(19)

8. WHO CAN TEACH RELIGION-SPIRITUALITY TO TRAINEES?

This topic can be taught by anyone with a passion for providing this education, with good clinical skills, experience with religious patients, a willingness to invest time in choosing and teaching a curriculum or single session, and a willingness to bring an even-handed nonsectarian approach to education. One need not be a published expert, an accomplished teacher, or researcher to teach religion-spirituality effectively. Moses succeeded in freeing the Israelite from Egypt despite his protestations of being a puny public speaker (Exod. 6:12, 30).(85) All teachers have to begin their development somewhere. This author began as an inexperienced junior faculty member teaching a short course for residents.

If you are interested in teaching this topic, don't let self-doubt stop you. You don't have to teach alone. Moses and Aaron teamed up with God to teach Pharaoh (Exod. 5–14).(86) Psychiatrists can gather a multidisciplinary team of clergy, psychologists, nurses, or other clinicians to develop and teach this topic. An interfaith group of teachers is ideal to avoid sectarian bias in education and maximize acceptance of an educational proposal. Use the array of resources now available in your area, including the *Model Curriculum*,(19) recent books,(46, 87, 88) and assessment instruments.(89) Resources are available to teach religion-spirituality in programs oriented toward psychoanalysis,(90–92) cognitive-behavioral treatments,(93) and psychobiology.(93) Programs and faculty in resource-poor situations can use the Internet for educational resources available from GWISH,(18) the Templeton Foundation,(37) and the WPA.(22)

9. DEALING WITH LIMITATIONS AND RESISTANCE TO CURRICULAR INTEGRATION

Faculty or clinicians who attempt to teach mental health clinicians about religion-spirituality will inevitably run into some resistance from students, faculty, program directors, or entire institutions. Most resistance is due to ignorance or countertransference issues. Ignorance can be countered with persistent education about the universality of religious-spiritual concerns in patients. Countertransference resistances in students and administrators alike generally fall into the categories of personal discomfort with this topic or unresolved religious-spiritual conflicts. Passive trainee resistance of "forgetting" to assess religion can be dealt with directly in individual supervision. Discussion of countertransference to this topic should also be part of individual supervision. Overt skepticism about religion-spirituality teaching by administrators can be countered with provision of data on religion-spirituality and mental health and by gently expressing wonderment that any scientist would be unwilling to look at data on any clinical topic. This author suggests maintaining an explicitly scientific approach to resistance to inclusion of religion-spirituality in curricula. Resistance to education on religion-spirituality must be addressed if educational efforts are to occur or be effective.

Be persistent in confronting resistance. Remember, Moses and Aaron did not succeed the first three times they asked Pharaoh to free the Israelite slaves (Exod. 5–14).(86) Several approaches may be necessary to get religion-spirituality into trainee or undergraduate curricula.(5, page 377).

ACKNOWLEDGMENT

The author thanks author and editor Letha Dawson Scanzoni for invaluable assistance with Internet research.

REFERENCES

1. World Psychiatric Association and World Federation for Medical Education (WPA-WFME). *Core Curriculum in Psychiatry for Medical Students.* Geneva: WPA; 1993–1999.
2. Larson DB, Hohmann AA, Kessler LG, Meador KG, Boyd JH, McSherry E. The couch and the cloth: the need for linkage. *Hosp Community Psychiatry.* 1988;39(10):1064–1068.
3. Beitman BD. Pastoral counseling centers: a challenge to community mental health centers. *Hosp Community Psychiatry.* 1982;33:486.
4. Regier DA, Goldberg JD, Taube CA. The de facto U.S. mental health services system: a public health perspective. *Arch Gen Psychiatry.* 1978;35:685–693.
5. Bowman ES. Integrating religion into the education of mental health professionals. In: Koenig HG, ed. *Handbook of Religion and Mental Health.* San Diego: Academic Press;1988:367–378.
6. Kroll J, Sheehan W. Religious beliefs and practices among 152 psychiatric inpatients in Minnesota. *Am J Psychiatry.* 1994;146:67–72.
7. Pargament, KI. *The Psychology of Religion and Coping.* New York: Guilford; 1997.
8. King DE, Bushwick B. Beliefs and attitudes of hospital inpatients about faith healing and prayer. *J Fam Pract.* 1994;39(4):349–352.
9. Koenig, HG, Cohen HJ, Blazer DG, et al. Religious coping and depression among elderly hospitalized medically ill men. *Am J Psychiatry.* 1992;149:1693–1700.
10. Accreditation Council for Graduate Medical Education (ACGME). *Special Requirements for Residency Training in Psychiatry.* Chicago: Accreditation Council for Graduate Medical Education; 1994:11–12, 18. http://www.acgme.org/. Accessed May 23, 2008.
11. Royal College of Physicians and Surgeons of Canada (RCPSC). *Specialty Training Requirements in Psychiatry.* Ottawa, ON: Royal College of Physicians of Canada; 2007a. http://rcpsc.medical.org/information/index.php?specialty=165&submit=Select. Accessed May 20, 2008.
12. Royal College of Physicians (RCP). *A Competency-Based Curriculum for Specialist Training in Psychiatry. Specialist Module in Adult Psychiatry.* London: Royal College of Psychiatrists; 2006.
13. American Psychological Association. *Guidelines and Principles for Accreditation of Programs in Professional Psychology.* Washington, DC: American Psychological Association; 2000.
14. American Psychiatric Association (APA). *Task Force Report No. 10: Psychiatrist's (sic) Viewpoints on Religion and Their Services to Religious Institutions and the Ministry.* Washington, DC: APA Press; 1975.
15. American Psychiatric Association (APA). Guidelines regarding possible conflict between psychiatrists' religious commitments and psychiatric practice. *Am J Psychiatry.* 1990;147:542.
16. American Psychiatric Association (APA). *The Principles of Medical Ethics With Annotations Especially Applicable to Psychiatry.* Arlington, VA:

APA; 2001. http://www.psych.org/MainMenu/PsychiatricPractice/Ethics/ResourcesStandards.aspx. Accessed May 31, 2008.

17. American Psychological Association. *Ethical Principles of Psychologists and Code of Conduct.* Washington, DC: APA, section 2.01b; 2002. http://www.apa.org/ethics/code2002.html#2_01. Accessed June 2, 2008.

18. George Washington Institute for Spirituality and Health (GWISH) (2008). *Curricular Awards to Medical Schools, Primary Care Residencies and Psychiatry Residencies.* http://www.gwish.org/. Accessed December 11, 2008.

19. Larson DB, Lu FG, Swyers JP, eds. *Model Curriculum for Psychiatry Residency Training Programs: Religion and Spirituality in Clinical Practice. A Course Outline.* Rockville, MD: National Institute for Healthcare Research; 1996, revised 1997. This curriculum is no longer in print. Locations of library copies may be found at http://www.worldcat.org/oclc/40562405&referer=brief_results. AccessedDecember 11, 2008.

20. Gartner J, Larson D, Allen G. Religious commitment and mental health: a review of the empirical literature. *J Psychol Theol.* 1991;19:6–25.

21. Koenig HG. Research on religion and mental health in later life: a review and commentary. *J Geriatr Psychiatry.* 1990;23:23–53.

22. World Psychiatric Association (WPA). 2008. http://www.wpanet.org/. Accessed June 1, 2008.

23. World Federation for Medical Education (WFME). The Edinburgh declaration. *Lancet.* 1988;ii:464.

24. World Federation for Medical Education (WFME). Proceedings, of the World summit on medical education. *Med Edu.* 1994;28:Suppl.1.

25. World Federation for Medical Education (WFME). Proceedings of the Eastern Mediterranean Regional Conference on Medical Education. *Med Edu.* 1995;29:Suppl.1.

26. World Psychiatric Association and World Federation for Medical Education (WPA-WFME). *Core Curriculum for Postgraduate Training in Psychiatry.* Geneva: WPA; 2002. http://www.worldpsychiatricassociation.org/education/core-curric-psych-stu.shtml. Accessed December 11, 2008.

27. American Psychiatric Association (APA). *Diagnostic and Statistical Manual of Mental Disorders,* 4th ed. Washington, DC: American Psychiatric Association; 1994: 685.

28. Royal College of Physicians and Surgeons of Canada (RCPSC). *Specific Standards of Accreditation for Residency Programs in Psychiatry.* Ottawa, ON: Royal College of Physicians and Surgeons of Canada; 2007b. http://www.rcpsc.medical.org/information/index.php?specialty=165&submit=Select. Accessed May 19, 2008.

29. Nemeth M, Underwood N, Howse J. Special report: The religion poll – God is alive. *MacLean's.* 2003:32–37.

30. Baetz M, Larson D, Marcoux G, Bowen R, Griffin R. Canadian psychiatric inpatient religious commitment: an association with mental health. *Can J Psychiatry.* 2002;47(2):159–166.

31. van Zyl LT, Davidson PR. Canadian psychiatry residency training programs: a glance at the management structure. *Can J Psychiatry.* 2006;51:377–381.

32. Grabovac AD, Ganesan S. Spirituality and religion in Canadian psychiatric residency training. *Can J Psychiatry.* 2003;48:171–175.

33. Sansone RA, Khatain K, Rodenhauser P. The role of religion in psychiatric education: a national survey. *Acad Med.* 1990;14:37–41.

34. Waldfogel S, Wolpe PR, Shmuley Y. Religious training and religiosity in psychiatry residency programs. *Acad Psychiatry.* 1998;22:29–35.

35. Bergin AE, Jensen JP. Religiosity of psychotherapists: a national survey. *Psychotherapy.* 1990;27(1):3–7.

36. Princeton Religious Research Center. *Religion in America 1993-1994.* Princeton, NJ: Princeton Religious Research Center; 1993.

37. Templeton Foundation. 2008. http://www.templeton.org/. Accessed June 7, 2008.

38. Accreditation Council for Graduate Medical Education (ACGME) 2008. For listing of accredited psychiatry residencies: http://www.acgme.org/. Accessed June 2, 2008.

39. Gallup, G. *Religion in America: 1990.* Princeton, NJ: Princeton Religion and Research Center; 1990.

40. Gallup Poll Church/Synagogue Membership. In: *Gallup Poll Monthly.* Princeton, NJ: Gallup Organization; 1991:57–58.

41. Gallup G. *Religion in America. Report No. 236.* Princeton, NJ: The Gallup Report; 1985.

42. Bergin AE. Religiosity and mental health: A critical revaluation and meta-analysis. *Prof Psychol Res Pract.* 1983;14:170–184.

43. Shafranske EJ, Maloney HN. Clinical psychologists' religious and spiritual orientation and their practice of psychotherapy. *Psychotherapy.* 1990;27:72–78.

44. Lannert, JL. Resistance and countertransference issues with spiritual and religious clients. *J Humanistic Psychol.* 1991;31:68–76.

45. Brawer PA, Handal PJ, Fabricatore AN, Roberts R, Wajda-Johnston VA. Training and education in religion/spirituality within APA-accredited clinical psychology programs. *Prof Psychol Res Pract.* 2002;33(2):203–206.

46. Shafranske EJ. *Religion and the Clinical Practice of Psychology.* Washington, DC: American Psychological Association; 1996.

47. Richards PS, Bergin AE. *Handbook of Psychotherapy and Religious Diversity.* Washington, DC: American Psychological Association; 1999.

48. Neeleman J, King MB. Psychiatrists' religious attitudes in relation to their clinical practice: a survey of 231 psychiatrists. *Acta Psychiatr Scand.* 1993;88:420–424.

49. Office of Population Censuses and Surveys. *National Opinion Poll UK Survey*. London: HMSO; 1985.

50. Peach HG. Religion, spirituality and health: how should Australia's medical professionals respond? *Med J Aust*. 2003;178(2):86–88.

51. Proceedings of the 1st Australian Conference on Spirituality and Health, Adelaide, 2005, July 28–29; *Med J Aust*. 2007;186(10):S41-S76.

52. Passmore, N. Religious issues in counselling: are Australian Psychologists "Dragging the Chain"? *Aust Psychol*. 2003;38(3):183–192.

53. Njenga, F. Focus on psychiatry in East Africa. *Br J Psychiatry*. 2002;181:354–359.

54. Uganda Ministry of Health. 2000. http://74.125.47.132/search?q=cache:2KDxSwR-wTFsJ:www.health.go.ug/rc/modules/smartsec-tion/item.php%3Fitemid%3D3+Butabika+Hospital+complex&hl=en&ct=clnk&cd=2&gl=us. Accessed December 11, 2008.

55. Muhimbili University of Health and Allied Sciences (MUHAS). 2008. www.muhas.ac.tz/. Accessed June 7, 2008.

56. Nairobi University School of Medicine (NUSOM), Department of Psychiatry. 2008. http://www.uonbi.ac.ke/departments/index.php?dept_code=JL&fac_code=61. Accessed December 11, 2008.

57. Ndetei DM, Lhasakhala L, Maru H, et al. Clinical epidemiology in patients admitted at Mathari psychiatric hospital, Nairobi, Kenya. 2008. *Social Psychiatry and Psychiatric Epidemiology* (5/9/08). http://www.springerlink.com/index/046p314616387n03.pdf. Accessed May 29, 2008.

58. British Broadcasting Company (BBC). Kenya's Mix and Match Mental Health Policy. 2003. http://news.bbc.co.uk/2/hi/africa/2998060.stm. Accessed May 26, 2008.

59. Moi University School of Medicine, Eldoret, Kenya. 2006. http://www.chs.mu.ac.ke/. Accessed May 27, 2008.

60. Emsley, R. Focus on psychiatry in South Africa. *Br J Psychiatry*. 2001;178:382–386.

61. Flisher AJ, Riccitelli G, Jhetam N, et al. A survey of professional activities of psychiatrists in South Africa. *Psychiatric Serv*. 1997;48:707–709.

62. Herzig H. Teaching psychiatry in poor countries: a description of how mental health is taught to medical students in Malawi, Central Africa. *Edu Health Change Learn Pract*. 2003;16(1):32–39.

63. Mohit, A. Mental health and psychiatry in the Middle East: historical development. *East Mediterr Health J*. 2001;7(3):336–347.

64. Muslim Mental Health Association (MMHA). 2008. http://www.muslimmentalhealth.com/. Accessed December 11, 2008.

65. World Islamic Association for Mental Health (WIAMH). 2008. http://www.geocities.com/wiamh2001/intro.html. Accessed June 6, 2008.

66. Sadek A. The Arabian identity of psychiatry. Paper presented at the Pan Arab Congress of Psychiatry, Manama, Bahrain, 9–11 February, 1999.

67. Naeem F, Ayub M. Psychiatric training in Pakistan. *Med Educ Online* [serial online]. 2004;9:19. http://www.med-ed-online.org/f0000092.htm. Accessed June 4, 2008.

68. El Rufaie O. UAE\ Universities & Technology Institutes\United Arab Emirates University\ College of Medicine and Health Sciences\ Department of Psychiatry and Behavioural Sciences. 2002. www.arabdecision.org/show_func_3_12_22_1_6_4160.htm. Accessed June 4, 2008.

69. Trappler B, Greenberg S, Friedman S. Treatment of Hassidic Jewish patients in a general hospital medical-psychiatric unit. *Psychiatric Serv*. 1995;46(8):833–835.

70. Israel Ministry of Health. 1999. http://www.mfa.gov.il/MFA/MFAArchive/1990_1999/1999/10/Ministry+of+Health.htm?DisplayMode=print. Accessed December 11, 2008.

71. Enosh (Israel Mental Health Association). 2008. http://members.tripod.com/Goldin_Yarik/about_amuta_e.htm. Accessed June 8, 2008.

72. Barak, P. Forensic psychiatry in Israel. *Psychiatr Bull*. 2002;26:143–145.

73. Tel Aviv University. *Sackler Faculty of Medicine*. Tel Aviv, Israel. 2008. http://med.tau.ac.il/cme/english.asp. Accessed June 4, 2008.

74. Hadassah University Medical Center. Jerusalem: Hadassah Hebrew University. 2008. http://www.hadassah.org.il/. Accessed May 31, 2008.

75. Blass DM. A pragmatic approach to teaching psychiatry residents the assessment and treatment of religious patients. *Acad Psychiatry*. 2007;31:25–31.

76. Lev-Ran S, Fennig S. Points to ponder regarding contemporary psychiatric training in Israel. *Israeli J Psychiatry Related Sci*. 2007;44(3):187–193.

77. Puchalski CM. Spirituality and medicine: curricula in medical education. *J Cancer Edu*. 2006;21(1):14–18; also, see *John Templeton Foundation Capabilities Report*. West Conshohocken, PA: Templeton Foundation; 2006:68.

78. Puchalski CM, Larson DP, Lu FG. Spirituality in psychiatry residency training programs. *Int Rev Psychiatry*. 2001;13:131–138.

79. Puchalski CM, Romer AL. Taking a spiritual history allows clinicians to understand patients more fully. *J Palliat Med*. 2000;3:129–137.

80. Battista JR. Offensive spirituality and spiritual defenses. In: Scotton BW, Chinen AB, Battista JR, eds. *Textbook of Transpersonal Psychiatry and Psychology*. New York: Basic Books, 1996: 250–260.

81. Meissner W. The phenomenology of religious psychopathology. *Bull Menninger Clinic*. 1991;55:281–298.

82. Fowler JW. *Stages of Faith*. San Francisco: Harper & Row; 1981.

83. Stillwell BA, Galvin M, Kopta SM, Padgett RJ. Moralization of attachment, a fourth domain of conscience functioning. *J Am Academy Child Adolescent Psychiatry*. 1997;36:1140–1147.

84. Gilligan C. *In a Different Voice*. Cambridge, MA: Harvard University Press; 1982.

85. American Bible Society. *In the Holy Bible*. New York: American Bible Society; 1995:70–71.

86. American Bible Society. In Hioly Bible. New york: American Bible Society; 1995: 68–81.

87. Miller WR. *Integrating Spirituality into Treatment. Resources for Practitioners*. Washington: American Psychological Association; 1999.

88. Koenig, HD. *Handbook of Religion and Mental Health*. San Diego: Academic Press; 1998.

89. Hill PC, Hood RW, eds. *Measures of Religiosity*. Birmingham, AL: Religious Education Press; 1999.

90. Meissner WW. *Psychoanalysis and Religious Experience*. New Haven, CT: Yale University Press; 1984.

91. Black DM, ed. *Psychoanalysis and Religion in the 21st Century*. New York: Routledge; 2006.

92. Jones JW, ed. *Contemporary Psychoanalysis and Religion*. New Haven, CT: Yale; 1991.

93. Finn M, Gartner J, eds. *Object Relations Theory and Religion*. Westport, CO: Praeger; 1992.

94. Newberg A, D'Aquili E, Rause V. *Why God Won't Go Away*. New York: Ballantine; 2001.

23 Conclusion: Summary of What Clinicians Need to Know

PHILIPPE HUGUELET AND HAROLD G. KOENIG

In editing this book, our desire was to provide clinicians with knowledge about religion and mental health that would be useful in the treatment of patients with psychiatric disorders. In addition, we thought that clinicians would also find useful information on more theoretical issues such as history, neurobiology, and theology as they relate to psychiatry.

1. OVERVIEW

A growing scientific literature based on religion and psychiatry has allowed rapid progress in the integration of religion into psychiatry. Despite this progress, the integration of relevant religious issues into clinical practice will likely meet resistance for many years to come. There is some question, however, about whether concepts such as well-being, meaning, or even recovery belong exclusively to the domain of conventional psychiatry.(1) In their description of the complex interactions between religion and psychiatry, Palouzian and Park (2) define a multilevel interdisciplinary paradigm, which, as mentioned in the introduction, should accommodate many dimensions of psychology and psychiatry, but also other domains like evolutionary biology, neurosciences, anthropology, philosophy, and other allied areas of science. A thorough discussion of these conceptual issues is far beyond the scope of the present book. However, this complexity and multidisciplinarity may be viewed as richness, which is reflected in the diversity of perspectives presented in this book.

Thus, we hope that, despite a certain level of subjectivity, the diversity of approaches expressed here has at least exposed readers to the multidisciplinary nature of this interaction between religion and mental health care. In the case of the treatments described, we do not endorse all approaches presented here. However, clinicians should know that these approaches exist so that they can refer patients for the appropriate treatment when necessary or be able to answer patients when they ask for advice about participating in such treatments.

Of course, because we are psychiatrists, we have put more emphasis on psychiatric issues (rather that anthropological, theological, or historical ones). This book has been written primarily for psychiatrists who want to know more about religion and how to integrate it into clinical practice. Other mental health professionals who interact with psychiatrists and treat those with mental illness, such as psychologists, counselors, sociologists, chaplains, or other members of the clergy, may also benefit from this book. We hope that it has been written in a way that will be useful to professionals from a variety of backgrounds. The goal is to help build bridges between all of that it will enhance the care of patients, who are unique in their humanness, suffering, and worldview.

With this in mind, let's recall and highlight the main points that readers should take away from each of the chapters in this book.

2. HISTORICAL CONSIDERATIONS

The first part of the book aims to provide knowledge about history, theology, and neurobiology. The chapter on historical considerations examines the relationships between insanity and religion, medicine and theology, treatment and ritual. Focusing primarily on care provided in Christian environments in Europe and North America, the author describes the way psychiatric illness is featured in the Bible and then reviews the worldview and healing practices of the ancient Greeks. Early church authors (for example, John Chrysostom) generally had a view of madness that incorporated a spiritual perspective, while also acknowledging the physical influences. Religious approaches to mental illness in the Middle Ages are detailed through a description of the Leechbook of Bald. This book distinguishes between demon possession and lunacy. The physician is encouraged to treat the demon-possessed, as well as lunatics, with herbal concoctions. During the Renaissance, those dealing with the mentally ill moved further away from solely relying on supernatural explanations. Reginald Scott in England, for example, explained that people who are sad or distressed suffer from a natural malady and not from supernatural influences. A more secular medical approach to mental illness developed later during the Enlightenment (eighteenth century). Those dealing with the mentally ill began separating religious causes from other causes. (For example, see Robert Burton's *Anatomy of Melancholy*, 1621.)(3) The nineteenth century was marked by the creation of asylums. Sometimes these reforms were driven by a religious motive – as in England at the York Retreat. In other cases, they were prompted by a rationalist/secular reform motive as in the case of Philippe Pinel and his reforms in France at the Salpetrière. Sometimes the reasons for humane reforms were a mixture of religious and secular motivation, as at the South Carolina Lunatic Asylum in Columbia, South Carolina. During the latter part of the nineteenth century, psychiatry in Europe and the United States began to lean toward a view of mental illness that was more rationalistic and focused on heredity and biology. The most important influence of the twentieth century was the work of Sigmund Freud (1856–1939), who viewed religion as a shared delusion, helpful for some, harmful for others, but ultimately something that was an indicator of psychological immaturity.

3. THEOLOGY

The chapter on theological considerations gives insight as to how a theologian may consider mental illness and the clinicians treating it. This provides clinicians with an idea of how mental illness might be understood by members of the clergy. According to the author, reductionism should be avoided and the religious backgrounds of patients considered in assessment and treatment. Religion should not be considered only for its therapeutic possibilities. An informed theological perspective on a patient's beliefs and dispositions may help the clinician better understand how such beliefs and dispositions relate to a particular patient's mental illness. Those beliefs and dispositions may follow "naturally" from the patient's religious commitments, or they may have become distorted and intertwined with their psychiatric pathology. One should not forget, however, that active mental illness of various kinds is not incompatible with orthodox religious belief. The author emphasizes that clinicians should address religion in its particularity, such as Judaism, Christianity, or Islam, rather than religion in general, even if many religious systems share some resemblances. The author describes two challenges facing clinicians confronted with Christianity. The first concerns the connotation that some religious patients have concerning the category "mental" illness. Indeed, clinicians may have to contend with religious patients who are suspicious of and even hostile toward the idea of modern psychiatry. Concepts understood in modern psychiatry such as the distinction between the spiritual and the physical, the body and the soul, or the natural and the supernatural, are, from the perspective of scripture, deeply problematic and useful only in a limited sense. The second challenge is the question of why suffering afflicts good and faithful people. In philosophy, this corresponds to the problem of theodicy (from the Greek *theos*, "god," and *dikē*, "justice"), which is typically posed in the form of a question: "Why does a benevolent, all-powerful God allow the innocent to suffer?" From the perspective of scripture, "why" questions about sickness and suffering are almost always the wrong place to begin. God is fundamentally supposed to be non-coercive with respect to the human will; God entices us by attraction rather than by pushing us from behind. The human capacity to choose God's will naturally implies the freedom to choose against God's will as well. Christian tradition calls the act of choosing against God's will *sin* and suggests that it is sin that is the cause of various forms of suffering. Thus, suffering is one of the most obvious effects of sin, not in the sense that God punishes sinners by making them suffer, but in the sense that sin is in a variety of ways its own punishment. In other words, the natural consequences of sin result in suffering and pain, not in the full and flourishing life that God intended.

4. THE BIBLE

The Bible is composed of many individual books written by men whom Jews and Christians believe were divinely inspired. Judaism and Christianity are Bible-based religions and neither could have survived by oral tradition alone. The Bible is the most globally influential and widely read book ever written. Thus, being such a vast and complicated book, it is important to provide clinicians with insight into these writings that are likely to influence their patients.

Many religions (including those based on the Bible) may use sin and guilt as methods that influence their members' behavior, as well as the way that symptoms of psychiatric illness are expressed.

The Judeo-Christian tradition has been a significant force in defining the "natural" role of Western women. Unfortunately, the Bible was written and edited over the course of more than a thousand years in a largely male-dominated society so that no consistent feminine "model" emerges (except figures such as Debra and Ruth in the Old Testament, and Mary in the New Testament). Overall, women in the Old Testament were valued primarily as mothers, as was typical in Middle Eastern society in the second millennium BC. Some negative portrayals of women, described as a man's possession whose role was to be silent or described as the seductive

and manipulative person are found throughout the "wisdom" literature of the Hebrews. Such scriptures have been used by men to rationalize abusive behavior, even in Western countries.

This chapter also discusses homosexuality, an issue that divides societies and families. The Book of Levitical Laws, as well as other scriptures, condemns homosexual behavior. Christians are not obligated to follow these laws, yet many continue to condemn homosexuality (based on the writings of the Apostle Paul), even though most psychiatrists no longer consider it to be a mental disorder.

The history of Christian religious healing is reviewed and demonstrates that sick individuals who participate in religious rituals may feel better psychologically and physically, at least temporarily. However, some self-serving Christian healers can also be viewed as charlatans. Due to its complexity, the Bible can often be interpreted to suit many purposes by those who wish to justify their actions or manipulate the actions of others for personal gain. Nevertheless, the mentally ill often read the Bible to reaffirm their faith in a God who personally cares for them and is always present for them. In their reading, they may discover a passage that relates to their experiences and has special meaning to them that helps them to continue living and enables them to function.

5. NEUROPSYCHIATRY

Emotions, thoughts, and behaviors have their origin in the brain. Besides questions about the relationship of the soul to the brain, it is important to know what neuroscientists have discovered about religion.

For example, brain-imaging studies have shown that regions of the brain associated with mystical and spiritual experiences are located in the frontal and temporal lobes. However, such research is not always consistent, and reports may differ depending on the particular research group reporting.

Neurotransmitters are chemicals that relay messages between the neurons in the brain across a gap called a synapse. Some benefits of praying and meditation on psychiatric disorders could be explained by a modulation of the neurotransmitter serotonin (5-HT). The involvement of the 5-HT system in spiritual experiences is supported by observations that drugs known to perturb the 5-HT system (LSD, psilocybin) can induce spiritual-like experiences. Given its importance in many personality traits, emotions such as anger, depression, and psychotic illness, the neurotransmitter dopamine has also been investigated as playing a role in spiritual experience. Of note, dopaminergic neurons are also under the control of the 5-HT system. Research has shown an activation of the dopaminergic receptors in the striatum during meditation, indicating an increased level of dopamine in this region during such religious activity. Some studies also show increased activity in GABA (the main inhibitory neurotransmitter in the brain) during meditation. This possibly reflects increased GABA activity in the brain linked to the deafferentation observed during meditation practice. From a genetic perspective, there is some evidence that human psychological traits, and possibly the capacity to have spiritual experiences, are stable over time and influenced by genetic factors. Not surprisingly, researchers have focused their analyses on genes and genetic polymorphisms mainly related to 5-HT and dopaminergic systems. Some researchers have postulated that religious beliefs could be genetically driven and, rightly or wrongly, have considered spirituality as a component of personality. For example, self-transcendence encompasses several aspects of religious behavior, subjective experience, and the way an individual perceives the world. There is evidence that the capacity of the person to experience self-transcendence may partly depend on genetic influences.

Recently, research has been focusing on gene-environment interactions is, or GxE, as part of a new comprehensive model of psychiatric disorders. GxE typically occurs when the effects of one environmental factor on the individual is dependant on his or her genotype. Spirituality and religiousness are examples of complex traits that could be understood in this way. Environmental factors, including hormone levels (as a reflection of gender), diet, drugs, geographical region of origin, and so on, may play a role in the expression of spirituality.

6. PSYCHOSIS

In this and following chapters we considered clinical issues as they relate to specific psychiatric conditions. Psychosis is an example where religion and mental illness may interact due to the fact that some patients have delusions with religious content. This may have led to the à priori conclusion that religion is harmful to patients with psychosis.

Yet recent research indicates that patients with illnesses such as schizophrenia, delusional depression, or bipolar disorder are able to reconstruct a life worth living despite their disabling delusions or negative symptoms. Religious involvement may help these patients find ways of regaining hope as well as developing meaningful activities and social roles.

Indeed, religious coping appears to be important for a large majority of patients with psychosis. Religion provides these patients with a positive sense of self, guidelines for interpersonal behavior, and resources to cope with their symptoms.

With regard to the negative effects of religion in psychotic disorder, it is possible that, at least in some cases, religion may predispose individuals to exacerbations of illness due to its arousal of intense emotional experiences (religious conversion, for example) that may be disorienting and worsen psychotic illness.

No specific guidelines exist in the scientific literature on how to incorporate religious issues into the individual care of patients with psychosis, although some clues on how to intervene have been provided as follows.

First, although it appears that many patients have religious beliefs and pray alone, they are often not involved in religious community activities. They repeat in religious settings what happens in other areas of their lives because they have problems creating and maintaining an interpersonal and social network. This area can be a focus of treatment, because these deficits could be overcome with proper treatment.

Psychotherapeutic work might also address other issues such as spiritual crisis, identity building, and meaning.

Group therapy approaches that involve spirituality have been developed, at least in the United States. Other programs may exist elsewhere, but they have not been reported in the literature. Some groups are more supportive and less organized and/or psychodynamically oriented; others are more structured, based on behavioral-cognitive principles. A group format has some advantages over individual treatment not only in terms of costs but also in terms of the opportunities for interaction among patients.

For psychotic disorders, perhaps even more than for other mental conditions, explanatory models may vary across culture and religious background. Assessing the patient's explanatory model is thus important to overcome barriers to treatment.

7. HALLUCINATIONS AND DELUSIONS

Hallucinations and delusions are considered in a separate chapter, because these symptoms may arise in various psychiatric disorders. A delusion is a false belief based on incorrect inferences about external reality, a false belief which is firmly held despite what almost everyone else believes and despite what constitutes incontrovertible and obvious evidence to the contrary. The discontinuity between pathology and normality has been challenged by epidemiological studies finding that delusions are present in the general population. It has been shown that 10 to 28 percent of the general population experiences delusions, whereas the prevalence of psychosis remains at around 1 percent.

Religious delusions have been described in all major cultures across the continents. However, prevalence differs according to the country and sociocultural context. The prevalence of religious delusions varies widely not only with geography, but also with time. Also, political change and technological progress impact the content of delusions. In the United States, among psychiatric patients hospitalized in emergency wards, the rate of religious delusions in one study was 36 percent for patients with schizophrenia, but these symptoms were also observed among patients with bipolar disorder (33 percent), other psychotic disorder (26 percent), alcohol or drug disorder (17 percent), and depression (14 percent).

Religious delusions may also lead to violent behavior. Aggression and homicides have been perpetrated by religiously deluded people, as they have been by nonreligiously deluded persons.

Religious delusions have also been associated with poorer outcome in some studies, although not in others. People with religious delusions have been found in some studies to be more severely ill, with more hallucinations for a longer period of time. However, the association between religious delusion and a poorer outcome seems to be controversial. Further research is needed to better understand this phenomenon. Is religious delusion in itself a marker of the severity of the pathology?

Abnormal perceptual experiences (that is, hallucinations) are not restricted to psychiatric patients either, and may occur in any sensory modality (for example, auditory, visual, olfactory, gustatory, and tactile). In the United Kingdom, the annual prevalence of auditory or visual hallucinations is 4 percent in the general population, with only one out of eight people with hallucinations meeting criteria for a psychiatric diagnosis. The basic mechanism of hallucinations lies in the inability to differentiate an internal from an external stimulus. Delusions and hallucinations often go together. This association may be partly due to the fact that some delusions come about in order to give meaning to hallucinations.

For clinicians, it is important to be able to differentiate religious delusions from "normal" faith. How can we distinguish a religious belief from a religious delusion?

The more implausible, unfounded, strongly held, not shared by others, distressing, and preoccupying a belief is, the more likely it is to be considered a delusion. Yet, disentangling beliefs from delusions may be tricky.

Three criteria can help to make this distinction:

1 The experience reported by the patient gives the impression that it is a delusion.
2 Other psychiatric symptoms are present.
3 The outcome of the experience seems more like the evolution of a mental illness, rather than that of a life-enhancing experience.

In the management of patients with religious delusions, clinicians need cultural sensitivity to be respectful and to differentiate between functional and dysfunctional beliefs. The question is not if the belief is true or false, because this is not the central question in delusions with religious content. Rather, the clinician has to decide if the behaviors associated with the delusion and/or hallucination are dysfunctional therapeutic intervention and require or not. If so, the treatment of the delusion should be standard for such symptoms, including medication, psychotherapy, and social support, while helping the individual determine what the belief means in his or her current life situation.

8. MOOD DISORDERS AND BEREAVEMENT

Religion can be related to depression in various ways, either increasing vulnerability or promoting recovery. Although studies rarely address clinical samples, there is evidence that religiousness may improve depression outcomes. However, more and more studies demonstrate that depressive symptoms are often accompanied by religious discontent manifested as negative feelings toward God or a sense of having been abandoned by God. Also, people involved in religion may be more likely to report feelings of guilt, even though this may reflect more about their perceived moral standards and religious upbringing than about pathological guilt.

In its myths and beliefs, religion has a great potential for helping people cope with the end of life bereavement, and with. In this context, the relationship with God may provide comfort if a loved one dies and help compensate for the lack of a love relationship. A meta-analysis on the relationship between religious and spiritual beliefs and bereavement showed that about half the studies reported benefits. Beyond a "direct effect," religious and spiritual beliefs could have an impact on other aspects besides depressive symptoms, such as autonomy, personal growth, or engagement in social activities.

The relationship between religiousness and the two poles of the bipolar disorder spectrum may follow the vulnerability-stress model. There is little evidence on how religiousness is related to the presentation and course of bipolar disorder. It is hypothesized that religiousness itself may become a subject of mood swings, but it could also evoke disillusionment in the patient and suspicion in the clinician. Regarding the relationship between facets of religiousness and bipolar disorder, four aspects deserve special mention:

1 *Symptom formation*: Do aspects of religiousness such as the religious tradition influence the emergence of religious insights and emotions during the manic state?
2 *Religious experiences during mania*: Bipolar patients sometimes cherish the memory of their enlightened state or spiritual discoveries, irrespective of the negative consequences of their manic episodes.
3 *Religious preoccupations as early signs*: When bipolar patients intensify their religious involvement, this may in turn lead to religious and spiritual preoccupations.
4 *Disillusionment with religion*: In the depressive state and the symptom-free interval, disillusionment with religion and spirituality may be experienced. This may interfere with a person's ability to cope with a chronic mental disorder and represent an additional loss in life, the loss of trust in one's religion.

Suicide statistics show that, to a limited extent, religiousness can be protective. Besides the role that social integration plays in lowering suicide rates in regions with higher levels of religious affiliation, religious beliefs are associated with limited tolerance of suicide. Yet it seems that only a few core religious beliefs (for example, in an afterlife) and prayer help prevent suicide.

Mental problems in general and mood disorders in particular often raise questions about the meaning of life. Without going into the field of theology, there are two practical ways to include religion and spirituality in clinical contacts with patients with mood disorders. The first is by examining whether religious or spiritual ideas manifest themselves as psychiatric symptoms or seem to color the expression of symptoms. The second is by establishing a mutual understanding of how spirituality and religiousness represent a relevant domain in life. This can facilitate the therapeutic relationship, and at some time in the treatment phase, may lead to a referral to a pastoral counselor.

9. SUBSTANCE ABUSE

Spirituality and religiosity are well-known protective factors that consistently predict lower rates of alcohol and drug abuse. Spirituality may reduce behavioral risks through the promotion of a healthier lifestyle and by expanding the social support network. The inverse relationship between spirituality and substance use is further supported by research on the role of spirituality in recovery. Substance use moves the individual away from rather than toward purpose in life and connection to others. Thus, one path out of addiction is to find meaning and purpose through involvement in religion. Hope can be found in the discovery of a power greater than one's self and an openness to that which is beyond the realm of human understanding.

In twelve-step programs such as Alcoholics Anonymous (AA), members engage in specific behaviors to facilitate spiritual growth. Learning through modeling occurs as members share their experiences of "strength and hope" and work with a sponsor who has an understanding of the spiritual nature of the program.

Research also supports the role of meditation, service to others, and celebration as an intervention in the treatment of addiction.

Spirituality directly affects substance use, and likewise, spirituality itself is enhanced by attending programs such as AA. Do preexisting spiritual/religious beliefs and practices enhance the likelihood that a person will use spiritual-based interventions? Recent evidence indicates that atheists attending AA may reap the same benefit as religious and spiritual alcoholics.

How can the issue of spirituality be raised in addiction treatment? Open questions are a good place to start. However, clinicians should keep in mind that spiritual exploration too early in treatment may be counterproductive. Indeed, the clinician often needs to address other needs first before moving on to spiritual aspects of care.

10. ANXIETY DISORDERS

When worry and tension are present over time and symptoms become so intense that they interfere with a person's ability to function at work or in social relationships, then an anxiety disorder is said to be present. The disorders addressed in this chapter include generalized anxiety disorder, panic disorder, posttraumatic stress disorder, obsessive-compulsive disorder, and phobia.

Some studies show that the greater the religious involvement, the greater the anxiety. This is particularly true when religion manifests itself as either extrinsic religiousness (where religious involvement is motivated by external concerns other than religion, such as economic or social goals) or as negative religious coping (where God is seen as punishing, distant, abandoning, or powerless). Whether it is the religion that is driving the anxiety, or the anxiety that is driving the religious expression is difficult to determine. In contrast, intrinsic religiosity, where religious involvement is an end in itself, is often inversely related to anxiety.

Thus, although religion can potentially increase anxiety, there is also evidence that suggests a protective effect for religion. Also, studies have found that anxiety symptoms may often decrease following religious conversion or rededication to religion.

Religious interventions appear to be effective in patients with a generalized anxiety disorder (according to three randomized, controlled trials involving religious interventions, two Muslim-based and one Tao-based).

For panic disorder, religious involvement may help to relieve panic symptoms, particularly when accompanied by traditional psychotherapy.

Religion is a source of coping for many persons suffering from severe trauma. Patients with posttraumatic stress disorder may have symptoms that are particularly persistent and unresponsive to therapy if their religious worldview has been affected and their faith weakened or lost (that is, spiritual injury), necessitating that this be addressed in therapy.

For obsessive-compulsive disorder (OCD), the role of religion warrants a careful examination. Indeed, like delusions, OCD symptoms may involve a religious dimension. Research shows that religiosity is significantly correlated with the severity of OCD symptoms. But there is no relationship between religiosity and general anxiety, social anxiety, or depressive symptoms, suggesting some degree of specificity for the relationship between religion and severity of OCD symptoms at least within OCD patients. Nevertheless, because such associations are reported almost exclusively in cross-sectional studies, it is not possible to say whether religiosity aggravates OCD symptoms in OCD patients or whether OCD symptoms lead to greater religiosity (and the measures of OCD severity, in these studies, may be confounded with items that tap traditional religious values). When religious obsessions and compulsions are present, these patients may have a worse prognosis. Although a form of faith-based cognitive therapy has been developed to help treat religious patients with OCD, it is not clear that this treatment is as effective in OCD patients with religious obsessions.

Beyond a careful spiritual assessment, clinicians should support the patient's religious beliefs unless obviously pathological. If appropriate, the therapist may provide the patient with a list of scriptures to meditate on or to repeat when facing situations that arouse anxiety. Certain scriptures within Christianity instruct people to dwell on the positive, not the negative. Other world religions have similar teachings that build confidence and may calm the anxious person. The type of therapy chosen, of course, should match the religion of the patient.

If religious beliefs are being used neurotically to obstruct needed changes or psychological insights, a different tact should be taken. After a therapeutic relationship has been established, the psychiatrist may need to gently challenge those beliefs. Before doing so, however, it may be best to seek consultation with or referral to a pastoral counselor with training to address such issues.

11. DISSOCIATIVE DISORDERS

Dissociative symptoms may occur in many psychiatric conditions. Due to the scope of this book, dissociative trance disorder has been emphasized. Although dissociative trance disorders, especially possession disorder, are common, little systematic research into this phenomenon has been carried out in psychiatry.

The experience of being "possessed" by another entity holds different meanings in different cultures. Explaining the phenomenon of possession as a dissociative symptom with religious content has contrasted with certain religious interpretations, which may describe possession as resulting from invasion of the body by spiritual forces. The *Diagnostic and Statistical Manual of Mental Disorders, Fourth Edition (DSM-IV)* places pathological possession in the category of possession trances under the diagnosis of dissociative disorder not otherwise specified (Code F 44.9).

Many societies around the world have one or more forms of possession belief. When a person in these societies complains of being possessed, the traditional intervention is exorcism or manipulation. Exorcism describes a ritual that is intended to expel the negative force or forces. Manipulation involves rituals that seek to integrate the negative forces within the personality. Exorcism can be understood as religious coping, with God, gods, or good spirits pitted against demons, whereas manipulation can be understood as a from of religious coping that involves compromise with those demons.

How can psychiatrists and religious authorities cooperate when treating such patients? What should the clergy or religious authority (priest, pastor, exorcist, or shaman) be responsible for and what should the psychiatrist be responsible for? The efficacy of the intervention largely depends on the extent to which the possessed person and his or her family accept the underlying explanation for the particular approach. The psychiatrist should attempt to establish links between the two worlds of meanings. The challenge is to include (if possible) the patient's worldview, the spiritual counselor's worldview, and the clinician's worldview in the discussion. An ethnopsychiatric consultation can also be helpful. During such a session, a psychiatrist and co-therapists from the patient's cultural-religious background meet with the patient to discuss his symptoms and specific problems. The goal is to allow both participants, the psychiatrist as well as the patient, to continue the treatment without each being locked into his or her own system of reference.

12. SELF-IDENTITY

The "self" represents how individuals think of themselves over the long term. The feeling of identity, the feeling of "being oneself," and the individual's self-image are the result of an ongoing process of construction. This process is ultimately culture dependent.

Parental figures are the first figures that the person identifies with. The attachment relationship is a foundation and a vector for the internalization of the parental figures. These parental figures are stable and formative in a secure attachment; they are much less formative when the forms of attachment are insecure and built on anxiety.

Later, religious figures can play the role of attachment figures, because they offer a secure relational bond. God, priests, pastors, or members of the religious community can be attachment

figures. Thus, in various religious traditions, exemplary figures contribute to the foundations of identity. For example, identity can be built by complete or partial appropriation of the figures found in religious belief systems or, on the contrary, by antagonistic reaction to these figures. Also, religious rites may influence identification.

Religion/spirituality can help restore identity when facing threatening conditions such as those experienced by patients with severe mental symptoms. However, religious experiences can also disturb and destabilize. Thus, keeping a critical eye on the role played by the religious dimension in identity construction is important. In a multicultural context, the medical treatment should aim to construct a therapeutic framework based on a conception of the self that is consistent with the cultural tradition of the patient.

13. PERSONALITY DISORDERS

A personality disorder (PD) represents a rigid and ongoing pattern of thoughts and behaviors that deviate markedly from the expectations of the patient's culture and social group. What is the relationship between personality disorders and religion?

There are many personality traits. Recent research has discovered that the majority of these traits cluster themselves around five broader dimensions. This is known as the *Five Factor Model of Personality* (FFM). Research has shown that spirituality and religiousness represent qualities that are distinct from the FFM domains.

What is the role of spirituality in treating PDs?

Patients with a *schizotypal PD* can be helped to foster a connection to the transcendent that helps them to gain a sense of self and develop a better sense of personal support. Involvement in supportive religious communities can also help break down the stigmas associated with having a psychiatric label and provide increased personal meaning.

Spiritual techniques can help to promote more internally stable emotional states in patients with *borderline and narcissistic PD* (for example, by using dialectical-behavior therapy techniques). Psychospiritual interventions can help these patients create for themselves an inner mental state that is dynamic, attractive, peaceful, and creative. For the *narcissistic PD*, developing a relationship with God could serve a useful intrapsychic object that provides personal security enabling him or her to counter the inner vulnerabilities that compromise the narcissist from developing and maintaining healthy interpersonal relationships.

Spiritually oriented psychotherapy could also be a powerful intervention for *antisocial PDs*. Spirituality can sometimes be useful in promoting authenticity, moral and social capacity, and a greater faith in life. Creating an awareness of social responsibility may work against the more manipulative, selfish orientation that characterizes this disorder.

Overall, spirituality can be a useful therapeutic resource for treating personality disorders because it serves as an antidote to narcissism. Committing to a larger vision allows individuals to find personal stability and coherence, even during times of difficulty.

Although addressing religious issues has a number of positive benefits, one must also be aware of the potential adverse affects it may have. Religious crisis may have an impact on psychosocial functioning. Spirituality is sometimes a source of pain, guilt, or exclusion. Some patients with antisocial traits may use spiritual information to manipulate others.

14. LIAISON PSYCHIATRY

Medical physicians consult psychiatrists in acute medical or surgical settings for patients suffering from anxiety, depression, psychosis, somatoform disorders, pain, PTSD, substance abuse, delirium, agitation, psychosis, and dementia. Given the many losses and life changes that physical illness can cause, it is not surprising that depressive disorders are common in hospital settings. Because emotional disorders in medical patients are often a direct result of inability to cope with those life changes and loss, mental health specialists should

seek out resources that can help patients adjust successfully.

In such a context, religion may be a powerful coping resource for some patients. Religious beliefs may help medical patients reframe their losses in a more positive light and give them a sense of purpose and meaning. Research has shown that religious coping is associated with more rapid adaptation to medical illness and disability.

In other cases, religious beliefs may be a symptom of depression or other emotional illness. For example, the medical patient may explain the extreme guilt and sadness stemming from a depressive disorder as the result of having committed an "unpardonable" sin. Also, religious beliefs may delay psychiatric care by encouraging treatments within the faith community, which may not recognize the need for professional psychiatric care.

Chronic medical illness is associated with high rates of suicide. Religious and spiritual beliefs often help people to cope with the pain and suffering that leads to suicidal thinking, and they provide hope and meaning that can prevent suicide. Also, religious involvement increases the likelihood that persons with suicidal thoughts will obtain timely psychiatric care. For the severely ill, spiritual well-being provides substantial protection against end-of-life despair. Patients with active religious beliefs are less likely to have positive attitudes toward assisted suicide.

Hospitalized patients with medical illness may have a variety of worries and fears. Religious worries may center on concerns about salvation, fear of hell, or guilt over becoming sick. Religious beliefs may influence the type and the severity of anxiety that patients experience. Some may become preoccupied by religious worries or become involved in religious behaviors such as compulsive prayer or repeated confessions. Others may use religious beliefs and behaviors in healthy ways to cope with the anxiety due to medical illness.

There is little systematic evidence for a relationship between somatization disorder and religious involvement, although cases where this occurs are highly publicized. Examples of physical manifestations of psychological conflicts related to religion include the phenomenon of stigmata, where a physical wound (or bleeding) appears spontaneously in the same location as the wounds suffered by Jesus, or the "faint" that occurs when someone is "slain in the spirit" at a Pentecostal healing service.

Religious beliefs – particularly if rigid and inflexible – may worsen pain, but more often, patients turn to religion in an attempt to cope with pain. In chronic pain patients, mindfulness meditation (a Buddhist practice) as part of a stress-reduction and relaxation program (SRRP) has produced a significant reduction in pain, mood disturbance, and other psychological symptoms. Religious involvement may also help to reduce the complications seen in chronic pain patients, including substance abuse and pain medication addiction.

When patients with dementia have a religious background, engaging the patient in rituals or prayers may help to reduce agitation and increase cooperation. Religion can also help patients cope with the stress involved in the development of dementia, especially during the early stages when patients still have insight into what is happening to them. There is also some surprising evidence that religious involvement may slow the development of cognitive impairment in Alzheimer's disease and perhaps even slow the natural progression of memory loss with aging.

What can liaison clinicians do? In a few words: Take a spiritual history; show respect for all religious or spiritual beliefs and practices that are supportive for patients; actively support healthy religious practices; anticipate religious resistance to psychiatric treatments; use religious beliefs in counseling, as appropriate; and if necessary, seek collaboration with chaplains, pastoral counselors, or community clergy.

15. COMMUNITY PSYCHIATRY

About one quarter of people with a psychiatric diagnosis will have first sought help from clergy. This warrants an understanding of the role that clergy play in counseling, as well as an attempt to collaborate with clergy when treating religious patients.

Barriers to psychiatric treatment include social stigma, self stigma, cost issues, or explanatory models outside the medical realm. Clinicians often have few relationships with religious professionals, and the reverse is also true. To overcome this problem, the author encourages the establishment of forums that invite leaders in the spiritual, psychiatric, and medical communities together to consider models of referral and collaboration.

Sometimes spiritual themes may help to reduce the stigma associated with mental illness (examples of depression in the Bible, for example). Conversely, some religious perspectives might add to stigma by (like some medical models) labeling the illness in a narrow and negative way (that is, depression resulting from not having sufficient faith in God).

Religious professionals can help to inform clinicians on various aspects of the patient's illness: Spiritual leaders might know some common practices within their own traditions that help; they may provide information about culture and regional norms influencing individual mental health; or a faith-based counselor may help with transference issues (for example, when asked about one's own spiritual orientation).

How is it possible to improve communication/referrals?

Both clinicians and spiritual leaders can be assisted by supervision (even if it is foreign to one or the other).

Training programs (for example, continuing education) that blend spiritual and psychological insight in training and case discussions are likely to help professionals on both sides.

Building referral networks can help individualize care. This involves knowing what the other thinks and knows about each other's respective domains.

More generally, professionals should be aware that healing usually stems from multiple elements, not only those of our field!

And finally, it should be remembered that pastoral counselors are professionals with specific training and a code of ethics.

16. SPIRITUAL ASSESSMENT

A spiritual assessment is the first step for the psychiatrist who wants to address or consider religious or spiritual issues in his or her practice. Most chapters of this book emphasize this point.

The reasons for assessing the religiousness/spirituality of patients are numerous. Religion and spirituality are considered cultural factors influencing the process of diagnosis and treatment. Religion and mental health depend heavily on one another. Sometimes, patients do not benefit from psychiatric treatment because the primary problem involves religious beliefs or spiritual crises that may have led to the emotional, behavioral, or social disturbances. Also, in a patient-centered approach, examining the individual's spiritual and religious history is a therapeutic tool in itself. Patients will appreciate the doctor's sensitivity and feel understood and respected.

Religion is a multidimensional construct, strongly influenced by the cultural context. During the screening phase of the spiritual assessment, clinicians should develop an outline of the patient's spiritual and religious history. Therefore, the following domains should be explored:

- religious background (patient and significant others)
- evolution of spirituality over the lifetime
- influence of psychiatric disorder on religion/spirituality
- current spiritual/religious beliefs and practices
- private religious practices
- religious preference (in the sense of a social or cultural identity)
- the patient's relationships with members of the religious community
- support received from the religious community
- subjective importance of religion in life

For patients in whom religion is important, addressing the following issues should determine how religion is used to cope with the illness:

- the spiritual meaning of the illness

- the role of religion in coping with symptoms
- religious coping style (for example, self-directing, deferral, or collaborative style)
- synergy/incompatibility of religious beliefs with psychiatric care

Of course, all spiritual orientations must be respected when addressing religion/spirituality with patients, including a professed absence of belief.

17. INTEGRATINGS SPIRITUALITY INTO THERAPY

This section of the book focuses in therapeutic issues. The first chapter examines the integration os spirituality into therapy, and is followed by a chapter discussing explanatory models of mental illness and then by three chapters describing different types of religious therapies from Christian, Muslim, and Buddhist perspectives.

Numerous treatment programs exist that include religious components. These can involve a comprehensive array of services, be in a group format, or involve individual (psycho-) therapy. Clinicians working on the front lines should be familiar with some of these approaches so that they can refer patients if needed or give advice regarding such treatments. When working with patients with severe mental disorders in Western countries, psychiatrists are often criticized for only giving medications without providing more whole person treatments. Patients sometimes complain that one or another specific approach is not available (for example, the so-called "Soteria paradigm"(4)). Knowing what the patient is talking about may improve the dialogue that clinicians have with patients. For instance, psychiatrists should know that the Buddhist-based "Windhorse" program involves taking medication, even if one of the aims of treatment is to minimize medication dose.

In many places, group interventions involving spirituality/religion have been conducted in community mental health practices. Research has provided some data on their efficacy. A number of hospitals and outpatient facilities have implemented a holistic and interdisciplinary model for therapy based on an "extended" bio-psycho-social model. In such settings, the pastoral/spiritual counselor may be involved in the interdisciplinary team, with rights and responsibilities similar to that of other therapists.

The chapter on integrating spirituality into therapy includes detailed information about one such program in Langenthal, Switzerland. Patients who request such treatment are provided with both state-of-the-art psychiatric and psychological treatment plus spiritual treatment, where the goals of therapy focus on regaining hope and meaning, strengthening the relationship with God, or working toward forgiveness in broken relationships. Psycho-educational group meetings are offered that focus on the integration of therapeutic and spiritual aspects of care, emphasizing the benefit and importance of religious and spiritual coping. There are also spiritual singing and music groups, art therapy, and discussion groups, often led by a pastoral counselor. Spiritual issues such as unhealthy beliefs are also challenged from both a spiritual and a psychotherapeutic view in counseling.

Families taking care of patients with mental disorders often face a heavy burden. Research has generally found that religiosity among caregivers is linked to enhanced adjustment. Family members often turn to religion to cope with the stress of caring for an ill family member. The author emphasizes how religiosity may contribute to the well-being of caregivers by expanding their capacity and motivation for self-care.

18. EXPLANATORY MODELS MENTAL ILLNESS AND ITS TREATMENT

Over the course of history, a number of theoretical issues concerning the causes of mental disorders (or explanatory models) have preoccupied the mental health field. People who are suffering tend to explain their disease according to collectively elaborated social constructions, which cannot be reduced to mere institutional or medical definitions. These explanations include several

dimensions of a religious, collective, existential, emotional, and sentimental nature.

When clinicians meet with their patients, there are actually two different cultural and spiritual perspectives to reconcile through communication, confrontation, and sometimes even negotiation. Furthermore, as compared with Western societies, people in developing countries (and minority groups living within developed countries) seem to attach more importance to the symbolic and spiritual side of the disease. The different understandings of the disease may influence treatment choices as they are developed by patients. Chronic mental disorders are a major reason why patients seek out alternative therapies.

Clinicians can deal with this issue by carefully considering patients' explanatory models for their psychiatric disorders. Religious beliefs can have either a positive or negative impact on adherence to the treatment. Sometimes, medical treatment may enter into conflict with the teachings of religious groups.

Even if the patient's account of the situation may be perceived as irrational or inconsistent, clinicians should try to build bridges between their own explanatory models and those of patients. Even neuropharmacology can be presented as related to God's creation. Nobody can prove it, but nobody can disprove it either! In this way, an explanatory model that takes both positions into account can be "negotiated" with the patient. This is especially important because evidence suggests that patients are more satisfied when their psychiatrist shares their model of understanding distress and treatment.

19. PSYCHOTHERAPY FROM A CHRISTIAN PERSPECTIVE

Christian forms of psychotherapy seek to transform the mind of the believer so that they can find meaning and purpose in their relationship with God. They use the teachings found in the Bible and integrate them with current secular concepts. Christian psychotherapy involves belief in a cosmology (an explanation as to why things are as they are, where it all comes from, and where we come from), a futurology (an extrapolation of the past into the future), values (what is good and what is evil), and knowledge. Christians believe that man is composed of three functional units: body, soul, and spirit.

Mental disorders are viewed as the consequence of man's alienation from God (that is, sin, either original sin or individual sin), which leads to an alienation from society as well. During therapy, the patient must be reconciled with God and continue to transform as he matures in his faith. Therapists consider that God's intervention makes it possible to heal wounds from events that have occurred in the past as they are relived in the present. Depending on the circumstances, the therapy can be short-term or long-term. The therapist has to learn about the patient's conscious and subconscious mental conflicts. By responding to the patient in ways that do not reward the behaviors that produce pain and anxiety, the therapist helps to bring about extinction or inhibition of such behaviors. He must then teach new behavioral patterns by using Biblical guidelines.

20. PSYCHOTHERAPY FROM AN ISLAMIC PERSPECTIVE

Because Muslims are a minority in most Western countries, they are usually stereotyped. Islam has different laws regarding some of the rights and duties of men and women, which may not be accepted by Western clinicians (for example, conditions for women). Therapists should have some knowledge of Islam, or admit to a lack of knowledge about the patient's culture or religion, to establish a positive therapeutic alliance.

From an Islamic perspective, religious psychotherapy may be used if religious conflicts are an important part of the patient's problems. Moreover, a religious technique should be truly meaningful to the patient. Concepts involving religious considerations, such as belief in an afterlife or guilt management, can be used.

Islamic concepts may be used by specialists in cognitive behavioral therapy (CBT) by

working with reference to religious themes to challenge dysfunctional beliefs in the same way that dysfunctional assumptions (or schemata) are modified in secular CBT. Both dysfunctional thoughts and behaviors can be altered according to these principles. For instance, Islamic rules stating that husbands should respect their wives and should not oppress them can be effectively used when treating abusive husbands.

21. PSYCHIATRIC CARE USING BUDDHIST PRINCIPLES

The Windhorse Therapy is an example of a comprehensive therapy based on the Buddhist understanding of fundamental health and wellness, while integrating applicable Western psychology. The goal of the treatment is recovery by "discovering and synchronizing with one's own fundamental health." To create a recovery environment, a team is assembled that is made up of the clinicians, the client, and whenever possible, the family. Clients live in a house with a housemate who is part of a treatment team. There are clinicians on the team who spend time with the client on a regularly scheduled basis, doing a wide variety of activities. These activities are elements of an individually tailored environment to help the person live in an ordinary and healthy way. The client may work, see friends and family, and be part of the normal community in which he or she lives. The schedule usually includes meeting with a psychotherapist and with a psychiatrist if medications are used. There is a system of meetings that all members of the team, including the client and his or her family, participate in. Most treatments last six months to two years. Windhorse Therapy is primarily designed for individuals with chronic disorders such as schizophrenia. Applying Buddhist principles such as those used in mindfulness,(5) patients learn to tolerate how it feels to be aware in the present moment and how it feels to be with whatever is going on in one's life without self-conscious judgment. With this come "islands of clarity," which may appear progressively in the midst of psychosis. Healthy self-love, a basic life energy, is supposed to be the result.

What can programs such as Windhorse Therapy bring to patients with severe mental disorders? The goal of current secular approaches for these disorders is recovery. With this kind of care, aiming at recovery is not always an easy task, because motivating patients often involves repetitive activities that are often felt to be stigmatizing. Also, antipsychotic medications, even second-generation antipsychotics, are sometimes poorly tolerated by patients. Environments like Windhorse can bring together the conditions that are likely to help patients initiate activities and reduce stress, which in turn is likely to reduce medication needs. As with Christian or Muslim psychotherapy, this treatment should only be used after explaining the underlying Buddhist principles on which it is based, and it should only be suggested for patients who would be willing to embark on such a therapy.

22. PSYCHIATRIC EDUCATION

Beyond reading books and papers, there should be education about religion for psychiatrists, as well as education about psychiatry/psychology for clergy and chaplains. Rationales for teaching religion-spirituality are detailed throughout this book. Currently, educational guidelines for psychiatry residents recommend teaching sensitivity to religious and cultural issues and training that ensures a minimum degree of competency in these areas. Education on this topic should take place early in the training curriculum for students and post-graduate trainees, to form life-long attitudes and habits. Training programs for psychiatrists, medical students, or psychologists exist in North America, in some parts of Europe, and in Australia. There is little information about training programs in most countries in Africa, the Middle East, and Asia.

All clinicians involved in mental health care should receive training on religion/spirituality. Three broad goals are: (1) to recognize and distinguish pathological from normal religious and spiritual expressions, (2) to acquire therapeutic skills, knowledge, and attitudes to deal with religion-spirituality issues in mental health care, and (3) to acquire clinical competence in addressing religion/spirituality in actual treatment settings. Essential content should include: (a) general information about research relating to religion/spirituality in health and (b) gathering and interpreting information about the religious/spiritual history. If possible, the curriculum could include more specific notions such as religious/spiritual development over the lifetime and techniques of addressing this topic in psychotherapy. Didactic courses and seminars are the most common formats, but other brief teaching formats can also be implemented, such as intermittent in-service training.

When trying to implement a training program on religion/spirituality, one may expect to run into some resistance from students, faculty, program directors, or entire institutions, most resistance being due to ignorance or countertransference issues.

REFERENCES

1. Holloway F. Is there a science of recovery and does it matter? *Advan Psychiatr Treat.* 2008;14:245–247.
2. Palouzian RF, Park CL. *Handbook of the Psychology of Religion and Spirituality.* New York: Guilford Press; 2005.
3. Burton R. *Anatomie de la Mélancolie, trad. fr. par B. Hoepffner, préface de J. Starobinsky, postface de J. Pigeaud,* Paris: José Corti; 2000.
4. Calton T, Ferriter M, Huband N, Spandler H. A systematic review of the Soteria paradigm for the treatment of people diagnosed with schizophrenia. *Schizophr Bull.* 2008;34:181–192.
5. Linehan MM. *Cognitive Behavioral Treatment of Borderline Personality Disorder.* New York: Guilford Press; 1993.

Index

Printed in the United States
By Bookmasters